CRC
HANDBOOK OF
Dietary Fiber
in Human
Nutrition
3rd Edition

CRC
HANDBOOK OF
Dietary Fiber
in Human
Nutrition
3rd Edition

Edited by
Gene A. Spiller, D.Sc., Ph.D.
Director
Health Research and Studies Center, Inc.
SPHERA Foundation
Los Altos, California

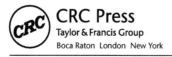

CRC Press
Taylor & Francis Group
Boca Raton London New York

CRC Press is an imprint of the
Taylor & Francis Group, an **informa** business

CRC Press
Taylor & Francis Group
6000 Broken Sound Parkway NW, Suite 300
Boca Raton, FL 33487-2742

First issued in paperback 2019

© 2001 by Taylor and Francis Group, LLC
CRC Press is an imprint of Taylor & Francis Group, an Informa business

No claim to original U.S. Government works

ISBN-13: 978-0-8493-2387-4 (hbk)
ISBN-13: 978-0-367-39721-0 (pbk)
Library of Congress Card Number 2001025278

Library of Congress Cataloging-in-Publication Data

CRC Handbook of dietary fiber in human nutrition / edited by Gene A. Spiller.--3rd ed.
     p. cm.
    Includes bibliographical references and index.
    ISBN 0-8493-2387-8 (alk. paper)
    1. Fiber in human nutrition-Handbooks, manuals, etc. I. Spiller, Gene A.

QP144.F52 C73 2001
613.2'8--dc21

2001025278
CIP

Visit the Taylor & Francis Web site at
http://www.taylorandfrancis.com

and the CRC Press Web site at
http://www.crcpress.com

Dedication

To Hugh Trowell and Denis Burkitt, who pioneered a new understanding of the role of plant fibers in human health. They have been to me teachers of science, medicine, and humility. They should be remembered not only as pioneers in medicine, but also for their selfless and total dedication to the prevention of disease and human suffering.

Preface to the First Edition

The *CRC Handbook of Dietary Fiber in Human Nutrition* is proof of the amazing growth in the study of dietary fiber during the 1970s and 1980s. When I first edited a book on dietary fiber, *Fiber in Human Nutrition*, in the mid-1970s, I was happy to find at least a few good investigators who could contribute chapters to it. It would have been impossible to find a large number of scientists that could have made a major contribution to that early book.

However, as work was beginning on this Handbook in 1982 and I was presenting the design at the Symposium on Fiber in Human and Animal Nutrition in New Zealand that year, not only was I able to find all the 50-plus authors I needed, but I had the sad task of omitting some outstanding names.

Interest in what used to be the disregarded Cinderella nutrient of the early 20th century has grown at a rate greater than almost any other nutrient. The plant cell wall and the gums and mucilages had found their well-deserved niche in nutrition and medicine.

Even though few people still believe that dietary fiber has not found the ultimate proof that makes it a required nutrient, the momentum is with the ones who have found valid uses for it in high-fiber foods in treating diseases such as type-II diabetes. The momentum is also with the epidemiologists who have found correlations with lower incidence of colorectal cancer, the ones that have found in high-fiber foods one of the best ways to prevent excessive fat and food intake. It is a list that can go on and on.

Has the ultimate study on the long-range effects of dietary fiber been published? Of course not. It is probably impossible to carry out the ultimate study on the correlation of nutrition to chronic diseases under present conditions: we must accept the pieces of evidence derived from good epidemiology, from controlled human studies and, of course, animal studies. The lifetimes of many of us would be needed to satisfy the purists who hope for the ultimate study, in this or any other field in which we deal with the lifetime of a human being.

There is more to complicate things: dietary fiber polymers are quite elusive, unlike vitamins that can be isolated or synthesized readily. Some of these polymers may change when torn apart from their complex structure in the cell wall. Thus, when we attempt to extract them, too often we isolate something quite different from the original material, perhaps useful, but most certainly different. This bothers many scientists who would like to use the pure form of nutrients for their investigations. There is more: dietary fiber is so interactive that other components of the diet probably vary its effect on humans. All this makes dietary fiber research so challenging and so difficult!

This book is proof that there are many dedicated scientists and clinicians that have given their best efforts to dietary fiber. There are many who could not be included here, as there is a point in an effort of this kind at which the editor must sadly stop asking for contributions and recognize that the book must be a finite number of pages. I owe a very special thanks to all the authors in this book, for, after all, it is their book.

The book presents a large volume of data. The reader is directed to the Table of Contents which illustrates the design of the book, a design that was conceived to make it as easy as possible to find the needed data. Chemistry, analytical methodologies, physiological and biochemical aspects, clinical and epidemiological studies, and consumption patterns are covered extensively. Tables with the dietary fiber content of various foods analyzed by different methods are given at the end of the book.

Gene A. Spiller
Los Altos, California — February 1985

Preface to the Second Edition

Dietary fiber research has seen a great deal of progress since the first edition of this Handbook. This new edition is revised and updated by individual authors and, with the exception of a few chapters, such as the Southgate and the crude fiber analytical methods, that are unchanged, new material is added. Some new authors and chapters have been added, including the new method of analysis by Englyst and Hudson (Chapter 3.3) and Bosello, Armellini, and Zamboni's chapter on fiber consumption in Italy. Hugh Trowell passed away in 1989; his chapter has been left untouched. A major addition in the second edition is the inclusion of more extensive tables of data on dietary fiber in foods. They are prepared by various authors to give the reader a chance to compare data from different sources or methods.

This new edition should give researchers, physicians, nutritionists, and other health professionals a useful and ready source of information, as a handbook should. Again, as in the first edition, we could not ask all the experts in this field to contribute, so we decided to stay with the original authors as much as possible. We hope that our efforts will make this work valuable to everyone interested in this topic.

Gene A. Spiller
Health Research and Studies Center, Inc.
SPHERA Foundation, Los Altos, California — January 1992

Preface to the Third Edition

Dietary fiber research has seen a great deal of progress since the first and second editions of this Handbook. This new edition has been revised and updated by individual authors, with the exception of a few chapters that either have historical value or have data that should be available in a handbook of this nature, even though it may have been written a few years before the publication. I like to define the latter as "classic" chapters that have an essential, timeless nature. Some new authors and chapters have been added, including a new section on cereal fiber that emphasizes the crucial role of associated phytochemicals.

Hugh Trowell passed away in 1989; his chapter has been left untouched. Denis Burkitt passed away soon after the publication of the second edition, in which he had written the opening chapter with me. I have chosen to expand this first chapter without changing the part published in the second edition of the Handbook. I have added a second part to that chapter to bring it up to date.

This new edition should give researchers, physicians, nutritionists, and other health professionals a useful and ready source of information, as a handbook should. Again, as in the other editions, we could not ask all the experts in this field to contribute.

We hope that our efforts will make this work valuable to everyone interested in this topic. One new chapter (2.8) discusses a fiber from animal sources. This is an interesting topic in fiber definitions, as dietary fiber is considered to be from plant sources.

With all the great progress we have made in the past 10 years in nutrition research, it is unfortunate that the past 10 years have also seen conflicting studies on fiber, as on other topics in nutrition. In the late 1970s, Hugh Trowell, during one of our many meetings, expressed to me his concern that in the earnest desire to do more research, the picture of the benefits of fiber may become "muddled." I would like to close this preface with an appeal to all fiber researchers to be careful in reaching sweeping conclusions before considering carefully the complexity and the interactivity of dietary fiber. Some major publications have reached conclusions on the effects of fiber after studying diets that were a long way from diets that could be called high-fiber diets.

Dietary fiber is a precious gift that plants bring to us. Let's research it and teach about it with care.

Gene A. Spiller
Health Research and Studies Center, Inc.
SPHERA Foundation, Los Altos, California — December 2000

Acknowledgments

The editor wishes to thank Monica Alton Spiller for her extensive assistance in all phases of editing, from the original design to the various stages of manuscript assessment and the final proofreading of the first edition of this Handbook.

For the second edition of this Handbook, the editor wishes to thank Rebecca Carr and Monica Alton Spiller for their assistance in the editing process.

For the third edition of this Handbook, the editor wishes to thank Rosemary Schmele, Connie Burton, and Len Marquart for their assistance.

Bunpei Mori, Ph.D.
Professor
Department of Life Science
Toita Women's College
Tokyo, Japan

David G. Oakenfull, Ph.D.
Hydrocolloids Research
Wahroonga, New South Wales,
Australia

Donald Oberleas, Ph.D.
Professor Emeritus
Texas Tech. University
Lubbock, Texas

Mark A. Pereira, Ph.D.
Department of Nutrition
Harvard School of Public Health
Department of Pediatrics
Division of Endocrinology
Children's Hospital
Boston, Massachusetts

Janet Pettit, B.S.
Database Nutritionist
Nutrition Coordinating Center
Division of Epidemiology
School of Public Health
University of Minnesota
Minneapolis, Minnesota

Joel J. Pins, M.P.H., M.S.
University of Minnesota
School of Medicine
Department of Family Practice and
  Community Health
Minneapolis, Minnesota

John D. Potter, M.D., Ph.D.
Head
Cancer Prevention Research Program
Fred Hutchinson Cancer Research Center
Professor of Epidemiology
University of Washington
Seattle, Washington

Kim M. Randles, B.S.
V.A. Medical Center and
  University of Kentucky
Lexington, Kentucky

Sally J. Record, M.A.C.S.
Consumer Science Program
Commonwealth Scientific and Industrial
  Research Organisation (CSIRO)
Health Sciences and Nutrition Division
Adelaide, Australia

James B. Robertson, Ph.D.
Department of Animal Science
Cornell University
Ithaca, New York

Sally F. Schakel, R.D.
Database Nutritionist
Nutrition Coordinating Center
University of Minnesota
Minneapolis, Minnesota

Barbara O. Schneeman, Ph.D.
Professor
Department of Nutrition
University of California
Davis, California

Zhi-Ping Shen, M.D.
Professor
Institute of Nutrition and Food Science
Chinese Academy of Preventive Medicine
Beijing, China

David A. T. Southgate, Ph.D.
Former Head
Nutrition, Diet and Health Department
AFRC Institute of Food Research
Norwich, England

Gene A. Spiller, D.Sc., Ph.D.
Director
SPHERA Foundation
Health Research and Studies Center
Los Altos, California

Monica Spiller, MS
SPHERA Foundation
Los Altos, California

Olof Theander, Dr. Techn.
Professor Emeritus - Organic Chemistry
Department of Chemistry
Swedish University of Agricultural Sciences
Uppsala, Sweden

Sherwood L. Gorbach, M.D.
Department of Family Medicine and
  Community Health
Tufts University School of Medicine
Boston, Massachusetts

Mary Beth Hall, Ph.D.
Assistant Professor
Department of Animal Science
University of Florida
Gainesville, Florida

Barbara F. Harland, Ph.D., R.D.
Professor
Department of Nutritional Sciences
College of Pharmacy
Nursing and Allied Health Sciences
Howard University
Washington, D.C.

John H. Himes, Ph.D., M.P.H.
Professor and Director
Nutrition Coordinating Center
Division of Epidemiology
School of Public Health
University of Minnesota
Minneapolis, Minnesota

Peter J. Horvath, Ph.D.
Department of Animal Science
Cornell University
Ithaca, New York

Geoffrey J. Hudson, Ph.D.
Cambridge, England

David R. Jacobs, Jr., Ph.D.
Division of Epidemiology
School of Public Health
University of Minnesota
Minneapolis, Minnesota

Mazda Jenab, Ph.D.
Department of Nutritional Sciences
University of Toronto
Toronto, Ontario, Canada

Alexandra Jenkins, R.D., C.D.E.
Clinical Nutrition and Risk Factor
  Modification Center
St. Michael's Hospital
Toronto, Ontario, Canada

David J. A. Jenkins, M.D., Ph.D., D.Sc.
Department of Nutritional Sciences
University of Toronto
Toronto, Ontario, Canada

Julie M. Jones, Ph.D.
Department of Family and Consumer
  Science
College of Saint Catherine
St. Paul, Minnesota

Heinrich Kasper, M.D.
Professor
Department of Internal Medicine
Medical University Clinic
University of Würzburg
Würzburg, Germany

Joseph Keenan, M.D.
Department of Family Practice and
  Community Health
University of Minnesota Medical School
Minneapolis, Minnesota

Hanako Kobayashi, M.S.
Department of Nutritional Science and
  Toxicology
University of California
Berkeley, California

Yves Le Quintrec, M.D.
Assistance Publique Hopitaux de Paris
Service de Gastro-enterologie et Pathologie
  Digestive Postoperatoire
Hospital Rothschild
Paris, France

Betty A. Lewis, Ph.D.
Division of Nutritional Sciences
Cornell University
Ithaca, New York

Leonard Marquart, Ph.D., R.D.
Nutrition Research Department
General Mills, Inc.
Minneapolis, Minnesota

(Harold E.) Gene Miller, Ph.D.
Principal Scientist
General Mills, Inc.
Minneapolis, Minnesota

Lilian Thompson, Ph.D.
Department of Nutritional Sciences
University of Toronto
Toronto, Ontario, Canada

Keisuke Tsuji, M.D., Ph.D.
Chief of Laboratory
The National Institute of Health
  and Nutrition
Tokyo, Japan

Peter J. Van Soest, Ph.D.
Professor
Animal Nutrition
Department of Animal Science
Cornell University
Ithaca, New York

Vladimir Vuksan, Ph.D.
Clinical Nutrition and Risk Factor
  Modification Center
St. Michael's Hospital
Toronto, Ontario, Canada

Alexander R. P. Walker, D.Sc.
Human Biochemistry Research Unit
The South African Institute for Medical
  Research
Johannesburg, South Africa

Eric Westerlund, Ph.D
Associate Professor in Organic Chemistry
Department of Chemistry
Swedish University of Agricultural Sciences
Uppsala, Sweden

Thomas M. S. Wolever, B.M., B.Ch., Ph.D.
Department of Nutritional Sciences
University of Toronto
Toronto, Ontario, Canada

Margo N. Woods, D.Sc.
Associate Professor
Department of Family Medicine and
  Community Health
Tufts University School of Medicine
Boston, Massachusetts

Mauro Zamboni, M.D.
Istituto di Clinica Medica
Policlinico di Borgo Roma
Università di Verona
Verona, Italy

Su-Fang Zheng, M.D.
Professor
Institute of Cancer
Chinese Academy of Medical Sciences
Beijing, China

Contributors

Abayomi O. Akanji, M.D., Ph.D.
Department of Pathology
Kuwait University Faculty of Medicine
Kuwait

Per Åman, Dr. Agr.
Professor of Plant Foods
Department of Food Science
Swedish University of Agricultural Sciences
Uppsala, Sweden

James W. Anderson, M.D.
Professor of Medicine and Clinical Nutrition
V.A. Medical Center and
  University of Kentucky
Lexington, Kentucky

Roger Andersson, Ph.D.
Department of Food Science
Swedish University of Agricultural
  Sciences
Uppsala, Sweden

Fabio Armellini, M.D.
Istituto di Clinica Medica
Policlinico di Borgo Roma
Università di Verona
Verona, Italy

Nils-Georg Asp, M.D.
Professor
Department of Food Chemistry
Chemical Center
University of Lund
Lund, Sweden

Katrine I. Baghurst, B.Sc., Ph.D.
Consumer Science Program
Commonwealth Scientific and Industrial
  Research Organisation (CSIRO)
Health Sciences and Nutrition Division
Adelaide, Australia

Peter A. Baghurst, B.Ag.Sci., Ph.D., M.Sc.
Consumer Science Program
Commonwealth Scientific and Industrial
  Research Organisation (CSIRO)
Health Sciences and Nutrition Division
Adelaide, Australia

Sheila Bingham, Ph.D.
Medical Research Council
Dunn Clinical Nutrition Centre
Cambridge, England

Ottavio Bosello, M.D.
Professor
Istituto di Clinica Medica
Policlinico di Borgo Roma
Università di Verona
Verona, Italy

John H. Cummings, M.D.
Department of Molecular and Cellular
  Pathology
Ninewells Medical School
University of Dundee
Dundee, Scotland

Hans N. Englyst, Ph.D.
Medical Research Council Southampton
East Leigh, Hants., England

Sharon E. Fleming, Ph.D.
Professor
College of Natural Resources
Agricultural Experiment Station
Department of Nutritional Sciences
University of California
Berkeley, California

Hugh J. Freeman, M.D.
Professor of Gastrointestinal Medicine
Department of Medicine
University of British Columbia
Vancouver, British Columbia, Canada

Wenche Frølich, D.Ph.
Lindebergveien 39
JAR, Norway

Ivan Furda, Ph.D.
Furda and Associates, Inc.
Wayzata, Minnesota

Daniel D. Gallaher, Ph.D.
Assistant Professor
Department of Food Science and Nutrition
University of Minnesota
St. Paul, Minnesota

The Editor

Gene A. Spiller is the director of the Health Research and Studies Center and of the SPHERA Foundation in Los Altos, California.

Dr. Spiller received a doctorate in chemistry from the University of Milan (Italy) and later a master's degree and a Ph.D. in nutrition from the University of California at Berkeley. He did additional studies at the Stanford University School of Medicine, Stanford, California. He is a Fellow of the American College of Nutrition, a Certified Nutrition Specialist, and a member of many professional nutrition societies.

In the 1970s, Dr. Spiller was head of Nutritional Physiology at Syntex Research in Palo Alto, California, where he did extensive research on dietary fiber and related topics. At the same time he edited many clinical nutrition books. He continued his work in clinical nutrition research and publishing in the 1980s and 1990s, as a consultant and as the director of the Health Research and Studies Center and of the SPHERA Foundation. Many human clinical studies, reviews, and other publications were the results of this work. Dr. Spiller has carried out clinical studies on the effect of dietary fiber and high-fiber foods including nuts, raisins, and whole grains. Other studies have focused on antioxidants and lipids. He is a lecturer in nutrition at Foothill College in the San Francisco Bay Area and earlier taught at Mills College in Oakland, California.

Dr. Spiller is the editor of many clinical nutrition books on fiber and other topics at the forefront of nutrition research, such as caffeine and lipids. Among his multi-author books on fiber are *Fiber in Human Nutrition* (Plenum, 1975), *Topics in Dietary Fiber Research* (Plenum, 1978), and *Medical Aspects of Dietary Fiber* (Plenum, 1980), followed by the *CRC Handbook of Fiber in Human Nutrition,* 1st and 2nd Editions (CRC Press, 1985 and 1992).

He has a special interest in lesser-known nutritional factors that may be beneficial to human health, though not essential to life, especially factors that are present in plant foods and that may work together with dietary fiber in the prevention of degenerative diseases.

Dr. Spiller has been responsible for organizing international workshops on dietary fiber, such as the International Nutrition Congress in Brazil in 1978 and in Brighton (U.K.) in 1985, and has chaired many symposia and sessions on this and related topics at national meetings of various scientific societies.

Contents

Section 4. Physiological and Metabolic Effects of Dietary Fiber

Section 5. Dietary Fiber in the Prevention and Treatment of Disease

Section 6. Effect of Whole Grains, Cereal Fiber, and Phytic Acid on Health

Section 7. Definitions and Consumption

Appendix: Tables of Dietary Fiber and Associated Substances Content in Food

SECTION 1

Overview

Dietary Fiber: From Early Hunter–Gatherers to the 1990s

Denis P. Burkitt and Gene A. Spiller

The decline in plant fiber consumption by humans over tens of thousands of years is shown in Figure 1.1.1. According to Kliks, the author of this figure, over the past 20,000 years the human diet has changed from one based on a coarse, plant-based regimen of greens, seeds, stalks, roots, flowers, pollen, and small amounts of animal products to a more limited, often monotypic diet in which the plant foods are primarily a few cereal grains, tubers, and legumes. Even though the study of specimens of coprolite from lower Pleistocene humans has proved difficult, this coprolite has been extremely valuable in the study of human diets of civilization dating back about 10,000 years.[1] These specimens of coprolite showed a high consumption of fibrous plant food.

In more recent history, the concept that coarse foods of plant origin help to combat constipation goes back to Hippocrates in the 4th century B.C., who commented on the laxative action of outer layers of cereal grains, an observation repeated over 1000 years later (9th century A.D.) by the Persian physician Hakim. Shakespeare referred to the action of cereal bran in his play Coriolanus in 1610.

In the early 19th century, Graham[2] and Burne[3] in the U.S. and, in the late 19th century and at the dawn of the 20th century, Allinson in Britain extolled the virtues of whole grains in improving health by combating constipation.

The history of dietary fiber and health in the first 50 years of the 20th century reveals occasional interest but very few scientific publications. Fiber was relegated to being the Cinderella of nutrients. Remember that these were the days of major discoveries in vitamins, minerals, and all the other digestible nutrients. Somehow the concept that a group of substances practically undigestible by human GI enzymes could be important to health did not appeal to nutritionists, physiologists, and physicians in those years.

In the 1920s, McCarrison[4] drew attention to the good health of tribesmen in North India, which he attributed to the consumption of whole grains little tampered with by modern technology. In the same decade, John and Harvey Kellogg were extolling the virtues of whole grains in the U.S. The convictions of the latter culminated in the development of the breakfast cereal industry. Cowgill and Anderson in the 1930s published well-controlled research that proved that "fiber" was responsible for the laxative action of wheat bran. At the same time, the British surgeon Albuthnot Lane, whose name is eponymously commemorated in anatomical anomalies and surgical instruments, recognized the "dangers" of stagnant fecal content in the colon. His first reaction was to remove the colon surgically, but fortunately he subsequently appreciated that the administration of bran

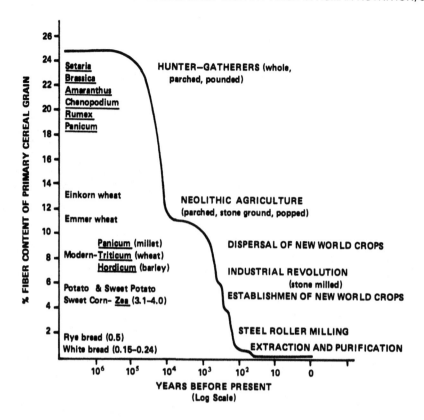

Figure 1.1.1 The decline in fiber consumption by humans. (From Kliks, M., in *Topics in Dietary Fiber Research*, Spiller, G. A. and Amen, R. J., Eds., Plenum Press, New York, 1978, 182. With permission.)

was altogether simpler, safer, and equally effective. In the late 1930s, Dimmock, a young British physician, reported his careful studies on the effectiveness of wheat bran in treating constipation and, in the late 1940s, Walker of South Africa was one of the first to appreciate the properties of plant fibers and to study them in a truly scientific manner.

In the years that followed, some epidemiological correlations by Cleave in Britain (1956 to 1966) and Trowell in Africa, with his 1960 book, *Non-Infectious Diseases in Africa*,[5] attributed protective effects to unrefined carbohydrates and "bulky" foods.

This, we could say, is the early history of fiber.

Other events took place in the 1970s and 1980s: the publication of a series of multiauthor books contributed to the clarification of the role of dietary fiber. As books are key steps in the growth of any field of science and as they become an intrinsic part of the history of science, it is worthwhile to recall some of their titles.

Some of the pioneering books appeared in 1975 to 1976: Burkitt and Trowell published *Refined Carbohydrate Foods and Disease*,[6] Reilly and Kirsner published *Fiber Deficiency and Colonic Disorders*,[7] and Spiller and Amen published *Fiber in Human Nutrition*.[8] They were followed in 1977 by Spiller and Amen, *Topics in Dietary Fiber Research*,[9] in 1978 by Heaton, *Dietary Fiber: Current Developments of Importance to Health*,[10] and in 1979 by Inglett and Falkenhag, *Dietary Fibers: Chemistry and Nutrition*.[11] In the 1980s, as dietary fiber became well established as a topic worthy of extensive research in human nutrition, more books on specific topics began to appear: Spiller and McPherson-Kay published *Medical Aspects of Dietary Fiber*,[12] the Royal College of Physicians wrote *Medical Aspects of Dietary Fiber*,[13] James and Theander wrote *The Analysis of*

Dietary Fiber in Food,[14] Vahouny and Kritchevsky wrote *Dietary Fiber in Health and Disease*,[15] and Trowell and Burkitt wrote *Western Diseases: Their Emergence and Prevention*.[16]

Many more books followed in the late 1980s and early 1990s, too many to list here. The pioneering days were over and *dietary fiber* had become an established, important factor in human nutrition and medicine.

It is interesting to realize that only 4 or 5 years before the publication of the first edition of this Handbook in 1986, it would have been quite difficult to find sufficient scientific and medical data to publish a Handbook such as this. This Handbook is proof of how rapidly the field of dietary fiber research is growing. Fast growth is exciting, but we should also take time to set up proper experiments and to review the literature carefully. In spite of all this growth, there are still conflicting views as to how dietary fiber should be defined (see Chapter 2.1) and there is less than precise use of terms in some publications. The complexity of dietary fiber and its tremendous interactions with other food components make its study a most difficult one indeed!

Since 1978 many major meetings that focused on various aspects of dietary fiber have taken place, meetings that have led to important debates on definition, functions, and health effects of dietary fiber. International congresses of nutrition in Brazil (1978), San Diego (1981), Brighton (U.K., 1985), and others began to include dietary fiber as an integral part of their programs. The National Institutes of Health sponsored a major international meeting in Washington, D.C. (1977) that appears to us now as a milestone in the history of dietary fiber. The proceedings were published in a special supplement of the *American Journal of Clinical Nutrition*[17] in 1978. In 1981 and 1984, two major symposia were also held in Washington at George Washington University. The Royal Society of New Zealand held a major symposium[18] in Palmerston North in 1982 which was reported in their Bulletin 20. Many other meetings have taken place in recent years, including several in analytical and chemical aspects of dietary fiber.

Notwithstanding all this progress and widespread interest by scientists, physicians, and health professionals on every continent, there are still many controversial aspects that will become evident to the reader of this Handbook, not the least of which is the definition of *dietary fiber*, and even the term *fiber* itself.

Since the first edition of this Handbook, the field of fiber research has also suffered the loss of two great pioneers in dietary fiber work. Hugh Trowell passed away in England in 1989, at the age of 85, after a lifelong dedication to medicine. During the last 20 years of his life, dietary fiber was the most important topic in his work, work he carried on to his very last days. And George Vahouny, who had developed many animal models for fiber research and who was an author in the first edition of this Handbook, passed away in Washington, D.C.

Denis Burkitt passed away in England soon after the publication of the second edition. I have left the preceding section unchanged as it was written with him. It has a great historical value and the insight that Denis Burkitt had in all his work. It is strange that some researchers remember him more for his Burkitt lymphoma than for his work with fiber. What follows is a brief update since 1992.

Since 1992, perhaps the most important development has been the tremendous amount of research on the hundreds of phytochemicals that are present in plant foods and how many of them are closely linked with fiber foods. Such phytochemicals range from many antioxidants with a variety of health benefits to tartaric acid, all working together with fiber. These phytochemicals, from antioxidants to tartaric acid, closely interact with fiber, and this is reflected in some of the new chapters in this edition.

As often happens in science, what was true is 1992 is still true now: there are still some controversial aspects of the effects of fiber that will become evident to the reader of this Handbook. Dietary fiber is so complex that it defies the reductionist scientist's desire to isolate a pure substance and study it in humans or animals. Too often fiber purification means major structural alterations. While we can study fiber concentrates, and while many of them have a valuable place in health maintenance, the ultimate purification of fiber often implies physical–chemical changes that need to be carefully remembered when studies are carried out.

The "Fiber Hypothesis" of Trowell and Burkitt is now beyond a hypothesis: it is a truth that can help people lead much healthier lives and prevent many chronic diseases.

REFERENCES

1 . Kliks, M., Paleodietetics: a review of the role of dietary fiber in preagricultural human diets, in *Topics in Dietary Fiber Research*, Spiller, G. A. and Amen, R. J., Eds., Plenum Press, New York, 1978, 181.
2. Graham, S., *Lectures on the Science of Human Life*, Capen, Lyon and Webb, Boston, 1829.
3. Burne, J., *Treatise on the Causes and Consequences of Constipation*, Haswell, Barrington and Haswell, New Orleans, LA, 1840.
4. McCarrison, R., *Studies in Deficiency Disease*, Frowde, Hodder and Stoughton, London, 1921.
5. Trowell, H., *Non-Infectious Diseases in Africa*, Edward Arnold, London, 1960.
6. Burkitt, D. P. and Trowell, H. C., *Refined Carbohydrate Foods and Disease*, Academic Press, New York, 1975.
7. Reilly, W. R. and Kirsner, J. B., *Fiber Deficiency and Colonic Disorders*, Plenum Press, New York, 1975.
8. Spiller, G. A. and Amen, R. J., *Fiber in Human Nutrition*, Plenum Press, New York, 1976.
9. Spiller, G. A. and Amen, R. J., *Topics in Dietary Fiber Research*, Plenum Press, New York, 1978.
10. Heaton, K. W., *Dietary Fiber: Current Developments of Importance to Health*, John Libbey, London, 1978.
11. Inglett, G. E. and Falkenhag, S. I., *Dietary Fibers: Chemistry and Nutrition*, Academic Press, New York, 1979.
12. Spiller, G. A. and McPherson-Kay, R., *Medical Aspects of Dietary Fiber*, Plenum Press, New York, 1980.
13. Royal College of Physicians, *Medical Aspects of Dietary Fiber*, Pitman Medical, Tunbridge Wells, Kent, U.K., 1980.
14. James, W. P. T. and Theander, O., *The Analysis of Dietary Fiber in Food*, Marcel Dekker, New York, 1981.
15. Vahouny, G. V. and Kritchevsky, D., *Dietary Fiber in Health and Disease*, Plenum Press, New York, 1982.
16. Trowell, H. C. and Burkitt, D. P., *Western Diseases: Their Emergence and Prevention*, Harvard University Press, Cambridge, MA, 1981.
17. Roth, H. P. and Mehlman, M. A., Eds., Proceedings: symposium on the role of dietary fiber, *Am. J. Clin. Nutr.*, 31S, 1978.
18. Wallace, G. and Bell, L., Eds., Proceedings: fiber in human and animal nutrition, *R. Soc. N.Z. Bull.*, 1983.

Definitions and Properties of Dietary Fiber

Definitions of Dietary Fiber

Gene A. Spiller

Term recommended and author	Definition
Dietary Fiber (DF) (Trowell)	Plant substances not digested by human digestive enzymes, including plant cell wall substances (cellulose, hernicelluloses, pectin, and lignin) as well as intracellular polysaccharides such as gums and mucilages. Largely identical to undigested (unavailable) carbohydrates plus lignin. The early definition by Trowell of "the remnants of plant cells resistant to hydrolysis by the alimentary enzymes of man" remains as a key definition, even though it may better apply to the dietary fiber complex defined below. A key contribution by Trowell was to emphasize the distinction between dietary fiber and crude fiber.
Dietary Fiber Complex (Trowell, Spiller)	Same as dietary fiber but defined to include other plant substances that are undigested by human digestive enzymes, such as waxes, cutins, and undigestible cell wall proteins. These are the substances that are normally associated with and concentrated around the plant cell wall.
Dietary Fiber (Southgate)	The sum of lignin and the polysaccharides that are not hydrolyzed by the endogenous secretions of the human digestive tract. Southgate considers this as a physiological and philosophical definition and feels that it is necessary to produce a definition that can be translated into purely analytical terms. This author suggests a chemical definition based on the fact that the sum of lignin and the non-α glucan polysaccharides (nonstarch polysaccharides) is the best index of dietary fiber in the diet.
Dietary Fiber (Furda)	Chemical definition: the sum of the plant nonstarch polysaccharides and lignin. Physiological definition: the remnant of plant foods resistant to hydrolysis by the alimentary enzymes of humans.

0-8493-2387-8/01/$0.00+$1.50
© 2001 by CRC Press LLC

Plantix (Spiller)	A term designed to represent dietary fiber as defined by Trowell but that avoids the word "fiber," since many of the substances defined may not, strictly speaking, be of a fibrous nature. In fact, cellulose is the only truly fibrous component of the plant cell wall. It also implies that the material is present in plants only. It includes the plant polysaccharides and lignin that are not digested by human digestive enzymes.
Plantix Complex (Spiller)	Suggested to replace dietary fiber complex, again to avoid the word "fiber." It includes undigestible parts of the plant cell that are not included in plantix, such as waxes, undigestible proteins, and others.
Purified Plant Fiber (Spiller)	Any highly purified single polymer derived from plants that is not digested by human digestive enzymes but that may be digested by microorganisms in the human intestinal tract. Examples are purified pectin and purified cellulose. This is a modification of an earlier definition that included more than one substance.
Unavailable Carbohydrate (McCance and Lawrence)	A classical term used in nutrition for many years to distinguish between available and nonavailable carbohydrate in humans. As originally defined it included lignin, which is not a carbohydrate. Furthermore, the fact that some of these carbohydates are digested by bacteria in the human intestine and produce fatty acids that are actually "available" makes the term "unavailable" ambiguous.
Edible Fiber (Trowel, Godding)	An expanded definition of dietary fiber as given above; other groups of undigested (human enzyme–undigested) polysaccharides and related substances are added: (1) animal fibers not digested by human digestive enzymes, e.g., aminopolysaccharides; (2) synthetic or partially synthetic polysaccharides not digested by human digestive enzymes, e.g., methylcelluloses; (3) polysaccharides that are not part of traditional foods and that are not digested by human digestive enzymes. These products may be of pharmaceutical importance.
Neutral Detergent Residues (NDR) (Van Soest)	A residue after special digestion (see Section 3) with detergents, essentially the sum of cellulose, hemicellulose, and lignin. Often called neutral detergent fiber (NDF).
Crude Fiber	The remnants of plant material after extraction with acid and alkali. The term should not be used with reference to dietary fiber. Old definition from the 19th century. Crude fiber values include only variable portions of the cellulose, hemicelluloses, and lignin present in dietary fiber.
Nonstarch Polysaccharides (NSP) (Englyst)	The carbohydrate plant cell wall material originally called *dietary fiber* less the lignin, analyzed in such a way as to eliminate any other plant substance that may appear as fiber in other analytical methods. Methods to determine NSP must be such that any *resistant starch* (see below) is not taken into account.
Resistant Starch (RS) (Englyst)	Starch that is not digested by human digestive enzymes and that reaches the colon, often acting in the same way as *fiber*.

Dietary Fiber Parts of Food Plants and Algae

David A. T. Southgate

The major portion of dietary fiber in foods is derived from the plant cell walls in foods.[1] A wide range of plant organs and types of tissue is consumed in the human diet, although highly lignified (woody) tissues are rejected during food preparation.[2]

The organization and detailed composition of the plant cell wall varies with the type of tissues, but the essential features are common to virtually all walls. This is a network of cellulose fibers in a matrix of non-cellulosic polysaccharides. The composition of the matrix varies with the maturity of the plant tissues, the plant species, and the major plant grouping.[3,4]

The nomenclature used to describe the detailed composition of the plant cell wall is based on the classical schemes for fractionating the components. The essential features of this scheme are given in Figure 2.2.1.[5]

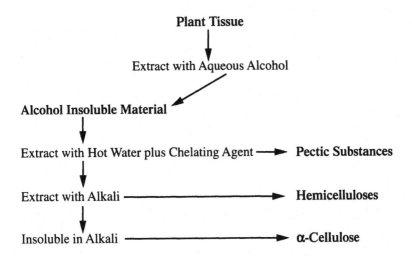

Figure 2.2.1 Schematic representation of the major stages in the classical scheme for the fractionation of the plant cell wall that forms the basis for the nomenclature used to describe the components of the plant cell wall.

0-8493-2387-8/01/$0.00+$1.50

The plant tissue was extracted with aqueous alcohol and the insoluble material was extracted first, with hot water. This often contained a chelating agent to disrupt the polysaccharides forming the intercellular middle lamellae. This gave a "pectic substances" fraction, which included, in addition to the rhamnogalacturonans (true pectins), arabinogalactans, β-glucans, and arabinoxylans.

The water-insoluble material was then extracted with increasing strengths of alkali to give the so-called hemicellulose fraction, which included a range of xylans, with arabinosyl and 4-0-methylglucuronyl substituents, gluco- and galactomannans, and xyloglucans. The material insoluble in the strongest alkali was designated the "α-cellulose," which contained cellulose and lignin.

Where a mature plant tissue that contained substantial amounts of lignin was being fractionated, it was necessary to oxidize the lignin before the hemicelluloses could be extracted.

It is known that the fractions obtained in the classical fractionation schemes are arbitrary and that artifacts are often produced. Although modern derivatives of this method[6] have refined the alkaline extraction stages to avoid some of the degradation from the alkali, Albersheim[7] proposed that the term "non-cellulosic polysaccharides" (NCP) should be used for this fraction, which would include a spectrum of polysaccharides which range from those rich in uronic acids to those poor in uronic acids.

Although lignin is an aromatic polymer and therefore not a carbohydrate, it is covalently linked to the polysaccharides and was included in the original definition of dietary fiber (see Trowell et al.[8]).

It important to recognize that the plant cell wall is a highly organized structure, not merely a collection of polysaccharides. These polysaccharides are linked together in what can be described as a supramolecular structure which confers additional properties on the wall.[6] Furthermore, plant tissues are highly organized structures which confer physical properties on these materials when they are consumed in foods.

Plant foods contain a range of water-soluble gums and mucilages. These have structures analogous to many cell wall components and are included in the non-cellulosic polysaccharides and the non-starch polysaccharides (NSP) of Englyst et al.[9]

The major components of dietary fiber are summarized in Table 2.2.1.

Table 2.2.1   Dietary Fiber Components of Foods

Classical Nomenclature	Solubility Characteristics	Classes of Polysaccharide	Nomenclature Used in Dietary Fiber Literature
Plant Cell Wall Components			
Pectic substances	Water-soluble	Rhamnogalacturonans, arabinogalactans, β-glucans, arabinoxylans	Included in non-cellulosic polysaccharides (NCP) and non-starch polysaccharides (NSP); soluble fiber
Hemicelluloses	Insoluble in water, soluble in dilute alkali	Arabinoxylans, galactomannans, xyloglucans	Included in NCP and NSP
α-Cellulose	Insoluble in alkali	Cellulose (and lignin where present)	Included in NSP
Lignin	Insoluble in 12M H_2SO_4	Aromatic polymer, non-carbohydrate	Lignin, and in total dietary fiber (AOAC method)
Non-Structural Components			
Gums and mucilages	Water-soluble or dispersible	Galactomannans, arabinogalactans, wide range of branched and substituted galactans	Included in NCP and NSP; soluble fiber

REFERENCES

1. Southgate, D. A. T., Fibre in nutrition, *Bibl. Nutr. Dieta*, 22, 109, 1975.
2. Southgate, D. A. T., The chemistry of dietary fiber, in *Fiber in Human Nutrition*, Spiller, G. A. and Amen, R. J., Eds., Plenum Press, New York, 1976, 31.
3. Brett, C. and Waldron, K., *Physiology and Biochemistry of Plant Cell Walls*, 2nd ed., Chapman and Hall, London, 1996.
4. Selvendran, R. R., The plant cell wall as a source of dietary fiber: chemistry and structure, *Am. J. Clin. Nutr.*, 39, 320, 1984.
5. Gaillard, B. D. E., A detailed summative analysis of the crude fibre and nitrogen-free extractives fraction of roughages. Proposed scheme of analysis, *J. Sci. Food Agric.*, 9, 170, 1958.
6. Selvendran, R. R. and O'Neill, M. A., Plant glycoproteins, in *Methods of Chemical Analysis*, Glick, D., Ed., John Wiley, New York, 1987, 32, 25.
7. Albersheim, P., Biogenesis of the cell wall, in *Plant Biochemistry*, Bonner, J. and Varner, J. E., Eds., Academic Press, 1965, 298.
8. Trowell, H., Southgate, D. A. T., Wolever, T. M. S., Leeds, A. R., Gassull, M. A., and Jenkins, D. A., Dietary fibre redefined, *Lancet*, 1, 967, 1976.
9. Englyst, H. N., Quigley, M. E., and Hudson, G. J., Determination of dietary fibre as non-starch polysaccharides, with gas-liquid chromatographic, high-performance chromatographic or spectrophotometric measurement of constituent sugars, *Analyst*, 119, 1511, 1994.

Food Components That Behave as Dietary Fiber

David A. T. Southgate

Dietary fiber exerts a wide range of physiological effects when consumed, and its complex nature is responsible for a range of physical and chemical properties that are responsible for these physiological effects. One characteristic property is that dietary fiber is not hydrolyzed by the endogenous enzymes of the human gastrointestinal tract.[1] It therefore escapes digestion in the small intestine and passes into the large intestine, where it provides a substrate for the microflora of the large intestine which can degrade many of the polysaccharides present.[2]

By convention, dietary fiber has been restricted to the indigestible polysaccharides and lignin,[1] although some proteins and fats in the human diet are also indigestible. Some authors have argued that all the indigestible components of the diet should be considered part of dietary fiber.[3,4] Table 2.3.1 lists various indigestible components of food other than dietary fiber.

Table 2.3.1   Food Components That Share Indigestibility with Dietary Fiber

Category	Dietary Sources	Occurrence
Indigestible components of plant cellular tissues	Lignin	Most mature plant tissues
	Cutin	Epidermal tissues of plants
	Suberin	Subepidermal tissues
	Waxes	Surfaces of fruits
	Protein, inorganic constituents	Virtually all plant tissues
Resistant starch	Crystal structure	Green banana
	Physically enclosed	Cereal grains, broken
	Retrograded amylose	Many heat-processed foods
Indigestible carbohydrates	Fructo-oligosaccharides, galacto-oligosaccharides	Many plants, especially vegetables and fruits
	Sugar alcohols	Added to processed foods
Non-structural carbohydrates	Gums, modified starches, semi-synthetic polymers	Many processed foods; used as ingredients
Non-assimilable components	Hydrocarbon oils, waxes	Contaminants
	Dyes	Processed foods
	Pigments	Natural and synthetic
	Chitin from exoskeleton	Insects and crustaceans
	Mucopolysaccharides, hair	Animal tissues

0-8493-2387-8/01/$0.00+$1.50

INDIGESTIBLE COMPONENTS OF PLANT CELLULAR TISSUES

In most human diets the plant cell wall material in the diet is the major source of indigestible polysaccharides; however, plants contain other substances that are indigestible. These include non-carbohydrate materials which are associated with or are integral parts of the plant cell wall structure, such as lignin, cutin, suberin, waxes, protein, and inorganic constituents. Most of these escape digestion in the small intestine either because they are intrinsically nondigestible or because the cell wall structures inhibit or prevent enzymatic attack.

RESISTANT STARCH[5]

This latter effect is also seen with starches that are contained within cellular structures. A few foods also contain starch grains with special crystalline structures that resist enzymatic hydrolysis.

Many starch-rich foods, especially those which have been processed by heat treatment in moist conditions and allowed to cool, contain retrograded amylose, which forms an insoluble crystalline material that is resistant to enzymatic hydrolysis.

These three types of enzymatically resistant starch are often grouped as "resistant starch," which refers to resistance to hydrolysis under physiological conditions.[6]

INDIGESTIBLE CARBOHYDRATES[7]

In addition to the carbohydrates in the plant cell wall, there are a range of indigestible carbohydrates in foods. These include fructan, inulin, and two series of oligosaccharides — those based on fructose and the galacto- series: raffinose, stachyose, and verbascose. These compounds are present at significant levels in many fruits and vegetables. The other major series of oligosaccharides in foods, the malto- series, are hydrolyzed to glucose very effectively by the brush-border enzymes of the small intestine.

Processed foods and a few raw foods also contain sugar alcohols that are only partially absorbed.

These carbohydrates are soluble in 80% v/v ethanol and therefore require additional stages to the NSP methods and total dietary fiber (AOAC) to measure them.[8]

NON-STRUCTURAL POLYSACCHARIDES

The fourth group includes polysaccharides which are not alpha-linked glucans (and therefore indigestible) that are present in foods but are not part of cell wall structures. These may occur naturally in plant foods or may be food ingredients of additives that have been added to processed foods. These ingredients include semi-synthetic, randomized polymers of glucose, such as poly-dextrose. Some exudate gums are used as ingredients in confectionery, and a range of other polysaccharides are used as food additives, usually to control or influence the physical properties of a food.[9]

HEAT-PRODUCED ARTIFACTS

A fifth group contains degraded carbohydrates, usually in the form of carbohydrate–protein complexes formed during the processing of foodstuffs.

NON-ASSIMILABLE COMPONENTS OF FOODS

Finally, there is a range of non-assimilable components of food, hydrocarbon oils, waxes and dyes, degraded connective tissue components, the exoskeleton of insects and crustacea, mucopolysaccharides, and hairs.[10]

All these substances can be said to behave as dietary fiber in the sense that they are indigestible. Many authors believe that most of these components are not considered appropriate to include in dietary fiber because they include a heterogeneous collection of materials far removed from the original conceptual definition of dietary fiber, which was not synonymous with indigestibility.[11]

REFERENCES

1. Trowell, H., Southgate, D. A. T., Wolever, T. M. S., Leeds, A. R., Gassull, M. A., and Jenkins, D. A., Dietary fibre redefined, *Lancet*, 1, 967, 1976.
2. Stephen, A. M. and Cummings, J. C., Mechanism of action of dietary fibre in the human colon, *Nature (London)*, 284, 283, 1980.
3. Hellendoorn, E. W., Some critical observations in relation to "dietary fibre," the methods of determination and the current hypotheses for the explanation of its physiological action, *Voeding*, 33, 230, 1978.
4. Saunders, R. M. and Betschart, A. A., The significance of protein as a component of dietary fiber, *Am. J. Clin. Nutr.*, 33, 960, 1980.
5. Gudmand-Hayer, E., *Methodological aspects of the in vivo methods for measurement of starch digestibility*, Euresta, Contract No. AGRF/0027, European Union, Brussels,1992.
6. Englyst, H. N., Kingman, S. M., and Cummings, J. C., Classification and measurement of nutritionally important starch fractions, *Eur. J. Clin. Nutr.*, 46, S33 (Suppl. 2), 1992.
7. Guillon, F. et al., Eds., Functional Properties of Non-Digestible Carbohydrates. *Profibre*, European Air Concerted Action, AIR3CT94-2203, Institut National de la Recherche Agronomique, Nantes, 1998.
8. Southgate, D. A. T., *Dietary Fibre Analysis*, Royal Society of Chemistry, Cambridge, 1995.
9. Glicksman, M., *Gum Technology in the Food Industry*, Academic Press, New York, 1969.
10. Southgate, D. A. T., Non-assimilable components of foods, in *Nutritional Problems in a Changing World*, Hollingsworth, D. F. and Russell, M., Eds., 1973, 199.
11. Englyst, H. N., Trowell, H., Southgate, D. A. T., and Cummings, J. H., Dietary fiber and resistant starch, *Am. J. Clin. Nutr.*, 46, 873, 1987.

Food Components Associated with Dietary Fiber

David A. T. Southgate

INTRODUCTION

Plant foods contain a wide range of substances and many of these are biologically active (for example, vitamins, phytoestrogens, glucosinolates, and polyphenolic substances). These phytochemicals are therefore consumed with dietary fiber components, and it is highly probable that they contribute to the protective effects of high-fiber diets. This section is, however, concerned with the components of plant foods that are intimately associated with dietary fiber (Table 2.4.1).

Table 2.4.1 Food Components Associated with Dietary Fiber

Component	Sources	Main Structural Features
Lignins	Found in all vascular plants; major component of woody tissues and some seeds	Complex aromatic polymers formed from coumaryl, guaiacyl, coniferyl, and sinapyl alcohols
Protein	Present in all cell walls	Often rich in hydroxyproline and linked to polysaccharides
Cutin	External surfaces of many fruits and leaves	Polymeric internal esters of C16 and C18 hydroxyaliphatic acids
Suberin	Sub-epidermal tissues of many plants, especially roots and tubers	Polymeric material from C20, C26 acids and alcohols with phenolics and dicarboxylic acids
Plant waxes	External surfaces of many fruits	Complex mixtures of hydrocarbons, ketones, ketols, etc.
Inorganic constituents	Virtually all walls	Ca, K, Mg salts and silicates common

The plant cell wall contains or is very closely associated with a range of non-carbohydrates. Some of these are integral to the cell wall structures, whereas others appear to be chance inclusions, and still others are closely associated with the walls on the exterior surfaces of the plants.[1] The non-carbohydrates are usually quantitatively minor components of the plant cell wall; nevertheless, they modify the physical and chemical properties of the wall polysaccharides and thereby can be expected to modify the physiological properties of dietary fiber when eaten.[2]

0-8493-2387-8/01/$0.00+$1.50
© 2001 by CRC Press LLC

LIGNIN

Although many authors consider the lignins (a wide range of structures are found in plants) as part of dietary fiber in a formal sense, it is more appropriate to consider lignin as an associated component, because it is only by conventional usage that lignin is included in dietary fiber.[3]

Lignin is the name given to a complex group of aromatic polymers formed by the condensation of aromatic alcohols, coumaryl, guaiacyl, coniferyl, and sinapyl alcohols. This condensation is, in the main, non-enzymatic, and this accounts for the very wide range of structures observed.

Lignification of the plant cell wall is an infiltration process of the matrix where the lignin forms a three-dimensional structure within the polysaccharide matrix and the wall expands in volume during the process.[4]

In many food plants, which are consumed relatively immature, the lignification is limited to the spiral and annular bands in the walls of the xylem vessels. As the plant matures the lignification spreads through the entire wall of the xylem and extends into supporting tissues.[5] In mature woody tissues the xylem walls are completely lignified. These woody tissues are most frequently not consumed as foods, especially in the developed world.

Lignified tissues are present in the cell walls of the seed coats of cereals, and lignified seeds are widely distributed in many fruits and vegetables. Pears contain clumps of lignified cells within their flesh.[5]

Lignification produces a hydrophobic region within the wall, and as lignin is highly resistant to bacterial and enzymatic attack, lignified tissues from foods are recoverable virtually intact from fecal material.

Analytical procedures for lignin are often nonspecific and depend on the resistance of lignin to chemical attack. Thus, insolubility in 12M H_2SO_4 is the basis of the measurement of "Klason" lignin.[6] In the Van Soest and Wine method the susceptibility to oxidation by alkaline permanganate is the basis of the determination.[7] Colorimetric procedures for some grass species have been described, but these are specific for the species concerned.

PROTEIN

Some protein is found in virtually all cell walls and may form up to 10% of the wall in immature plants. The proportion falls as the wall matures and proportionately more polysaccharides are deposited in the wall. The cell wall proteins appear to play an important structural role and are in some tissues characteristically rich in hydroxyproline.[8] The proteins are often covalently linked to polysaccharide side chains.

The cell wall proteins in some tissues appear to have an intrinsically lower digestibility, and for this reason some authors believe that these proteins should be considered part of the dietary fiber complex.[9]

CUTIN, SUBERIN, AND PLANT WAXES[1,5]

These substances are complex lipid materials present in many plant tissues.

Cutin

Many external surfaces of plants are covered with a waxy layer which includes a range of complex substances containing long-chain hydroxy aliphatic acids which form internal esters. This material is highly hydrophobic and intimately associated with the cell wall at the plant surface.

Cutinized tissues are resistant to hydrolysis and degradation in the intestine and frequently can be recovered from fecal material. In some analytical schemes the cutin is analyzed with the lignin unless the material is extracted with a lipid solvent. The detergent fiber procedures of Van Soest provide an extension which provides a method for measurement of cutin.[6]

Suberin

Suberin is also a complex mixture with a composition analogous to cutin which includes phenolic components. Suberin is characteristically deposited in sub-epidermal layers in many plant tissues, particularly in underground organs such as roots and tubers, but it is also found in the skins of some fruits. Suberinized tissues are also hydrophobic and resistant to degradation in the intestine and usually are analyzed with lignin.

Waxes

Complex hydrocarbon waxes are found in many plants in very small quantities. The waxes are mixtures of ketones, esters, phenolic esters, and alcohols. These waxes coat external surfaces of many fruits with a hydrophobic layer. Although these materials are hydrolyzed by lipases in the presence of bile salts, their degradation in the intestine appears to be limited.

INORGANIC MATERIALS

Most plant cell walls contain inorganic material. In some plants the inorganic material apparently has structural significance, this being especially true for silica and silicates.[10] Calcium is also closely involved in the structure of the pectic components of the middle lamellae between cells and the integrity of plant tissues. Other inclusions of potassium and magnesium salts with phosphates and oxalates are quite common.

REFERENCES

1. Bonner, J. and Varner, J. E., Eds., *Plant Biochemistry*, 2nd ed., Academic Press, New York, 1977.
2. Southgate, D. A. T., The structure of dietary fibre, in *Dietary Fiber in Health and Disease*, Kritchevsky, D. and Bonfield, C., Eds., Eagan Press, St. Paul, MN, 1995, 26.
3. Trowell, H., Southgate, D. A. T., Wolever, T. M. S., Leeds, A. R., Gassull, M. A., and Jenkins, D. A., Dietary fibre, *Lancet*, 1, 967, 1976.
4. Brett, C. and Waldron, K., *Physiology and Biochemistry of Plant Cell Walls*, 2nd ed., Chapman and Hall, London, 1996, 58.
5. Cutting, E. G., *Plant Anatomy, Experiment and Interpretation*, part 2, Edward Arnold, London, 1971.
6. Goering, H. K. and Van Soest, P. J., *Forage Fiber Analysis (Apparatus Reagents, Procedures and Some Applications)*, Agricultural Handbook No. 379, U.S. Department of Agriculture, Washington, D.C., 1970.
7. Van Soest, P. J. and Wine, R. H., Determination of lignin and cellulose in acid detergent fiber by oxidation with permanganate, *J. Assoc. Off. Analyt. Chem.*, 52, 780, 1968.
8. Selvendran, R. R. and O'Neill, M. A., Plant glycoproteins, in *Plant Carbohydrates*, Loewus, F. A. and Tanner, W., Eds., Springer-Verlag, Basel, 1982, 575.
9. Saunders, R. M. and Betschart, A. A., The significance of protein as a component of dietary fiber, *Am. J. Clin. Nutr.*, 33, 960, 1980.
10. Jones, L. H. P., Mineral components of plant cell walls, *Am. J.Clin. Nutr.*, 31, 594, 1978.

Polysaccharide Food Additives That Contribute to Dietary Fiber

David A. T. Southgate

A variety of polysaccharides are added to processed foods. While none are synthetic in the true sense, many of them have been extensively modified chemically to enhance specific properties or to reduce undesirable characteristics.[1,2] A few are prepared biosynthetically using microorganisms, but the majority are derived from plant polysaccharides and many from cell wall polysaccharides. The polysaccharides all share one common structural feature: they do not contain α-glucosidic links (i.e., they are nonstarch polysaccharides) and are, therefore, not hydrolyzed by mammalian digestive enzymes. For this reason, they fall within the most commonly used definition of dietary fiber.[3] Many have been, and still are, used as models for cell wall components of dietary fiber in experimental physiological studies. They fall into a number of distinct categories.

MODIFIED CELL WALL POLYSACCHARIDES

These native structures have been chemically modified to improve their solubility or capacity to form gels. They are added to foods to modify or control the physical properties of foods.

Pectins

The additives are selected from high-methoxyl varieties which have higher gelling properties. Amidation also improves the gelling capacity, and amidated pectins are used in low-sugar jams and as emulsifiers and stabilizers.

Cellulose

A relatively simple modification involves the reduction in the chain lengths of the polymers by ball milling; this produces water-dispersible celluloses which are used as fillers. Chemical modification involves the introduction of methyl and methoxyl groups which create a range of dispersible compounds which are used as emulsifiers and stabilizers.

Modified Starches

The chemical modifications include the introduction of phosphate groups or isopropyl groups and a variety of other substituents primarily aimed at preventing retrogradation in heat-processed foods where the introduced groups prevent association of the amylose chains.

INDIGESTIBLE FRUCTOSE POLYMERS AND OLIGOSACCHARIDES

Many vegetable foods such as Jerusalem artichokes and chicory contain the fructan *inulin*. Modern extraction techniques have made inulin available as an ingredient. Fructan is an indigestible carbohydrate and contributes substrate to the large intestinal flora.[4]

A range of fructose oligosaccharides which are also indigestible is available as ingredients with claimed probiotic properties.

GUMS

Several exudate gums — for example, gum Arabic and gum tragacanth — are used as additives and food ingredients. The most widely used gums are the galactomannan gums, guar and carob (locust) bean gums which are used as thickeners in soups and other foods.

ALGAL POLYSACCHARIDES

Algae provide a range of polysaccharides used in processed foods. Agar is used as a thickening agent in a wide range of foods. Alginates, extracted from brown algae and modified alginates, are also used as thickening agents. Carrageenans, extracted from Irish moss and other algae, are used in many milk products because of the ability to associate with milk proteins.

SEMISYNTHETIC POLYMERS

These polymers include xanthan gum produced biosynthetically and are used as gelling agents.

A number of randomized glucose polymers have been prepared which are resistant to small intestinal digestion, and polydextrose is in use as an ingredient in "low-calorie" yogurts and similar products.

Table 2.5.1 summarizes the major types of polysaccharides in use. In most foods the concentration of the additives is less than 1% by weight and usually less than 0.5%. Some exudate gums and some randomized glucose polymers are used as ingredients at higher concentrations.

These polysaccharides make a minor contribution to the total intake of dietary fiber[5] but have been fed at much higher levels of intake in experimental studies.

Table 2.5.1   Polysaccharide Food Additives That Contribute to Dietary Fiber

Major Category	Polysaccharides	Major Types Used	Main Structural Features
Modified cell wall components	Pectins	High methoxyl	Methoxyl esters of rhamnogalacturonans
		Amidated	Amidated rhamnogalacturonans
	Cellulose	Methyl, methoxyl	Both ether and ester derivatives are used
Modified starches	Cross-linked	Phosphate, isopropyl	Cross-linked to prevent association between amylose chains
Indigestible fructose polymers	Fructans	Inulin	Relatively low molecular weights
	Fructo-oligosaccharides	Range of polymers	Range of oligosaccharides
Gums	Exudate gums	Arabic, tragacanth	Complex heteropolysaccharides
	Galactomannan gums	Guar, carob (locust) bean	Variable proportions of glucose substituents
Algal polysaccharides	Agar	Two major polymers	Linear polymer of D-galactose and L-anhydrogalactose
	Alginates	Salts of copolymers	Salts of D-mannuronic and L-gluronic acid
	Carrageenans	Range of different polymers	Polymers of anhydro-galactose, sulfated galactose, and sulfated anhydro-galactose
Semi-synthetic polymers	Bacterial synthesis	Xanthan gum	Backbone of glucose with alternating trisaccharide side chains of mannose and glucuronic acid, with terminal pyruvic acid and acetyl groups
	Randomized glucans	Polydextrose is an example	Thermally randomized polymers

REFERENCES

1. Glicksman, M., *Gum Technology in the Food Industry*, Academic Press, New York, 1969.
2. Guillon, F. et al., Eds., *Functional Properties of Non-Digestible Carbohydrates*, Institut National de la Recherche Agronomique, Nantes, 1998.
3. Trowell, H., Southgate, D. A. T., Wolever, M. S., Leeds, A. R., Gassull, M. A., and Jenkins, D. A., Dietary fibre redefined, *Lancet*, 1, 967, 1976.
4. Gibson, G. R., Beatty, E. B., Wang, X., and Cummings, J. H., Selective simulation of bifidobacteria in the human colon by oligofructose and iulin, *Gastroenterology*, 108, 975, 1995.
5. Wirths, W., Aufnahme an Hydrocolloiden in der Bundersrepublick Deutschland, in *Pflanzenfasen-Ballastoffe in der menschlichen Ernahrung*, Rottka, H., Ed., Thieme Verlag, Stuttgart, 1980, 76.

Glossary of Dietary Fiber Components*

David A. T. Southgate and Gene A. Spiller

Acid detergent fiber (ADF) — The cellulose plus lignin in a sample; it is measured as the residue after extracting the food with a hot dilute sulfuric acid solution of the detergent, cetyl trimethylammonium bromide (CTAB). See Chapter 3.2.

Agar — A mixture of polysaccharides occurring as the cell wall constituents of certain red marine algae Rhodophytaceae, e.g., *Gelidium* sp., from which it can be extracted with hot water. It gels on cooling at a concentration as low as 0.5%. Agarose, the main constituent, is a neutral polysaccharide containing 3,6-anhydro-L-galactose and D-galactose as the repetitive unit. Agaropectin is a minor constituent polysaccharide and contains carboxyl and sulfate groups. It is not hydrolyzed by mammalian digestive enzymes and is, therefore, part of dietary fiber when used as a thickening agent in foods; it is a laxative. The chief use, however, is as a solid medium for cultivating microorganisms, since it is undigested by almost all of them.

Algal polysaccharides — The extract from the tissues of algae, divided into two groups: (1) reserve polysaccharides which are water soluble and (2) structural polysaccharides which are not. They are not hydrolyzed by the mammalian digestive enzymes and are therefore part of dietary fiber.

Alginates — Algal polysaccharides not hydrolyzed by mammalian digestive enzymes and, therefore, part of dietary fiber. Commercial algin is sodium alginate: it is slowly soluble in water, forming an extremely viscous solution. It is used as a stabilizer for ice cream and other food products.

Alginic acid — Water-insoluble algal polysaccharide, polymannuronic acid, which can be extracted from certain dried seaweeds, as a water-soluble alginate with aqueous alkali metal hydroxides or carbonates, and precipitated by the addition of an acid. Alginic acid is not hydrolyzed by mammalian digestive enzymes and is, therefore, part of dietary fiber.

Arabinans — Polysaccharides that give L-arabinose on hydrolysis. They are present in wood cellulose, are associated with pectin, and have been isolated from the pectic substances of mustard seed and sugar beet.

Arabinogalactans — Substituted galactans that form part of the hemicellulose complex in many tissues. Although most emphasis has been given to arabinogalactans from woody tissues, polymers of this type are widely distributed. The water-soluble arabinogalactan of larch has received considerable study.

---

* Adapted from Southgate, D. A. T., *Medical Aspects of Dietary Fiber*, Spiller, G. A. and Kay, R. M., Eds., Plenum Press, New York, 1980. With permission.

0-8493-2387-8/01/$0.00+$1.50
© 2001 by CRC Press LLC

Arabinoxylans — Have a main chain composed of $(1 \rightarrow 4)$ β-D-xylopyranosyl units with an occasional branching in some preparations. The arabinose is present as single- or double-residue side chains. Arabinoxylans are widely distributed in the cell walls of many materials, although they are uncommon in woody tissues; they have been isolated from the husks of many grains.

Carrageenan — An algal polysaccharide chiefly composed of polymerized sulfated D-galacto-pyranose units, but with other residues also present. It is the dried extract from certain red marine algae Rhodophytaceae, and often from the species *Chrondus crispus* (carrageenan, Irish moss). The ability of carrageenan to react with milk protein has led to its widespread use in preparations containing milk and chocolate. It has been shown to be a potent cholesterol-lowering agent but, unlike almost any other plant polysaccharide, has an adverse effect on the gut. Ulceration of the cecum of both rats and guinea pigs has been demonstrated when carrageenan was added to the diet.

Cellulose — Best known, most widely distributed, and only truly fibrous component of the plant cell wall. It is a polymer of glucose and the glucoside linkage is β. The β-linkages in cellulose are not hydrolyzed by the enzymes present in man; cellulose is therefore part of dietary fiber. Cellulose also has the property of taking up water (0.4 g water per gram of cellulose), and this explains its ability to increase fecal weight when added to the diet.

Crude fiber — Residue left after boiling the defatted food in dilute alkali and then in dilute acid. The method recovers 50 to 80% of cellulose, 10 to 50% of lignin, and 20% of hemicellulose. Inconsistent results are obtained, and it should not be used as a method for the determination of dietary fiber.

Cutin — A complex polymer of mono-, di-, tri-, and polyhydroxy fatty acids, it is a lipid component of the waterproof covering and cuticle on the outer cellulose wall of plants. Cuticular substances are extremely resistant to digestion and in turn are thought to impair the digestibility of the other cell wall constituents. Their resistance to digestion means they appear in the feces and may constitute a large proportion of the fecal fat. Cutins may account for a substantial part of the increased fecal fat seen in subjects on a high cereal-fiber diet.

Dietary fiber — Includes all the polymers of plants that cannot be digested by the endogenous secretions of the human digestive tract, i.e., cellulose, pectins, hemicellulose, gums, mucilages, and lignin; see also Chapter 2.1.

Galactans — Polysaccharides which, on hydrolysis, give galactose. They occur in wood and in many algae. The most important galactan is agar.

Galactomannans — Polysaccharides that have both galactose and mannose in the chain, in varying proportions. Guar gum (guaram) is a representative example. Galactomannans are part of the hemicellulose fraction of the plant cell wall.

Glucofructans — Linear polymers with both fructose and glucose in the chain. They are found in the hemicellulose section of the cell wall and form the storage polysaccharides in many temperate-climate grasses.

Glucomannans — Appear to be linear polymers with both mannose and glucose in the chain. The ratio of mannose to glucose is between 1:1 and 2.4:1. Hardwood glucomannans appear to contain no galactose and are relatively insoluble, but the glucomannans from gymnosperms have galactose side chains and a higher mannose-to-glucose ratio (3:1). The presence of side chains tends to make these polysaccharides more soluble in water, possibly because the side chains prevent the formation of intermolecular hydrogen bonding. Glucomannans are part of the hemicellulose fraction of the plant cell wall.

Glucoronoxylans — Have a main "backbone" chain of $(1 \rightarrow 4)$ linked β-D-xylopyranosyl residues, containing side chains of 4-*O*-methyl-α-D-glucopyranosyluronic acid and, in some annual plants, unmethylated D-glucuronic acid. Glucuronoxylans are found in the hemicellulose fraction of all land plants and most plant organs.

Glycan — Generic name for a polysaccharide; from glycose, a simple sugar, and the ending -an signifying a polymer.

Glycuronans — Generic name for the polymers of uronic acids; e.g., galacturonan is a polymer of galacturonic acid and is therefore, a glycuronan.

Guar gum (guaran) — A neutral polysaccharide, a D-galacto-D-mannan, that is isolated from the ground endosperm of guar seed, a leguminous vegetable cultivated in India for animal feeds. In small amounts it finds widespread use in the food and pharmaceutical industries as a thickener and stabilizer in, for example, salad dressing and ice cream, as well as in nonfood items such as toothpaste.

Gum (exudates and seed gums) — Complex polysaccharides, each containing several different sugar molecules and uronic acid groups. The true plant gums, gum acacia and gum tragacanth, are the dried exudates from various plants obtained when the bark is cut or the plant is otherwise injured. They are soluble in water to give very viscous colloidal solutions, sometimes called mucilages, and are insoluble in organic solvents. These are not part of the cell wall structure but are generally indigestible and are thus considered a part of dietary fiber. Guar and locust bean gums are examples of gums derived from seeds.

Hemicelluloses — A wide variety of polysaccharide polymers, at least 250 of which are known. The largest group consists of pentosans such as the xylans and arabinoxylans; a second group consists of hexose polymers such as the galactans. The acidic hemicelluloses which contain galacturonic acid or glucuronic acid form a third group of hemicelluloses. Hemicelluloses are those polymers extractable from plants by cold aqueous alkali. They are not precursors of cellulose and have no part in cellulose biosynthesis but represent a distinct and separate group of plant polysaccharides. Together with pectin, the hemicelluloses form the matrix of the plant cell wall in which are enmeshed cellulose fibers. The hemicelluloses are not digested in the small intestine but are broken down by microorganisms in the colon more readily than cellulose.

Heteroglycans — Polysaccharides that hydrolyze to two, three, or more monosaccharides. They have prefixes of di-, tri- , and so on to indicate the number of different types of sugar residues.

Hexoses — Monosaccharides with each molecule containing six carbon atoms. Glucose, fructose, galactose, and mannose are all hexoses.

Homoglycan — Polysaccharide containing only one type of sugar unit and hence on hydrolysis giving only one monosaccharide type. The most abundant polysaccharides are of this type, e.g., starch and cellulose.

Lignin — An aromatic polymer of molecular weight of about 10,000 based on coniferyl and sinapyl alcohols; it occurs in woody plant tissues. Since it is virtually indigestible, lignin is usually classified as part of dietary fiber. It is a commercial source of vanillin and other aromatic chemicals.

Mannans — Polysaccharides made up of mannose units, found in the hemicellulose fraction from many cell walls. They seem to be storage polysaccharides.

Middle lamella — Develops from the cell plate that forms between the daughter nuclei of the plant cell wall and extends to meet the existing wall, and therefore is the structure between adjacent cell walls. It appears to be rich in galacturonans, which are characteristically part of the pectic substances.

Mucilages — Polysaccharides usually containing galactose, galacturonic acid residues, and often xylose and arabinose. Structurally, they resemble the hemicelluloses and are water soluble, being obtained as slimy, colloidal solutions. They are found mixed with the endosperm or storage polysaccharides or in special cells in the seedcoat. They retain water and so protect the seed against desiccation.

Neutral detergent fiber (NDF) — That part of food remaining after extraction with a hot neutral solution of the detergent sodium lauryl sulfate. It is a measure of the cell wall constituents of vegetable foodstuffs. The method for determining NDF was designed to divide the dry matter of feeds very nearly into those constituents which are nutritionally available for the normal digestive process and those which depend on microbial fermentation for their availability. See Chapter 3.2.

Noncellulosic polysaccharides — Another term for hemicelluloses, which include all the matrix polysaccharides from the cell wall, other than cellulose.

Nonstarch polysaccharides (NSP) — A term suggested by Englyst and co-workers for the carbohydrate plant cell wall material originally called *dietary fiber* less the lignin; considered by the authors to be a better definition than *fiber.*

Oligosaccharides — Collective term for di-, tri-, and tetrasaccharides; processed foods may contain oligosaccharides with up to 9 residue.

Pectic substances — Mixtures of acidic and neutral polysaccharides that can be extracted with water from plant tissues. They are characteristically rich in galacturonic acid and are galacturonans with a variable degree of methyl esterification.

Pectin — General term designating those water-soluble pectinic acids of varying methyl ester content and degree of neutralization which are capable of forming gels with water and acid under suitable conditions. Pectin is found in the primary cell wall and intracellular layer. It changes from an insoluble material in the unripe fruit to a much more water-soluble substance in the ripe fruit. Its ability to form gels and its ion binding capacity may be important in human nutrition. Also see pectic substances.

Pectinic acid — Groups of pectins in which only a portion of the acidic groupings are methylated.

Pentoses — Monosaccharides with each molecule containing five carbon atoms. Pentose sugars most commonly present in human foods are L-arabinose and D-xylose, which are widely distributed in the polysaccharides in plants. Pentoses are present in small amounts in all cell walls whether animal, plant, or bacterial. Dietetically, the five-carbon sugars are of little importance as a source of energy for the body.

Plantix — A term coined from "plant" and "matrix" to replace dietary fiber to avoid the uncertain and diversified meaning of the term fiber. It includes the same polymers found in dietary fiber from plants.

Primary plant cell wall — The cellulose fibers of the primary cell wall are laid down in a random network on the middle lamella. The fibrils are surrounded by an amorphous matrix of hemicellulose.

Protopectin — Term applied to the water-insoluble parent pectic substance which occurs in plants, and which upon hydrolysis yields pectinic acid.

Resistant starch — Starch that is not digested by human digestive enzymes and that reaches the colon, often acting in the same way as *fiber.*

Sclerenchyma — Tissue forming the hard parts of plants such as nutshell or seedcoat.

Secondary cell wall — Polysaccharide in nature and apparently amorphous. It is formed after the cell has reached maturity and is laid down inside the primary cell wall, either as a continuous layer or as localized thickenings or bands.

Silica — Deposited in the plant cell wall, usually in the aerial part of the plant. The amount varies according to the species, the silica content of the soil, and the maturity of the plant. The ash content of the cell wall, particularly of wheat, may be as high as 10%; of this, the principal element present is often silicon. Silica has the capacity to impair the digestibility of cell wall materials.

Suberin — A cutin-like substance found in cork. It is a plant lipid that cannot be extracted with a simple solvent but needs saponification before extraction.

Uronic acids — Present in the pectic substances and the hemicellulose portion of the plant cell wall. They are found in about half the known plant polysaccharides, the most common being D-galacturonic and D-glucuronic acids. Uronic acids are derived from sugars by oxidation of the terminal $-CH_2OH$ to $-COOH$ and, when present as glycosides, behave like simple hydrocarboxylic acids, forming metal salts, amides, and alkyl and methyl esters.

Water-holding capacity — Amount of water that can be taken up by unit weight of dry fiber to the point at which no free water remains. A close relationship exists between acid detergent fiber content of vegetable dietary fiber and water-holding capacity, but there is no such relationship between lignin content and water-holding capacity.

Water-soluble fraction — Fraction of dietary fiber soluble in water; it includes pectic substances, gums, mucilages, and some polysaccharide food additives.

Xylans — Groups of polymers having a main chain of $(1 \rightarrow 4)$ β-D-xylopyranosyl residues; arabinose and 4-O-methyl glucuronic acid are the most usual substituents. A few D-xylans are neutral molecules containing D-xylose residues only. Xylans are found in the hemicellulose portion of the plant cell wall in all land plants and in most plant organs.

Xylem — Water-conducting elements of plant tissues, usually made up of cells with lignified walls. In mature woody tissues, the walls of xylem vessels are completely lignified; in less mature tissues, the lignification is partial and localized.

REFERENCES

1. Southgate, D. A. T., White, M., Spiller, G. A., and Kay, R. M., Glossary, in *Medical Aspects of Dietary Fiber,* Spiller, G. A. and Kay, R. M., Eds., Plenum Press, New York, 1980.
2. Smith, F. and Montgomery, R., Eds., *The Chemistry of Plant Gums and Mucilages and Some Related Polysaccharides,* Reinhold, New York, 1959.
3. Butler, G. W. and Bailey, R. W., *Chemistry and Biochemistry of Herbage,* Vol. 1, Academic Press, New York, 1973.
4. Windholz, M., Budavari, S., Stroumtsos, L. Y., and Fertig, M. N., Eds., *The Merck Index,* 9th ed., Merck, Rahway, NJ, 1976.

Physical Chemistry of Dietary Fiber

David Oakenfull

INTRODUCTION

As explained in other parts of this Handbook, dietary fiber is a complex mixture of polysaccharides with many different functions and activities as it passes through the gastrointestinal tract. Many of these functions and activities depend on its physical chemistry.

This chapter outlines how physical chemistry impacts with chemical composition and influences the many different roles of dietary fiber at the various stages in its passage through the gut — from its role in influencing what we eat to its role in easing defecation.

FOOD PREFERENCES

Dietary fiber often has a negative impact on food preference. (If this were not so, consumption of fiber-rich foods would have increased by far more than it actually has in response to fiber's clear health benefits.) Most people, for example, prefer white bread to wholemeal bread and white rice to brown rice. One reason for this may be that fiber-rich foods often require considerable effort to chew. A study comparing breakfast cereals suggested that the energy required to break the product down into small pieces (the comminution energy) increases with its dietary fiber content. Further, the popularity of these products (reflected by sales in supermarkets) was inversely proportional to the comminution energy, as shown in Figure 2.7.1.[1] Apparently, we prefer foods that require little chewing.

A positive effect of fiber on food preference can be seen in the use of non-starch polysaccharides as texture-modifying agents by the food industry. The remarkable ability of polysaccharides to thicken or gel aqueous solutions is exploited in numerous food products ranging from dessert jellies to oil-free salad dressings. Through subtle adjustment to formulation and processing methods, these materials can greatly enhance the consumer appeal of otherwise unattractive products. For example, a great deal of attention is currently being paid in the use of polysaccharides to mimic the texture of fat. There are already a number of polysaccharide-based products available which their manufacturers claim can be used to formulate low-fat versions of traditionally high-fat products such as ice cream (see also, for example, Ward[2]). Although not usually added to foods at significantly high levels, these additives significantly boost our intake of dietary fiber.

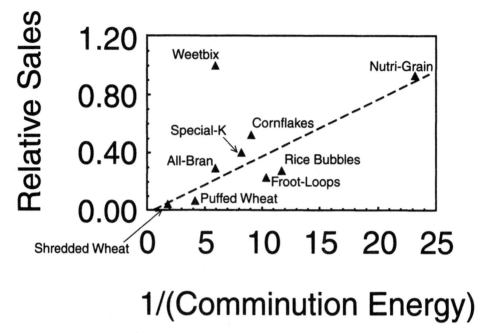

Figure 2.7.1 Relative sales in Australia of breakfast cereals plotted against the reciprocal of the comminution energy as determined from the electrical energy required to grind the cereal to fine particles in a small hammer mill (see text).

SATIETY

How Dietary Fiber Influences Satiety

Not surprisingly, physical factors are also significant in the influence of dietary fiber on satiety and hence energy intake. Because distension of the stomach is believed to be one of the signals to stop eating, several investigators have speculated that the bulk associated with high-fiber foods induces a feeling of satiety and thus reduces meal size and food intake. Experimentally, though, conflicting results have been reported. Some workers have found that fiber decreases energy intake[3,4]; others have found that it has no effect.[5,6]

A numerical measure of the satiating effects of different foods has recently been developed called the *satiety index* (SI).[7] The SI compares how full (on average) different foods made a group of volunteers feel for the same intake of energy. White bread is given a score of 100, and the SI for all other foods is based on this standard. A plot of satiety index against dietary fiber content for a broad range of different foods (Figure 2.7.2) shows no correlation (the correlation coefficient is –0.0864.). This is perhaps not surprising, because energy density has a strong effect on satiety[8] and may well swamp any effect of fiber on SI. Nonetheless, the high-satiety foods tend to have bulky, fibrous, or crunchy textures which make them relatively more difficult to chew or swallow.[9]

Fiber appears to influence satiety when other, more dominant, influences are more or less equal — and it seems that solubility and viscosity are critical factors. A supplement of psyllium gum, which is rich in soluble fiber, decreased spontaneous energy intake in a group of 12 women, whereas wheat bran had no effect.[10] Studies in experimental animals and in humans have suggested that viscous polysaccharides can slow the rate of gastric emptying.[11] Furthermore, consumption of fiber in a meal appears to reduce energy ingested at a subsequent meal.[12] Blundell and his colleagues[13] have recently found that soluble and insoluble fiber behave differently. Soluble fiber reduced appetite a longer time after eating than insoluble fibers, but there was no difference between

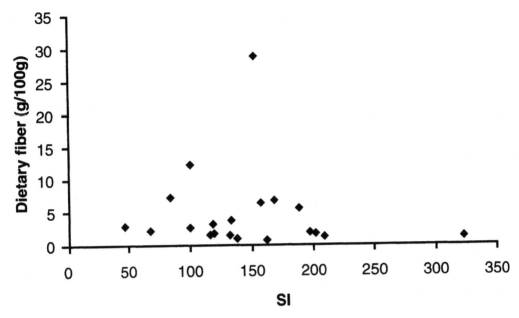

Figure 2.7.2 Dietary fiber content (g/100 g) for a range of different foods plotted against the corresponding satiety index.

how the two types affected total energy intake. Solubility and viscosity both depend on the chemical composition of the fiber and the molecular structure of its component polysaccharides.

Solubility

Solubility is a major factor in the nutritional properties of dietary fiber, generally speaking. So what determines whether a particular fiber fraction is soluble or insoluble? The key to understanding why some polysaccharides are soluble in water and others are not is molecular structure.[14] Polysaccharides are composed of linked monosaccharide units, of which the most common is D-glucose (Figure 2.7.3). Many different structures are possible with different linkage geometries and different monosaccharide units. But physical properties (such as solubility) are determined more by the linkages than by the nature of the monosaccharide units.[14]

This is illustrated by comparing two forms of poly-D-glucose familiar from other chapters of this book — cellulose, which is insoluble, and the water-soluble β-glucans from barley and oat bran. Cellulose has exclusively β(1–4) linkages, whereas the β-glucans have mixed β(1–4) and β(1–3) linkages. Cellulose's regularity enables it to adopt ordered crystalline structures of polysaccharide chains held together by hydrogen bonds.[14,15] These ordered structures are insoluble.[14] In contrast, the irregular structure of the β-glucans prevents the formation of ordered crystalline structure, so these polysaccharides tend to be water soluble. Branched structures, as in the arabinoxylans in wheat, are similarly unable to adopt ordered crystalline structures, and these compounds are also water soluble. Polysaccharides with charged groups (COO^- or SO_3^-), such as the pectins and carrageenans, are also often water soluble, in this case because electrostatic repulsion prevents the molecules from packing close together in ordered structures.[14]

Viscosity

Almost all water-soluble polysaccharides produce viscous solutions. Viscosity is caused by physical interactions between polysaccharide molecules in solution — in simple terms, by the

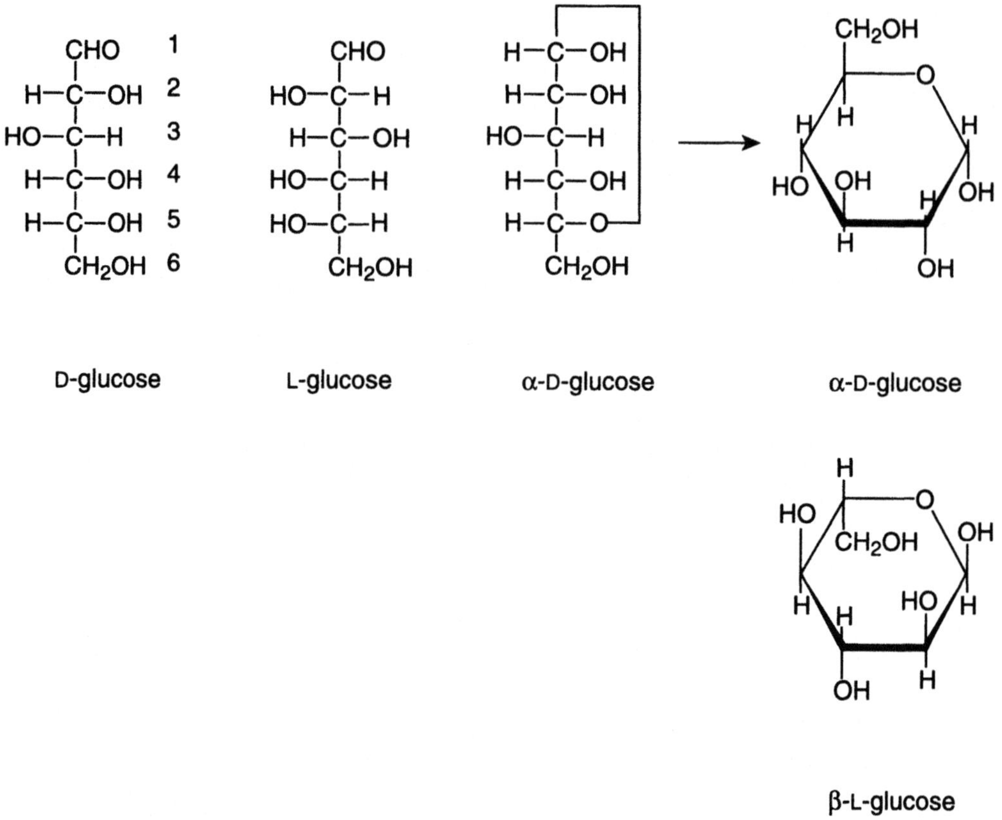

Figure 2.7.3 Representations of D- and L-glucose in open chains and α-D-glucose and β-L-glucose in ring forms.

molecules becoming entangled.[16] At low concentrations the molecules are well separated from each other and free to move independently. At a critical concentration ($c*$) the molecules become sufficiently crowded to start to interpenetrate one another and form a tangled network.[16] (This is shown diagrammatically in Figure 2.7.4.) The viscosity then increases sharply with concentration and becomes more dependent on the rate of shear (this means, in effect, the rate at which the liquid is stirred). Polysaccharide solutions usually show "shear thinning" — the apparent viscosity decreasing with increasing rate of shear.[17,18]

ABSORPTION OF NUTRIENTS FROM THE SMALL INTESTINE

Effects of Viscosity

Viscous polysaccharides or polysaccharides which form a gel matrix may slow absorption by trapping nutrients, digestive enzymes, or bile acids in the matrix and by slowing mixing and diffusion in the intestine.[19] In an *in vitro* model using dialysis tubing, Johnson and Read[20] showed that guar gum appears to inhibit absorption by resisting the convective effects of intestinal contractions. Polysaccharides that give viscous solutions seem to be those most effective in lowering plasma cholesterol concentrations (Table 2.7.1).

Thus, it is not unreasonable to suppose that viscous, soluble fiber inhibits absorption of cholesterol and bile acids from the small intestine.[20,21,22] Newman and her colleagues,[23] for example, have suggested that the cholesterol lowering observed in rats fed high β-glucan barley fractions is related to the increased viscosity in the small intestine, and Tietyen and colleagues[24] found that

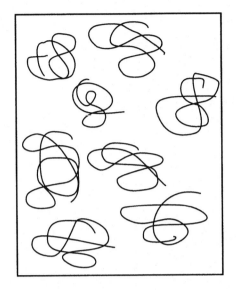

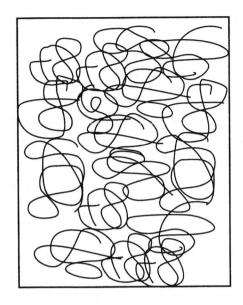

Low Concentration   High Concentration

Figure 2.7.4 Random coil molecules — at low concentrations the molecules move independently through the solution; at higher concentrations (greater than the critical overlap concentration, c^*) they become entangled, giving very viscous solutions.

Table 2.7.1   Effect of Fiber from Different Sources on Plasma Cholesterol Concentrations

Source of Fiber	Quantity Ingested (g/day)	Change in Plasma Cholesterol (%)
Cellulose	16	0
Wheat bran	17	+1
Whole oats[a]	15	−11
Oat bran[a]	27	−17
Pectin[a]	25	−13
Guar gum[a]	24	−16
Beans[a,b]	30	−19

[a] Composed of or containing viscous polysaccharides.
[b] Would also contain saponins which have cholesterol-lowering activity.

Source: Data from Chen and Anderson.[19]

reducing the viscosity of oat bran fiber (by treatment with enodo-β-glucanse from *Bacillus subtilis*) reduced its ability to lower plasma cholesterol. In a study using everted sacs of rat jejunum, Johnson and Gee[25] found that viscous gums (guar and carboxymethyl cellulose) increased the thickness of the unstirred layer overlying the mucosa (Table 2.7.2). But the relevance of the unstirred layer has been questioned,[26] and in an experiment in which rats were fed methylcelluloses of different viscosity grades, no differences between plasma or liver cholesterol concentrations were observed.[27] In another study, in which guar gum, locust bean gum, and fenugreek gum were compared, reduction of plasma cholesterol was again not related to viscosity (Table 2.7.3).[28] Viscosity does, however, appear to influence glucose absorption, and guar gum and pectin have proved beneficial in controlling hyperglycemia.[29] Ellis and his colleagues[30] have shown that guar gum inhibits glucose absorption in inverse proportion to the viscosity of the digesta. Also, high dietary intakes of pectin (6 and 8% of the diet) decrease the availability of vitamin E in rats.[31] But, in contrast, gum acacia, which is

Table 2.7.2   Apparent Thickness of Mucosal Unstirred Layer in Jejunal Sacs Preincubated with and without Guar Gum or Carboxymethylcellulose

Polysaccharide	Unstirred Layer Thickness (µm)	
	Control	With Polysaccharide
Guar gum (viscosity 16 cP)	317 ± 15	468 ± 25
Carboxymethycellulose	346 ± 12	402 ± 12

Source: Data from Tietyen et al.[24]

Table 2.7.3   Relationship between Viscosity and Cholesterol-Lowering — Comparison of Three Galactomannans and α-Cellulose in the Cholesterol-Fed Rat

Fiber	Viscosity	Total Plasma Cholesterol (mM)
α-Cellulose	(Insoluble)	4.60 ± 0.34
Guar gum	High	3.26 ± 0.09
Locust bean gum	Medium	3.46 ± 0.12
Fenugreek gum	Low	3.16 ± 0.09

Source: Data from Topping et al.[27]

not viscous, also improves glucose tolerance[32] and viscosity is not predictive of glycemic response.[33] Eastwood and Morris[34] have concluded that there is, in fact, little evidence to suggest that viscous polysaccharides inhibit transport across the small intestinal epithelia. This is obviously a complex and controversial area.

Adsorption of Bile Acids

Another questionable concept is the frequently cited ability of fiber to bind bile acids.[35,36] The cholesterol-lowering effect of dietary fiber, it is suggested, can (at least in part) be explained by adsorption of bile acids to fiber in the small intestine. Bile acids are thereby diverted from the enterohepatic cycle, lost by fecal excretion, and the loss is made good by conversion of cholesterol into bile acids by the liver.[35,36] Although dietary fiber (for example, oat bran) can indeed increase fecal excretion of bile acids, adsorption of bile acids to fiber preparations *in vitro* is so small as to be trivial when expressed quantitatively in terms of µmoles adsorbed per gram of fiber.[37] Moreover, pectin also causes increased fecal excretion of bile acids, and adsorption of bile acids onto pectin is physically unlikely because both molecules are negatively charged at gut pH.[38,39]

FERMENTATION IN THE COLON

Effects of Physical Properties and Structure on the Fermentability of Fiber

Although, by definition, fiber is not broken down by the enzymes of the gastrointestinal tract, virtually all fiber fractions are broken down to some extent by the microorganisms in the colon. Pectin, gum arabic, and guar gum disappear almost completely during transit; in humans, about 40% of dietary cellulose is broken down.[40] Fermentation depends on the accessibility of the polysaccharide molecules to the microorganisms, which depends, in turn, on chemical structure and physical properties, particularly solubility. The chemical properties of the polysaccharide also appear to influence the types of microbial activity present in the large intestine.[40] Soluble fiber fractions are very accessible and ferment rapidly in the proximal colon; insoluble fiber fractions ferment much more slowly in a process that is continuous during transit. The extent of breakdown may also be related to the physical structure of the plant — fiber from fruits and vegetables appears to be more fermentable than that from cereals.[41] Thus, physical effects have a profound effect on the kinetics of release of metabolically important metabolites such as short-chain fatty acids. It is often suggested that short-chain fatty acids may be factors in controlling cholesterol metabolism, although some evidence suggests otherwise,[27] and short-chain fatty acids, particularly butyrate, may influence the development of colorectal cancer.[40,42] In this connection, the kinetics of fermentation appears to be a particularly important factor.

Animal studies have shown that readily fermented fiber, such as guar gum and pectin, offer little protection from colorectal cancer. In contrast, slowly fermented fiber, such as wheat bran, has the more protective effect.[43,44] These studies are summarized in Table 2.7.4. The explanation seems to be that readily fermented fiber produces a short-lived burst of metabolites, confined to the proximal colon, whereas slowly fermented fiber produces a sustained release of metabolites along the full length, reaching the distal colon.[44] The fermentation pattern also seems to be important. In a series of rat studies with partially hydrolyzed guar gum, Weaver and colleagues[45] found that propionate as a fermentation product promotes the development of cancer, whereas butyrate was confirmed as having a protective effect.

Table 2.7.4 Summary of Published Reports on Effects of Dietary Fibers on Tumorigenesis in Rat Models of Large Bowel Cancer

Fiber Type	Effect on Tumorigenesis			Total Number
	Protective	Equivocal	Enhanced	
Poorly fermentable:				
Cellulose	8	3	0	11
Lignin	2	0	0	2
Slowly fermentable:				
Wheat bran	7	9	0	16
Rapidly fermentable:				
Guar	0	2	1	3
Pectin	0	2	3	5
Oat bran	0	0	1	1

Source: Data from Young.[44]

Particle Size and Porosity

Particle size particularly affects fermentation. The range of particle sizes depends on the types of plant cell walls present in the foods and on their degree of processing. Particle size may vary during transit through the gut as a result of chewing, grinding in the stomach, and bacterial degradation in the colon. Some components involved in the cohesiveness of the fiber matrix may be progressively solubilized. Thus, particle size before ingestion of the food is not necessarily related to the subsequent behavior of the fiber during transit.[46] Porosity and surface area are also relevant factors in controlling susceptibility to bacterial and enzymic attack. Again, these factors are related to origin and processing history. Chemical composition may be another significant factor here, and it is possible that pectins have a dominant role in determining cell wall porosity.[47]

Microstructure — Resistant Starch

Resistant starch (discussed in more detail in other chapters of this Handbook) behaves functionally as dietary fiber because it resists digestion by the enzymes of the stomach and small intestine. This is a case in which microstructure has a powerful effect on physiological properties. Starch is poly-D-glucose in a complex structure — a mixture of linear amylose and highly branched amylopectin. Amylose has α(1–4) linkages which introduce a twist in the molecule, leading to the formation of helical structures; amylopectin has mixed α(1–4) and α(1–6) linkages, giving rise to its highly branched structure. In the plant, the starch is mostly packaged as starch granules, but the majority of starch-rich foods have been processed by a combination of heat and moisture which disrupts the native granular structure and causes partial solubilization of the starch polysaccharides. Starch that has been gelatinized by heating in water is readily hydrolyzed by the amylolytic enzymes. However, on cooling to room temperature the solubilized polysaccharides can reassociate or "retrograde."[48] Retrograded amylose is more than 70% resistant to amylolysis *in vitro*[49] and restricts access of the enzyme to the starch substrate as a whole *in vivo*.[50] Gidley and his colleagues[51] have investigated the molecular structure of resistant starch in great detail using a combination of physicochemical techniques. They have shown that resistant starch has substantial segments of the amylose chains in the form of double helices loosely arranged into aggregates. Single-chain material is also present as imperfections in helices or as chains trapped between aggregates. The double-helical conformation appears to be the primary barrier to enzyme action.[51]

Water-Holding Capacity

Polysaccharides are hydrophilic molecules; they have numerous free hydroxyl-groups which can form hydrogen bonds with water. Consequently, soluble and insoluble polysaccharides alike have the ability to hold water. The most obvious demonstration of the ability of soluble polysaccharides to hold water is the phenomenon of gelation.[52] A relatively small amount of polysaccharide, such as 1% agarose, can be enough to entrap the water in which it is dissolved in a three-dimensional network of polysaccharide molecules. The water is held within the polysaccharide matrix, unable to flow away, and the system has the semisolid properties characteristic of a gel.[52] Insoluble fibers can also absorb water but more in the manner of a sponge. They also form a hydrophilic matrix in which water is entrapped — but where the quasi-crystallinity of the polysaccharide remains and water fills the interstices, often causing considerable swelling.

Measurement of water-holding capacity is surprisingly problematic for such an apparently simple parameter. A recent European collaborative study[53] addressed this problem. Its authors reported that a method based on centrifugation gave tolerably consistent results across different laboratories, but the results were dependent on the sample weight used. (The percentage of water retained by the hydrated fiber pellet was measured. This probably depends on sample size because of a proportionate increase in the contribution from soluble material retained by the pellet at increased sample weight.)

Absorption of Small Molecules and Ions

In addition to binding water, polysaccharides have the ability to bind other polar molecules and ions. The reduced mineral availability and electrolyte absorption associated with some diets high in fiber appear to be due to binding of metal ions.[41,54] The number of free carboxyl groups and particularly the uronic acid content seem to be the major factors determining the ability of polysaccharides to bind metal ions. It is possible, though, that these ions are subsequently released and absorbed as fiber is broken down in the colon. It has been reported that absorption of zinc and iron are actually enhanced by sugar beet fiber and that the inhibition of absorption observed with wheat bran is caused by phytate.[55]

LAXATION

The huge displays of laxatives to be seen in any supermarket or pharmacy testify to popular concern with this topic. Feces are approximately 25% water and 75% dry matter. The major components are undigested residues plus bacteria and bacterial cell debris. These form a sponge-like, water-holding matrix which conditions fecal bulk and consistency.[56] Thus, the effect of fiber on laxation depends not only on the undegraded fiber residue but also on bacterial cell mass. The ability of different fiber types to increase fecal bulk depends on a complex relationship between the chemical and physical properties of the fiber and the bacterial population in the colon. Cereal fibers are highest in pentoses and therefore have the greatest fecal bulking power.[56,57] This is illustrated by comparing the results from studies of increased fecal bulk in response to various fiber supplements (Table 2.7.5).

Table 2.7.5   Effect of Fiber Supplements on Fecal Bulk

Fiber Supplement	Increase in Fecal Wet Weight (%)
Oat bran	15
Pectin	16–35
Guar gum	20
Apple	40
Carrot	59
Cabbage	67
Cellulose	75
Wheat bran, coarse	80–127
Wheat bran, fine	24

Source: Data from Cummings.[41]

The physical form of the fiber is also important. Coarsely ground wheat bran is a very effective fiber source in increasing fecal bulk, whereas finely ground wheat bran has little or no effect — and may even be constipating.[58] Additionally, some laxation effects may be due to the short-chain volatile fatty acids produced by fermentation,[41,57] and it is probably for this reason that resistant starch has a mild laxative effect.[59,60] Osmotic effects may be important in a way that is not yet well defined. Kinetic effects may also be significant again here, with rapidly fermented fiber different in its effects from slowly fermented fiber which gives a sustained release of low molecular weight (osmotically active) metabolites along the full length of the colon.[61]

CONCLUSIONS

The physiological functions of dietary fiber change as it progresses through the gastrointestinal tract. These functions depend to a large extent on physical properties which also change. Thus, we are dealing with a highly complex kinetic system which is still not well understood. Although the chemistry of dietary fiber is now well defined, it does not in itself predict biological activity. Biological activity depends on physical properties which do not relate in any simple way to crude chemical composition. The polysaccharides of which dietary fiber is mostly composed are complex structures in which the geometry of the linkage between monomer units largely defines physical properties. This means that we cannot assume that any material which falls within the chemical definition of dietary fiber, and analyzes as dietary fiber by the usual methods, will necessarily be of significant health benefit to consumers.

REFERENCES

1. Parker, N. S. and Oakenfull, D. G., Comminution energy and the sales of breakfast cereals, *Proc. Nutr. Soc. Aust.*, 11, 119, 1986.
2. Ward, F.M., Hydrocolloid systems as fat mimetics in bakery products: Icings glazes and fillings, *Cereal Foods World*, 42, 386, 1995.
3. Porikos, K. and Hagamen, S., Is fiber satiating? Effects of a high fiber diet preload on subsequent food intake of normal-weight and obese young men, *Appetite*, 7, 162, 1986.
4. Mickelsen, O., Makdani, D. D., Cotton, R. H., Titcomb, S. T., Colmey, J. C., and Gatty, R., Effects of a high fiber bread diet on weight loss in college-age males, *Am. J. Clin. Nutr.*, 32, 1703, 1979.
5. Bryson, E., Dore, C., and Garrow, J. S., Wholemeal bread and satiety, *J. Hum. Nutr.*, 34, 113, 1980.
6. Russ, C. S. and Atkinson, R. L., Use of high fiber diets for the out-patient treatment of obesity, *Nutr. Rep. Internat.*, 32, 193, 1985.
7. Holt, S. H. A., Brand Miller, J. C., Petocz, P., and Farmakalidis, E., A satiety index of common foods, *Eur. J. Clin. Nutr.*, 49, 675, 1995.
8. Rolls, B. J., The role of energy density in the overconsumption of fat, *J. Nutr.*, 130, 268S, 2000.
9. Holt, S., The satiety index: a new method to measure the filling powers of foods, *Food Aust.*, 51, 74, 1999.
10. Stevens, J., Levitsky, D. A., van Soest, P. J., Robertson, J. B., Kalkwarf, H. J., and Roe, D. A., Effect of psyllium gum and wheat bran on spontaneous energy intake, *Am. J. Clin. Nutr.*, 46, 812, 1987.
11. Leeds, A. R., Gastric emptying, fibre and absorption, *Lancet*, 1, 872, 1979.
12. Schwartz, S. E., Levine, R. A., Singh, A., Schneidecker, J. R., and Track, N. S., Sustained pectin ingestion delays gastric emptying, *Gastroenterology*, 83, 812, 1982.
13. Delargy, H. J., O'Sullivan, K. R., Fletcher, R. J., and Blundell, J. E., Effects of amount and type of dietary fibre (soluble and insoluble) on short-term control of appetite, *Int., J. Food Sci. Nutr.*, 48, 67, 1987.
14. Oakenfull, D., Polysaccharide molecular structures, in *Polysaccharide Association Structures in Food*, Walter, R. H., Ed., Marcel Decker, New York, 1998, 15.
15. Rees, D. A., *Polysaccharide Shapes*, Chapman and Hall, London, 1977.
16. Morris, E. R., Polysaccharide solution properties: origin, rheological characterization and implications for food systems, in *Frontiers in Carbohydrate Research — 1: Food Applications*, Millane, R. P., BeMiller, J. N., and Chandrasekaran, R., Eds., Elsevier, London, 1989, 132.
17. Graessley, W. W., The entanglement concept in polymer rheology, *Adv. Polymer Sci.*, 16, 1, 1974.
18. Morris, E. R., Cutler, A. N., Ross-Murphey, S. B., Rees, D. A., and Price, J., Concentration and shear rate dependence of viscosity in random coil polysaccharide solutions, *Carbohydrate Polym.*, 1, 5, 1981.
19. Chen, W.-J. L. and Anderson, J. W., Effects of plant fiber in decreasing plasma total cholesterol and increasing high density lipoprotein cholesterol, *Proc. Soc. Exp. Biol. Med.*, 162, 310, 1979.
20. Johnson, I. T. and Read, N. W., Do viscous polysaccharides slow absorption by inhibiting diffusion or convection? *Eur. J. Clin. Nutr.*, 42, 307, 1988.
21. Gee, J. M.,Blackburn, N. A., and Johnson, I. T., The influence of guar gum on intestinal transport in the rat, *Brit. J. Nutr.*, 50, 215, 1983.
22. Superko, H. R., Haskell, W. L., Sawrey-Kubicek, L., and Farquhar, J. W., Effects of solid and liquid guar gum on plasma cholesterol and triglyceride concentrations in moderate hypercholesterolemia, *Am. J. Cardiol.*, 62, 51, 1988.
23. Danielson, A. D., Newman, R. K., Newman, C. W., and Berardinelli, J. G., Lipid levels and digesta viscosity of rats fed a high-fiber barley milling fraction, *Nutr. Res.*, 17, 515–522, 1997.
24. Tietyen, J. L., Nevins, D. L., Schoemaker, C. F., and Schneeman, B. O., Hypocholesterolemic potential of oat bran treated with an endo-β-D-glucanase from *Bacillus subtilis*, *J. Food. Sci.*, 60, 558, 1995.
25. Johnson, I. T. and Gee, J. M., Effect of gel-forming gums on the intestinal unstirred layer and sugar transport *in vitro, Gut*, 22, 398, 1981.
26. Smithson, K. W., Millar, D. B., Jacobs, G., and Gray, M., Intestinal diffusion barrier: Unstirred layer or membrane surface mucous coat, *Science*, 214, 1241, 1981.
27. Topping, D. L., Oakenfull, D., Trimble, R. P., and Illman, R. J., A viscous fibre (methylcellulose) lowers blood glucose and plasma triacylglycerols and increases liver glycogen independently of volatile fatty acid production in the rat, *Brit. J. Nutr.*, 59, 21, 1988.

28. Evans, A. J., Hood, R. L., Oakenfull, D. G., and Sidhu, G. S., Relationship between structure and function of dietary fibre: a comparative study of the effects of three galactomannans on cholesterol metabolism in the rat, *Brit. J. Nutr.*, 68, 217, 1991.

29. Jenkins, D. J. A., Leeds, A. R., Wolever, T. M. S., Goff, D. V., Alberti, K. G. M. M., Gassull, M., and Hockaday, T. D. R., Dietary fibres, fibre analogues, and glucose tolerance: Importance of viscosity, *Brit. Med. J.*, 1, 1392, 1978.

30. Ellis, P. R., Roberts, F. G., Low, A. G., and Morgan, L. M., The effect of high-molecular weight guar gum on net apparent glucose absorption and net apparent insulin and gastric inhibitory polypeptide production in the growing pig: relationship to rheological changes in jejunal digesta, *Brit. J. Nutr.*, 74, 539, 1995.

31. Schaus, E. E., de Lumen, B. O., Chow, F. I., Reyes, P., and Omaye, S. T., Bioavailability of vitamin E in rats fed graded levels of pectin, *J. Nutr.*, 115, 263, 1985.

32. Sharma, R. D., Hypoglycemic effect of gum acacia in healthy human subjects, *Nutr. Res.*, 5, 1437, 1985.

33. Carrington-Smith, D., Collier, G. R., and O'Dea, K., Effect of soluble dietary fibre on the viscosity of gastrointestinal contents and the acute glycaemic response in the rat, *Brit. J. Nutr.*, 71, 563, 1994.

34. Eastwood, M. A. and Morris, E. R., Physical properties of dietary fiber that influence physiological function: a model for polymers along the gastrointestinal tract, *Am. J. Clin. Nutr.*, 55, 436, 1992.

35. Eastwood, M. A. and Hamilton, D., Studies on the adsorption of bile salts to non-absorbed components of diet, *Biochim. Biophys. Acta*, 152, 165, 1968.

36. Kritchevsky, D. and Story, J. A., Binding of bile salts *in vivo* by non-nutritive fiber, *J. Nutr.*, 104, 458, 1974.

37. Oakenfull, D. G. and Fenwick, D. E., Adsorption of bile salts from aqueous solution by plant fibre and cholestyramine, *Br. J. Nutr.*, 40, 299, 1978.

38. Hoagland, D. D. and Pfeffer, P. E., Role of pectin in binding of bile acids to carrot fiber, in *Chemistry and Function of Pectins*, Fishman, M. L. and Jen, J. J., Eds., ACS Symposium Series, 310, 1986, pp. 266-274.

39. Oakenfull, D. G. and Sidhu, G. S., Effects of pectin on intestinal absorption of glucose and cholate in the rat, *Nutr. Rep. Internat.*, 30, 1269, 1986.

40. Topping, D. L. and Illman, R. J., Bacterial fermentation in the human large bowel: time to change from the roughage model of dietary fibre?, *Med. J. Aust.*, 144, 307, 1986.

41. Cummings, J. H., *The Large Intestine in Nutrition and Disease*, Institut Danone, Bruxelles, 1997.

42. Schneeman, B. O., Dietary fiber: physical and chemical properties, methods of analysis and physiological effects, *Food Technol.*, 40, 104, 1986.

43. Burkitt, D. P., Dietary fiber and cancer, *J. Nutr.*, 118, 531, 1988.

44. Young, G. P., Dietary fibre and bowel cancer: which fibre is best? *Cereals International. Proceedings of an International Conference held in Brisbane Australia*, Royal Australian Chemical Institute, Melbourne, 1991, 379.

45. Weaver, G. A., Tangel, C. T., Krause, J. A., Alpern, H. D., Jenkins, P. L., Parfitt, M. R., and Stragand, J. J., Dietary guar gum alters colonic microbial fermentation in azoxymethane-treated rats, *J. Nutr.*, 126, 1979, 1996.

46. Guillon, F. and Champ, M., Structural and physical properties of dietary fibres, and consequences of processing on human physiology, *Food Res. Internat.*, 33, 233, 2000.

47. Guillon, F., Auffret, A., Robertson, J. A., Thibault, J.-F., and Barry, J.-L., Relationships between physical characteristics of sugar beet fibre and its fermentability by human faecal flora, *Carbohydr. Polym.*, 37, 195, 1998.

48. Miles, M. J., Morris, V. J., Orford, P. D., and Ring, S. G., The roles of amylose and amylopectin in the gelation and retrogradation of starch, *Carbohydr. Res.*, 135, 271, 1985.

49. Ring, S. G., Gee, J. M., Whittam, M. A., Orford, P. D., and Johnson, I. T., Resistant starch: its chemical form in foodstuffs and effect on digestibility in vitro, *Food Chem.*, 28, 97, 1988.

50. Botham, B. L., Morris, V. J., Noel, T. R., and Ring, S. G., A study on the *in vivo* digestibility of retrograded starch, *Carbohydr. Polym.*, 29, 347, 1996.

51. Gidley, M. J., Cooke, D., Darke, A. H., Hoffmann, R. A., Russell, A. L., and Greenwell, P., Molecular order and structure in enzyme-resistant retrograded starch, *Carbohydr. Polym.*, 28, 23, 1995.

52. Oakenfull, D., Gelation mechanisms, *Food Ingredients J. Jpn.*, 167, 48, 1996.

53. Robertson, J. A., de Monredon, F. D., Guillon, F., Thibault, J.-F., Amado, R., and Dysseler, P., Hydration properties of dietary fibre and resistant starch: a European collaborative study, *Lebesnm.-Wiss. u.-Technol.*, 33, 72, 2000.

54. Schneeman, B. O., Dietary fiber: physical and chemical properties, methods of analysis and physiological effects, *Food Technol.*, 40, 104, 1986.

55. Fairweather-Tait, S. J. and Write, A. J. A., The effects of sugar beet fibre and wheat bran on iron and zinc absorption in rats, *Brit. J. Nutr.*, 64, 547, 1990.

56. Stephen, A. M. and Cummings, J. A., Mechanism of action of dietary fibre in the human colon, *Nature*, 284, 283, 1980.

57. Cummings J. H., Southgate, D. A. T., Branch, W., Houston, H., Jenkins, D. J. A., and James, W. P. T., Colonic response to dietary fibre from carrot, cabbage, apple, bran and guar gum, *Lancet*, I, 5, 1978.

58. Oakenfull, D. and Topping, D. L., The nutritive value of wheat bran, *Food Tech. Aust.*, 39, 288, 1987.

59. Topping, D. L., Soluble fiber polysaccharides: effects on plasma cholesterol and colonic fermentation, *Nutr. Rev.*, 49, 195, 1991.

60. Cummings, J. H., Beatty, E. R., Kingman, S. M., Bingham, S. A., and Englyst, H. N., Digestion and physiological properties of resistant starch in the human large bowel, *Brit. J. Nutr.*, 75, 733, 1996.

61. Edwards, C. A., Bowen, J., and Eastwood, M. A., Effect of isolated complex carbohydrates on cecal and fecal short chain fatty acids in stool output in the rat, in *Dietary Fiber: Chemical and Biological Aspects,* Southgate, D. A. T., Waldron, K., Johnson, I. T., and Fenwick, G. R., Eds., Royal Society of Chemistry, London, 1990, 273.

Chitin and Chitosan — Special Class of Dietary Fiber

Ivan Furda

STRUCTURE AND DEFINITION

Chitin and chitosan are natural aminopolysaccharides which consist of linear chains containing N-acetyl-D-glucosamine and D-glucosamine units which are linked together by (1–4)-β glycosidic linkages. While the chitin contains predominantly N-acetyl-D-glucosamine units, chitosan is based primarily on D-glucosamine units. In chitin, the typical content of N-acetyl-D-glucosamine is 70–95%, and the reverse is true with chitosan, which usually contains 70–95% of D-glucosamine. Although there is no sharp distinction between these two biopolymers, it is generally accepted that chitin is highly acetylated, while chitosan is extensively deacetylated.

The unique structural feature of these polysaccharides, unlike other fibers, is the presence of amino groups in their molecules. Therefore, they are basic, or polycationic, while polysaccharides of common dietary fibers are either neutral or acidic (polyanionic).[1]

ORIGIN AND SOURCES

Unlike other common dietary fibers which are of plant origin, chitin and chitosan are predominantly of animal origin but could also be of plant origin. Chitin is mainly present in exoskeletons of arthropods such as insects, crabs, shrimp, lobsters, and other shells of shellfish, but it is also present in many fungal cell walls and yeasts.[2] Chitosan had been also found in different fungal cell walls, namely Mucorales, such as *Mucor rouxii*,[3,4] cell walls of the green alga *Chlorella*,[4] and others. Mucorales are used for preparation of numerous oriental fermented foods such as tempeh, sufu, ragi, and a few others.[3]

NUTRITIONAL AND PHYSIOLOGICAL PROPERTIES

Since chitin and chitosan have the same glycosidic linkages in their molecules as cellulose, they cannot be hydrolyzed by enzymes secreted in humans. In the gastrointestinal tract, therefore, they are not hydrolyzed in the small intestine and are partially degraded by the microbial flora in the large intestine. Chitin behaves as typical insoluble dietary fiber, while chitosan has a unique solubility profile. When ingested, chitosan is insoluble; however, in the stomach, due to low pH, it becomes fully or partially solubilized, depending on the particle size, concentration, and other factors. In the small intestine, due to the neutral pH, chitosan precipitates and thus becomes again insoluble. The polycationic nature and the unique *in vivo* solubility of chitosan may be responsible for special physiological attributes of this biopolymer.

Chitin and chitosan are biopolymers of very low toxicity. According to Arai et al.,[5] the LD_{50} of chitosan in laboratory mice is 16 g/kg of body weight. This is similar to that of salt or sugar.

Since the late 1970s, it has been repeatedly reported that chitosan has strong hypocholesterolemic and hypolipidemic properties. The initial studies were conducted in experimental animals such as rats,[6,7] mice,[8] rabbits,[9,10] and broiler chickens,[11,12] to mention a few. Lately, a number of clinical studies confirmed the results previously observed in experimental animals.[13–17] In addition, it was shown in animals and in humans that chitosan can augment high-density lipoproteins[13–15,18] and act as an effective lipid binder *in vivo*.[19–23]

The binding and reduction of absorption and utilization of lipids should lead to weight loss. This effect has been observed in recent studies in which a controlled low-calorie diet in placebo and in test groups was combined with ingestion of chitosan during main meals by overweight subjects. These studies lasted on average 4 weeks, and the subjects consumed 2 to 3 g of chitosan per day.[14,15,24,25] The studies in which free-living diets with no restrictions were used showed conflicting results. In one such study, which lasted 12 weeks, two-thirds of the subjects showed significant weight loss, while one-third of the subjects did not respond.[26] In two similar studies, one lasting 4 weeks[27] and one 8 weeks,[17] no weight loss was observed. There are a few plausible explanations why the studies using free-living diets did not always result in weight loss.

Unlike strong anion exchangers such as cholestyramine, chitosan did not show adverse effects on the morphology of the gastrointestinal tract when tested in experimental animals at moderate levels.[7,28] In the clinical studies no adverse effects have been reported, except for a few transient effects such as constipation.[13–17,24,25]

In order to explain chitosan activity, a number of mechanisms have been proposed and investigated. They have been reviewed, and at this time it is believed that a few mechanisms working sequentially may be involved.[29]

Since important benefits may be gained from using chitosan in oral applications, this area is currently under detailed investigation.

REFERENCES

1. Furda, I., Aminopolysaccharides — Their potential as dietary fiber, in *Unconventional Sources of Dietary Fiber*, Furda, I., Ed., American Chemical Society, Symposium Series, Vol. 214, Washington, D.C., 1983, chap. 8.
2. Muzzarelli, R. A. A., Enzymic synthesis of chitin and chitosan, in *Chitin*, Muzzarelli, R. A. A., Ed., Pergamon Press, Oxford, 1978, chap. 1.
3. Fenton, D., Davis, B., Rotgers, C., and Eveleigh, D. E., Enzymatic hydrolysis of chitosan, in *Proceedings of the First International Conference on Chitin/Chitosan*, Muzzarelli, R. A. A., and Pariser, E. R., Eds., Massachusetts Institute of Technology, Cambridge, MA, 1978, 525.
4. Mihara, S., Change of glucosamine content of *Chlorella* cells during their life cycle, *Plant Cell Physiol.*, 2, 25, 1961.
5. Arai, K., Kinumaki, T., and Fujita, T., Toxicity of chitosan, *Bull. Tokai Reg. Fish Res. Lab.*, 56, 89, 1968.
6. Sugano, M., Fujikawa, T., Hiratsuji, Y., and Hasegawa, Y., Hypocholesterolemic effects of chitosan in cholesterol fed rats, *Nutr. Rep. Int.*, 18, 531, 1978.
7. Vahouny, G. V., Satchithanandam, S., Cassidy, M. M., Lightfoot, F. B., and Furda, I., Comparative effect of chitosan and cholestyramine on lymphatic absorption of lipids in the rat, *Amer. J. Clin. Nutr.*, 38, 278, 1983.
8. Miura, T., Usami, M., Tsuura, Y., Ishida, H., and Seino, Y., Hypoglycemic and hypolipidemic effect of chitosan in normal and neonatal *Streptozotocin* — induced diabetic mice, *Biol. Pharm. Bull.*, 18, 11, 1995.

9. Hirano, S., Itakura, C., Seino, H., Akiyama, Y., Nonaka, I., Kanbara, N., and Kawakami, T., Chitosan as an ingredient for domestic and animal feeds, *J. Agric. Food Chem.*, 38, 1214, 1990.

10. Hirano, S. and Akiyama, Y., Absence of hypocholesterolemic action of chitosan in high-serum-cholesterol rabbits, *J. Sci. Food Agric.*, 69, 91, 1995.

11. Razdan, A. and Pettersson, D., Effect of chitin and chitosan on nutrient digestibility and plasma lipid concentrations in broiler chickens, *Brit. J. Nutr.*, 76, 387, 1994.

12. Razdan, A. and Pettersson, D., Broiler chicken body weights, feed intakes, plasma lipid and small-intestinal bile acid concentrations in response to feeding of chitosan and pectin, *Brit. J. Nutr.*, 78, 283, 1997.

13. Maezaki, Y., Tsuji, K., Nakagawa, Y., Kawai, Y., Akimoto, M., Tsugita, T., Takekawa, W., Terada, A., Hara, H., and Mitsuoka, T., Hypocholesterolemic effect of chitosan in adult males, *Biosci. Biotech. Biochem.*, 57, 1439, 1993.

14. Veneroni, G., Veneroni, F., Contos, S., Tripodi, S., DeBernardi, M., Guarino, C., and Marletta, M., Effect of a new chitosan dietary integrator and hypocaloric diet on hyperlipidemia and overweight in obese patients, *Acta Toxicol. Ther.*, 17, 1, 53, 1996.

15. Sciutto, A. M. and Colombo, P., Lipid lowering effect of chitosan dietary integrator and hypocaloric diet in obese subjects, *Acta Toxicol. Ther.*, 16, 4, 215, 1995.

16. Jing, S. B., Li, L., Ji, D., Takiguchi, Y., and Yamaguchi, T., Effect of chitosan on renal function in patients with chronic renal failure, *J. Pharm. Pharmacol.*, 49, 721, 1997.

17. Wuolijoki, E., Hirvela, T., and Ilitalo, P., Decrease in serum LDL cholesterol with microcrystalline chitosan, *Methods Find. Exp. Clin. Pharmacol.*, 21(5), 357, 1999.

18. Sugano, M., Fujikawa, T., Hiratsuji, Y., Nakashima, K., Fukuda, N., and Hasegawa, Y., A novel use of chitosan as a hypocholesterolemic agent in rats, *Amer. J. Clin. Nutr.*, 33, 787, 1980.

19. Furda, I., Nonabsorbable lipid binder, *U.S. Patent* 4,223,023, 1980.

20. Deuchi, K., Kanauchi, O., Imasato, Y., and Kobayashi, E., Decreasing effect of chitosan on the apparent digestibility by rats fed on a high-fat diet, *Biosci. Biotech. Biochem.*, 58, 1613, 1994.

21. Kanauchi, O., Deuchi, K., Imasato, Y., Shizukuishi, M., and Kobayashi, E., Mechanism for the inhibition of fat digestion by chitosan and for the synergistic effect of ascorbate, *Biosci. Biotech. Biochem.* 59(5), 786, 1995.

22. Han, L.-K., Kimura, Y., and Okuda, H., Reduction of fat storage during chitin-chitosan treatment in mice fed a high-fat diet, *Int. J. Obes. Relat. Metab. Disorders*, 23, 174, 1999.

23. Nauss, J. L., Thompson, J. L., and Nagyvary, J. J., The binding of micellar lipids to chitosan, *Lipids*, 18, 10, 714, 1983.

24. Macchi, G., A new approach to the treatment of obesity: chitosan's effect on body weight reduction and plasma cholesterol levels, *Acta Toxicol. Ther.*, 17(4), 303, 1996.

25. Giustina, A. and Ventura, P., Weight-reducing regimens in obese subjects: effect of new dietary fiber integrator, *Acta Toxicol. Ther.*, 16(4), 199, 1995.

26. Wadstein, J., Thom, E., Heldman, E., Gudmunsson, S., and Lilja, B., Biopolymer L 112, a chitosan with fat binding properties and potential as a weight reducing agent: a review of *in vitro* and *in vivo* experiments, in *Chitosan Per Os: From Dietary Supplement to Drug Carrier*, Muzzarelli, R. A. A., Ed., Atec, Grottammare, 2000, 65.

27. Pittler, M. H., Abbot, N. C., Harkness, E. F., and Ernst, E., Randomized, double-blind trial of chitosan for body weight reduction, *Eur. J. Clin. Nutr.*, 53, 379, 1999.

28. Jennings, C. D., Boleyn, K., Bridges, S. R., Wood, P. J., and Anderson, J. W., A comparison of the lipid-lowering and intestinal morphological effects of cholestyramine, chitosan and oat gum in rats, *Proc. Soc. Exp. Biol. Med.*, 189, 13, 1988.

29. Furda, I., Reduction of absorption of dietary lipids and cholesterol by chitosan and its derivatives and special formulations, in *Chitosan Per Os: From Dietary Supplement to Drug Carrier*, Muzzarelli, R. A. A., Ed., Atec, Grottammare, 2000, 41.

Methods of Analysis for Dietary Fiber

Enzymatic Gravimetric Methods

Nils-Georg Asp

INTRODUCTION

Enzymatic gravimetric methods date back to the 19th century. In the 1930s, McCance et al.[1] measured total unavailable carbohydrates in fruits, nuts, and vegetables by determining the residue insoluble in 80% ethanol. This was corrected for starch measured after enzymatic hydrolysis with taka-diastase and for protein. Similar procedures have been used more recently.[2,3] The main limitation of this approach is that the protein correction gives an unacceptable error in samples with low dietary fiber and high protein content.

METHODS MEASURING INSOLUBLE DIETARY FIBER

Methods employing both amylolytic and proteolytic treatment and separation of an insoluble undigestible residue are listed in Table 3.1.1. Weinstock and Benham[4] used the enzyme preparation Rhozyme S with high amylase activity. Thus, starch was removed efficiently, whereas a considerable protein residue remained associated with the fiber.[5,6] Thomas[7] improved the method by adding a pancreatin step. Later on, Elchazly and Thomas[8] omitted the crude Rhozyme preparation and used amyloglucosidase or takadiastase and trypsin or pancreatin. These authors also introduced special centrifugation tubes with fritted glass filters for separation of the insoluble fiber from the enzyme digest.

Table 3.1.1 Enzymatic Gravimetric Methods Measuring Insoluble Fiber

Agents for Protein and Starch Solubilization	Incubation Time (h)	Ref.
Rhozyme S	24	4
Pancreatin	5	7
Rhozyme or other amylase	18	
Amyloglucosidase or	3	8
takadiastase	18	
Trypsin or pancreatin	18	
Pepsin	18	9
Pancreatin	1	

Hellendoorn et al.[9] used only physiological enzymes, pepsin plus pancreatin. This analytical method is therefore related to a physiological dietary fiber definition.[10,11] The residues of protein and starch associated with the dietary fiber after enzymatic treatment[6,12] were even considered an advantage, representing *in vivo* undigestible material.[13] Saunders and Betschart[14] also suggested that indigestible protein could play a significant role in the physiological effects of dietary fiber. However, the protein and starch residues are dependent upon the choice of enzymes and the conditions for enzymatic digestion,[12–14] and it is impossible to define exactly the degree of hydrolysis obtained *in vivo*. This fact has led most workers to prefer a more "chemical" definition of dietary fiber, i.e., the sum of undigestible polysaccharides and lignin.[15] However, in practice the delimitation is always related to a method involving enzymatic degradation of starch *in vitro*, which may be more or less related to *in vivo* conditions.

METHODS MEASURING INSOLUBLE AND SOLUBLE DIETARY FIBER

Soluble dietary fiber components constitute a considerable fraction of the total dietary fiber in mixed diets[5,6] and include polysaccharides such as pectins and gums with important physiological effects. It is generally agreed that soluble components should be included in the definition and determination of dietary fiber.[15–18] Table 3.1.2 lists developments of enzymatic methods, also measuring soluble dietary fiber components.

Table 3.1.2   Enzymatic Gravimetric Methods Measuring Both Soluble and Insoluble Fiber

Agents for Protein and Starch Solubilization	Incubation Time	Ref.
B. subtilis amylase and protease	16–18 h	19, 20
Pepsin	20 h	21
Pancreatin + glucoamylase	18 h	
Pepsin	18 h	6
Pancreatin	1 h	
Termamyl	15 min	12
Pepsin	1 h	
Pancreatin	1 h	
Amyloglucosidase	3 h	22
Pancreatin/trypsin	15–18 h	
Termamyl	15–30 min	23
B. subtilis protease	30 min	
Amyloglucosidase	30 min	

Furda[19,20] used *Bacillus subtilis* amylase and protease in a single overnight incubation at neutral pH. Soluble dietary fiber components were recovered by precipitation with 4 vol of 95% (v/v) ethanol. Both insoluble and precipitated soluble fiber were separated by filtration in crucibles with glass wool as a filtering aid.

The methods of Schweizer and Würsch[21] and Asp et al.[6,12] are developments of Hellendoorn et al.[9] using the physiological enzymes pepsin and pancreatin. Soluble dietary fiber is precipitated with ethanol. Two of these methods[6,21] employ long (19- to 38-h) incubation times and repeated centrifugations to recover the dietary fiber fractions. In the more recent modification of Asp et al.,[12] enzyme incubation time was reduced to 2 h, and separation of both insoluble and precipitated soluble fiber — either separately or together — was carried out by filtration using Celite as a filtering aid. The main steps of this method are shown in Figure 3.1.1.

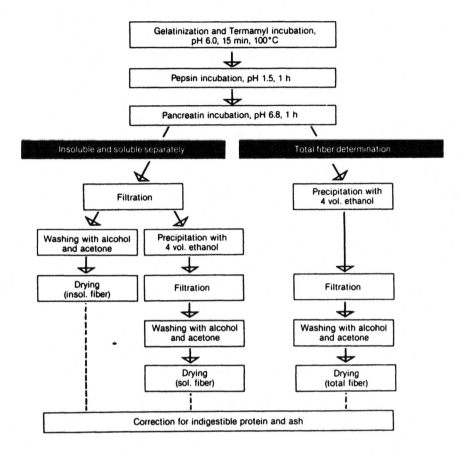

Figure 3.1.1 Flow diagram of the method of Asp et al.[12]

Meuser et al.[22] developed a method based on the enzymatic method of Elchazly and Thomas,[8] using membrane ultrafiltration to separate the soluble dietary fiber components from the enzyme digest.

The AOAC method[23–26] is based on the common experience of three groups that have developed enzymatic gravimetric methods for the assay of total dietary fiber.[12,20,21] The main steps are shown in Figure 3.1.2, and a detailed step-by-step description is given at the end of this chapter. This method employs the short technique, incubation times, and filtration introduced by Asp et al.[12] but with other enzymes. A modification of the AOAC method with further simplifications has recently been tested collaboratively by Lee et al.[27] and approved.

The separate determination of soluble and insoluble dietary fiber was suggested in the different enzymatic gravimetric methods[6,12,19–22] (Figure 3.1.1) and has been tested collaboratively for the AOAC method.[25,27] The solubility of the dietary fiber polysaccharides is method dependent, and the experimental conditions giving a solubility closest to that in the intestinal content have not yet been defined. Furthermore, physiological effects on plasma lipid levels and postprandial glucose and hormone response, attributed to soluble fiber, seem to be related to the properties of the soluble fiber, especially the viscosity.

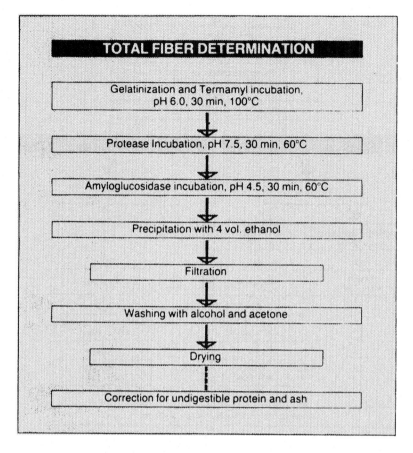

Figure 3.1.2   Flow diagram of the AOAC method for total dietary fiber.[23–27]

DISCUSSION OF VARIOUS STEPS IN ENZYMATIC GRAVIMETRIC METHODS

Sample Preparation

Milling to small particles is essential for proper enzyme action. Usually, milling to pass a 0.3- to 0.5-mm screen is recommended, but it is recognized that milling to such a small particle size may present difficulties with some materials.

Defatting is usually recommended and may be necessary for proper milling. In the AOAC method,[23,31,32] simple defatting with petroleum ether at room temperature is recommended whenever the fat content exceeds 10%. It should be noted, however, that Asp et al. were able to analyze dietary fiber with their method[12] in samples with 20% fat without defatting. Probably much of the fat melts at the high temperature during the starch gelatinization step, and any fat residue will be dissolved by the alcohol and acetone washing of the dietary fiber residue after filtration.

Starch Gelatinization and Hydrolysis

Whereas some authors[21, 22] employ autoclaving for starch gelatinization, Asp et al.[12] demonstrated that a 15-min. heating in a boiling waterbath in the presence of the thermostable α-amylase Termamyl gave sufficient gelatinization and prehydrolysis of the starch. Even in starchy materials such as wheat flour and potatoes, which are recognized as difficult in this respect, only a small amount of starch available to glucoamylase remained in the dietary fiber residue.[12,28]

"Resistant starch," i.e., starch available to glucoamylase only after solubilization with 2 M KOH, remained associated with the dietary fiber in bread,[26] similarly as found with a gas-chromatographic method[30] using 1-h boiling for starch gelatinization. The total starch remaining in the dietary fiber residue prepared with an enzymatic gravimetric method can be differentiated into one fraction available to glucoamylase without alkali solubilization ("residual starch") and another fraction available only after solubilization in 2 M KOH or dimethylsulfoxide, DMSO ("resistant starch").[31]

The resistant starch in the fiber residue is mainly retrograded amylose.[32] This fraction is resistant to degradation also in the small intestine of both rat[33] and man.[34]

Recently it has been suggested that the term resistant starch be used in a broader sense, representing all the starch escaping digestion and absorption in the human small intestine.[35]

Different methods employ either only α-amylases[6,9,12] or only glucoamylase,[19,20] or a combination of both types of amylase.[21-27] An advantage with glucoamylase is that it degrades the starch to free glucose, which can easily be analyzed in the filtrate to measure starch.

It is essential that all enzyme preparations used are free from contaminating activities hydrolyzing dietary fiber. This can be checked most conveniently by running samples of known polysaccharide preparations through the whole procedure.[23] The reason why the crude Termamyl preparation can be used is the high temperature employed, inactivating contaminating activities. Thus, heating should be performed immediately after Termamyl addition to avoid hydrolysis of dietary fiber components.

Protein Hydrolysis

At very acidic pH (around 1) as originally used by Hellendoorn et al.,[9] acid-labile groups of dietary fiber polysaccharides, such as arabinose residues in cereal pentosans, may be hydrolyzed. By increasing the pH to 1.5 and reducing the incubation time to 1 h, Asp et al.[12] were able to use pepsin without measurable loss of dietary fiber constituents. The AOAC method[23-27] employs the *B. subtilis* protease originally used by Furda[19,20] at neutral pH.

To be consistent with the definition of dietary fiber as the sum of undigestible polysaccharides and lignin, values obtained with enzymatic gravimetric methods need to be corrected for undigestible protein associated with the fiber. This can be done by analyzing the dietary fiber residue for nitrogen with the Kjeldahl method.[12,23-27] The universal protein conversion factor 6.25 should be used, since the true correct factor of the undigestible protein is not known. It may differ from that in the original protein.

Recovery of Soluble Dietary Fiber Constituents

Most methods employ precipitation with 78–80% (v/v) ethanol to separate soluble fiber components from the enzyme digest. The precipitate is recovered by centrifugation[21] or filtration using glass wool[19,20] or Celite[12,23-27] as a filtering aid. Procedures using ultrafiltration[22] or dialysis have not been documented to be more selective. The 80%-ethanol precipitation is an arbitrary delimitation between polysaccharides included in dietary fiber and oligosaccharides not included. Polysaccharides with DP (degree of polymerization) >10 are usually precipitated, but in some cases larger polysaccharides will stay in solution, especially if highly branched. This has been demonstrated for arabinans and pectic substances in sugar beet fiber.[37]

Coprecipitation of minerals may be a problem when using alcohol precipitation.[38,39] Although correction for ash is recommended,[12,23-27] the buffer strength of the incubation medium should be kept low enough to avoid excessive ash precipitation and thus an unnecessary source of variability between samples.

INTERLABORATORY STUDIES

Enzymatic gravimetric methods have been compared and evaluated vs. other methods. In the EEC/IARC study conducted in 1978, three groups participated with enzymatic methods. Although incompletely developed at that time, the enzymatic methods gave comparatively consistent results and good agreement with gas chromatographic methods.[40]

Raw and processed wheat and potato products were analyzed in another interlaboratory study.[28] Enzymatic methods showed good agreement with each other and with gas chromatographic methods. The AOAC method[23] and the method of Asp et al.[12] showed good agreement on these samples and also on the samples analyzed in the first AOAC collaborative study (Figure 3.1.3). Similar results have been obtained when comparing the component analysis methods of Theander et al. and the enzymatic gravimetric method of Asp et al. for both processed and unprocessed cereals and vegetables.[37] The lower values obtained with the Englyst method can generally be explained by the fact that this method does not include lignin and resistant starch.

The first interlaboratory study with the AOAC method for total dietary fiber (TDF)[23] was the biggest collaborative effort reported so far. It identified a number of problems that were corrected in the second study, after which the method was approved by the AOAC.[24] A Swiss collaborative study with a slightly modified TDF method[26] reported the best precision measures obtained so far. These modifications were introduced and approved in the third AOAC study.[25] Insoluble fiber determination also showed satisfactory results in that study, and soluble fiber determination was approved as the difference between total and insoluble fiber. Later on, direct determination of soluble fiber was approved, as well.[27]

All the collaborative studies reported so far — both with enzymatic gravimetric methods and with the method of Englyst et al. — have recently been calculated in the same way and compared.[41] The gravimetric AOAC method has been tested on a wider range of foods with more variable dietary fiber content and has generally shown reproducibility values as good as or better than the Englyst method.

The AOAC method has been officially approved in Switzerland, Germany, Denmark, Finland, Iceland, Norway, Sweden, and The Netherlands. It is recommended in several other countries. Gravimetric dietary fiber values, both with and without correction for protein, have recently been introduced in the Japanese food tables.[42]

CONCLUSION

Enzymatic gravimetric methods using alcohol precipitation of soluble dietary fiber components are suitable for assay of total dietary fiber or insoluble and soluble fiber separately. Correction for undigestible protein and ash associated especially with the soluble fiber should be made to conform with currently accepted definitions of dietary fiber. Once a protein correction is accepted, a somewhat higher protein residue obtained at the very short incubation time in the protease step(s) can be accepted, as well as some variation in the residue due to choice of enzymes.

Alcohol precipitation is the most rapid way to separate soluble dietary fiber components from the enzyme digest. Ultrafiltration and especially dialysis are much slower processes and have not been documented to be more selective and complete.

Filtration in glass filter crucibles can be used to recover both insoluble and alcohol-precipitated soluble components if a filtering aid such as Celite is used. Centrifugation is an alternative, especially to recover very viscous types of fiber that can give filtration problems.

Enzymatic methods are useful as preparatory steps before detailed analysis of dietary fiber composition. The enzymatic treatment removes material that might interfere in later steps, and the

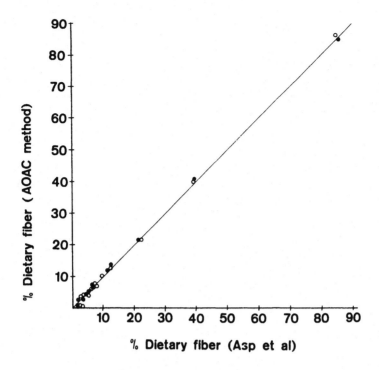

Figure 3.1.3 Comparison of the methods of Asp et al.[12] and Prosky et al.[23] using different enzymes on samples in the first interlaboratory study of the AOAC method. The different symbols denote two different laboratories.

total fiber value obtained in the gravimetric assay can serve as a control of the standardization of detailed analyses. The efficiency of starch removal and presence of resistant starch can be checked by analyzing the dietary fiber residue.

THE DETERMINATION OF TOTAL DIETARY FIBER IN FOODS AND FOOD PRODUCTS: APPROVED AOAC METHOD OF PROSKY ET AL.[24,25]

Procedure

Duplicate samples of dried foods, fat extracted if containing more than 10% fat, are gelatinized with Termamyl (heat stable α-amylase), then enzymatically digested with protease and amyloglucosidase to remove the protein and starch present. Then 4 vol of 95% ethanol (v/v) is added to precipitate the soluble dietary fiber. The total residue is filtered, washed with 78% ethanol, 95% ethanol, and acetone. After drying, the residue is weighed. One of the duplicates is analyzed for protein, and the other is incinerated at 525°C and the ash determined. Total dietary fiber is the weight of the residue less the weight of the protein and ash present.

Apparatus

1. Balance, analytical, capable of weighing to 0.1 mg.
2. Fritted crucible, porosity #2. Clean thoroughly, ash at 525°C, soak in distilled water, and rinse in same. Add approximately 0.5 g of Celite 545 to dried crucibles before drying to obtain constant weight. Dry at 130°C for 1 h, cool, and store in desiccator until used. The fritted crucible is a Pyrex 32940, Course ASTM 40 to 60 μm, and may be purchased from Scientific Products Co., C-8525-1; V. W. R. Scientific Co., 23863-040; Fisher Scientific Co., 08237-1A; Sargent Welch Co., F-243-90-B or F-243-90-C, depending on size needed.

   Crucibles indicated in the procedure may not be available in Europe. Porosity #2 in Europe signifies pores of 40 to 90 μm, whereas it means 40 to 60 μm in the U.S. Several collaborators have reported breakage of crucibles when the temperature was raised to 525°C and have recommended Corning No. 36060 Buchner, fritted disk, Pyrex, 60-ml ASTM 40 to 60, which seems to have less breakage and gives the same results.
3. Vacuum source: a vacuum pump or aspirator equipped with an inline double vacuum flask should be used to prevent contamination in case of water backup.
4. Vacuum oven at 70°C and desiccator; alternatively, an air oven capable of operating at 105°C can be used.
5. Boiling water bath.
6. Constant-temperature water bath adjustable to 60°C and equipped to provide constant agitation of the digestion flasks during enzymatic hydrolysis. This can be accomplished with either a multistation shaker or multistation magnetic stirrer.
7. Vortex mixer.
8. Beaker (tall form) 400 ml.

Reagents

1. Distilled water (DW).
2. 95% ethanol (v/v)—technical grade.
3. 78% ethanol: mix one volume of distilled water with four volumes of 95% ethanol.
4. Acetone—reagent grade.
5. Phosphate buffer 0.08 M pH 6.0: dissolve to 1.400 g of sodium phosphate dibasic anhydrous (or 1.753 g of the dihydrate) and 9.68 g sodium phosphate monobasic monohydrate (or 10.99 g of the dihydrate) in approximately 700 ml of DW. Dilute to 11 with DW. Check pH.
6. Termamyl (heat-stable α-amylase) solution: 120 L (Novo Laboratories Inc.). Store the enzyme solution in refrigerator after each use.
7. Protease P-3910 (Sigma Chemical Co.): refrigerate the dry enzyme after each use.
8. Amyloglucosidase A-9913 (Sigma Chemical Co.): keep refrigerated when not in use.
9. Sodium hydroxide solution (0.275 N): dissolve 11.00 g sodium hydroxide AR in approximately 700 ml DW in 1-1 volumetric flask. Dilute to volume with DW.
10. Hydrochloric acid solution (0.350 N): dilute a stock solution with known titer, e.g., 350 ml of 1 M HCl to 11 with distilled water. Dilute to volume with DW.
11. Celite 545 (Fisher Scientific Co.). Acid washed. Equivalent to Celite C-211.

Determination

1. Run a blank through the entire procedure along with the samples to measure any contribution from reagents to the residue.
2. Weigh, in duplicate, 1 g of sample accurate to 0.1 mg (sample weight should not differ by more than 20 mg) into 400-ml tall form beakers. Add 50 ml of pH 6.0 phosphate buffer to each beaker. Check pH. Adjust to pH 6.0 ± 0.2 with 0.275 N NaOH if necessary.
3. Add 100 µl Termamyl solution.
4. Cover beaker with aluminum foil and place in boiling waterbath for 15 min. Shake gently at 5-min intervals. Increase the length of incubation time when the number of beakers added to the boiling waterbath makes it difficult for the beaker contents to reach an internal temperature of 100°C; 30 min should be sufficient.
5. Cool. Adjust to pH 7.5 ± 0.1 by adding 10 ml of 0.275 N NaOH solution.
6. Add 5 mg of protease. Since protease sticks to the spatula, it may be preferable to make an enzyme solution just prior to use with a small amount of (about 100 µl) phosphate buffer and pipette the required amount.
7. Cover with aluminum foil. Incubate at 60° for 30 min with continuous agitation.
8. Cool. Add 10 ml of 0.350 M hydrochloric acid solution to adjust pH to 4.0 to 4.6.
9. Add 0.3 ml of amyloglucosidase solution.
10. Cover with aluminum foil. Incubate at 60°C for 30 min with continuous agitation.
11. Add 280 ml of 95% ethanol preheated to 60°C. Measure volume after heating.
12. Allow precipitate to form at room temperature for 60 min.
13. Tare crucible containing Celite to nearest 0.1 mg. After taring the crucible containing the Celite, redistribute the bed of Celite in the crucible using a stream of 78% ethanol from a wash bottle. Suction is then applied to the crucible to draw the Celite onto the fritted glass as an even mat. When the fiber is filtered, i.e., Step 14, the Celite effectively separates the fiber from the fritted glass of the crucible, allowing for easy removal of the crucible contents.
14. Filter enzyme digest from Step 12 through crucible.
15. Wash residue successively with three 20-ml portions of 78% ethanol, two 10-ml portions of 95% ethanol, and two 10-ml portions of acetone. With some samples a gum is formed, trapping the liquid. If the surface film that develops after the addition of the sample to the Celite is broken with a spatula, filtration is improved. Long filtration times can be avoided by careful intermittent suction throughout the filtration. Normal suction can be applied at washing. Back-bubbling of air is another way of speeding up filtrations, if available.
16. Dry crucible containing residue overnight in a 70°C vacuum oven or a 105°C air oven.
17. Cool in desiccator and weigh crucible, Celite, and residue to nearest 0.1 mg.
18. Analyze the residue from one sample of the set of duplicates for protein. Protein is probably most easily analyzed by carefully scraping the Celite and the fiber mat onto a suitable piece of filter paper which can then be folded shut and analyzed for protein. A piece of filter paper should be analyzed to assure that it will not affect the protein value obtained. Collaborators should use the Kjeldahl analysis as specified in "Official Methods of Analysis" of the AOAC. Use 6.25 for the protein factor.
19. Incinerate second sample of the duplicate for 5 h at 525°C.
20. Cool in desiccator. Weigh crucible containing Celite and ash to nearest 0.1 mg. (See flow diagram in Figure 3.1.4 and formula for calculating "total dietary fiber" from the data in Figure 3.1.5.)

Sample preparation (10g), dry, pulverized and if more than 10% lipids
extracted with 25 mL petroleum ether to remove the lipids.

Repeat extraction 2 times with 25 mL petroleum ether.
Weighing of duplicate samples, 1g.
Addition of 50 mL 0.08 M phosphate buffer, pH 6.0.
Addition of Termamyl for gelatinization, 100 μl.

Incubation, boiling water bath, 15–30 min, shaking at 5 min intervals
Adjustment to pH 7.5 with 0.275 N NaOH.
Addition of Protease, 5 mg.

Incubation, 60° C, 30 min, continuous agitation.
Adjustment to pH 4.5 with 10 mL 0.350 M hydrochloric acid.
Addition of Amyloglucosidase, 0.3 mL.
Incubation, 60 °C, 30 min, continuous agitation.
Addition of 280 mL, 95% ethanol, preheated to 60°C.

Formation of precipitate, 60 min.

Filtration through bed containing
0.5 g Celite 545. Washing with three 20 mL
portions of 78% ethanol, two 10 mL portions of 95%
ethanol and two 10 mL portions of acetone.

Drying of crucibles, 70°C vacuum oven or 105°C air oven, overnight.

Cooling and weighing of crucibles.

Protein determination,   Ash determination
use entire crucible   525°C, 5 hrs.,
contents, Factor = 6.25   cool and weigh

+---+
| Calculation of Total Dietary Fiber |
| TDF = weight of residue, minus weight of protein, |
| minus weight of ash, minus weight of blank |
+---+

Figure 3.1.4 Sequences in the analysis of total dietary fiber by the official AOAC method.[24,25]

$$\% \text{ TDF} = \frac{\dfrac{R_1 + R_2}{2} - P - A - B}{\dfrac{M_1 + M_2}{2}} \times 100$$

TDF = Total Dietary Fiber
R_1 and R_2 = Residue weights (mg)
P = protein, A = ash, B = blank corrections (mg)
M_1 and M_2 = sample weights (mg)

Figure 3.1.5 Calculation of percentage dietary fiber from data obtained by official AOAC method.[24,25]

REFERENCES

1. McCance, R. A., Widdowson, E. M., and Shackleton, L. R. B., The nutritive value of fruits, vegetables and nuts, *Med. Res. Counc. (G.B.) Spec. Rep. Serv.*, 213, 32, 1936.
2. Katan, M. B. and van de Bovenkamp, P., Determination of total dietary fiber by difference and of pectin by colorimetry of copper titration, in *The Analysis of Dietary Fiber in Food*, James, W. P. T. and Theander, O., Eds., Marcel Dekker, New York, 1981, 217.
3. Sandberg, A.-S., Hallgren, B., and Hasselblad, C., Analytical problems in the determination of dietary fibre, *Näringsforskning*, 4, 132, 1981.
4. Weinstock, A. and Benham, G. H., The use of enzyme preparations in the crude fibre determination, *Cereal Chem.*, 28, 490, 1951.
5. Asp, N.-G., Critical evaluation of some suggested methods for assay of dietary fibre, in *Dietary Fibre: Current Developments of Importance of Health*, Heaton, K. W., Ed., John Libbey, London, 1978, 21.
6. Asp, N.-G. and Johansson, C.-G., Techniques for measuring dietary fiber: principal aims of methods and a comparison of results obtained by different techniques, in *The Analysis of Dietary Fiber in Food*, James, W. P. T. and Theander, O., Eds., Marcel Dekker, New York, 1981, 173.
7. Thomas, B., Enzymatische Rohfaserbestimmung in Getreideprodukten, *Getr. Mehl Brot.*, 29, 115, 1975.
8. Elchazly, M. and Thomas, B., Über eine biochemische Methode zum Bestimmen der Ballaststoffe und ihrer Komponenten in pflanzlichen Lebensmitteln, *Z. Leb-ensm. Unters. Forsch.*, 162, 329, 1976.
9. Hellendoorn, W., Noordhoff, M. G., and Slagman, J., Enzymatic determination of the indigestible residue of human food, *J. Sci. Food Agric.*, 26, 1461, 1975.
10. Trowell, H. C., Crude fibre, dietary fibre and atherosclerosis, *Atherosclerosis*, 16, 138, 1972.
11. Trowell, H. C., Definitions of fibre, *Lancet*, 1, 503, 1974.
12. Asp, N-G., Johansson, C.-G., Hallmer, H., and Siljeström, M., Rapid enzymatic assay of insoluble and soluble dietary fiber, *J. Agric. Food Chem.*, 31, 476, 1983.
13. Hellendoorn, E. W., Some critical observations in relation to 'dietary fibre', the methods for its determination and the current hypotheses for the explanation of its physiological action, *Voeding*, 39, 230, 1978.
14. Saunders, R. M. and Betschart, A. A., The significance of protein as a component of dietary fiber, *Am. J. Clin. Nutr.*, 33, 965, 1980.
15. Trowell, H., Southgate, D. A. T., Wolever, T. M. S., Leeds, A. R., Gassull, M. A., and Jenkins, D. A., Dietary fibre redefined, *Lancet*, 1, 967, 1976.
16. Southgate, D. A. T., Hudson, G. J., and Englyst, H., The analysis of dietary fibre—the choices for the analyst, *J. Sci. Food Agric.*, 29, 979, 1978.
17. Theander, O. and Aman, P., Studies on dietary fibres, *Swed. J. Agric. Res.*, 9, 97, 1979.

18. Cummings, J. H., What is fiber?, in *Fiber in Human Nutrition*, Spiller, G. A. and Amen, R. J., Eds., Plenum Press, New York, 1976, 5.

19. Furda, I. Fractionation and examination of biopolymers from dietary fiber, *Cereal Foods World*, 22, 252, 1977.

20. Furda, I., Simultaneous analysis of soluble and insoluble dietary fiber, in *The Analysis of Dietary Fiber in Food*, James, W. P. T. and Theander, O., Eds., Marcell Dekker, 1981, 163.

21. Schweizer, T. F. and Würsch, P., Analysis of dietary fibre, *J. Sci. Food Agric.*, 30, 613, 1979.

22. Meuser, F., Suckow, P., and Kulikowski, W., Analytische Bestimmung von Ballaststoffen in Brot, Obst und Gemuse, *Getreide Mehl Brot.*, 37, 380, 1983.

23. Prosky, L., Asp, N.-G., Furda, I., DeVries, J., Schweizer, T. F., and Harland, B., Determination of total dietary fiber in foods, food products and total diets: interlaboratory study, *J. Assoc. Off. Anal. Chem.*, 67, 1044, 1984.

24. Prosky, L., Asp, N.-G., Furda, I., DeVries, J. W., Schweizer, T., and Harland, B., Determination of total dietary fiber in foods and food products: collaborative study, *J. Assoc. Off. Anal. Chem.*, 68, 677, 1985.

25. Prosky, L., Asp, N.-G., Schweizer, T. F., DeVries, J. W., and Furda, I., Determination of insoluble soluble and total dietary fiber in foods and food products: inter-laboratory study, *J. Assoc. Off. Anal. Chem.*, 71, 1017, 1988.

26. Schweizer, T. F., Walter, E., and Venetz, P., Collaborative study for the enzymatic, gravimetric determination of total dietary fibre in foods, *Mitt., Geb. Lebensmitte-lunters. Hyg.*, 79, 57, 1988.

27. Lee, S., Prosky, L., and DeVries, J., Determination of total, soluble, and insoluble dietary fiber in foods. Enzymatic-gravimetric method, MES-TRIS buffer: collaborative study, *J. Assoc. Off. Anal. Chem.*, 75, 395, 1992.

28. Varo, P., Laine, R., and Koivistoinen, P., Effect of heat treatment on dietary fiber: interlaboratory study, *J. Assoc. Off. Agric. Chem.*, 66, 933, 1983.

29. Johansson, C.-G., Siljeström, M., and Asp, N.-G., Dietary fibre in bread and corresponding flours—formation of resistant starch during baking, *Z. Lebensm. Unters. Forsch.*, 179, 24, 1984.

30. Englyst, H. N., Anderson, V., and Cummings, J. H., Starch and non-starch polysaccharides in some cereal foods, *J. Sci. Food Agric.*, 34, 1434, 1983.

31. Siljeström, M. and Asp, N.-G., Resistant starch formation during baking—effect of baking time and temperature and variations in the recipe, *Z. Lebensm. Unters. Forsch.*, 181, 4, 1985.

32. Siljeström, M., Eliasson, A. C., and Björck, I., Characterization of resistant starch from autoclaved wheat starch, *Starch/Staerke*, 41, 147, 1989.

33. Björck, I. Nyman, M., Pedersen, B., Siljeström, M., Asp, N.-G., and Eggum, B., On the digestibility of starch in wheat bread, *J. Cereal. Sci.*, 4, 1, 1986.

34. Schweizer, T. F., Andersson, H., Langkilde, A. M., Reimann, S., and Torsdottir, I., Nutrients excreted in ileostomy effluents after consumption of mixed diets with beans or potatoes. II. Starch, dietary fibre and sugars, *Eur. J. Clin. Nutr.*, 44, 567, 1990.

35. Englyst, H. N. and Kingman, S. M., Dietary fiber and resistant starch. A nutritional classification of plant polysaccharides, in *Dietary Fiber*, Kritchevsky, D., Bonfield, C., and Anderson, J. W., Eds., Plenum, New York, 1990, 49.

36. Jeraci, J. L., Lewis, B. A., Van Soest, R. J., and Robertsson, J. B., Urea enzymatic dialysis procedure for determination of total dietary fiber, *J. Assoc. Off. Anal. Chem.*, 72, 677, 1989.

37. Asp, N.-G., Delimitation problems in definition and analysis of dietary fiber, in Furda, I. and Brine, C. J., Eds., *New Developments in Dietary Fiber*, Plenum Press, New York, 1990, 227.

38. Schweizer, T. F., Frolich, W., DeVedovo, S., and Besson, R., Minerals and phytate in the analysis of dietary fiber from cereals. I, *Cereal Chem.*, 61, 116, 1984.

39. Frølich, W., Asp, N.-G., and Schweizer, T. F., Minerals and phytate in the analysis of dietary fiber from cereals. II, *Cereal Chem.*, 61, 357, 1984.

40. James, W. P. T. and Theander, O., Eds., *The Analysis of Dietary Fiber in Food*, Marcel Dekker, New York, 1981.

41. Asp, N.-G., Schweizer, T. F., Southgate, D. A. T., and Theander, O., Dietary fiber analysis, in *Dietary Fibre—A Component of Food—Nutritional Function in Health and Disease*, Eastwood, M., Edwards, C., Mauron, J., and Schweizer, T., Eds.. Springer, London, 1992, 57.

42. Nishimune, T., Sumimoto, T., Yakusiji, T., Kunita, N., Ichikawa, T., Doguchi, M., and Nakahara, S., Determination of total dietary fiber in Japanese foods. *J. Assoc. Off. Anal. Chem.*, 74, 350, 1991.

Detergent Analysis of Foods

James B. Robertson and Peter J. Horvath

The use of detergents to isolate plant cell walls of low nitrogen content from forages was proposed in 1963. The detergent systems are neutral solutions of sodium lauryl sulfate[1] for cell wall analysis and an acidic medium containing cetyltrimethylammonium bromide for isolation of the less fermentable fraction of low hemicellulose content from forages.[2,3] Thus, the detergent system has a nutritional basis for the fractionation of food components.[4] The neutral detergent (ND) system has undergone many changes from its inception for use with ruminant forages to human foods. A major advantage of the ND procedure for dietary fiber analysis is that microbial material is soluble.[5] Fecal analysis by the detergent system is not complicated by microbial mass produced during colonic fermentation.[6] The primary drawback of ND is that soluble dietary fiber, primarily pectic substances and soluble hemicelluloses, is not recovered. However, it is normally totally digested.[7]

The original acid detergent (AD) system has not changed much for human food analysis. Baker[8] suggested buffering the AD (pH 1.5 to 2.0) to reduce cellulose loss. This buffered AD system recovered more material. However, some of this additional residue was hemicellulose[9] and pectic substances.[10] ADF has usually been used as a starting material for lignin determination, so hemicellulose should be removed to avoid the production of artifact lignin.[11] Pectin can also undergo Maillard reactions. Because of these problems, a preliminary extraction with ND before refluxing with AD has been suggested.[12,13] ADF has also been used to predict cell wall digestibility, and for this purpose removal of the insoluble hemicellulose and recovery of the AD-soluble cellulose may not be desirable.[14] These "celluloses" are easily fermentable and the linear hemicelluloses are of low fermentability.[15] The decision to obtain an ADF of low fermentability or an ADF composed of cellulose and lignin, free from hemicellulose, depends on how the ADF will be used.

A complex system of detergent extractions and subsequent hydrolysis and oxidation has been developed for a gravimetric component analysis of insoluble dietary fiber.[16] Figure 3.2.1 shows a flow diagram for this system. The classification of fiber components and how they can be determined is displayed in the center of Figure 3.2.1. Typically, the detergent system has been used as a gravimetric method. Sugar analysis of the NDF and ADF has been progressing.[17–19] One problem with a gravimetric method is that small samples or components in low concentration are difficult to weigh accurately. A semimicro method has been developed for samples of 0.2 g.[20] For very small samples, a sugar component analysis may be useful. Lignin is usually present in low amounts and can be assayed in other ways.

Other problems with the detergent systems include difficulty in starch removal, lipid and protein interference, and difficulty in filtration. Starch in low concentrations is solubilized in the ND, but

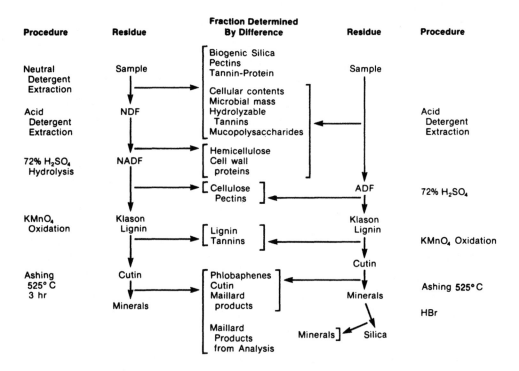

Figure 3.2.1 Flow diagram for fiber analysis by the detergent system. (The quantity of each fraction is measured as either the amount of residue or the weight loss after each procedure. The materials measured by weight loss are shown in brackets.)

certain types (modified or retrograded) and high concentrations can lead to filtration problems and an overestimation of dietary fiber (as currently defined). The problem of starch removal has been explored by many workers. In most cases treatment during ND extraction with an amylase from *Bacillus subtilis* is adequate.[6,21] Other procedures have been compared by Mascarenhas-Ferreira et al.[22] Some studies suggested a mammalian or fungal enzyme and a protease, but Marlett and Lee[23] found little difference in results from these methods. They found that temperature, not the length of incubation, is most important. Heat-stable bacterial amylase might be the fastest and easiest.[24,25]

Difficulty with filtration can also occur when other polysaccharides such as β-glucan are present. β-glucanase has been used to remove these glucans.[26] This may not be desirable because β-glucans are included in the dietary fiber complex as water-soluble unavailable carbohydrates.

Lipids and proteins interfere when in amounts that exceed the capacity of the reagents. The limits are about 10% of dry matter for lipid and 30% for protein. Preextraction with ethanol or ether will remove lipids. Detergent-stable proteases are available to hydrolyze protein for removal.

The sample is usually dried before it is ground. Both drying and particle size can affect the values. Heller et al.[27] found that as particle size was decreased, NDF decreased with other fractions varying nonuniformly. Drying above 60°C or in a microwave oven can increase NDF, ADF, and lignin values.[28,29] Freeze-drying may be the optimum way to dry the sample for grinding.

The reagents used for detergent extractions have undergone important changes since 1970.[14] Cellosolve (2-ethoxy ethanol) is an eye and mucous membrane irritant and could adversely affect the kidneys, liver, and central nervous system. It has the potential to cause adverse reproductive effects in males and females and embryotoxic effects including teratogenesis in the offspring of the exposed, pregnant female. *Consequently, 2-ethoxy ethanol should no longer be used in the neutral detergent solution.* Since cellosolve was included in the original reagent because it facilitates the solution of starch, it can be omitted if only forages are being analyzed. However, in starch containing feeds and foods, a volume-for-volume substitution of cellosolve with triethylene glycol produces identical analytical values. Decalin has been omitted from both detergent solutions to eliminate filtering problems and the consequent high fiber values. Sulfite, which was used to reduce the nitrogen content of the NDF, has been shown to cause a significant loss of lignin[21] and should be omitted in sequential analysis. The permanganate solution is essentially unchanged.[3] If a detailed analysis of the ADF is done, it is recommended that hydrolysis with 72% H_2SO_4 without the use of asbestos[30] be carried out before lignin oxidation. Cutin can be determined as the residue lost upon ashing.[14]

Detailed instructions and procedures are described in Robertson and Van Soest[16] and Van Soest et al.[25] A summary of total dietary fiber and detergent values is given in Table 2 of the Appendix.

REFERENCES

1. Van Soest, P. J., Use of detergents in the analysis of fibrous feeds. I. Preparation of fiber residues of low nitrogen content, *J. Assoc. Off. Agric. Chem.*, 46, 825, 1963.
2. Van Soest, P. J., Use of detergents in the analysis of fibrous feeds. II. A rapid method for the determination of fiber and lignin, *J. Assoc. Off. Agric. Chem.*, 46, 829, 1963.
3. Van Soest, P. J. and Wine, R. H., Use of detergents in the analysis of fibrous feed. IV. Determination of plant cell-wall constituents, *J. Assoc. Off. Anal. Chem.*, 50, 50, 1967.
4. Robertson, J. B., The detergent system of fiber analysis, in *Topics in Dietary Fiber Research,* Spiller, G. A. and Amen, R., Eds., Plenum Press, New York, 1978, 1.
5. Mason, V. C., Some observations on the distribution and origin of nitrogen in sheep feces, *J. Agric. Sci. Camb.*, 73, 99, 1969.
6. McQueen, R. E. and Nicholson, J. W. G., Modification of the neutral-detergent fiber procedure for cereals and vegetables by using alpha-amylase, *J. Assoc. Off. Anal. Chem.*, 62, 676, 1979.
7. Cummings, J. H., Southgate, D. A. T., Branch, W. J., Wiggins, H. S., Houston, D. J. A., and Jenkins, D., Digestion of pectin in the human gut and its effect on calcium absorption and large bowel function, *Br. J. Nutr.*, 41, 477, 1979.
8. Baker, D., Determining fiber in cereals, *Cereal Chem.*, 54, 360, 1977.
9. Morrison, I. M., Hemicellulose contamination of acid detergent residues and their replacement by cellulose residues in cell wall analysis, *J. Sci. Food Agric.*, 31, 639, 1980.
10. Belo, P. S., Jr. and De Lumen, B.O., Pectic substance content of detergent-extracted dietary fibers, *J. Agric. Food Chem.*, 29, 370, 1981.
11. Goering, H. K., Van Soest, P. J., and Hemken, R. W., Relative susceptibility of forages to heat damage as affected by moisture temperature and pH, *J. Dairy Sci.*, 56, 137, 1973.
12. Bailey, R. W. and Ulyatt, M. J., Pasture quality and ruminant nutrition. II. Carbohydrate and lignin composition of detergent-extracted residues from pasture grasses and legumes, *N.Z. J. Agric. Res.*, 13, 591, 1970.
13. Testolin, G., Bossi, E., Vercesi, P., Porrini, M., Simonetti, P., and Ciappellano, S., A rapid method for the analysis of alimentary fiber, *Nutr. Rep. Int.*, 25, 859, 1982.
14. Goering, H. K. and Van Soest, P. J., Forage fiber analysis (apparatus, reagents, procedures and some applications), Agricultural Handbook 379, U.S. Department of Agriculture, Washington, D.C., 1970.
15. Gaillard, B. D. E., The relationship between the cell-wall constituents of roughages and the digestibility of the organic matter, *J. Agric. Sci. Camb.*, 59, 369, 1962.
16. Robertson, J. B. and Van Soest, P. J., The detergent system of analysis and its application to human foods, in *The Analysis of Dietary Fiber in Foods,* James, W. P. T. and Theander, O., Eds., Marcel Dekker, New York, 1981, 123.
17. Bittner, A. S. and Street, J. C., Monosaccharide composition of alcohol- and detergent-insoluble residues in maturing reed canary grass leaves, *J. Agric. Food Chem.*, 31, 7, 1983.
18. Slavin, J. L. and Marlett, J. A., Evaluation of high-performance liquid chromatography for measurement of the neutral saccharides in neutral-detergent fiber, *J. Agric. Food Chem.*, 31, 467, 1983.
19. Windham, W. R., Barton, F. E., and Himmelsbach D. S., High pressure liquid chromatographic analysis of component sugars in neutral-detergent fiber for representative warm- and cool-season grasses, *J. Agric. Food Chem.*, 31, 471, 1983.

20. Sills, V. E. and Wallace, G. M., A semi-micro neutral-detergent fiber method for cereal products, in *Fiber in Human and Animal Nutrition*, Bulletin 10, Royal Society of New Zealand, Wellington, N.Z., 1983, 116.

21. Robertson, J. B. and Van Soest, P. J., Dietary fiber estimation in concentrated feedstuffs, *J. Anim. Sci.*, 45(Suppl. 1), 254 (Abstr.), 1977.

22. Mascarenhas-Ferreira, A., Kerstens, J., and Gasp, C. H., The study of several modifications of the neutral-detergent fibre procedure, *Anim. Feed Sci. Technol.*, 9, 19,1983.

23. Marlett, J. A. and Lee, S. C., Dietary fiber, lignocellulose and hemicellulose contents of selected foods determined by modified and unmodified Vap Soest procedures, *J. Food Sci.*, 45, 1688, 1980.

24. Jeraci, J. L., Hernandez, T. H., Lewis, B. A., Robertson, J. B., and Van Soest, P. J., New and improved procedure for neutral-detergent fiber, *J. Anim. Sci.*, 66 (Suppl. 1), 351 (Abstr.), 1988.

25. Van Soest, P. J., Robertson, J. B., and Lewis, B. A., Methods for dietary fiber, neutral detergent fiber, and nonstarch polysaccharides in relation to animal nutrition, *J. Dairy Sci.*, 74, 3583, 1991.

26. Roth, N. J. L., Watts, G. H., and Newman, C. W., Beta-glucanase as an aid in measuring neutral-detergent fiber in barley kernels, *Cereal Chem.*, 58, 245, 1981.

27. Heller, S. N., Rivers, J. M., and Hackler, L. R., Dietary fiber: effect of particle size and pH on its measurement, *J. Food Sci.*, 42, 436, 1977.

28. Van Soest, P. J., Use of detergents in analysis of fibrous feeds. III. Study of effects of heating and drying on yield of fiber and lignin in forages, *J. Assoc. Off. Agric. Chem.*, 48, 785, 1965.

29. Darrah, C. H., Van Soest, P. J., and Fick, G. W., Microwave treatment and heat damage artifacts in forages, *Agron. J.*, 69, 120, 1977.

30. Van Soest, P. J., Collaborative study of acid-detergent fiber and lignin, *J. Assoc. Off. Anal. Chem.*, 56, 781, 1973.

Dietary Fiber Analysis as Nonstarch Polysaccharides (NSPs)

Hans Englyst and Geoffrey Hudson

INTRODUCTION

There is a steadily growing body of evidence that both the amounts and the types of dietary carbohydrates are important for the promotion and maintenance of public health. As a consequence, scientists, nutritionists, health professionals, and the compilers of food tables and databases have argued strongly for the acquisition of specific analytical values for dietary carbohydrates, including dietary fiber.[1-3] In 1998, FAO/WHO[3] presented a list of recommendations on the role of carbohydrates in nutrition, proposing "that the analysis and labeling of dietary carbohydrates, for whatever purpose, be based on the chemical divisions recommended. Additional groupings such as polyols, resistant starch, non-digestible oligosaccharides and dietary fiber can be used, provided the included components are clearly defined." The methods that we have developed for the specific measurement of chemically identified carbohydrate fractions, including nonstarch polysaccharides (see Table 3.3.1), are in keeping with these requirements.

The term "dietary fiber" was coined as a description of the plant cell wall material that was recognized as the common characteristic of the unrefined plant foods that composed a naturally "high-fiber" diet.[4-8] The main component (approximately 90%) of the cell walls of the plant foods in the human diet is carbohydrate, specifically, polysaccharides that do not have α-glucosidic linkages, collectively termed nonstarch polysaccharides (NSPs).[9,10] NSP values provide a reliable marker of a naturally high-fiber diet, which justifies their use for food labeling for dietary fiber, and this has repeatedly been recommended by the U.K. Committee on Medical Aspects of Food and Nutrition Policy (COMA).[11,12]

For more than 15 years, the widely used McCance and Widdowson Food Tables[13] have contained values for dietary fiber measured as NSP.[14,15] The food industry is at liberty to use appropriate values from these tables without carrying out or commissioning its own analysis. The NSP content of cooked foods can be calculated from analytical values for the raw ingredients, since the NSP content of a food is not dependent on processing, such as heating, cooling, and drying.

The classification and measurement scheme for dietary carbohydrates shown in Table 3.3.1 has evolved in a virtually unbroken chronological sequence from the work of McCance and Widdowson,[16] then Southgate,[17] and, more recently, Englyst,[18] and their colleagues. The classification scheme is complete, but not immutable, and analytical procedures are available for all of the major categories of dietary carbohydrates so far identified. A cornerstone of this classification

Table 3.3.1   Classification of Dietary Carbohydrates

	Main Components	Comments
Free sugars		(Soluble in 80% ethanol; ≤ 2 sugar units)
Mono- and disaccharides	Glucose, fructose, sucrose, maltose, lactose	Glucose, maltose, and sucrose rapidly digested. Fructose and lactose may, in part, escape digestion and absorption in the small intestine. Physiological response depends on identity
Sugar alcohols		(Soluble in 80% ethanol; ≤ 2 sugar units)
Mono- and disaccharides	Sorbitol, inositol, mannitol, galactitol, maltitol	Poorly absorbed in the small intestine. May reach the large intestine.
Short-chain carbohydrates		(Soluble in 80% ethanol; > 2 sugar units)
Maltodextrins	α-Glucans	Partly hydrolyzed starch. Normally included in the measurement of starch
Resistant short-chain carbohydrates (non-digestible oligosaccharides)	Fructo-oligosaccharides, galacto-oligosaccharides, pyrodextrins, polydextrose	Escape digestion in the small intestine and are fermented to different extents. Some may stimulate growth of bifidobacteria. Physiological effect largely unknown
Polysaccharides		(Insoluble in 80% ethanol)
Starch	α-Glucans	The most abundant dietary carbohydrates.
Rapidly digestible starch (RDS)	Rapidly released glucose	Rapidly digested in the small intestine.
Slowly digestible starch (SDS)	Slowly released glucose	Slowly digested in the small intestine.
Resistant starch (RS)	RS_1 (physically inaccessible), RS_2 (resistant granules), RS_3 (retrograded amylose)	The three types of RS escape digestion in the small intestine and are fermented to different extents. Physiological effect largely unknown
Nonstarch (NSPs)	Many different types of polysaccharides	Escape digestion in the small intestine and are fermented to different extents.
Plant cell-wall NSPs	Main constituents: arabinose xylose, mannose, galactose glucose, uronic acids	Encapsulate and slow absorption of nutrients. Good marker for naturally high-fiber diets for which health benefits have been shown
Other NSPs	Many types of constituents	Food additives. Minor components of the human diet. The amounts added to foods are known and regulated

scheme is the measurement of chemically identified components, which, on the basis of current knowledge of the relation between dietary carbohydrates and health, may be grouped into categories of specific nutritional importance. The information on the composition, fate, and physiological properties of the various types of dietary carbohydrates shown in Table 3.3.1 is useful when considering the definition and measurement of dietary fiber.

The link between the ingestion of unprocessed foods and good health is chronicled as far back as Hippocrates (4th century B.C.), who recommended the eating of wholemeal bread for its "salutary effects upon the bowels." The term dietary fiber was used first by Hipsley.[8] The dietary fiber hypothesis, which was put forward by Cleave, Burkitt and Trowell,[5] was related to the health benefits consequent upon the ingestion of a diet rich in unrefined plant foods and was specifically related to the plant cell wall. The plant cell wall encapsulates and thus controls the release of nutrients, including free sugars and starch, from the plant tissue and thereby influences the glycemic response. This ability to influence digestion and absorption, and thus the physiological effects of other nutrients, was seen at an early stage to be an important property of dietary fiber. The other main properties associated with dietary fiber were its abilities to increase fecal bulk and reduce transit time.

There is convincing evidence and a general consensus that (1) naturally high-fiber diets, i.e., those rich in fruit, vegetables, and whole grains, are beneficial to health, and (2) at least some of the benefits to health may reflect the fact that such diets tend to be rich in vitamins, minerals, and antioxidants, and are often low in fat.

A naturally high-fiber diet has been suggested to be protective against (1) coronary heart diseases (CHD), (2) diabetes, and (3) colon cancer. The evidence for the first two, CHD and diabetes, is convincing. However, this is not the case for colon cancer, as a considerable number of studies have failed to show a protective effect of dietary fiber, and some studies even suggest that fiber supplementation and RS may promote colon cancer. On the basis of its extensive review of the scientific evidence, the FDA has stated the following (10 October 2000):

FDA has concluded from this review that the totality of the publicly available scientific evidence not only demonstrates lack of significant scientific agreement as to the validity of a relationship between dietary fiber and colorectal cancer, but also provides strong evidence that such a relationship does not exist.

The weight of the evidence for a health claim about dietary fiber and colorectal cancer is outweighed by the evidence against such a claim. Therefore, FDA has determined that health claims relating dietary fiber and reduced risk of colorectal cancer are inherently misleading.

The use of such health claims is therefore prohibited by the Federal Food, Drug, and Cosmetic Act. A dietary supplement that bears a claim about dietary fiber and reduced risk of colorectal cancer will be subject to regulatory action as a misbranded food under 21 U.S.C. § 343.

It is clear that (1) the material measured as dietary fiber must be a reliable marker for the type of naturally high-fiber diet for which benefit to health has been shown, and that (2) lack of digestion in the small intestine is not a characteristic on which to base the definition of dietary fiber. In unrefined and minimally processed foods, the plant cell walls encapsulate and moderate the release of nutrients, including sugar and starch. This property is related to the integrity of the cell wall structure, which is not a characteristic of RS, non-digestible digosaccharides (NDO), or any fiber supplement. The main component (approximately 90%) of the cell walls of the plant foods in the human diet is carbohydrate, specifically, polysaccharides that do not have α-glucosidic linkages, collectively termed *nonstarch polysaccharides* (NSPs). NSPs therefore, provide a reliable marker of a naturally high-fiber diet for which benefit to health is shown, and this justifies the use of NSP values for food labeling for dietary fiber. The measurement of NSP is described here.

INTERNATIONAL COLLABORATIVE TRIALS

MAFF-organized trials. The Englyst procedure has been the subject of a series of international collaborative trials organized by the U.K. Ministry of Agriculture, Fisheries & Food. In the MAFF IV study,[19] 37 laboratories from 11 countries took part to compare the accuracy and precision of the Englyst gas-liquid chromatographic (GLC) and colorimetric procedures. This series of trials culminated in the publication of the GLC and the colorimetry techniques as MAFF-approved methods.[20,21]

Certification of Reference Materials

EC-organized trials. As the result of a large international trial of methodology, following rigorous study of stability of the test materials, five BCR-certificated reference materials (CRMs) are available for the Englyst GLC and colorimetry NSP procedures:[22] (1) dried haricot bean powder, CRM 514; (2) dried carrot powder, CRM 515; (3) dried apple powder, CRM 516; (4) full fat soya flour, CRM 517; and (5) dried powdered bran breakfast cereal, CRM 518. These CRMs can be used to check the performance of the analytical method and as quality control of analytical measurements for nutritional labeling.

Methods and Principles of Measurement

The Englyst procedure measures dietary fiber as NSP, using enzymatic chemical methods, and has evolved from the principles laid down by McCance and Southgate. Starch is completely removed enzymatically, and NSPs are measured as the sum of the constituent sugars released by acid hydrolysis. The sugars may be measured by gas–liquid chromatography (GLC) or by high-pressure liquid chromatography (HPLC) to obtain values for individual monosaccharides, or a single value for total sugars may be obtained by colorimetry. Values may be obtained for total, soluble, and insoluble NSP, and a small modification allows cellulose to be measured separately.

The Englyst procedure allows measurement of total, soluble, and insoluble NSP in plant food products within an 8-hour working day using the colorimetric endpoint, or within 1.5 working days with the chromatography procedures. Preparation of the hydrolyzate for analysis is virtually a single-tube procedure, and no special skill or equipment is needed for the colorimetric version.

The procedure as described here provides the following options: (1) GLC procedure that measures NSP as the sum of neutral sugars obtained by GLC and uronic acids measured separately; (2) HPLC procedure: measures NSP as the sum of neutral sugars and uronic acids; (3) colorimetric procedure that measures NSP as reducing sugars; and (4) colorimetric procedure with separate measurement of uronic acids.

PRINCIPLE

1. Dry/defat sample if necessary
2. Disperse (DMSO) and hydrolyze starch enzymatically
3. Precipitate NSP in acidified aqueous ethanol
4. Disperse and hydrolyze NSP with sulfuric acid
5. Measure released constituent sugars by:

Option 1	GLC*
Option 2	HPLC*
Option 3	Colorimetry**

*   Values for individual constituent sugars of insoluble and total NSP. Soluble NSP calculated as the difference between insoluble and total NSP.

** Single values for insoluble and total NSP. Soluble NSP calculated as the difference between insoluble and total NSP.

THE PROCEDURE

Apparatus and Reagents

High-purity reagents and distilled, deionized water, or water of equivalent purity, should be used throughout the method.

Reagents Common to the GLC, Colorimetric, and/or HPLC Procedures

All sugars used for standards should be dried to constant mass under reduced pressure with phosphorus pentoxide before use.

Acidified ethanol, absolute and 85% (v/v). Add 1 mL of 5 *M* hydrochloric acid per liter of ethanol.

Dimethylphenol solution. Dissolve 0.1 g of 3,5-dimethylphenol in 100 mL of glacial acetic acid.

Dimethylsulfoxide (DMSO).

Enzyme solution I. Take 2.5 mL of heat-stable amylase (EC 3.2.1.1: Termamyl), make to 200 mL with pre-equilibrated sodium acetate buffer, mix, and keep it in a 50°C waterbath. Prepare the solution immediately before use.

Enzyme solution II. Take 1.2 g of pancreatin into a 50-mL tube, add 12 mL of water, vortex-mix initially, and then mix for 10 min with a magnetic stirrer. Vortex-mix again, then centrifuge for 10 min. Take 10 mL of the (cloudy) supernatant, add 2.5 mL of pullulanase (EC 3.2.1.41: Promozyme), and vortex-mix. Prepare the solution immediately before use and keep it at room temperature.

Glass balls, 2.5 to 3.5 mm diameter.

Sand, acid-washed, 50–100 mesh.

Sodium acetate buffer, 0.1 *M*, pH 5.2. Dissolve 13.6 g of sodium acetate trihydrate and make to 1 L with water. Adjust to pH 5.2 with 0.1 *M* acetic acid. To stabilize and activate enzymes, add 4 mL of 1 *M* calcium chloride to 1 L of buffer.

Sodium chloride–boric acid solution. Dissolve 2 g of sodium chloride and 3 g of boric acid in 100 mL of water.

Sodium phosphate buffer, 0.2 *M*, pH 7. Adjust 0.2 *M* Na_2HPO_4 to pH 7 with 0.2 *M* NaH_2PO_4.

Sulfuric acid, 12 *M*.

Sulfuric acid, 2 *M*. Add 5 mL of 12 *M* sulfuric acid to 25 mL of water. Allow to cool to room temperature before use.

Sulfuric acid, 2.4 *M*. Add 5 mL of 12 *M* sulfuric acid to 20 mL of water and mix.

Reagents Used Only in the GLC Procedure

Acetic anhydride.

Ammonium–sodium tetrahydroborate solution. A solution of 6 *M* ammonium hydroxide, containing 200 mg/mL of sodium tetrahydroborate [$NaBH_4$]. Prepare immediately before use.

Benzoic acid, saturated. Prepare a saturated solution of benzoic acid at room temperature. Add 0.5 g of benzoic acid per 100 mL of water; some benzoic acid should remain undissolved after overnight stirring. The saturated solution is stable at room temperature for long periods.

Bromophenol blue solution, 0.4 g/L.

GLC internal standard solution, 1 mg/mL. Weigh to the nearest 1 mg: 500 mg of allose. Dissolve in water, add 250 mL of saturated benzoic acid, and make to 500 mL with water to give a 1 mg/mL solution. The solution is stable at room temperature for several months.

Glacial acetic acid.

GLC stock sugar mixture. Weigh to the nearest 1 mg: 0.52 g of rhamnose, 0.48 g of fucose, 4.75 g of arabinose, 4.45 g of xylose, 2.3 g of mannose, 2.82 g of galactose, 9.4 g of glucose, and 2.79 g of galacturonic acid (or 3.05 g of galacturonic acid monohydrate). Dissolve together in water, add 500 mL of saturated benzoic acid, and make to 1 L with water. The solution is stable at room temperature for several months.

1-Methylimidazole.

Reagents Used Only in the HPLC Procedure

HPLC neutral sugars internal standard solution. Weigh to the nearest 1 mg: 10,000 mg of deoxy-galactose. Add 10 mg of thiomersal ($C_2H_5 \cdot Hg \cdot S \cdot C_6H_4 \cdot COONa$) as preservative and make to 1 L with water.

HPLC neutral sugars stock sugar mixture. Weigh to the nearest 1 mg: 0.52 g of rhamnose, 0.48 g of fucose, 4.75 g of arabinose, 4.45 g of xylose, 2.3 g of mannose, 2.82 g of galactose, and 9.4 g of glucose. Dissolve together in water, add 10 mg of thimerosal as preservative, and make to 1 L with water. Store at 4°C.

HPLC uronic acids internal standard solution. Weigh to the nearest 1 mg: 0.0454 g of mannuronic acid lactone. Dissolve in water, add 1 mg of thimerosal as preservative, and make to 100 mL with water. Store at 4°C.

HPLC uronic acids stock sugar mixture. Weigh to the nearest 1 mg: 0.0930 g of galacturonic acid (or 0.102 g of galacturonic acid monohydrate) and 0.0233 g of glucuronic acid. Dissolve together in 2 M sulfuric acid, and make to 100 mL with 2 M sulfuric acid. Store at 4°C.

Pectinase solution (EC 3.2.1.15: Novo Nordisk). Add 25 volumes of water to 1 volume of pectinase.

Reagents Used Only in the Colorimetric Procedure

Color reagent. Dissolve 10 g of 3,5-dinitrosalicylic acid and 300 g of sodium/potassium tartrate in approx. 300 mL of water plus 400 mL of 1 M NaOH. Dissolve by stirring (overnight) and make to a final volume of 1 L with water. Sparge for 10 min with helium or nitrogen, or degas using an ultrasonic bath. Store in well-capped opaque bottles, and keep for 2 days before use. The reagent is stable at room temperature for at least 6 months.

Dimethylglutaric acid solution, 0.5 M. Add 98.5 g of 5 M NaOH to 8.0 g (weighed to the nearest 1 mg) of dimethylglutaric acid (DMG) and make to 100 mL with water at room temperature. [Note: since the purity of DMG varies between lot numbers, it is essential that the pH is checked. A portion of the DMG solution should be diluted 1:1 (v/v) with 2 M sulfuric acid; the pH should be 3.75 (±0.15) at room temperature. If the pH is greater than 3.9, add 1 mL of water to the stock solution and check the pH again. If the pH is less than 3.9, add 1 mL of 5 M NaOH to the stock solution and check the pH again. Repeat as necessary.]

Color stock sugar mixture. Make the color stock sugar solution by weighing to the nearest 1 mg: 10.185 g of arabinose, 5.145 g of glucose, and 2.16 g of galacturonic acid (or 2.36 g of galacturonic acid monohydrate). Dissolve together in water, add 500 mL of saturated benzoic acid, and make to 1 L with water. The solution is stable at room temperature for several months.

Pectinase solution (EC 3.2.1.15: Novo Nordisk). Add 9 volumes of water to 1 volume of pectinase.

Sample Preparation

All samples must be finely divided (to pass a 0.5-mm mesh) so that representative subsamples may be taken. Foods with a low water content (<10 g per 100 g of sample) may be milled, and foods with a higher water content may be homogenized wet or milled after freeze-drying. Analysis of three subsamples, A, B, and C, allows separate values to be obtained directly for total NSP, insoluble NSP, and cellulose, respectively. Soluble NSP is determined as the difference between total and insoluble NSP. Portions A and B are treated identically throughout the procedure, except in steps 3 and 4. The third portion, C, is needed only if a separate value for cellulose is required; carry it through steps 1, 2, and 3 of the procedure; then go to step 5.2.

Step 1.1 Weigh, to the nearest 1 mg, between 50 and 1000 mg, depending on the water and NSP content of the sample (to give not more than 300 mg of dry matter; e.g., 300 mg is adequate for most dried foods but smaller amounts should be used for bran and purified fiber preparations), into 50–60 mL screw-top glass tubes. Add 300 (±20) mg of acid-washed sand and approximately 15 glass balls to each. If the sample is dry (85–100 g of dry matter per 100 g of sample) and contains less than 10 g of fat per 100 g of sample, proceed to step 2.1; otherwise, go to step 1.2. All analyses should be done in duplicate.

Step 1.2 Add 40 mL of acetone, cap the tubes, and mix several times over 30 min. Centrifuge at 1000g for 10 min to obtain a clear supernatant and remove as much of the supernatant liquid as possible without disturbing the residue. Vortex-mix vigorously to ensure that the residue is dispersed thinly around the bottom 5 cm of the tube. Place the rack of tubes in a pan of water at 75°C in a fume-cupboard. Remove the tubes singly and vortex-mix vigorously at frequent intervals until the tubes and residues are dry.

Isolation and Hydrolysis of NSP

Dispersion and Enzymatic Hydrolysis

Pre-equilibrate sufficient acetate buffer at 50°C (8 mL required per sample).

Step 2.1 Add 2 mL of dimethylsulfoxide (DMSO) to the dry sample, cap the tube, and immediately mix the contents using a vortex-mixer, treating each tube in turn. It is essential that all the sample is wetted and no material is encapsulated or adhering to the tube wall before proceeding. When DMSO has been added to all the tubes, vortex-mix three or four times for 5 min. Vortex-mix and immediately place 2 tubes into a boiling waterbath. Remove after 20 s, vortex-mix, and immediately replace the tubes in the bath. Repeat this for subsequent pairs of tubes until all the tubes are in the bath; leave them for 30 min from that time. During this period, prepare enzyme solutions I and II (see Step 4.1; the volumes given are suitable for 24 samples).

Step 2.2 Remove one tube at a time, vortex-mix, uncap, and immediately add 8 mL of enzyme solution I (kept at 50°C), cap the tube, vortex-mix thoroughly — ensuring that no material adheres to the tube wall — and replace it in the boiling waterbath. Leave the tubes there for 10 min, timed from the last addition of enzyme. Transfer the rack of tubes to the 50°C waterbath. After 3 min, add 0.5 mL of enzyme solution II to each tube and mix the contents thoroughly to aid distribution of the enzyme throughout the sample. Replace the tubes in the 50°C waterbath and leave them there for 30 min. Mix the contents of each tube continuously or after 10 min, 20 min, and 30 min. Transfer the rack of tubes to the boiling waterbath and leave them there for 10 min.

Precipitation and Washing of the Residue for Measurement of Total NSP

Only sample portion A is given this treatment.

Step 3.1 Cool the samples by placing in ice water. Add 0.15 mL of 5 M hydrochloric acid and vortex-mix thoroughly 2 or 3 times for 5 min with samples being replaced in the ice water. Add 40 mL of acidified absolute ethanol and mix well by repeated inversion, then leave in ice water for 30 min. Centrifuge at 1500 g for 10 min to obtain a clear supernatant liquid. Remove as much of the supernatant liquid as possible, without disturbing the residue, and discard it.

Step 3.2 Add approximately 10 mL of acidified 85% ethanol to the residue and vortex-mix. Make to 50 mL with acidified 85% ethanol, mix thoroughly by repeated inversion. Centrifuge and remove the supernatant liquid as above. Repeat this stage using 50 mL of absolute ethanol.

Step 3.3 Add 30 mL of acetone to the residue and vortex-mix thoroughly to form a suspension. Centrifuge and remove the supernatant liquid as described in step 3.1.

Step 3.4 Place the rack of tubes in a pan of water at 75°C in a fume-cupboard or a TurboVap (Zymark Ltd.) at 65°C. Remove the tubes singly and vortex-mix vigorously at frequent intervals, to ensure that the residue in each tube is finely divided, until each tube and residue appears dry. Place the rack of tubes in a fan oven at 80°C for 10 min to remove any last traces of acetone. It is essential that the residues and tubes are completely free of acetone.

Extraction and Washing of the Residue for Measurement of Insoluble NSP

Only sample portion B is given this treatment.

Step 4.1 After the treatment with enzymes in step 2, add 40 mL of sodium phosphate buffer. Place the capped tubes in a boiling waterbath for 30 min. Mix continuously or a minimum of three times during this period. Remove the tubes and equilibrate to room temperature in water. Centrifuge and remove the supernatant liquid as described in step 3.1.

Step 4.2 Add approximately 10 mL of water and vortex-mix. Make to approximately 50 mL with water and mix well by repeated inversion. Centrifuge and remove the supernatant liquid as described in step 3.1. Repeat this stage using 50 mL of absolute ethanol. Proceed as described for steps 3.3 and 3.4.

Acid Hydrolysis of the Residue from Enzymatic Digestion

Step 5.1 Add 5 mL of 12 M sulfuric acid to one tube and immediately vortex-mix vigorously; ensure that all the material is wetted. Repeat this for each tube in turn. Once the acid has been added to all the tubes, vortex-mix again and place all the tubes into a waterbath at 35°C. Leave the tubes at 35°C for 30 min with vigorous vortex-mixing after 5, 10, and 20 min to disperse the cellulose. Add 25 mL of water rapidly and vortex-mix. Place into a boiling waterbath and leave for 1 hour, timed from when boiling recommences; mix after 10 min. Cool the tubes in tap water.

Step 5.2 A modification allowing the separate measurement of cellulose and non-cellulosic polysaccharides (NCPs). To portion C, after steps 1 through 3, add 30 mL of 2 M sulfuric acid, and mix. Place in a boiling waterbath and leave for 1 hour, timed from when boiling recommences, stirring continuously or after 10 min. The value for cellulose is obtained as the difference between glucose (measured by GLC or by glucose oxidase) for sample portions A and C. NCP is calculated as the difference between total NSP and cellulose.

Breaks in the Procedure

The procedure may be halted at the following stages. (1) After precipitation, washing, and drying the starch-free residue in steps 3 and 4. The residue may be stored for long periods. (2) After the hydrolysis with 2 M sulfuric acid in step 5. The hydrolysate may be kept at 4°C for 48 hours.

Determination of Constituent Sugars by GLC

This assay includes the measurement of neutral sugars by GLC and the separate measurement of uronic acids by colorimetry.

Measurement of Neutral NSP Constituents by GLC

Preparation of the standard sugar mixture. Mix 1.0 mL of the GLC stock sugar solution and 5 mL of 2.4 M sulfuric acid. Treat 2 × 1.0 mL of this standard sugar mixture for calibration in parallel with the hydrolysates from step 5 of the procedure.

Prepare the alditol acetate derivatives for chromatography as follows. Add 0.50 mL of GLC internal standard (1 mg/mL allose) to 1.0 mL of the cooled hydrolysates from step 5 and to 2 × 1 mL of the standard sugar mixture; vortex-mix. Place the tubes in ice water, add 0.4 mL of 12 M ammonium solution, and vortex-mix. Test that the solution is alkaline (add a little more ammonium solution if necessary, but replace the ammonium solution if more than 0.1 mL extra is required), then add approximately 5 µL of the antifoam agent octan-2-ol and 0.1 mL of the ammonium–sodium borohydride solution; vortex-mix. Leave the tubes in a heating block or in a waterbath at 40°C for 30 min, then remove and add 0.2 mL of glacial acetic acid, and mix again. Remove 0.5 mL to a 30 mL glass tube and add 0.5 mL of 1-methylimidazole and 5 mL of acetic anhydride. Vortex-mix, then leave the tubes for 10 min for the reaction to proceed (the reaction is exothermic and the tubes will become hot). Add 0.9 mL of absolute ethanol, vortex-mix, and leave for 5 min. Add 10 mL of water, vortex-mix, and leave for 5 min. Add 0.5 mL of bromophenol blue solution. Place the tubes in ice water and add 5 mL of 7.5 M potassium hydroxide; a few minutes later add a further 5 mL of 7.5 M potassium hydroxide, cap the tubes, and mix by inversion. Leave until the separation into two phases is complete (10 to 15 min) or centrifuge for a few minutes. Draw part of the upper phase into the tip of an automatic pipette; if any of the blue lower phase is included, allow it to separate, then run it out of the tip before transferring a portion of the upper phase alone to a small (auto-injector) vial. Inject 0.5 to 1 μL of the alditol acetate derivatives.

GLC Conditions

Injector temperature, 275°C; column temperature, 220°C; detector temperature, 275°C; carrier gas, helium; flow rate, 8 mL/min. Under these conditions, a GLC chromatograph fitted with flame ionization detector, auto-injector, and computing integrator, using a Supelco SP-2330 wide-bore capillary column (30 m × 0.75 mm) or a Supelco SP-2380 wide-bore capillary column (30 m × 0.53 mm), will allow accurate determination of the individual sugars in the GLC standard sugar mixture within 8 min. Carry out conventional GLC measurement of the neutral sugars. At the beginning of each batch of analyses, equilibrate with the isothermal elution conditions for at least 1 hour. Do several calibration runs to check that the response factors are reproducible.

Table 3.3.2   Calibration Ratios for GLC Standard Sugar and GLC Internal Standard Combination

Sugar	Actual (mg/mL)	Recovery (%)	Apparent (mg/mL)	Calibration Ratio
Rhamnose	520	52	1000	1
Fucose	480	96	500	0.5
Arabinose	4750	95	5000	5
Xylose	4450	89	5000	5
Mannose	2300	92	2500	2.5
Galactose	2820	94	3000	
Glucose	9400	94	10,000	10
Allose (Int. std.)				3

In Table 3.3.2, the calibration ratios are shown for the combination of the GLC standard sugar mixture and GLC internal standard (allose). The Actual column shows the amount of each sugar in the mixture, and the Apparent column shows the values to be used for calibration, taking into account the recovery of NSP constituents. The calibration ratio column gives the ratio of sugars to the internal standard after the addition of allose to the standard sugar mixture, as described in the text. (The experimental evidence for the recovery values has been published and is discussed in detail below.)

Calculation of Neutral Sugars

The amount of each individual sugar (expressed as grams of polysaccharide per 100 g of sample) is calculated as

$$\text{Sugar} = \frac{A(t) \times W(i) \times 100 \times R(f) \times 0.89}{A(i) \times W(t)} \qquad (3.3.1)$$

where $A(t)$ and $A(i)$ are the peak areas of the sample and the internal standard, respectively; $W(i)$ is the weight (in mg; here 15: total hydrolysate 30 ml × 0.5 mg allose) of the internal standard; $W(t)$ is the weight (mg) of the sample; $R(f)$ is the response factor for individual sugars obtained from the calibration run with the sugar mixture and internal standard (allose) treated in parallel with the samples; and 0.89 is the factor for converting experimentally determined values for monosaccharides to polysaccharides.

Measurement of Uronic Acids by Colorimetry

Make the standard solutions as follows. The GLC standard sugar mixture in 2 M sulfuric acid contains, for the purpose of calibration, 500 µg/mL of galacturonic acid. To prepare the uronic acid standard solutions, take 0.5 mL, 2.0 mL, and 3.0 mL of this sugar mixture into separate tubes, and make to 10 mL with 2 M sulfuric acid to give standards of 25, 100, and 150 µg/mL of galacturonic acid.

Place into separate tubes (40–50 mL capacity) 0.3 mL of blank solution (2 M sulfuric acid), 0.3 mL of each of the standard solutions, and 0.3 mL of the sample hydrolysates, diluted if necessary (with 2 M sulfuric acid) to contain no more than 150 µg/mL of uronic acids (e.g., no dilution for flour, 1:2 for bran, 1:5 for most fruits and vegetables). Add 0.3 mL of sodium chloride–boric acid solution and mix. Add 5 mL of concentrated sulfuric acid and vortex-mix immediately. Place the tubes into a heating block at 70°C for 40 min. Remove the tubes and cool to room temperature in water (the tubes may be kept in the water for up to 1 hour). Add 0.2 mL of dimethylphenol solution and vortex-mix immediately. After 15 min measure the absorbance at 400 nm and at 450 nm in the spectrophotometer against the blank solution. The timing for measurement of the absorbance of standards and samples should be identical. In practice, this is achieved by adding the color reagent at 1-min intervals. Subtract the absorbance reading at 400 nm from that at 450 nm, to correct for interference from hexoses. A straight line should be obtained if the differences in absorbance for the standards are plotted against concentration. Only the 100 µg/mL standard is required for routine analysis, and it may be kept at 5°C for several weeks.

Calculation of Uronic Acids

The amount of uronic acids (expressed as grams of polysaccharide per 100 g of sample) is calculated as

$$\text{Uronic acids} \ = \ \frac{A(t) \times V(t) \times D \times C \times 100 \times 0.91}{A(s) \times W(t)} \tag{3.3.2}$$

where $A(t)$ is the difference in absorbance of the sample solution; $V(t)$ is the total volume of sample solution (mL, here 30); D is the dilution of the sample solution; C is the concentration of the standard (here 0.1 mg/mL); $A(s)$ is the difference in absorbance of the 100 µg/mL standard; $W(t)$ is the weight (mg) of the sample; and 0.91 is the factor for converting experimentally determined values for monosaccharides to polysaccharides.

Calculation of NSP

The amount of total, soluble, and insoluble NSP (in grams per 100 g of sample) is calculated as

Total NSP   = Neutral sugars calculated for portion A
                     + Uronic acids calculated for portion A
Insoluble NSP = Neutral sugars calculated for portion B
                     + Uronic acids calculated for portion B
Soluble NSP   = Total NSP – Insoluble NSP

It is recommended that a sample be taken for determination of the dry matter as the loss in weight after overnight incubation at 104°C. Results may then be expressed as grams of polysaccharides per 100 g of dry matter.

Breaks in the GLC Procedure

The procedure may be halted at either of the following stages: (1) after acidification of the reduced samples (see Determination of Constituent Sugars by GLC section); the samples may be stored at room temperature for 2 to 3 days; or (2) the acid hydrolysate from Step 5 may be kept at 5°C for several weeks before the measurement of uronic acids.

Determination of Constituent Sugars by HPLC

This assay includes dilution of one subsample of the hydrolysate and direct measurement of the neutral sugars, and the separate measurement of uronic acids in a second subsample of the hydrolysate subjected to treatment with pectinase.

Measurement of Neutral Sugars by HPLC

Preparation of the HPLC standard sugar mixture. Mix 1.0 mL of the HPLC stock sugar mixture and 5 mL of 2.4 M sulfuric acid. Treat 2×0.15 mL of this standard sugar mixture for calibration of HPLC in parallel with the hydrolysates from step 5 of the procedure.

To 0.15 mL of hydrolysate or the HPLC standard sugar mixture, add 5 mL of the neutral sugars internal standard solution (deoxygalactose) and mix well. Inject 25 μL for analysis.

HPLC Conditions

A Dionex model PAD 2 detector may be used with the following pulse potentials and durations: $E_1 = 0.05$ V ($t_1 = 300$ ms); $E_2 = 0.60$ V ($t_2 = 120$ ms); $E_3 = -0.60$ V ($t_3 = 60$ ms), and with a response time of 1 s and the detector output set at 1000 nA.

A Dionex AG-5 guard column, an inert high-pressure valve, and a CarboPac PA-1 column are placed in series. The AG-5 column and inert high-pressure valve are used to retain and bypass sulfate ions around the analytical column. Elute with the following: 23% (v/v) solution 1 (0.020 M NaOH) from 0 to 3.5 min; a gradient from 23% to 1% (v/v) solution 1 from 3.5 to 4.5 min; and 1% (v/v) solution 1 from 4.5 to 30 min at a flow rate of 1 mL/min. Re-equilibrate with the starting conditions for at least 6 min between runs. Add 0.30 M NaOH at a flow rate of 0.5 mL/min to the column effluent before the PAD cell to minimize baseline drift and increase the analytical signal. Saturate the eluent with helium (Dionex Eluent De-gas module) to minimize CO_2 absorption. Under the conditions described here, sulfate ions are retained for 80 s on the AG-5 guard column, and column switching (via the inert high-pressure valve) is applied after 60 s to prevent sulfate ions from reaching the analytical column. Sulfate ions are purged from the guard column within 19 min, well within the total run time. To regenerate the PA-1 column at the end of the chromatographic run, wash with 0.10 M NaOH–0.60 M sodium acetate for 1 hour at a flow rate of 1 mL/min. Then wash with 1 M NaOH (1 mL/min) for 1 hour but, to avoid contamination of the internal reference solution, do not allow this solution to pass through the detector.

Table 3.3.3   Calibration Ratios for HPLC Standard Sugar and HPLC Internal Standard Combination

Sugar	Actual (mg/mL)	Recovery (%)	Apparent (mg/mL)	Calibration Ratio
Rhamnose	520	52	1000	1
Fucose	480	96	500	0.5
Arabinose	4750	95	5000	5
Xylose	4450	89	5000	5
Mannose	2300	92	2500	2.5
Galactose	2820	94	3000	3
Glucose	9400	94	10,000	10
Deoxygalactose (Int. std.)				2

Table 3.3.3 shows the calibration ratios for the combination of the standard sugar mixture and deoxygalactose and the HPLC internal standard; the Actual column shows the amount of each sugar in the mixture, and the Apparent column shows the values to be used for calibration, taking into account the recovery of NSP constituents.

The amount of each individual sugar (in grams per 100 g of sample) is calculated as

$$\text{Sugar} = \frac{A(t) \times W(i) \times 100 \times R(f) \times 0.89}{A(i) \times W(t)} \tag{3.3.3}$$

where $A(t)$ and $A(i)$ are the peak areas of the sample and the HPLC internal standard, respectively; $W(i)$ is the weight of the internal standard if added to the whole sample (in mg, here 25); $W(t)$ is the weight of the sample (mg); $R(f)$ is the response factor for individual sugars obtained from a calibration run with the sugar mixture treated in parallel with the samples; and 0.89 is the factor for converting experimentally determined values for monosaccharides to polysaccharides. It is recommended that a sample be taken for the analysis of the dry matter as the material remaining after overnight incubation at 104°C. Results may then be expressed as grams of polysaccharides per 100 g of dry matter.

Measurement of Uronic Acids by HPLC

To 0.5 mL of hydrolysate or calibration mixture, add 0.5 mL of the HPLC uronic acid internal standard solution (mannuronic acid lactone), 0.5 mL of dimethylglutaric acid solution (8 g/100 mL), and 2.1 mL of 1 M NaOH. After vortex-mixing, the pH must be between pH 3.5 and 4.0. (If the pH is not correct, prepare fresh DMG solution and repeat). Add 0.1 mL of pectinase solution, vortex-mix, and place the tubes into a waterbath at 50°C for 20 min. Cool the tubes, remove 0.5 mL, and add 0.1 mL of phenol red indicator solution (1 mg/mL); add sufficient (approximately 2 mL) freshly prepared 0.017 M NaOH until the pH is between 7 and 8. Inject 25 μL onto the chromatography column. Baseline separation of galacturonic acid (GalA), glucuronic acid (GlcA), and mannuronic acid is achieved isocratically within 13 min using 25% solution 2 (0.10 M NaOH, 0.6 M sodium acetate) and 75% water at a flow rate of 1.0 mL/min. Use the following ratios for the calibration mixture for the calculation of the response factors: 0.5 for GalA, 0.125 for GlcA, and 0.25 for mannuronic acid to take into account losses during hydrolysis. The values for the calculation of response factors take into account 7% loss of both GalA and GlcA and the hydrolysis of mannuronic acid lactone to mannuronic acid, as described above.

The amount of uronic acids (in grams per 100 g of sample) is calculated as

$$\text{Uronic acids} = \frac{A(t) \times W(i) \times 100 \times R(f) \times 0.91}{A(i) \times W(t)} \tag{3.3.4}$$

where $A(t)$ and $A(i)$ are the peak areas of the test and the internal standard, respectively; $W(i)$ and $W(t)$ are the weight of the internal standard (in mg; here 15) and the mass of the test sample (mg), respectively; $R(f)$ is the response factor for individual uronic acids obtained from the calibration mixture; and 0.91 is the factor for converting the experimentally determined values for monosaccharides to polysaccharides.

Determination of Constituent Sugars by Colorimetry

Preparation of the Standard Sugar Mixture

Take 0.5 mL of the colorimetry stock sugar mixture into a glass tube, add 2.5 mL of 2.4 M sulfuric acid, and mix to give 3 mL of 3 mg/mL color sugars standard solution in 2 M sulfuric acid. The colorimetric reaction is linear up to 3 mg/mL sugar. The absorbance of the test samples should not exceed that of the standard.

Measurement of Total Reducing Sugars

Place into separate glass tubes: 0.5 mL of the standard sugar solution and 0.5 mL of the hydrolysate from step 5; and place into each of two tubes (blanks 1 and 2): 0.5 mL of 2 M sulfuric acid. Add 0.5 mL of DMG solution and vortex-mix. Check the pH of 1 drop of blank 1; it should be between 3.5 and 4. If it is different from this, check the preparation of the 2 M and the 12 M sulfuric acid, and the DMG solution. If the pH is correct, add 0.1 mL of diluted pectinase solution, vortex-mix, and place all the tubes into a waterbath at 50°C for 20 min. Cool the tubes to room temperature, add 0.1 mL of 3 M sodium hydroxide, vortex-mix, and leave for 5 min. Add 1 mL of the dinitrosalicylate reagent to each tube and vortex-mix. Place all the tubes together into a briskly boiling waterbath for 5 min. Remove the rack of tubes and cool to room temperature in water. Add 10 mL of water (at room temperature) and mix well by inversion (do not use a vortex-mixer at this stage). Measure the absorbance at 530 nm against blank 2.

Note: Sample blanks may be prepared by diluting the hydrolysates as described above, replacing the color reagent with water, and reading the absorbance against water. Alternatively, and more conveniently, the absorbance of the undiluted hydrolysate can be measured against water and the value divided by 24.4 (the dilution of the hydrolysate after addition of the color reagent and water). The absorbance of the test sample is then calculated by subtracting this value. When the hydrolysate is colorless and the NSP content is more than 5%, the sample blank is not required.

Calculation of NSP

The amount of total NSP (portion A) and of insoluble NSP (portion B), in grams of polysaccharide per 100 g of sample, is calculated as

$$\text{NSP} = \frac{A(t) \times V(t) \times D \times F \times C \times 100 \times 0.89}{A(s) \times W(t)} \tag{3.3.5}$$

where $A(t)$ is the absorbance of the sample solution (minus the absorbance of the hydrolysate blank if measured); $V(t)$ is the total volume of the sample solution (in mL, here 30); D is the dilution of the sample solution ($D = 1$ if no dilution); F is the factor correcting the difference between the composition of monosaccharides in the standard sugar mixture and that in NSP of various types of plant foods (for the calculation of NSP in cereals (except oats), $F = 0.95$; for fruit and nonstarchy vegetables, $F = 1.05$; and for starchy vegetables, oat products, and unknown samples, $F = 1$; using the standard sugar mixture as specified and these factors makes corrections for the 2 to 4% hydrolytic losses); C is the concentration (in mg/mL sugars) of the standard; $A(s)$ is the absorbance of the standard; $W(t)$ is the weight (mg) of sample taken for analysis; and 0.89 is the factor for converting experimentally determined monosaccharides to polysaccharides. The amount of soluble NSP is calculated as the difference between total NSP and insoluble NSP. It is recommended that a sample be taken for the analysis of the dry matter as the material remaining after overnight incubation at 104°C. Results may then be expressed as grams of polysaccharides per 100 g of dry matter.

Correction Based on Separate Measurement of Uronic Acids

When a sample, e.g., pectin, has a high content of uronic acids, a more accurate value for NSP may be obtained if uronic acids are measured separately. The color standard sugar mixture contains 12.5% (w/v) uronic acids, and it has been determined (data not shown) that this leads to 17% underestimation of NSP when the sample contains only uronic acids (using $F = 1$). Correction for the underestimation is straightforward if a separate value for uronic acids is obtained. If the sample contains 12.5% monomeric uronic acids, the color standard sugar mixture is entirely appropriate and no correction is required; otherwise, the correction required is an increment or decrement to the NSP value obtained by colorimetry equivalent to 17% of the uronic acid content that is in excess of or less than 12.5% of the sample, respectively.

The percentage of the NSP value to be corrected for is the difference (Δ) between the value for uronic acids (Z; expressed as a percentage of the NSP value, X) and 12.5, and it is calculated as

$$\Delta = (Z/X \times 100) - 12.5 \tag{3.3.6}$$

and the correction factor Y is calculated as

$$Y = 0.17\,(X/100 \times \Delta) \tag{3.3.7}$$

which may be reduced to $0.17Z - 0.021X$, and the value for total NSP after correction is $X + Y$.

Breaks in the Colorimetry Procedure

The procedure may be halted at either of the following stages: (1) after precipitation, washing and drying the starch-free residue (see step 3.4); the residue may be stored for long periods; or (2) after the hydrolysis with 2 M sulfuric acid; the hydrolysate may be kept at 4°C for 48 hours.

QUALITY CONTROL

The certificated reference materials (CRMs) may be used as part of a complete quality control procedure.

Trouble Shooting for the Common Hydrolysis Steps

1. Variation between replicate analyses may be due to inaccurate pipetting (test/calibrate dispensers by weighing replicates of water) or to incomplete removal of acetone in step 3.4.
2. If values for glucose are too high for samples of known composition and/or variable for replicates, this may be due to incomplete wetting of sample with DMSO in step 2.1. Mix vigorously immediately after addition of DMSO.
3. If values for glucose and uronic acids for samples of known composition are too low and/or are variable for replicates, this may be due to incomplete wetting of samples with 12 M sulfuric acid in step 5. Vortex-mix vigorously before and after addition of sulfuric acid and at intervals during the incubation.

Trouble Shooting for the GLC Procedure

1. Extra peaks on the chromatogram may be due to incomplete reduction of monosaccharides. Ensure alkaline pH before adding $NaBH_4$. Replace old $NaBH_4$; do not compensate for loss of activity by adding more $NaBH_4$.
2. Variation between replicate analyses may be caused by nonreproducible pipetting of the internal standard or hydrolysates. Test/calibrate dispensers by weighing 1-mL replicates of water.
3. If the response factors are not reproducible, this may be due to inaccurate pipetting of the sugar mixture and/or internal standard. Test/calibrate dispensers by weighing replicates of water.

Trouble Shooting for the HPLC Procedure

1. If retention times vary during chromatography, regenerate the analytical columns as described in the section on Determination of Constituent Sugars by HPLC.

Trouble Shooting for the Colorimetry Procedure

1. Variation between replicate analyses may be due to inaccurate pipetting (test/calibrate dispensers by weighing replicates of water) or to incomplete removal of acetone in step 3.4.
2. If no color is produced for standards and/or samples, this may be due to an error in the preparation of the sulfuric acid or sodium hydroxide solutions. Make new reagents. Test that the pH of the solution is between 7 and 8 before adding the color reagent solution.

REFERENCES

1. Southgate, D. A. T. and Greenfield, H., Principles for the Preparation of Nutritional Databases and Food Composition Tables, Siminopoulos, A. P., Butrum, R. R., Eds., International Food Data Bases and Information Exchange, *World Rev. Nutr. Diet.*, 68, 27, 1992.
2. Koivistoinen, P. E., Asp, N.-G., Englyst, H. N., Hudson, G. J., Hyvönen, L., Kallio, H., and Salo-Väänänen, P. P., Memorandum on terms, definitions, and analytical procedures of protein, fat and carbohydrates in food for basic composition data: issues and recommendations, *Food Chem.*, 57, 33, 1996.
3. FAO, Carbohydrates in Human Nutrition. Report of a Joint FAO/WHO Expert Consultation, Rome, 14-18 April 1997. FAO Food and Nutrition Paper 66. Food and Agriculture Organization of the United Nations, Rome.
4. Trowell, H., Ischemic heart disease and dietary fibre, *Am. J. Clin. Nutr.*, 25, 926, 1972.
5. Trowell, H., Dietary fibre; a paradigm, in *Dietary Fibre, Fibre-Depleted Foods and Disease*, Trowell, H. C., Burkitt, D., and Heaton, K. W., Eds., Academic Press, London, 1985, 1–20.
6. Cleave, T. L., Campbell, G. D., and Painter, N. S., *Diabetes, Coronary Thrombosis and the Saccharine Disease*, John Wright, Bristol, 1969.
7. Burkitt, D. P. and Trowell, H., Eds., *Refined Carbohydrate Foods and Disease. Some Implications of Dietary Fibre*, Academic Press, New York, 1975.
8. Hipsley, E. H., Dietary fibre and pregnancy toxaemia, *Br. Med. J.*, ii, 420, 1953.
9. Englyst, H. N., Wiggins, H. S., and Cummings, J. H., Determination of the nonstarch polysaccharides in plant foods by gas–liquid chromatography of constituent sugars as alditol acetates, *Analyst*, 107, 307, 1982.
10. Englyst, H. N., Trowell, H., Southgate, D. A. T., and Cummings, J. H., Dietary fiber and resistant starch, *Am. J. Clin. Nutr.*, 46, 873, 1987.
11. COMA Committee News, *Dietary Fibre*. Food Safety Information Bulletin, No. 97, June 1998.
12. COMA Committee News, *Definition of Dietary Fibre for Labelling Purposes*. Food Safety Information Bulletin, No. 109, June 1999.
13. Holland B., Welch, A. A., Unwin, I. D., Buss, D. H., Paul, A. A., and Southgate, D. A. T., *McCance & Widdowson's The Composition of Foods*, 5th ed., Ministry of Agriculture Fisheries & Food and Royal Society of Chemistry, Cambridge and London, 1991.
14. Englyst, H. N., Bingham, S. A., Runswick, S. A., Collinson, E., and Cummings, J. H., Dietary fibre (nonstarch polysaccharides) in fuit, vegetables and nuts, *J. Hum. Nutr. Dietet.*, 1, 247, 286, 1988.
15. Englyst, H. N., Bingham, S. A., Runswick, S. A., Collinson, E., and Cummings, J. H., Dietary fibre (nonstarch polysaccharides) in cereal products, *J. Hum. Nutr. Dietet.*, 2, 253, 1989.
16. McCance, R. A., Widdowson, E. M., and Shackleton, L. R. B., The nutritive value of fruits,vegetables and nuts. Special Report Series, MRC, London, No. 213, HMSO, London, 1936.
17. Southgate, D. A. T., Determination of carbohydrates in foods. II. Unavailable carbohydrates, *J. Sci. Food Agric.*, 20, 331, 1969.

18. Englyst, H. N. and Hudson, G. J., The classification and measurement of dietary carbohydrates, *Food Chem.*, 57, 15, 1996.
19. Wood, R., Englyst, H. N., Southgate, D. A. T., and Cummings, J. H., Determination of dietary fibre in foods — collaborative trials. IV. Comparison of Englyst GLC and colorimetric measurement with the Prosky procedure, *J. Assoc. Publ. Analysts*, 29, 57, 1993.
20. V39, Dietary fibre: Englyst procedure for determination of dietary fibre as nonstarch polysaccharides: measurement of constituent sugars by gas–liquid chromatography, *J. Assoc. Publ. Analysts*, 33, 127, 1997.
21. V40, Dietary fibre: Englyst procedure for determination of dietary fibre as nonstarch polysaccharides: measurement of constituent sugars by colorimetry, *J. Assoc. Publ. Analysts*, 33, 145, 1997.
22. Pendlington, A. W., Meuree-Vanlaethem, N., and Brookes, A., The Method Specific Certification of the Mass Fraction of Dietary Fibre in Lyophilised Haricot Beans, Carrot, Apple, Full Fat Soya Flour and Bran Breakfast Cereal Reference Materials, CRMs 514, 515, 516, 517 & 518. Office for Official Publications of the European Communities, Luxembourg, 1996.

The Southgate Method of Dietary Fiber Analysis

David A. T. Southgate

INTRODUCTION

This method, strictly speaking for the measurement of unavailable carbohydrates,[1,2] was developed in the late 1950s in connection with a major study for the evaluation of the energy conversion factors used to calculate the energy value of the human diet.[3] In this study we were concerned about the factor which should be used for available carbohydrates[1] as compared with carbohydrate "by difference"[4] as used in the classical Atwater system of factors.[5] The protocol for the study also required us to measure all the carbohydrates, and therefore, a method was required for unavailable carbohydrates.

The conceptual basis for the method was the method used by McCance et al.[6] and aimed to measure the carbohydrates in the alcohol-insoluble residue.

I also decided to introduce a number of constraints: first, to develop a procedure that measured all the carbohydrates in the same analytical sample, to avoid measuring a fraction twice; second, to attempt to use specific methods for the carbohydrates; and third, to start with a sample of a sufficient size because of the problems of taking a representative sample of many foods.

STAGES OF THE METHOD

The stages are summarized in Figure 3.4.1.

Initial Extraction of the Sample

Preparation of Alcohol-Insoluble Residue

(Two analytical portions of the food are taken through the whole scheme.)

The analytical samples should be of sufficient size (at least 5–10 g) to be representative and thoroughly mixed. The volume of alcohol added depends on the moisture content of the mixture and is about 85% v/v with respect to methanol; the mixture is brought to a boil with constant stirring (later versions of the method used ethanol at 80% v/v[7]). After filtering the residue is extracted with three further portions of aqueous alcohol. The alcoholic filtrates are combined and used for the measurement of free sugars.

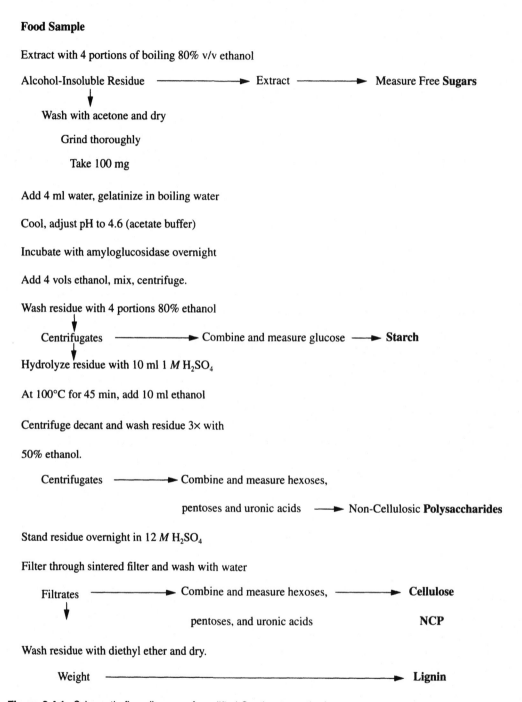

Food Sample

Extract with 4 portions of boiling 80% v/v ethanol

Alcohol-Insoluble Residue ——————————▶ Extract ——————————▶ Measure Free **Sugars**

    Wash with acetone and dry

      Grind thoroughly

        Take 100 mg

Add 4 ml water, gelatinize in boiling water

Cool, adjust pH to 4.6 (acetate buffer)

Incubate with amyloglucosidase overnight

Add 4 vols ethanol, mix, centrifuge.

Wash residue with 4 portions 80% ethanol

    Centrifugates ——————————▶ Combine and measure glucose ———▶ **Starch**

Hydrolyze residue with 10 ml 1 M H_2SO_4

At 100°C for 45 min, add 10 ml ethanol

Centrifuge decant and wash residue 3× with

50% ethanol.

    Centrifugates ——————▶ Combine and measure hexoses,

                      pentoses and uronic acids ———▶ Non-Cellulosic **Polysaccharides**

Stand residue overnight in 12 M H_2SO_4

Filter through sintered filter and wash with water

    Filtrates ——————————▶ Combine and measure hexoses, ——————————▶ **Cellulose**

                      pentoses, and uronic acids   **NCP**

Wash residue with diethyl ether and dry.

    Weight ——————————————————————————————▶ **Lignin**

Figure 3.4.1 Schematic flow diagram of modified Southgate method.

Enzymatic Hydrolysis of Starch

The alcohol-insoluble residue is extracted with diethyl ether and allowed to air-dry and weighed. The residue is finely ground and portions are taken for the measurement of polysaccharides. These portions are gelatinized with water in tubes immersed in a boiling waterbath for at least 10 min. After cooling the pH is adjusted with acetate buffer, amyloglucosidase enzyme is added, and the mixture is incubated at 37°C overnight (about 18 h). In the original method, a commercial Taka-diastase for analysis on talc (Parke Davis) was used; this preparation had some proteolytic activity which assisted in starch hydrolysis. This preparation is no longer available.

Four volumes of ethanol are added and the mixture is centrifuged to recover unchanged polysaccharides. After removal of the centrifugate, the residue is washed and recentrifuged with three portions of 80% v/v ethanol. The centrifugates are combined and glucose is measured to give a starch value.

Dilute Acid Hydrolysis (for Non-Cellulosic Polysaccharides, NCP)

The residue after enzymatic hydrolysis is suspended in 10 ml 1 M H_2SO_4 and heated for 2.5 h in a boiling waterbath. 10 ml of ethanol are added and the mixture is filtered. The residue is washed with three portions of 50% ethanol. The combined filtrates are analyzed for hexoses, pentoses, and uronic acids[4] to give a measure of the composition of the NCP.

Hydrolysis in Strong Acid

The residues are washed in ethanol followed by diethyl ether, and the ether is allowed to evaporate; 12 M H_2SO_4 are added and the mixture is stirred and left overnight. The mixture is filtered through a tared sintered glass filter and washed with water. The combined filtrates are made to volume and analyzed for hexoses, pentoses and uronic acids.

Measurement of Residual Lignin

The residue on the filter is washed with ethanol followed by diethyl ether and dried and weighed. The residue is taken as lignin.

Expression of Results

The colorimetric values for hexoses, pentoses, and uronic acids are not totally specific and need to be corrected for cross-interference.[8] The values are expressed as monosaccharides and are approximately 10% higher than if expressed as polysaccharides.

RETROSPECTIVE

This method is now really only of historical interest, having been superseded by more specific gas–liquid chromatographic (GLC) and high-performance liquid chromatographic (HPLC) methods for measuring the component sugars and uronic acids in the hydrolysates.[4] The method did, however, provide a quantitative direct measure of those components that approximated the original concept of dietary fiber[9] and showed that the composition of dietary fiber varied between the major classes of foods.[10]

REFERENCES

1. Southgate, D. A. T., Determination of carbohydrates in foods. I Available carbohydrates, *J. Sci. Food Agric.*, 20, 326, 1969
2. Southgate, D. A. T., Determination of carbohydrates in foods. II Unavailable carbohydrates, *J. Sci. Food Agric.*, 20, 331, 1969.

3. Southgate, D. A. T. and Durnin, J. V. G. A., Calories conversion factors. An experimental assessment of the factors used in calculation of the energy value of human diets, *Br J. Nutr.*, 24, 517, 1970.
4. Southgate, D. A. T., *Determination of Food Carbohydrates*, 2nd ed., Chapman and Hall, 1992.
5. Merrill, A. L. and Watt, B. K., *Energy Value of Foods. Basis and Derivation.* Agriculture Handbook No. 74, U.S. Department of Agriculture, 1955.
6. McCance, R. A., Widdowson, E. M., and Shackleton, L. R. B., The nutritive value of fruits, vegetables, and nuts, *Spec. Rep. Ser. Med., Res., Coun., no. 213*, HMSO, London. 1936.
7. James, W. P. T. and Theander, O., Eds., *The Analysis of Dietary Fibre in Foods*, Marcel Dekker, New York, 1981.
8. Hudson, G. J. and Bailey, B. S., Mutual interference effects in the colorimetric methods used to determine the sugar composition of dietary fibre, *Food Chem.*, 5, 201, 1980.
9. Southgate, D. A. T. and Englyst, H., Dietary fibre: chemistry, physical properties and analysis, in *Dietary Fibre, Fibre-Depleted Foods and Disease*, Trowell, H., Burkitt, D., and Heaton, K., Eds., Academic Press, London, 1985, 31.
10. Southgate, D. A. T., Bailey, B., Collinson, E., and Walker, A. F., A guide to calculating intakes of dietary fibre, *J. Human Nutr.*, 30, 303, 1976.

Determination of Total Dietary Fiber and Its Individual Components by the Uppsala Method

Olof Theander, Eric Westerlund, Roger Andersson, and Per Åman

INTRODUCTION

In recent years, it has become apparent that our understanding of the nutritional effects of dietary fiber (DF) has been considerably hampered by the lack of an appropriate definition of DF and, consequently, a lack of adequate analytical methods. In the original version of our methodology, Theander and Åman proposed that DF could be defined as the sum of nonstarch (amylase-resistant) polysaccharides and Klason lignin and, in conjunction with this chemical definition, published a gas-chromatographic method for analysis and characterization of DF.[1] In this method, the degree of polymerization of the nonstarch polysaccharides was intended to be the same as that defined by the International Union of Pure and Applied Chemistry (IUPAC), that is, greater than 10. This original method has now gained merit as a Current Contents Citation Classic.[2]

Enzyme-resistant starch, defined as the starch that resists hydrolysis with the thermostable α-amylase and the amyloglucosidase used in the method, is included in the dietary fiber polysaccharides, but not oligosaccharides or fructans. When human foods are analyzed, the value of Klason lignin includes native lignin but also other components such as tannins, cutins, and some proteinaceous products as well as Maillard reaction products in heat-treated foods. The latest version of the method, the Uppsala method,[3] has been studied in a collaborative study and is now approved as an official method by the Association of Official Analytical Chemists (AOAC-method 994.13), the American Association of Cereal Chemists (AACC-method 32-25), and the Nordic Committee on Food Analysis (NMKL-method 162).

The Uppsala method for total DF analysis, two AOAC enzymatic gravimetric methods, and a U.K. method were evaluated in an intercomparision and certification study organized by the Community Bureau of Reference, Commission of the European Communities.[4] The results showed that the five samples in the study could be accepted as standards for all four methods. The Uppsala method and the AOAC enymatic gravimetric methods often give similar results because they use a similar definition for DF, while the U.K. procedure that only includes plant cell wall nonstarch polysaccharides in the analysis generally gives lower values.

Today it is often proposed to expand the definition of dietary fiber to include other components — for example, oligosaccharides and fructans — in the analysis. AACC recently suggested DF be defined as follows: "DF consists of the remnants of edible plant cell, polysaccharides, lignin, and associated substances resistant to (hydrolysis) digestion by the alimentary enzymes of humans."[5,6] In accordance with a broader definition, we recently published a method for analysis of human digesta, which, besides dietary fiber polysaccharides and Klason lignin, also will include oligosaccharides, sugar alcohols, and fructans.[7] In Europe, however, efforts to agree upon a common definition on DF have not been successful, so far.

BACKGROUND

Our understanding of the chemical composition of DF in foods was to a large extent pioneered by Southgate, whose studies are based on the fractionation and colorimetric assay of the hexose, pentose, and uronic acid constituents.[8] This method, despite its complexity, is still not specific in regard to individual sugars, and the starch is incompletely removed. This was demonstrated at the meeting on DF analysis in Cambridge, U.K. in 1978,[9] where results from analyses of different types of food samples by Southgate's and other methods were presented. A large variability in results of the method between different laboratories was shown, although the agreement within laboratories seemed to be good.[10,11] In the Cambridge study, which initiated several new collaborative studies and further developments in the field of DF analysis, rapid gravimetric methods, as well as more comprehensive, informative ones, were also explored. These included two fractionation methods for soluble and insoluble fibers devised by Englyst[12] and Theander and Åman.[1,13] In both methods starch is removed enzymatically, but with different systems, and a direct gas–liquid chromatographic (GLC) assay is used for the neutral sugar constituents of the fiber fractions. The Englyst method has undergone a number of modifications,[14–17] including the development of a colorimetric procedure.[18] The original method of Theander and Åman[1] was later developed into two modifications[19,20] for analysis of total DF. The main differences between the present method[3] for total DF, developed by the Uppsala group, and that of the U.K. method of Englyst[17] are shown in Table 3.5.1.

The U.K. group used extraction with dimethylsulfoxide (DMSO) in combination with enzymatic treatments to remove not only the enzymatically available starch but also the so-called enzyme-resistant starch. We, as well as the scientists who have developed the enzymatic gravimetric AOAC method for analysis of DF, on the other hand, consider such enzymatically nonavailable starch as part of the DF complex.[21] In a comparison between the U.K. and Uppsala methods,[22] there was a rather good agreement in total DF when the values for enzyme-resistant starch and Klason lignin, obtained by the Uppsala method, are added to the values for nonstarch polysaccharides found by the U.K. method (Table 3.5.2). There was, however, a trend that these sums were slightly lower in the latter method. One possible explanation for this may be that the presence of DMSO partly hampers the precipitation of soluble DF polysaccharides.[23]

Marlett's group has made extensive studies on measurement of DF using a modification of the Uppsala methodology (see Marlett[24] and references therein). Another method, which is related to the Uppsala methodology but which uses DMSO for solubilization of starch, is that of Faulks and Timms.[25] A group that has been actively engaged in studies of individual fiber components — in particular, the preparation of cell wall materials — is that of Selvendran.[26,27] Their method involves extensive ball milling, gelatinization at pH 7 and 85 to 90°C, enzymatic treatments with α-amylase and pullulanase, GLC determination of sugar constituents, and colorimetric uronic acid determination. Selvendran has also published a review of methods for DF analysis which is recommended for further reading,[28] as well as the previously cited book by James and Theander.[9]

A more detailed description of the Uppsala methodology, including a critical discussion of the various steps and of alternative methods, is given below. For several polysaccharides, there is generally no sharp distinction between water-extractable (or removable) and water-unextractable fractions; the ratio between them is dependent on the choice of conditions during the pretreatment

Table 3.5.1 Comparison of Main Steps in Total Dietary Fiber Determination by GLC with the Latest Modifications of the Uppsla Method[3] and the U.K. Method[17]

Procedure	Uppsala method	U.K. method
Sample size (dry matter)	250–500 mg	50–300 mg
Fat removal	Extraction with petroleum ether when content exceeds 5%	Extraction with acetone when content exceeds 10%
Removal of low molecular weight carbohydrates	Extraction with 80% ethanol when content is very high	
Starch removal	1. Termamyl (0.5 h, boiling waterbath) in acetate buffer (0.1 M, pH 5.0) 2. Amyloglucosidase (16 h, 60°C)	1. Dimethylsulfoxide (DMSO) (0.5 h, boiling waterbath) 2. Termamyl (10 min, boiling waterbath) in acetate buffer (0.08 M, pH 5.2) 3. Pancreatin and pullulanase (0.5 h, 50°C + 10 min, boiling waterbath)
Precipitation of soluble fiber	80% (v/v) ethanol (1 h, 4°C)	80% (v/v) ethanol (0.5 h, ice water) at pH 2
Analysis of neutral sugars	1. 12 M H_2SO_4 (1 h, 30°C) 2. Addition of internal standard myo-inositol 3. 0.4 M H_2SO_4 (1 h, 125°C) 4. Alditol acetate preparation by sodium borhydride reduction and 1-methyl-imidazole/acetic anhydride treatment 5. Individual correction factor for each sugar	1. 12 M H_2SO_4 (0.5 h, 35°C) 2. 2 M H_2SO_4 (1 h, 100°C) 3. Addition of internal standard allose 4. Alditol acetate preparation by sodium borhydride reduction and 1-methyl-imidazole/acetic anhydride treatment 5. Individual correction factor for each sugar
Analysis of uronic acids	Colorimetry with 3,5-dimethylphenol (Scott, 1979)	Colorimetry with 3,5-dimethylphenol (Scott, 1979)
Lignin	Gravimetrically as Klason (sulfuric acid) lignin including ashing	Not determined

[a] Theander et al.[3]
[b] Englyst et al.[17]

Table 3.5.2 Content of Dietary Fiber (DF), Klason Lignin (KL), and Enzyme-Resistant Starch (RS) as Determined by the Uppsala Method, Nonstarch Polysaccharides (NSP) as Determined by the U.K. Method, and the Sum of NSP, KL, and RS for Comparison

	Uppsala Method[a]			U.K. Method[b]	NSP + KL + RS
Product	DF	KL	RS	NSP	(% dry matter)
Corn flakes	2.7	0.3	1.5	0.8	2.6
Bread crust	3.7	0.3	0.5	2.7	3.5
Bread crumb	3.8	0.3	0.8	2.7	3.8
Rye crisp	23.2	2.1	0.2	20.0	22.3
Green peas	14.5	0.3	0.3	12.8	13.4
Soybean	16.8	0.8	nd[c]	15.1	15.9
Deskinned onion	20.1	1.0	nd	19.2	20.2
Sugar-beet fiber	64.7	1.3	nd	67.0	68.3

[a] Theander et al.[3]
[b] Englyst and Cummings.[15]
[c] Not detected.

and solubilization procedure. These conditions are, however, never identical with *in vivo* conditions. Polysaccharides such as arabinoxylans, mixed-linkage β-glucans, and pectins (including associated neutral polysaccharides) are found both as water-soluble and water-insoluble components in plant materials. The yield of these components can vary considerably with the fractionation conditions used (physical pretreatment, enzymatic treatment, temperature, time, and so on). Thus, studies[29,30] have shown that the yield and composition of soluble fibers are very dependent on extraction conditions used. The use of DMSO in the U.K. method can be expected to increase the solubility of DF, since the reagent is an excellent solvent for hemicellulose polysaccharides.[23]

Recently, the Uppsala method (Figure 3.5.1) for routine analysis of total DF was tested in a collaborative study.[3] This method has been applied to a number of divergent samples, including foods, feeds, digesta, and feces, and has proven to be rugged, reproducible, adaptable, and accurate. A skilled analyst can run over 40 samples per week by this improved procedure. The Uppsala method is not much more time-consuming than the gravimetric enzymatic methods,[31,32] in which protein in the residue must be analyzed.

CRITICAL DISCUSSION OF VARIOUS STEPS IN DETERMINATION OF DIETARY FIBER

Removal of Free Sugars and Lipids

It is important that the samples are representative and homogeneous. Foods with low water content (<15%) are ground in a Cyclotec Sample Mill (Foss Tecator AB, Höganäs, Sweden) fitted with a 0.5-mm screen.[3] Materials with high water contents are generally freeze-dried, and samples which also have high sugar contents, like fruits and vegetables, are preferably extracted with 80% aqueous ethanol in an ultrasonic waterbath. If the lipid content of the sample exceeds 5%, extraction with petroleum ether at room temperature is efficient for most lipids.

Removal of Starch

Enzymatic removal of starch is a crucial operation in the Uppsala method in order not to overestimate the DF glucans. Starch is removed by incubations with a thermostable α-amylase (Termamyl) and amyloglucosidase. This enzyme system has proved to be very effective for various types of starch-containing fiber sources and products. The powerful Termamyl enzyme causes a rapid hydrolysis of starch during gelatinization. In the present procedure, the sample is treated with Termamyl for 30 min in a boiling waterbath. For practical reasons, the incubation with amyloglu-cosidase is then left to stand overnight, although complete hydrolysis to glucose is reached after about 6 h.[33] We usually quantify the glucose by a glucose oxidase reagent (Megazyme Int. Ireland Ltd., Bray, Ireland). Under the conditions used, neither of the enzymes liberated detectable amounts of sugars from purified barley grain β-glucan, barley straw arabinoxylan, or cotton cellulose.[1] The specificity of the Termamyl enzyme is probably explained by a rapid inactivation, at the high temperature used, of any nonstarch polysaccharide-degrading enzymes present. It is imperative that the enzymes used are free from fiber-degrading activity. Unfortunately it would appear that some commercial amyloglucosidase preparations at present have, for example, β-glucanase activity and will thus give low values for the fiber contents in, for instance, cereal samples. All enzyme preparations and batches should, therefore, be checked for such activities. Commercially available fractions of arabinoxylan, oat β-glucan, and citrus pectin are recommended for such use in the Uppsala method.

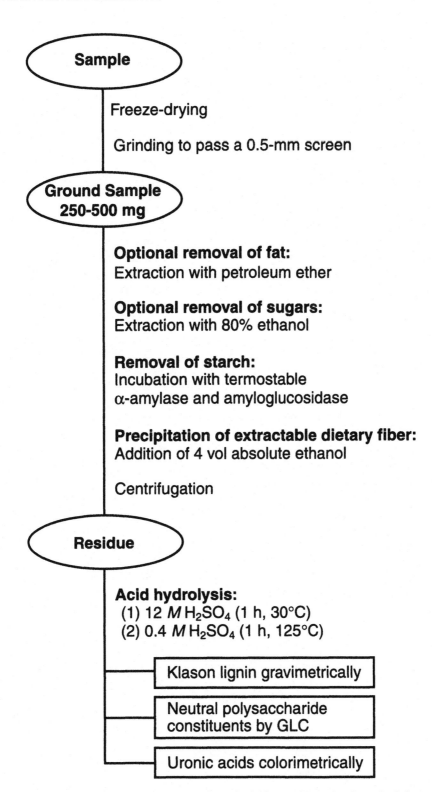

Figure 3.5.1 Analysis of dietary fiber by the Uppsala method. (*Source:* Theander, O. et al., *J. Assoc. Off. Anal. Chem.*, 78, 1030, 1995. With permission.)

Batey[34] reported that the gelatinization and solubilization of starch with a thermostable α-amylase prior to amyloglucosidase treatment resulted in higher starch values than those obtained after 8 M hydrochloric acid, DMSO or potassium hydroxide treatments. He pointed out that the good reproducibility of the analytical values using thermostable α-amylases — which is also our experience from various types of food products — is due to the rapid degradation of starch to lower molecular oligomers, which eliminates the phenomenon of retrogradation. The main advantage of using such enzymes — both for removal of starch in the DF determination and for direct starch analysis — is that autoclaving is not needed. Holm et al.[35] have studied *in vitro* and *in vivo* enzymatic digestibility of amylose–lipid complexes and found, among other things, that the use of Termamyl in combination with pancreatin almost completely hydrolyzed the complex. A number of other reactions and modifications of starch are conceivable during various normal heat treatments of food such as extrusion cooking, autoclaving, baking, frying, and so on. The two main routes whereby the amount of enzymatically available starch may decrease (and the DF glucan may consequently increase) are (1) retrogradation and (2) chemical modification of the starch structure.

It is well established that, after heat treatment, part of the starch in foods may be resistant to α-amylase hydrolysis and that a solution of gelatinized starch may retrograde on cooling and drying.[14,27] In connection with DF analysis, Englyst et al.[14] solubilized this retrograded enzyme-resistant starch with 2 M potassium hydroxide solution or DMSO[16] before hydrolysis with amyloglucosidase to glucose. They have applied this technique on a large series of cereal foods and reported values of enzyme-resistant starch in the range of 0.1 to 1.2% (except for one breakfast cereal having 3.1%).[36] We, as well as several others working in this field, regard this enzymatically nondegradable starch as a DF constituent and call it enzyme-resistant starch.

We have found that starch under food-technical conditions can also to some extent be modified nonreversibly via fragmentation to saccharides with 1,6-anhydroglucose end units, which can via further transglucosidation form enzyme-resistant, branched polysaccharide structures.[37,38] These modifications are, among other factors, dependent on the extent of heat treatment, the moisture content, and other factors. In the interlaboratory Helsinki study,[39] there was a slight but significant increase for the DF glucan values of extruded wheat flour and whole meal samples as well as for various heat-treated potato samples. Another factor contributing to the DF increase is from the Maillard reaction, which will be discussed below under the lignin determination.

A study[40] in our laboratory has shown that the formation of enzyme-resistant starch decreased from crumb to outer crust during baking (Table 3.5.3). This progressive decrease was probably due to water and temperature gradients formed in the bread during heating. The total content of dietary fiber glucans (enzyme-resistant starch is not included), on the other hand, increased from crumb to outer crust, mainly as a result of increasing contents of water-soluble glucans. This observation strongly suggested that formation of nonstarch glucans had, at least in part, occurred

Table 3.5.3   Content (g/100 g dry sample) of DF Polysaccharides and Enzyme-Resistant Starch in Dough and White Bread Fractions

	Dough	Crumb	Inner crust	Outer crust
Fraction yield	100	44	44	12
Soluble DF glucan	0.11	0.08	0.10	0.21
Insoluble DF glucan[a]	0.49	0.60	0.65	0.65
Soluble arabinoxylan	0.72	0.58	0.64	0.86
Insoluble arabinoxylan	1.20	1.09	1.03	0.70
Resistant starch	0.09	1.02	0.62	0.30

[a] Enzyme-resistant starch is not included.

Source: Westerlund, E. et al., *J. Cereal Sci.*, 10, 149, 1989.

via fragmentation of starch and subsequent reactions of the fragments. The content of insoluble arabinoxylans decreased during baking, particularly in the outer crust. This decrease was partly accompanied by an increase in the content of water-soluble arabinoxylans. The total dietary fiber content was higher in the bread fractions than in the dough, mainly due to the formation of RS.

Precipitation of Soluble Polysaccharides

In previous studies on rapeseed flour,[41,42] we found that some polysaccharides may remain in solution after precipitation with 80% ethanol. In the Uppsala method, it is a key point to reach as complete a recovery as possible of soluble DF on their precipitation in 80% aqueous ethanol. We have previously shown[20] that such precipitation losses did not exceed 3% of the total DF polysaccharides of, e.g., wheat flour, raw potato, carrot, and wheat bran. Recently in a detailed study using gel filtration of the ethanolic supernatant,[43] the polysaccharide fraction (DP > 10) escaping precipitation was analyzed in various foods. The amounts of soluble fiber polysaccharides not recovered were low: 1–6% (Table 3.5.4). These losses of the total fiber content of the original sample were observed, with the highest values found for the most severe heat-treated sample (bread crust). This indicates that the solubility of DF polysaccharides may be changed by thermal treatment, probably by depolymerization.[40]

Table 3.5.4   **Amounts of Neutral Polysaccharide Residues Not Recovered on Precipitation of Soluble Fiber with 80% Ethanol in Samples Analyzed by the Uppsala Procedure (% of total fiber content)**

Sample	Rhamnose	Arabinose	Xylose	Mannose	Galactose	Glucose	Total
Corn flakes	0.2	0.2	0.2	0.5	0.5	1.0	2.6
Bread crust	0.2	0.2	0.2	0.7	0.5	3.8	5.6
Bread crumb	0.2	0.2	0.2	1.1	0.2	1.9	3.8
Rye crisp	0.1	0.1	0.1	0.3	0.1	1.1	1.8
Green peas	0.1	0.1	0.1	0.1	traces	0.3	0.7
Soybean	0.2	0.1	0.2	0.3	0.3	0.4	1.5
Deskinned onion	0.5	0.1	0.1	0.3	0.2	1.1	1.9
Sugar-beet fiber	0.1	0.5	0.1	0.1	0.1	0.1	1.0

Source: Theander, O. et al., *J. AOAC Int.*, 77, 703, 1994.

Determination of Neutral Polysaccharide Constituents

Treatments with 12 M sulfuric acid aiming to effect dissolution of cellulose, followed by a secondary hydrolysis in dilute acid for hydrolysis of lignocellulosic materials in combination with Klason lignin determination as originally developed by Hägglund et al.[44] and later modified by, for example, Saeman et al.,[45] are widely used (see below). Such a method is used for the hydrolysis of the polysaccharides in the Uppsala method, namely pretreatment with 12 M sulfuric acid at room temperature for 2 h, dilution to 0.4 M, and hydrolysis for 6 h under reflux[1] or to gain time for 1 h at 125°C[20] (in an autoclave, essentially according to Sloneker[46]). It is important that the hydrolysis step with dilute sulfuric acid is sufficient to hydrolyze sulfate ester groups introduced in the first step. Figures 3.5.2 and 3.5.3, from an investigation made at the Swedish Forest Research Laboratories on the polysaccharide analysis, show an example of the sugar yield and rate of sulfate ester removal after different times of hydrolysis for xylose and glucose.[47] They illustrate the well-known higher rates of degradation with acids for pentoses (in particular xylose) and also why we choose 6 h for the posthydrolysis step to ensure hydrolysis of sulfate ester groups (also 1 h at 125°C is enough). In a preparative experiment in which the cellulose was hydrolyzed for only 4 h, we isolated part of the original cellulose as glucose-6-sulfate.[48] It is notable that Neilson and Marlett,[49] when

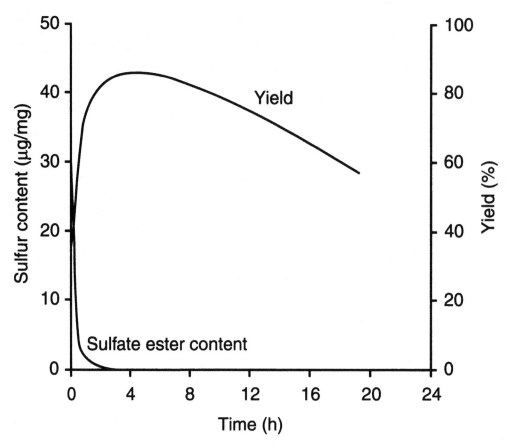

Figure 3.5.2   Yield and sulfate ester decomposition of xylose by reflux in 0.4 *M* sulfuric acid hydrolysis after pretreatment (30°C, 1 h) with 12 *M* sulfuric acid. (*Source:* Bethge, P. O. et al., *Kvantitativ Kolhydratbestämning — en detaljstudie*, Communication No. 63B, Swedish Forest Products Laboratory, Stockholm, 1971. With permission.)

comparing a modified neutral detergent fiber method with a modified Uppsala procedure with only 3 h in the second hydrolysis step, found appreciable amounts of cellobiose (around 10% of total sugars) in the hydrolysates of the latter method. Using the autoclaving conditions, the amounts of cellobiose or other oligosaccharides in our hydrolyzed fractions are negligible. The efficiency of our conditions for hydrolysis of crystalline cellulose has been demonstrated by eight independent analyses of purified cotton linter. On average, a cellulose content of 99.0% (SD 1.3) and a xylan content of 0.25% were found.[22] The effect of particle size and different prehydrolysis conditions to achieve optimum hydrolysis yield has been investigated.[50]

In the Uppsala method we have not, as have certain other workers in the field, attempted to estimate the noncellulose component of the insoluble DF separately from the cellulose by using an extra heterogeneous hydrolysis step with dilute sulfuric acid, since varying amounts of noncrystalline cellulose (depending on the source of the sample) may also be hydrolyzed under these conditions. Further, part of the hemicellulose fraction may be difficult to get into solution. It has been reported that for materials such as carrot, cabbage, and soybean, part of the xylose- and mannose-containing polymers need pretreatment with strong sulfuric acid to be completely hydrolyzed with the dilute acid.[14] The so-called β-glucans (containing β-1,4-linked glucose units interdispersed with β-1,3-linkages) are important components of some oat and barley products and can be determined by separate methods.[51]

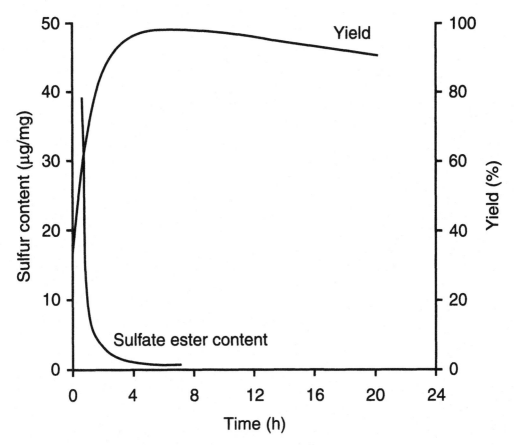

Figure 3.5.3 Yield and sulfate ester decomposition of glucose by reflux in 0.4 *M* sulfuric acid hydrolysis after pretreatment (30°C, 1 h) with 12 *M* sulfuric acid. (*Source:* Bethge, P. O. et al., *Kvantitativ Kolhydratbestämning — en detaljstudie,* Communication No. 63B, Swedish Forest Products Laboratory, Stockholm, 1971. With permission.)

GLC, particularly on capillary columns, is the method of choice for an efficient separation and accurate determination of the sugar constituents in hydrolysates. The sugars are first converted to the volatile alditol acetate derivatives,[1] essentially as described by Sloneker.[52] Hydrolysates containing appreciable amounts of uronic acids must be carefully neutralized and the pH adjusted to the slightly alkaline side with, for instance, dilute ammonium hydroxide (without causing any epimerization of sugars) in order to open any uronolactones, which would otherwise be reduced with borohydride to alditols in the subsequent reduction step. The reduction is left to stand at 40°C for 1 h, but most sugars are probably transformed into alditols much quicker. We have, however, not found any epimerization of hexoses or pentoses under the conditions used. In the original procedure (see, e.g., References 1, 47, and 52), the borate from the borohydride, after acidification, has usually been removed as the volatile trimethylborate by repeated evaporation with methanol. This is essential, since borate forms complexes with the alditols and interferes with the subsequent acetylation with acetic anhydride and the commonly used catalyst pyridine. Connors and Pandit[53] introduced the use of 1-methylimidazole as an effective catalyst for rapid acetylation of polyhydroxy compounds, and later Blakeney et al.[54] reported the use of this catalyst for the quantitative and rapid acetylation of alditols in the presence of borate (at room temperature for 10 min). This technique, which we now generally use, facilitates and shortens the derivatization step considerably. A procedure for direct acetylation of aldoses in the acidic hydrolysate (without previous reduction)

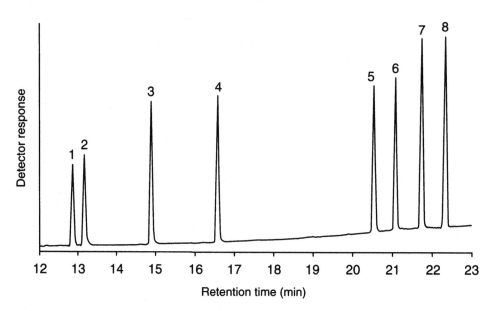

Figure 3.5.4 GLC-analysis of a monosaccharide reference mixture as alditol acetates. Capillary fused silica column (25 m × 0.25 mm). Peak 1, rhamnitol; 2, fucitol; 3, arabinitol; 4, xylitol; 5, mannitol; 6, galactitol; 7, glucitol; and 8, *myo*-inositol (internal standard).

was developed in our laboratory.[55] So far this procedure has been tested on only a limited number of samples, but the agreement is good compared with the Uppsala method.

In the GLC separation, *myo*-inositol is added as internal standard before the hydrolysis step with dilute sulfuric acid. Figure 3.5.4 shows a typical GLC separation of alditol acetates derived from a reference mixture, and Figure 3.5.5 shows the corresponding separation from a wheat bran concentrate. Correction factors for hydrolysis losses, derivatization yields, and GLC responses for the individual sugars have been applied. As the ratio between the different sugars may influence these factors, reference sugar mixtures, typical for the DF composition of the food sample in question, are also analyzed concomitantly. In these correction factors are also included the factors 0.88 and 0.90 used to convert the pentose/deoxyhexose and hexose contents, respectively, to polysaccharides. Capillary column chromatography has been a key factor in the separation of these complex mixtures, and the so-called bonded phase (BP) columns, in which the liquid phase is covalently bonded to the column, imparting good thermal stability and prolonged life, have introduced a further degree of efficiency into the chromatographic operations.

High-performance liquid chromatography (HPLC) offers an alternative procedure for analyzing aldoses in polysaccharide hydrolysates but has not so far proved to be as powerful a technique as GLC. The choice of method is, however, governed by the requirements of the investigation. An advantage of HPLC is that the preparation of derivatives is obviated, although derivatization has, in fact, often been used in HPLC in order to enhance resolution and detection of the components and to shorten the analysis time. Comprehensive reviews[56–58] on HPLC with various applications in the carbohydrate field have been published, including the use of amperometric determination[59] of monosaccharides, which seems promising. Automated procedures using ion-exchange resins have also been successfully employed for the separation of monosaccharides.[60,61]

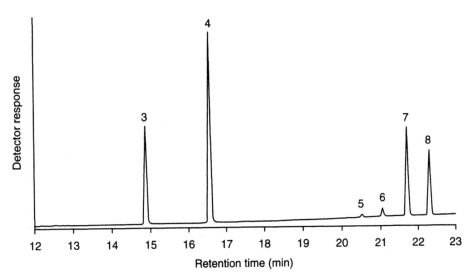

Figure 3.5.5 GLC-analysis of the monosaccharides in a hydrolysate of wheat bran concentrate as alditol acetates. Conditions and peak numbering as in Figure 3.5.4.

Determination of Uronic Acid Residues in DF Polysaccharides

The determination of uronic acid constituents in DF by GLC presents a greater problem than in the case of the neutral sugar constituents.[62] Although free, low-molecular uronic acids may be readily analyzed by GLC in the presence of neutral sugars,[63] the release of these acids in acceptable yields from the polymers is complicated by the high stability of glycosyl uronic acid linkages toward acid hydrolysis — resulting often in the formation of aldobiouronic acids. Further, the monomeric uronic acids when released are degraded to noncarbohydrate products more rapidly than the neutral sugars. A useful technique has been developed for the separation and analysis of individual monomeric uronic acids by partition chromatography of ion-exchange resins unmodified[64] (including oligomeric acids) or after transformation to aldonic acids.[65]

Most workers in the DF field have used colorimetric assays and, in particular, the modified carbazole method according to Bitter and Muir.[66] Common disadvantages with colorimetric methods are the sensitivity to reaction conditions, interference from absorbing compounds resulting from neutral sugars, proteins, phenols, and other components present, and the inability to distinguish between individual uronic acids. The introduction of 3-phenylphenol by Blumenkrantz and Asboe-Hansen[67] and later 3,5-dimethylphenol by Scott,[68] who also compared the use of different phenol derivatives for colorimetric determination of uronic acids in plant materials, offers certain advantages. The rate of formation of 5-formyl-2-furancarboxylic acid, on which the colorimetric determination is based, was shown to be faster for galacturonic than for glucuronic acids.[68] The Uppsala group uses galacturonic acid for calibration because of this and the fact that galacturonic acid is more predominant in most DF samples (pectins) compared to glucuronic acid. The latter phenol reagents seem to suffer less interference from hexoses and have a greater sensitivity than the carbazole reaction. In the Cambridge study, Katan and Van de Bovenkamp[69] used a copper-binding method for determining the uronide content. They also calculated the methyl ester content from the binding of copper to the sample before and after saponification. Methanol released by such a treatment can also be determined by GLC.

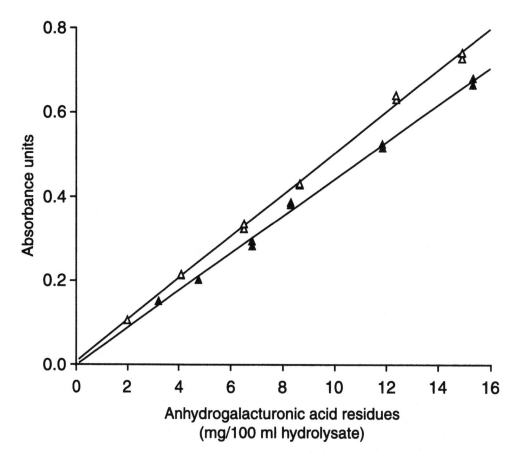

Figure 3.5.6 Differences in absorbance obtained by colorimetric determination of uronic acids in autoclaved hydrolysates of citrus pectin (upper line) and galacturonic acid (lower line).

In the Uppsala procedure, the degradation of D-galacturonic acid is compared with that of a well-characterized citrus pectin treated under identical acidic conditions (0.4 M sulfuric acid, 125°C, 1 h) to account for observed differences in the degradation rate[70] of polygalacturonic acid residues and that of the free monomer. Different amounts of rhamnogalacturonan from citrus with a well-determined content of polygalacturonic acid residues (analyzed by titration and corrected for the presence of acetyl groups) and the D-galacturonic acid were subjected to acid treatment in separate experiments.[62] The straight lines through the origin (Figure 3.5.6) showed that the rate of degradation of the uronic acid–containing samples was reproducible. Thus, if the calculated content of uronic acid residues is based on the degradation observed for the monomer, polyuronide values have to be multiplied by 0.88 to compensate for the lower degree of acid degradation of citrus pectin compared to that of the free monomer. One should be aware of the fact that variations in the pectic polysaccharide structure and molecular mass as well as experimental conditions may influence the value of this factor.

The decarboxylation method for uronic acid determination does not suffer from the interference problems which are incurred with the colorimetric methods. We have established that the decarboxylation method developed by Bylund and Donetzhuber[71] for woods and pulps also affords a rapid, accurate, and reproducible method for DF samples, even those with low uronic acid contents.[1,13,19] The sample, containing 1 to 20 mg uronic acid, is refluxed for 30 min with hydroiodic acid under nitrogen. The carbon dioxide released is trapped in a cell containing dilute sodium hydroxide, and the conductivity changes are registered by means of a potentiometric recorder. We have found that the uronic acid determination gives essentially the same result whether it is performed before or after the extraction with organic solvent and starch removal.[20] Different types of uronic acids, such as D-galacturonic acid, D-glucuronolactone, the aldobiouronic acid 2-O-(4-O-methyl-α-D-glucopyranosyluronic acid)-D-xylose, and pectic acid give the same change in conductivity per mole of hexuronic acid.[1] This method, like the colorimetric methods, does not estimate the amount of individual uronic acid constituents but only the sum of uronic acids. If the uronide content mainly comprises pectin, acidic xylan constituents, or alginate, paper electrophoresis of the polysaccharide hydrolysate from the sugar analysis (even though the uronides are not completely hydrolyzed) affords a rapid, rough estimate of the ratio between the corresponding galacturonic, glucuronic (or its 4-O-methyl ether), and mannuronic acids.[72]

Determination of Lignin

There is no specific method for the determination of lignin, the complex polymer of phenyl-propane units — at least, if one wishes to avoid laborious and time-consuming procedures. We have applied an oxidation/methylation technique to determine the lignin contents of different light- and dark-colored turnip rapeseed cultivars without interference from condensed tannins.[73] The acetyl bromide method, originally introduced by Johnson et al.[74] for wood and wood products, has been further developed and applied to forage crops by Morrison.[75] This method has the advantage of being rapid and requires only about 50 mg of material. The sample is extracted with water and organic solvents, and the lignin content is measured by dissolving the residue in 25% acetyl bromide in acetic acid and measuring the absorption at 280 nm. Eastwood and colleagues, however, considered the method inappropriate and not directly applicable to foods.[76,77] More recently, Selvendran et al.[28] pointed out that the acetyl bromide procedure can be used only to compare the lignin contents of different organs from the same plant or samples from similar species, since different species require different conversion factors.

We have, like many others working with lignified plant materials, chosen the sulfuric acid method, which was first applied by Klason[78] at the beginning of this century, but which has since been further modified.[79] Essentially, it involves removal of extractives and polysaccharides and the gravimetric determination of the residue as lignin after washing and drying. In the present Uppsala method, an ashing step is also included. It is conveniently combined with the determination of the neutral polysaccharide constituents of the DF.[1,22] When applied to human foods, however, the values in most cases represent not only native lignin but also tannins, cutin, and some proteinaceous products. From heat-treated foods, the residue may also contain products of the Maillard reaction and caramelization reactions. These constituents of the Klason lignin residue most likely represent food components, which, like lignin, are unavailable to human enzymes. We therefore propose that *the Klason lignin value will be designated the "noncarbohydrate" part of the DF.*

The lignin content determined according to Goering and Van Soest[80] by $KMnO_4$ oxidation of the ADF (acid detergent fiber) residue is probably generally closer to the amount of native lignin. Van Soest has demonstrated for some forages and feeds that high-temperature treatment increases the amount of crude protein and Klason lignin of the ADF residue.[81] We have found a similar increase of the Klason lignin residues and their crude protein contents with the extent of heat treatment for potato and cereals[37,39] (see Table 3.5.5 for some examples). A brown water-insoluble polymer was obtained (together with low molecular weight furans, phenols, pyrroles, pyridines, carboxylic acids, and lactones) by refluxing a slightly acidic aqueous solution of glucose and glycine.[82] It analyzed as 90% Klason lignin with a recovery of 84% of the original nitrogen.[83] The crude protein contents which one finds in the Klason lignin residue from heat-treated foods, besides originating from such Maillard reaction products, might also originate from protein-tannin

Table 3.5.5 Klason Lignin Values in Heat-Treated Cereals and Potato Samples

Sample	Klason Lignin (%)	Crude Protein in the Klason Lignin (% of original protein)
Wheat Flour		
Untreated	0.2	0.3
Extruded at 168°C	0.4	2.3
Wheat Whole Meal		
Untreated	1.4	4.7
Extruded at 180°C	2.8	11.0
Potato		
Raw	0.4	—
Boiled	1.2	—
Pressure-cooked	2.6	—

Sources: Theander, O. and Westerlund, E., Stärke, 39, 88, 1987. Varo, P. et al., J. Assoc. Off. Anal. Chem., 66, 933, 1983.

complexes, cell wall protein, and other nitrogen-containing components. In residues from unprocessed foods, however, we do not find more than 1 to 5% of the nitrogen of the original food. For brans, which represent a very lignin-rich food ingredient, this corresponds to not more than about 10% of the Klason lignin residue, when calculated as crude protein (N × 6.25).

The chemistry of DF polysaccharides, lignin, and other nondigestible substances associated with plant cell walls, which may be included in a broader definition of the term dietary fiber, is discussed in Theander and Åman,[84] Theander,[85] and Selvendran.[86] Cell wall proteins, cutin, waxes, polyphenols other than lignin, phytic acid, silica, and compounds such as acetic acid and phenolic acids, which are present as ester-linked substituents to DF polysaccharides and/or lignin, may be included in this group. So far, the importance of such plant fiber substituents, as well as lignin, has been discussed mainly in connection with digestion of plant materials by the rumen microflora. It is very likely, however, that phenolic acids, lignin, and other phenolic compounds may also play an important role relative to the microbial fermentation in the human gut, although generally present in only small amounts in human food. Acetyl and phenolic acid substituents in grasses can be analyzed by GLC methods.[87] Hartley and Haverkamp[88] reported the presence of 0.02% p-coumaric acid and 0.66% ferulic acid in wheat bran, as determined by HPLC after removal by alkali. Recently, the contents of these components were determined[22] in some high-fiber products (Table 3.5.6). The acetyl constituents were quantified as 1-acetylpyrrolidin by GLC[89] and phenolic acids, after release by alkaline treatment by HPLC.[90]

Table 3.5.6 Content of Ester Substituents in Some High-Fiber Products (% of dry matter)

Product	Dietary Fiber	Coumaroyl Groups	Feruloyl Groups	Acetyl Groups
Maize bran	76.4	0.2	2.4	1.5
Wheat bran	37.2	trace	0.2	0.3
Potato fiber	71.9	trace	trace	0.7
Sugar beet fiber	70.8	trace	0.5	1.6

Source: Theander, O. et al., in New Developments in Dietary Fiber, Furda, I. and Brine, C. J., Eds., Plenum Press, New York, 1990, 273.

Markwalder and Neukom[91] have isolated dehydrodiferulic acid from wheat flour, where it is thought to be a possible cross-link in pentosans. Maize bran is rich in phenolic acid residues.[92] By using controlled mild acid hydrolysis it was possible to release oligosaccharides with ester-linked phenolic residues still attached. Three main feruloylated saccharides were identified, which all had the same basic unit with an arabinofuranosyl residue esterified on position O-5 by ferulic acid. From this unit the other two saccharides were built by adding one xylopyranosyl residue on position 2 of the arabinose residue, and further one galactopyranosyl residue on position 4 of the xylose residue. These saccharides are probably side chains of the heteroxylan which have been released by the cleavage of the acid-labile glycosidic bonds of the arabinofuranosyl residues attached to the main xylan backbone. Both ferulic acid (2.9%) and dehydrodimers of ferulic acid (2.5%) were released from maize bran by alkaline treatment. The 5-5', 8-O-4' and 8-5' dimers dominated, but the 8-8' dimer was also present. Recently, the same group has also isolated and structurally elucidated two new 5-5'-diferuloyl oligosaccharides, which were also released by mild acid hydrolysis of maize bran.[93] In one of the oligosaccharides, both phenolic acids of the dimer were esterified to arabinose, and in the other oligosaccharide one phenolic acid was esterified to arabinose and the other to arabinose, which was further substituted with a 2-linked xylose residue. The structure of these saccharides indicates that the heteroxylans in maize bran are covalently cross-linked through dehydrodiferulates.

COLLABORATIVE STUDY OF THE UPPSALA METHOD

The Uppsala method for DF analysis has been successfully applied to the analysis of a number of divergent samples and tested in a collaborative AOAC/AACC study.[3] The study was completed by nine laboratories, four from North America and five from Europe, and eight unknown products were analyzed for total DF and DF constituents in duplicate by each collaborator. The samples — wheat bran concentrate, Potex (an enriched potato fiber product), carrot, oat bran, apple, green peas, rye bread and wheat bread — were selected to represent a wide range in the content and composition of DF and to represent important foods with significance for the intake of DF. The values determined for average total DF contents of these samples, calculated on a dry matter basis, varied from 4.6% for wheat bread to 84.3% for wheat bran concentrate, with generally small differences between laboratories (Figure 3.5.7).

Method performance for determination of total DF was good (Table 3.5.7), both for repeatability within laboratories (RSD_r) and reproducibility among laboratories (RSD_R). The average RSD_R value was 8.4% (range 4.8–11.1%), which is good considering that this enzymatic–chemical method is based on the determination of several analytes, i.e., the individual neutral sugar residues, uronic acid residues, and Klason lignin. The content of neutral polysaccharide residues ranged from 3.8 to 64.1% with an average RSD_R value of 7.5%. Individual sugar residues (rhamnose, arabinose, xylose, mannose, galactose, and glucose) generally also had good RSD_R values when present above 1%, whereas corresponding values for uronic acid residues and Klason lignin were higher. A collaborative study on an enzymatic gravimetric AOAC method has shown a similar range of RSD_R values (0.9–12.2%) for food samples with a total DF content of 13.1–71.8% of dry samples.[32]

APPLICATIONS

An obvious advantage of the Uppsala method is that the content of individual sugar residues and Klason lignin of the DF is determined. Such information is valuable, for instance, when properties of DF are to be investigated and predicted. A gravimetric method for determination of

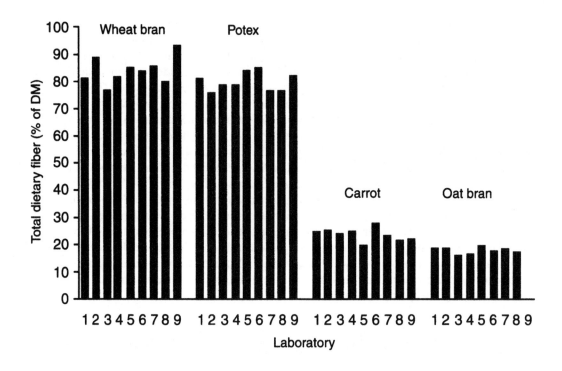

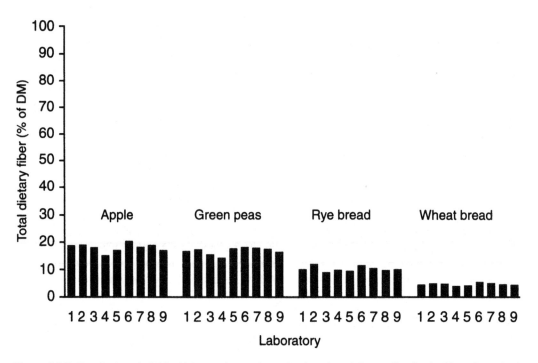

Figure 3.5.7 Results from individual laboratories on determination of total dietary fiber by the Uppsala method. Figures given are a percentage of dry matter as an average of duplicate analysis. (*Source:* Theander, O. et al., *J. Assoc. Off. Anal. Chem.*, 78, 1030, 1995.)

Table 3.5.7   **Method Performance for Determination of Total Dietary Fiber by the Uppsala Method**

Sample	Mean (% DM)	s_r	s_R	RSD_r	RSD_R
Wheat bran	84.3	1.52	4.90	1.8	5.8
Potex	80.4	2.88	3.86	3.6	4.8
Carrot	24.1	1.16	2.50	4.8	10.4
Oat bran	18.4	1.04	1.42	5.6	7.7
Apple	17.9	0.90	1.58	5.0	8.8
Green peas	16.7	0.93	1.43	5.6	8.6
Rye bread	10.3	0.48	1.02	4.7	9.9
White bread	4.6	0.32	0.52	6.9	11.1

Source: Theander, O. et al., J. Assoc. Off. Anal. Chem., 78, 1030, 1995.

total DF can never provide such information. The Uppsala method consequently provides a tool to determine the DF content and composition for the purposes of research, quality control, and labeling.

Total DF results published from our applications during many years using the Uppsala methodology on batches and/or varieties of cereals, vegetables, fruits, and products thereof are given in Table 3.5.8. In cereal products total DF ranged from 2.7% in corn flakes to 84.9% in enriched wheat bran. Also, for products of legume seeds, potatoes, vegetables, and fruits, large variations in content were found. The large ranges in total DF within the different sources demonstrate that care must be taken when generalizing from a single analysis of a certain DF source. This variation is due to cultivar as well as growing and processing conditions.

Contents of individual dietary fiber components are presented in Table 3.5.9.[3] In concentrated wheat bran arabinoxylans (arabinose and xylose residues), cellulose (glucose residues) and Klason lignin dominate. Major components in Potex, carrot, apple, and green peas are pectin (uronic acid residues), cellulose (glucose residues), and xyloglucan (glucose and xylose residues). Galactose residues in Potex and arabinose residues in peas, both probably part of the pectic polysaccharide complex, were also notably high in content. In oat bran, rye bread, and white bread arabinoxylan, mixed-linkage β-glucan (glucose residues) and cellulose are important DF components, together with Klason lignin, mainly in the two former samples, and enzyme-resistant starch, mainly in the two latter samples.

The application of the Uppsala methodology on a series of fiber-rich foodstuffs, namely wheat bran, rye bran, whole potato, carrot, pea, white cabbage, lettuce, and apple, is presented in Table 3.5.10.[1] The figures based on dry matter are in the range of 1 to 4% for water-soluble DF and 8 to 34% for insoluble DF. On a fresh weight basis, the brans are particularly rich fiber sources. The great differences in chemical composition among the different foods are notable, and one would therefore also expect great differences among the physical, biological, and nutritional properties of the different DF sources. The analyses thus indicate that brans have the highest Klason lignin values and are rich in arabinoxylans and cellulose but have a low proportion of uronic acid constituents. The other sources have higher cellulose contents and also more pectic and associated substances (galacturonic acid, rhamnose, arabinose, and galactose being typical constituents) than brans. The high galactan content is also typical for potatoes.

Table 3.5.8   Contents of Dietary Fiber (% of dry matter) in Products of Cereals, Legume Seeds, Potato Products, Vegetables, and Fruits as Determined by the Uppsala Method

Samples	Total Dietary Fiber	n	Range
Cereal Products			
Corn flakes	2.7	1	
White bread crust	3.2	5	2.9–3.7
White bread crumb	3.3	3	2.9–3.2
White flour	3.5	49	2.7–4.7
White bread	4.6	1	
Corn	9.4	1	
Rye bread	10.3	1	
Whole winter wheat	10.5	15	9.2–11.6
Dehulled oats	10.7	1	
Oat bran bread	10.9	1	
Whole spring wheat	11.3	14	9.9–13.8
Whole triticale	13.1	10	10.0–15.0
Rolled barley flakes	13.7	6	12.0–14.5
Rye biscuit	13.9	2	13.8–13.9
Whole rye	14.7	6	13.4–16.5
Rye crisp bread	15.1	2	7.1–23.1
Dehulled barley	15.9	12	12.3–18.2
Whole barley	18.8	18	15.9–24.8
Oat bran	19.8	4	19.7–20.5
Rye bran	25.8	2	23.5–28.1
Whole oat	29.6	16	19.8–38.7
Wheat bran	40.0	8	36.5–46.0
Wheat bran concentrate	84.9	10	81.0–89.0
Legume Seeds			
Dehulled broad bean	8.1	1	
Dehulled yellow peas	8.2	34	6.8–9.5
Dehulled dark peas	8.3	6	7.6–9.0
Dehulled soy bean	11.8	13	10.5–14.5
Dehulled brown bean	13.0	1	
Green peas	15.6	2	14.5–16.7
Soy bean	16.8	1	
Frozen green peas	22.3	2	21.3–23.3
Mung bean	23.0	1	
Brown bean	23.9	1	
Chick pea	24.0	1	
Potato Products			
Raw potato	5.9	14	4.5–7.9
Potato powder	6.0	1	
Enriched potato pulp	73.2	12	68.4–80.4
Vegetables			
Deskinned onion	20.1	1	
White cabbage	20.7	1	
Lettuce	21.1	2	16.2–26.0
Carrot	25.3	5	23.8–28.1
Sugar beet fiber	78.2	7	64.7–83.5
Fruits			
Apple pulp	10.2	1	
Apple	17.7	2	17.5–17.9
Citrus pectin	84.0	1	

Table 3.5.9   Content and Composition of Dietary Fiber in Some Food Products

	Wheat Bran	Potex	Carrot	Oat Bran	Apple	Green Peas	Rye Bread	White Bread
Individual sugar residues								
Rhamnose	—	1.5	0.6	—	—	—	—	—
Arabinose	14.8	4.6	1.4	1.7	1.7	3.2	1.7	0.7
Xylose	29.4	1.9	0.4	2.6	1.0	1.3	2.8	1.0
Mannose	0.7	1.3	0.8	0.5	0.6	0.4	0.5	0.4
Galactose	1.3	20.4	2.2	0.4	1.1	0.9	0.4	0.3
Glucose	17.8	26.0	6.9	9.8	5.0	6.5	3.4	1.5
Uronic acids	4.4	22.4	11.1	1.0	6.5	3.7	0.6	0.4
Klason lignin	15.5	2.6	0.9	1.9	1.7	0.6	0.9	0.4
Total dietary fiber	84.3	80.4	24.1	18.4	17.9	16.7	10.3	4.6

Source: Theander, O. et al., *J. Assoc. Off. Anal. Chem.*, 78, 1030, 1995.

Table 3.5.10   Chemical Characterization of Water-Extractable and Water-Unextractable Dietary Fibers in Various Foods

	Wheat Bran	Rye Bran	Potato (whole)	Carrot	Pea	White Cabbage	Lettuce	Apple
Water-extractable fraction								
Neutral sugar residues	2.1	2.3	3.1	0.9	0.6	0.9	0.3	0.5
Uronic acid residues	0.2	0.2	1.2	2.0	0.5	1.9	0.5	2.3
Relative composition of neutral sugar residues								
Glucose	41.8	36.9	45.9	14.0	24.1	tr[a]	8.9	10.8
Galactose	3.4	8.3	45.3	40.1	17.4	38.9	40.0	26.2
Mannose	tr	tr	tr	tr	tr	tr	5.0	tr
Xylose	20.8	30.3	tr	1.9	3.7	8.3	10.3	tr
Arabinose	34	24.5	5.8	28.2	51.9	40.9	34.3	58.2
Rhamnose	tr	tr	2.0	15.8	2.8	11.9	1.5	4.8
Fucose	—	—	1.0	—	—	—	—	—
Water-unextractable fraction								
Neutral sugar residues	28.3	21.1	6.2	15.1	15.9	14.3	8.6	11.1
Uronic acid residues	1.2	0.6	0.4	5.5	1.7	2.7	4.5	2.3
Klason lignin	4.7	3.9	0.9	1.5	2.6	0.9	2.3	1.3
Relative composition of neutral sugar constituents								
Glucose	31.3	28.2	46.1	60.5	69.0	62.8	63.5	46.0
Galactose	3.7	1.8	34.5	12.5	1.0	9.1	9.7	9.5
Mannose	1.3	tr	1.5	5.4	tr	4.3	4.2	2.8
Xylose	39.2	39.5	6.3	6.3	5.7	9.6	9.1	10.9
Arabinose	24.5	30.5	10.0	11.3	23.3	9.6	9.0	27.5
Rhamnose	tr	tr	1.4	3.8	1.0	3.4	4.5	1.6
Fucose	tr	tr	0.2	0.2	tr	1.2	tr	1.7
Total DF content	36.5	28.1	11.8	25.0	21.3	20.7	16.2	17.5

Note: All figures, except composition of neutral sugars, are given as a percentage of dry matter.

[a] Traces.

Source: Theander, O. and Åman, P., *Swedish J. Agric. Res.*, 9, 97, 1979.

REFERENCES

1. Theander, O. and Åman, P., Studies on dietary fibres. 1. Analysis and chemical characterization of water-soluble and water-insoluble dietary fibres, *Swedish J. Agric. Res.*, 9, 97, 1979.

2. Theander, O. and Åman, P., Informative analysis of dietary fibre, *Current Contents, Agriculture, Biology & Environmental Sciences, Citation Classic*, 22, 9, 1991.

3. Theander, O., Åman, P., Westerlund, E., Andersson, R., and Pettersson, D., Total dietary fiber determined as neutral sugar and uronic acid residues, and lignin (The Uppsala method): collaborative study, *J. Assoc. Off. Anal. Chem.*, 78, 1030, 1995.

4. Pendlington, A. W., Meuree-Vanlaethem, N., and Brookes, A., The method specific certification of the mass fraction of dietary fibre in lyophilised haricot beans, carrot, apple, full fat soya flour and bran breakfast cereal reference materials, *European Commision, BCR Information, Reference Materials*, Report EUR17451EN, Brussels, 1996.

5. Gordon, D. T., Defining dietary fiber — A progress report, *Cereal Foods World*, 44, 336, 1999.

6. Miller Jones, J., New AACC dietary fiber definition sets the stage for annual meeting technical round tables, *Cereal Foods World*, 45, 404, 2000.

7. Åman, P., Sundberg, B., and Andersson, R., Analysis of cabohydrates in ileal excreta from humans, in *Proceedings of the Profibre symposium: Plant polysaccharides in human nutrition: Structure, function, digestive fate & metabolic effects*, Guillon, F. et al., Eds., European Air Concerted Action AIR3CT94-2203, Nantes, 1997, 32.

8. Southgate, D. A. T., Determination of carbohydrates in foods. II. Unavailable carbohydrates, *J. Sci. Food Agric.*, 20, 331, 1969.

9. James, W. P. T. and Theander, O., Eds., *The Analysis of Dietary Fiber in Food*, Marcel Dekker, New York, 1981.

10. Southgate, D. A. T. and White, M. A., Commentary on results obtained by the different laboratories using the Southgate method, in *The Analysis of Dietary Fiber in Food*, James, W. P. T. and Theander, O., Eds., Marcel Dekker, New York, 1981, chap. 4.

11. Theander, O., A review of the different analytical methods and remaining problems, in *The Analysis of Dietary Fiber in Food*, James, W. P. T. and Theander, O., Eds., Marcel Dekker, New York, 1981, chap. 16.

12. Englyst, H., Determination of carbohydrate and its composition in plant materials, in *The Analysis of Dietary Fiber in Food*, James, W. P. T. and Theander, O., Eds., Marcel Dekker, New York, 1981, chap. 6.

13. Theander, O. and Åman, P., Analysis of dietary fibers and their main constituents, in *The Analysis of Dietary Fiber in Food*, James, W. P. T. and Theander, O., Eds., Marcel Dekker, New York, 1981, chap. 5.

14. Englyst, H., Wiggins, H. S., and Cummings, J. H., Determination of the nonstarch polysaccharides in plant foods by gas-liquid chromatography of constituent sugars as alditol acetates, *Analyst*, 107, 307, 1982.

15. Englyst, H. N. and Cummings, J. H., An improved method for the measurement of dietary fibre as nonstarch polysaccharides in plant foods, *J. Assoc. Off. Anal. Chem.*, 71, 808, 1988.

16. Englyst, H. N. and Cummings, J. H., Nonstarch polysaccharides (dietary fiber) and resistant starch, in *New Developments in Dietary Fiber*, Furda, I. and Brine, C. J., Eds., Plenum Press, New York, 1990, 205.

17. Englyst, H. N., Quigley, M. E., and Hudson, G. J., Determination of dietary fibre as nonstarch polysaccharides with gas-liquid chromatographic, high-performance liquid chromatographic or spectrophotometric measurement of constituent sugars, *Analyst*, 119, 1497, 1994.

18. Englyst, H. N. and Hudson, G. J., Colorimetric method for routine measurement of dietary fibre as nonstarch polysaccharides. A comparison with gas-liquid chromatography, *Food Chem.*, 24, 63, 1987.

19. Theander, O. and Åman, P., Studies on dietary fibre. A method for the analysis and chemical characterisation of total dietary fibre, *J. Sci. Food Agric.*, 33, 340, 1982.

20. Theander, O. and Westerlund, E., Studies on dietary fiber. III. Improved procedures for analysis of dietary fiber, *J. Agric. Food. Chem.*, 34, 330, 1986.

21. Asp, N.-G., Furda, L., Schweizer, T. F., and Prosky, L., Dietary fiber definition and analysis, *Am. J. Clin. Nutr.*, 48, 688, 1988.

22. Theander, O., Åman, P., Westerlund, E., and Graham, H., The Uppsala method for rapid analysis of total dietary fiber, in *New Developments in Dietary Fiber,* Furda, I. and Brine, C. J., Eds., Plenum Press, New York, 1990, 273.

23. Hägglund, E., Lindberg, B., and McPhersson, J., Dimethylsulphoxide, a solvent for hemicelluloses, *Acta Chem. Scand.,* 10, 1160, 1956.

24. Marlett, J. A., Measuring dietary fiber, *J. Anim. Feed Sci. Technol.,* 23, 1, 1989.

25. Faulks, R. M. and Timms, S. B., A rapid method for determining the carbohydrate component of dietary fibre, *Food Chem.,* 17, 273, 1985.

26. Selvendran, R. R. and Du Pont, M. S., Simplified methods for the preparation and analysis of dietary fibre, *J. Sci. Food Agric.,* 31, 1173, 1980.

27. Selvedran, R. R., Ring, S. G., and Du Pont, M. S., Determination of the dietary fiber content of the EEC samples and a discussion of the various methods of analysis, in *The Analysis of Dietary Fiber in Food,* James, W. P. T. and Theander, O., Eds., Marcel Dekker, New York, 1981, chap. 7.

28. Selvendran, R. R., Verne, A. V. F. V., and Faulks, R. M., Methods for analysis of dietary fibre, in *Plant Fibers: Modern Methods of Plant Analysis,* vol. 10, Linskens, H. F. and Jackson, J. F., Eds., Springer Verlag, Berlin, 1989, 234.

29. Graham, H., Grön Rydberg, M.-B., and Åman, P., Extraction of soluble dietary fiber, *J. Agric. Food Chem.,* 36, 494, 1988.

30. Marlett, J. A., Chesters, J. G., Longaere, M. J., and Bogdanske, J. J., Recovery of soluble dietary fiber is dependent on the method of analysis, *Am. J. Clin. Nutr.,* 50, 479, 1989.

31. Prosky, L., Asp, N.-G., Furda, L, Devries, J. W., Schweizer, T., and Harland, B. F., Determination of total dietary fiber in foods, food products and ingredients: collaborative study, *J. Assoc. Off. Anal. Chem.,* 67, 1044, 1984.

32. Lee, S. C., Prosky, L., and DeVries, J. W., Determination of total, soluble and insoluble dietary fiber in foods — Enzymatic gravimetric method, mes-tris buffer — Collaborative study, *J. AOAC Int.,* 75, 395, 1992.

33. Åman, P. and Hesselman, K., Analysis of starch and other main constituents of cereal grains, *Swed. J. Agric. Res.,* 14, 135, 1984.

34. Batey, I. L., Starch analysis using thermostable alfa-amylases, *Stärke,* 34, 125, 1982.

35. Holm, J., Björck, I., Ostrowska, S., Eliasson, A.-C., Asp, N.-G., Larsson, K., and Lundquist, L., Digestibility of amylose-lipid complexes in-vitro and in-vivo, *Stärke,* 35, 294, 1983.

36. Englyst, H. N., Andersson, V., and Cummings, J. H., Starch and nonstarch polysaccharides in some cereal foods, *J. Sci. Food Agric.,* 34, 1434, 1983.

37. Theander, O. and Westerlund, E., Studies on chemical modifications in heat-processed starch and wheat flour, *Stärke,* 39, 88, 1987.

38. Siljeström, M., Björck, I., and Westerlund, E., Transglycosidation reactions following heat treatment of starch. Effects on enzymic digestibility, *Stärke,* 41, 95, 1989.

39. Varo, P., Laine, R., and Koivistonen, P., Effect of heat treatment on dietary fiber: interlaboratory study, *J. Assoc. Off. Anal. Chem.,* 66, 933, 1983.

40. Westerlund, E., Theander, O., Andersson, R., and Åman, P., Effects of baking on polysaccharides in white bread fractions, *J. Cereal Sci.,* 10, 149, 1989.

41. Larm, O., Theander, O., and Åman, P., Structural studies on a water-soluble arabinan isolated from rapeseed *(Brassica napus), Acta Chem. Scand. B.,* 29, 1011, 1975.

42. Larm, O., Theander, O., and Åman, P., Structural studies on a water-soluble arabinogalactan isolated from rapeseed *(Brassica napus), Acta Chem. Scand. B,* 30, 627, 1976.

43. Theander, O., Åman, P., Westerlund, E., and Graham, H., Enzymatic/chemical analysis of dietary fiber, *J. AOAC Int.,* 77, 703, 1994.

44. Hägglund, E., *Chemistry of Wood,* Academic Press, New York, 1951, 326.

45. Saeman, J. F., Moore, W. E., and Millet, M. A., Sugar units present. Hydrolysis and quantitative paper chromatography, in *Methods in Carbohydrate Chemistry,* vol. 3, Whistler, R. L., Ed., Academic Press, New York, 1963, chap. 12.

46. Sloneker, J. H., Determination of cellulose and apparent hemicellulose in plant tissue by gas-liquid chromatography, *Anal. Biochem.,* 43, 539, 1971.

47. Bethge, P. O., Rådeström, R., and Theander, O., *Kvantitativ kolhydratbestämning — en detaljstudie,* Communication No. 63B, Swedish Forest Products Laboratory, Stockholm, 1971 (in Swedish).

48. Hardell, H.-L. and Theander, O., Quantitative determination of carbohydrates in cellulosic materials — losses as sulphates, *Svensk Papperstidn.*, 73, 291, 1970.
49. Neilson, M. J. and Marlett, J. A., A comparison between detergent and non-detergent analyses of dietary fiber in human foodstuffs, using high-performance liquid chromatography to measure neutral sugar composition, *J. Agric. Food Chem.*, 31, 1342, 1983.
50. Hoebler, C., Barry, J. L., David, A., and Delort-Laval, J., Rapid acid hydrolysis of plant cell wall polysaccharides and simplified quantitative determination of their neutral monosaccharides by gas-liquid chromatography, *J. Agric. Food Chem.*, 37, 360, 1989.
51. Åman, P. and Graham, H., Analysis of total and insoluble mixed-linked (1-3), (1-4)-beta-D-glukans in barley and oats, *J. Agric. Food Chem.*, 35, 704, 1987.
52. Sloneker, J. H., Gas-liquid chromatography of alditol acetates, in *Methods in Carbohydrate Chemistry*, vol. 6, Whistler, R. L. and BeMiller, J. N., Eds., Academic Press, New York, 1972, chap. 4.
53. Connors, K. A. and Pandit, N. K., N-Methylimidazole as a catalyst for analytical acetylations of hydroxy compounds, *Anal. Chem.*, 50, 1542, 1978.
54. Blakeney, A. B., Harris, P. J., Henry, R. J., and Stone, B. A., A simple and rapid preparation of alditol acetates for monosaccharide analysis, *Carbohydr. Res.*, 113, 291, 1983.
55. Hämiläinen, M., Theander, O., Nordkvist, E., and Ternrud, I., Multivariate calibration in the determination of acetylated aldoses by g.l.c., *Carbohydrate Res.*, 207, 167, 1990.
56. Verhaar, L. A. T. and Kuster, B. F. M., Liquid chromatography of sugars on silica-based stationary phases, *J. Chromatogr.*, 220, 313, 1981.
57. Honda, S., High-performance liquid chromatography of mono- and oligosaccharides, *Anal. Biochem.*, 140, 1, 1984.
58. Hicks, K. B., High-performance liquid chromatography of carbohydrates, *Adv. Carbohydr. Chem. Biochem.*, 46, 17, 1988.
59. Lee, Y. C., High-performance anion-exchange chromatography for carbohydrate analysis, *Anal. Biochem.*, 189, 151, 1990.
60. Samuelson, O., Partition chromatography on ion-exchange resins, in *Methods in Carbohydrate Chemistry*, vol. 6, Whistler, R. L. and BeMiller, J. N., Eds., Academic Press, New York, 1972, chap. 9.
61. Mopper, K., Improved chromatographic separations on anion-exchange resins. 1. Partition chromatography of sugars in ethanol, *Anal. Biochem.*, 85, 528, 1978.
62. Westerlund, E., Andersson, R., Åman, P., and Theander, O., Determination of uronic acids as components of dietary fibre polysaccharides, in *Recent Progress in the Analysis of Dietary Fibre*, European Commision, Brussels, 1994, 163.
63. Lehrfeld, J., Differential gas-liquid chromatography method for determination of uronic acids in carbohydrate mixtures, *Anal. Biochem.*, 115, 410, 1981.
64. Johnson, S. and Samuelson, O., Automated chromatography of uronic acids on anion-exchange resins, *Anal. Chim. Acta*, 36, 1, 1966.
65. Samuelson, O. and Thede, L., Automated ion exchange chromatography of organic acids in acetate media, *J. Chromatogr.*, 30, 556, 1967.
66. Bitter, T. and Muir, H. M., A modified uronic acid carbazole reaction, *Anal. Biochem.*, 4, 330, 1962.
67. Blumenkrantz, N. and Asboe-Hansen, G., New method for quantitative determination of uronic acids, *Anal. Biochem.*, 54, 484, 1973.
68. Scott, R. W., Colorimetric determination of hexuronic acids in plant materials, *Anal. Chem.*, 51, 936, 1979.
69. Katan, M. B. and Van de Bovenkamp, P., Determination of total dietary fiber by difference and of pectin by colorimetry or copper titration, in *The Analysis of Dietary Fiber in Food*, James, W. P. T. and Theander, O., Eds., Marcel Dekker, New York, 1981, chap. 14.
70. Selvendran, R. R., March, J. F., and Ring, S. G., Determination of aldoses and uronic acid content of vegetable fibre, *Anal. Biochem.*, 96, 282, 1979.
71. Bylund, M. and Donetzhuber, A., Semimicro determination of uronic acids, *Svensk Papperstidn.*, 15, 505, 1968.
72. Carlsson, B., Samuelsson, O., Popoff, T., and Theander, O., Isomerisation of D-glucuronic acid in neutral aqueous solution, *Acta Chem. Scand.*, 23, 261, 1969.
73. Theander, O., Åman, P., Miksche, G. E., and Yasuda, S., Carbohydrates, polyphenols, and lignin in seed hulls of different colors from turnip rapeseed, *J. Agric. Food Chem.*, 25, 270, 1977.

74. Johnson, D. B., Moore, W. E., and Zank, L. C., The spectrophotometric determination of lignin in small wood samples, *TAPPI*, 44, 793, 1961.

75. Morrison, I. M., A semi-micro method for the determination of lignin and its use in predicting the digestibility of forage crops, *J. Sci. Food Agric.*, 23, 455, 1972.

76. McConnell, A. A. and Eastwood, M. A., A comparison of methods of measuring "fibre" in vegetable material, *J. Sci. Food Agric.*, 25, 1451, 1974.

77. Robertson, J. A., Eastwood, M. A., and Yeoman, M. M., An investigation of lignin extraction from dietary fibre using acetyl bromide, *J. Sci. Food Agric.*, 30, 1039, 1979.

78. Klason, P., Die Verfahren der Holzzellstoff-Fabrikation. Aussprache, in *Verein der Zellstoff and PapierChemiker and Ingenieure*, Hauptversammlung, Berlin, 1908, 52.

79. Browning, B. L., Determination of lignin, in *Methods of Wood Chemistry,* vol. 2, Interscience, New York, 1967, chap. 34.

80. Goering, H. K. and Van Soest, P. J., Forage fiber analyses, U.S. Dept. Agric. Agricultural Handbook No. 379, U.S. Government Printing Office, Washington, D.C., 1970.

81. Van Soest, P. J., Use of detergents in analysis of fibrous feeds. III. Study of effects of heating and drying on yield of fiber and lignin in forages, *J. Assoc. Off. Anal. Chem.*, 48, 785, 1965.

82. Olsson, K., Pernemalm, P.-A., and Theander, O., Formation of aromatic compounds from carbohydrates, VII. Reaction of D-glucose and glycine in slightly acidic, aqueous solution, *Acta Chem. Scand. B,* 32, 249, 1978.

83. Theander, O., Advances in the chemical characterisation and analytical determination of dietary fibre components, in *Dietary Fibre,* Birch, G. G. and Parker, K. J., Eds., Applied Science, London, 1983, chap. 6.

84. Theander, O. and Åman, P., The chemistry, morphology, and analysis of dietary fiber components, in *Dietary Fibers: Chemistry and Nutrition,* Inglett, G. E. and Falkehag, S. I., Eds., Academic Press, New York, 1979, chap. 15.

85. Theander, O., The chemistry of dietary fibres in different sources, in *Nahrungsfasern Dietary Fibres,* Amado, R. and Schweizer, T., Eds., Academic Press, London, 1986, 13.

86. Selvendran, R. R., The chemistry of plant cell walls, in *Dietary Fibre,* Birch, G. G. and Parker, K. J., Eds., Applied Science Publishers, London, 1983, 95.

87. Theander, O., Udén, P., and Åman, P., Acetyl and phenolic acid substituents in timothy of different maturity and after digestion with rumen microorganisms or a commercial cellulase, *Agric. Environ.,* 6, 127, 1981.

88. Hartley, R. D. and Haverkamp, J., Pyrolysis-mass spectrometry of the phenolic constituents of plant cell walls, *J. Sci. Food Agric.*, 35, 14, 1984.

89. Månsson, P. and Samuelsson, B., Quantitative determination of O-acetyl and other O-acetyl groups in cellulosic material, *Svensk Papperstidn.*, 84, R15, 1981.

90. Ternrud, I. E., Lindberg, J. E., and Theander, O., Continuous changes in straw carbohydrate digestion and composition along the gastro-intestinal tract in ruminants, *J. Sci. Food Agric.*, 41, 315, 1987.

91. Markwalder, H. V. and Neukom, H., Diferulic acid as a possible crosslink in hemicelluloses from wheat germ, *Phytochemistry,* 15, 836, 1976.

92. Saulnier, L. and Thibault, J.-F., Review: Ferulic and diferulic acids as components of sugar-beet pectins and maize bran heteroxylans, *J. Sci. Food Agric.*, 70, 396, 1999.

93. Saulnier, L., Crepeau, M.-J., Lahaye, M., Thibault, J.-F., Garcia-Conesa, M., Kroon, P., and Williamson, G., Isolation and structural determination of two 5,5'-diferuloyl oligosaccharides indicate that maize heteroxylan are covalently crosslinked by oxidatively coupled ferulates, *Carbohydr. Res.*, 320, 82, 1999.

CHAPTER **3.6**

The Crude Fiber Method[1]

Ivan Furda

Crude fiber is the loss of ignition of dried residue remaining after digestion of a sample with 1.25% sulfuric acid and 1.25% sodium hydroxide solutions under specific conditions. The principle of the method is that a finely ground air-dried sample of the food is extracted with ether to remove lipids and that this dry sample is then extracted successively with boiling acid and alkali. The residue is filtered off and washed. After drying and weighing, the residue is ashed and residual inorganic matter is measured. The method is applicable to grains, cereals, flours, feeds, and any fiber-bearing material from which fat can be extracted to leave workable residue.

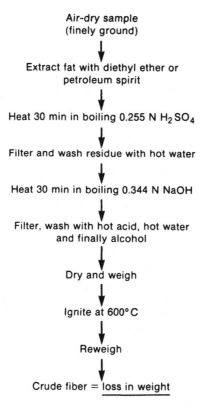

Figure 3.6.1 Flow chart for determining crude fiber.

0-8493-2387-8/01/$0.00+$1.50

REFERENCE

1. Horwitz, W., Ed., Official Methods of Analysis of the Association of Official Analytical Chemists, 13th ed., AOAC, Washington, D.C., 1980, 132.

Newer Methods for Phytate Analysis

Donald Oberleas and Barbara F. Harland

Good analytical methods, both qualitative and quantitative, are necessary for the study and understanding of phytate. There are no known reagents specific for the identification of phytate. The nature of the compound with its saturated ring does not lend itself to absorption within the ultraviolet (UV) or visible spectra. Therefore, many methods were tested throughout the twentieth century to achieve accurate identification and quantitation of phytate. These methods have been reviewed by Oberleas,[1] Cosgrove,[2] Cheryan,[3] Maga,[4] Oberleas,[5] and Oberleas and Harland.[6] By current standards and technology, some methods now have little more than historic value. The reader interested in the history of phytate analytical methods is directed to the above references for details.

QUALITATIVE METHODS

A detection system was devised by Wade and Morgan[7] that takes advantage of the strong complexation of inositol phosphates with the ferric ion. This paper chromatographic technique separated phosphate esters that were sprayed with a mixture of ferric ions in dilute acid. The chromatograms were then sprayed with an alcoholic solution of sulfosalicylic acid. Where free ferric ions were present, ferric sulfosalicylate formed a colorful complex, and where ferric ion was complexed with phosphate or phosphate esters, color did not develop. A later modification of this procedure by Sobolev and Vyskrebentseva[8] utilized ammonium thiocyanate as the colored iron-complexing reagent with similar results.

Anion exchange columns were employed in the separation and identification of phytate and inositol phosphates even before the principles and benefits of this technology were fully understood. Smith and Clark[9] selected a weak-anion exchange resin (60–80 mesh) in a 1.25×24 cm resin bed and used a step gradient elution of 0.1 to 0.8 N HCl. The elution was 32 mL per hour with 1-hour fraction collection for up to 280 h. Nine distinct fractions were separated and identified, but this represented an impractical analytical technique.

Other qualitative separations were effected by Tomlinson and Ballou[10] using Dowex 1 (Cl form). Extensive efforts were made by Cosgrove,[2,11,12] whose earliest efforts used Dowex 1 (X8, Cl form, 200–400 mesh) with a non-linear gradient of water and 1.5 N HCl. Anion-exchange techniques are available for the separation of mixtures of isomeric inositol polyphosphates.[13–15] A long column packed with Dowex 1 and eluted with 0.48 N HCl worked well. This concentration of acid is just sufficient for the elution of inositol hexakisphosphate and the subtle differences in isomeric configuration effects the differences in separation.[12,13,16,17]

QUANTITATIVE METHODS

Quantitative analytical methods underwent a considerable evolution within the twentieth century. The original method reported by Heubner and Stadler[18] was based on the principle that phytate was the only phosphate compound found in nature that formed an insoluble complex with ferric iron in dilute acid. Titration with a standard ferric iron solution against a sensitive ferric ion indicator identified the endpoint in this method. Several modifications of this original method are recorded in the reviews cited above. Phytate contains phosphate that can be quantified, but this is not specific and can be expressed only as phytate equivalent or phytate phosphorus. Phytate does complex heavy metals with some specific characteristics. Most of these complexes are pH-sensitive, and with careful separation and specific reagents, the properties of these metals and their complexing characteristics can be made quantitative for phytate and other inositol phosphates. With modern HPLC technology, it is possible to separate, identify, and quantify the various inositol phosphates simultaneously.

The quantification of phytate may be divided into three phases. Being a natural compound in plant seeds, some roots and tubers, and some fruits, the sample must be extracted from a complex set of matrices. It must then be separated from other soluble and thus extractable constituents. Finally, it must be detectable either *in toto* or some component that is proportional to the concentration in the original foodstuff. A reliable standard must always be considered important in quantitative analytical procedures and is essential for phytate analysis.

Extraction Methods

Phytic acid and its sodium and potassium salts are hydrophilic and hygroscopic. Though the salts are slow to dissolve in water, they are readily soluble. Free phytic acid is not found in plants because it is too strong an acid and phytate will complex with several minerals at neutral or slightly acidic pHs. Yet, for accuracy in any quantitative technique, assurance of complete extraction is the imperative first step in the analytical process. Heubner and Stadler[18] titrated isolated phytate samples in 0.6% HCl worked with isolated phytate rather than phytate extracted from foodstuffs. This has served as a working acid concentration, defining a dilute acidic solution, by many investigators as opposed to an extraction solution. Rather[19] recommended 1.2% HCl for extraction from food samples, whereas Averill and King[20] reported slightly better results with 2% HCl with a 25/1 (v/w) ratio and a 3-hour extraction time. In all cases, the acid concentration was diluted to 0.6% for titration against an ammonium thiocyanate indicator. Latta and Eskin[21] indicated that 2.4% HCl (0.66 mol/l) gave a more complete extraction in a 1-hour extraction of phytate from rapeseed.

De Lange et al.[22] used 5% TCA with centrifugation and re-extraction of the residue. Wheeler and Ferrel[23] extracted wheat and high-protein flour concentrates with 3% TCA and compared these results with 0.6 mol/l HCl with extractions of 30 to 45 min of shaking. Cilliers and van Niekerk[24] reported that 3% TCA was the preferred extractant. Tangendjaja et al.[25] selected this extraction procedure when they attempted their pioneering studies of adapting an HPLC procedure to phytate analysis. Bos et al.[26] reported that extraction with 0.8 mol/L HCl provided consistently higher extraction rates. Several other acids, in various concentrations, have been used by investigators for specific extractions. There appears to be little agreement with regard to the type or concentration of acid appropriate for extraction. Thus, any of the above conditions may be appropriate for a specific group of foodstuffs. Little effort has been extended toward finding an appropriate acid and concentration that can be utilized universally in all situations. Also, the addition of water-soluble sodium phytate or acid-soluble barium phytate (Wheeler and Ferrel[23]) to samples for measurement of recoveries is totally inadequate. It should be obvious that these salts would be recovered under the mildest of conditions. Table 3.7.1 shows the results of one effort for comparison among an almost endless variety of possible combinations.

Table 3.7.1   Evaluation of Various Extraction Acids of Wheat Cereals for Phytate Analysis (mg phytate/kg air dry cereal)

Sample Name	Shredded Grain	Bran	Fortified	Shredded Mini Wheat
3% TCA	4798.6	3270.3	914.2	2965.6
5% TCA	4717.9	3833.4	1009.1	2686.8
10% TCA	8014.5	6299.8	1506.7	5214.7
0.5 mol/L HCl	6557.3	6623.2	1627.7	3775.4
0.66 mol/L HCl	6379.1	5783.2	1706.4	5085.1

Notes: All extractions were for 3 h with gentle, continuous shaking. Paired "*t*" statistical analysis indicated that 3% and 5% TCA is not as effective as other extractions; 10% TCA, 0.5 and 0.66 mol/L HCl were not different.

Regardless of the extraction method, the hydrophilic nature of phytate dictates that an aqueous acid is necessary and that the fat content of the sample may interfere with the extraction process. Thus, the fat content of samples must be low or reduced before extraction with aqueous acid. Though no designed formal studies of fat content have been made, experience has shown that fat content less than about 5% poses no problem with the acid extraction process. Fat extraction may be done with diethyl ether[27] or petroleum ether[28] for 1 h or more. The lipophobic nature of phytate will preclude any loss of sample during fat extraction.

Extraction Time

Extraction time is another important consideration for which very little objective data are available. First, extraction is the dissociation and acid solubilization of phytate from its native matrix, whether that be as mixed salts or associated with proteins. Thus, "vigorous" physical agitation of the mixtures does not improve the chemical solubility or separation of the phytate from the organic matrix (foodstuff). Second, once solubilized, the phytate is stable in the acid for several days at room temperature. Thus, overextension or overextraction does not occur. The phytase activity inherent in the foodstuff would be inactivated by the acid and would not become a factor in the extraction process. The important aspect of extraction is to recover as much of the phytate as possible from all possible sample matrices with the conditions utilized.

The shortest extraction time reported was the 5-min blending of potato or other plant tissue with 100 mL of 10% TCA in a Waring Blender.[29] Averill and King[20] analyzed a large number of foodstuffs using a 3-hour extraction period under their conditions. McCance and Widdowson[30] used a 2-hour extraction period for their analyses, whereas Young[31] did not address the extraction time issue for her analytical method. Oberleas[27] suggested that overnight extractions would represent an 8- to 16-hr extraction time. Since too much extraction is a non-issue, certainly the extraction time was not a factor in the analyses; however, in retrospect, this lengthy extraction time was not essential. When incorporating the anion-exchange concept into quantitative phytate analysis, Harland and Oberleas[32] considered a 2-hour extraction period appropriate. With the introduction of HPLC to the analysis of phytate, Tangendjaja et al.,[25] Camire and Clydesdale,[33] and Cilliers and van Niekerk[24] each used a 2-hour extraction time with 3% TCA as the extracting reagent. Graf and Dintzis[28] used 2 hours, but extraction was with 0.5 *N* HCl. In none of these studies were objective data provided indicating an ideal extraction time. Only Young[31] indicated subjectively that repeated extractions did not improve the analysis. The best extraction time remains to be determined. With ideal conditions, it appears that 2 hours is the minimum extraction time that can be recommended and 3 hours may be optimum.

Sample-To-Solvent Extraction Ratio

Another factor to be considered is the ratio of the sample weight to the volume of the appropriate solvent. Averill and King[20] were the first investigators to analyze a large number of foodstuffs. They used a sample-to-solvent ratio of 1:25 of 2% HCl. Earley and DeTurk[34] and Earley[35] used a sample-to-solvent ratio of 1:20. Haug and Lantzsch[36] varied the sample size from 0.005 to 0.06 g of sample, depending on an estimated phytate content and extracted with 10 mL of extractant. This provides sample-to-solvent ratios from 167 to 2000, but, unfortunately, they were extracting with 0.2 N HCl, a solvent concentration that would not provide consistently reliable extractions. McCance and Widdowson[30] used a more casual 5–10 g of dried, finely ground material with 100 mL 0.5 N HCl, giving a sample-to-solvent ratio of between 10 and 20. The standard appeared to be 20 for several years,[27,32] until high-performance liquid chromatography (HPLC) entered the analytical scene. Tangendjaja et al.[25] used a 1:10 ratio with 3% TCA, and this was followed quickly by others who tested their method.[24] Graf and Dintzis[28] performed their analyses following extraction with a 1:20 sample-to-solvent ratio of 0.5 N HCl. Samples in Table 3.7.1 were extracted with 1:10 sample-to-solvent ratios.

In the final analysis, when developing an analytical method for quantitation of phytate, the following considerations appear to be important for extraction of the samples: (1) an adequate concentration of an appropriate acid, either 0.5 or 0.66 mol/l HCl or 10% TCA, (2) gentle agitation for a period of at least 2 and possibly 3 hours, and (3) a sample-to-solvent ratio of at least 1:10 (w/v).

Purification Methods

With consideration of the multitude of possible food matrices, extraction with one of the appropriate extraction acids includes several acid-soluble compounds. Each of these compounds will react according to its chemical nature within the reaction system. This was shown by Heubner and Stadler[18] when the precipitation of white ferric phytate in their titration system made the observation of the pink titration endpoint difficult and thus compromised the accuracy and sensitivity of that original method. This observation was repeated subsequently by Rather,[19] Averill and King,[20] McCance and Widdowson,[30] and Young.[38] This caused Earley and DeTurk[34] to modify the analytical method to precipitate acid-insoluble ferric phytate in dilute acid and collect the resulting precipitate on asbestos pads in Gooch crucibles which could then be dry-ashed. The resulting phosphate was eluted with acid and quantified colorimetrically. Modifications of the iron precipitation purification were then developed. Oberleas[27] conducted the ferric phytate precipitation in a 50-mL centrifuge tube, washed the precipitate with dilute acid, and wet-ashed prior to colorimetric phosphate analysis.

Detection Methods

It has been acknowledged that because of the nature of the phytate molecule, no useful UV or visible spectra are available. Dependence on wet chemistry methods and improved technology has provided alternatives that have served well, though some methods were nonspecific and most were laborious.

HPLC has the potential to become the panacea for phytate and inositol phosphate ester analysis, both qualitative and quantitative. The differential refractive index detector was the first successful detector to be applied to HPLC analysis of phytate.[25] However, this detector has several disadvantages. First, it is the least sensitive of the detectors available; second, it must be used in an isocratic system; and third, it is nonspecific because it detects only a change in the refractive index. This could be caused by any substance not present in the mobile phase. Using a reverse phase, C-18 column, most phytate peaks elute with the void volume in 2 to 4 min, depending on the flow rate.[25,28,33,37] Lee and Abendroth[38] were concerned by the lack of retention and thus added tetrabutylammonium hydroxide as an ion pair. In this system the void volume was 1.3 min, whereas phytate elution could be varied from 4.75 min to 11.3 min. The higher the concentration of the ion pair, the shorter was the elution time. The detection limit was reported at 2 ng and linearity was reported up to 40 μg of phytate. Other HPLC methodology variations include the isocratic anion exchange columns with post column derivatization.[39,40] These methods were non-specific for phytate.

A unique gradient HPLC method was reported by Rounds and Nielsen.[41] This method provides both a specific separation and quantitative detection to about 3–5 nmol. This can be adapted to provide both qualitative and quantitative detection of phytate and other inositol phosphates. It is being described in greater detail because the described modification of this method is being pursued for submission to AOAC International for consideration as an "Official Method."

FERRIC IRON-TO-SULFOSALICYLIC ACID HPLC PHYTATE ANALYSIS METHODS

Equipment

The following equipment is necessary when using this method for the analysis of phytate. Brand names are not used because several brands are available that are equally effective. A typical layout of the instrumentation is shown in Figure 3.7.1.

1. A pumping unit capable of creating a gradient.
2. A UV/Vis detector capable of monitoring specific wavelengths. In this method that wavelength is 500 nm (Figure 3.7.2). This detector may be connected to a recorder, a digital printout or single computer with appropriate software, or a computer network with appropriate analytical software.
3. An autosampler is not essential but is a convenient component to the system. The autosampler usually may be programmed for injection volume and the multiple number of injections per sample. The system may be programmed for a large number of samples, allowing the analyses to be performed over an extended period of time without close monitoring.
4. Some means of recording the output for analysis is essential. This may be as simple as an analog recorder. There is computer software capable of digitizing the output data, analyzing these data, and printing the results. An analog/digital converter between the detector and the computer network allows the data to be transmitted to a centralized network server unit.
5. A secondary pump is necessary for pumping Wade's reagent, which is used for post column reaction with phytate and inositol phosphates.

Several accessory items are needed to complete the HPLC system for the analyses of phytate.

1. Inline check valve (two required). These are absolutely necessary because of the pressure differentials that may be generated between the gradient pump and the reagent pump. These check valves require very small (i.e., 1.5 psi) breaking pressure and must sustain a sizeable (i.e., 5000 psi) reverse pressure. This is necessary so that at any time, gradient reagents do not back up into the Wade's reagent and vice versa.
2. A mixing tee, mixing cross, or similar device is needed for the initial mixing of all reagents combined to complete the analytical reaction.
3. A sample loop, mixing loop, web, etc. of the same dimensions (0.020" [0.5 mm] ID × 1/16" OD by 200 cm) as the operating tubing. This mixing loop is used to obtain thorough mixing of the post-column reactants.
4. PEEK or similar tubing, 0.020" [0.5 mm] ID × 1/16" OD, was adequate for connecting all of the necessary components of the system.

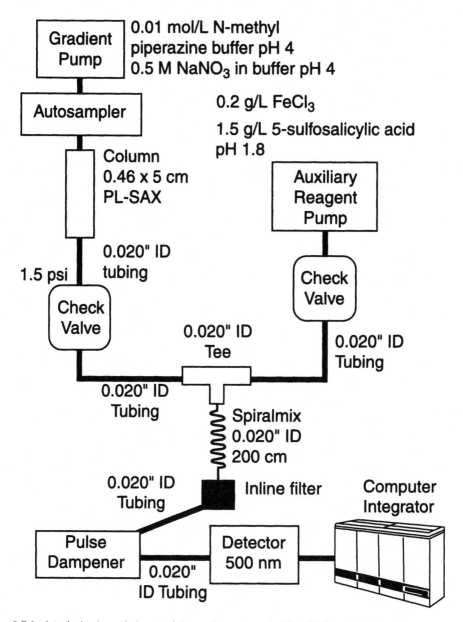

Figure 3.7.1 A typical schematic layout of the equipment needed for HPLC analysis for phytate.

5. PEEK or similar fittings and ferrules with appropriate thread pattern to connect the tubing with the HPLC system.
6. An inline filter with 0.45-μm filter frits that can be easily removed and the frits exchanged as frequently as needed. The frits should be easy to replace and may be recycled by sonication with detergent or, when necessary, 30% HNO_3, then rinsed by sonication with water. Clogged filter frits may create considerable noise in the analytical curves.
7. A pulse damper is necessary to smooth the flow following passage through the inline filter. This should be a low-volume damper.
8. A PL SAX (50 × 4.6 mm, particle size 8 μm, 100 nm pore type) or equivalent anion exchange column. This column is suitable for 20 μL injections of sample. A smaller column, 8 μm, 1000 Å, stainless steel, 50 × 2.1 mm, is available and may be successful with some HPLC systems. With this smaller column, 5 μL samples may be used.

Peak: IP6

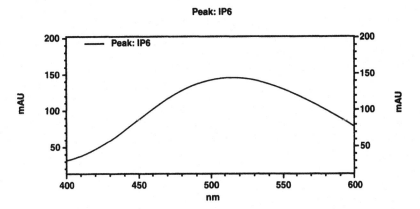

Figure 3.7.2 A visible spectrum of the ferric sulfosalicylate complex for the analysis for phytate.

Reagents

1. N-methyl piperazine (FW100.17) (corrosive, toxic, hygroscopic, combustible), pK about 4.3.
2. Sodium nitrate (FW 84.99) (strong oxidizer, toxic irritant, hygroscopic) or sodium chloride (FW 58.44) (irritation, systemic toxicity), reagent grade.
3. Ferric chloride (FW 270.30) (harmful solid, corrosive, hygroscopic), reagent grade.
4. 5-sulfosalicylic acid (FW 239.25) (corrosive), reagent grade.
5. Trichloroacetic acid, reagent grade or hydrochloric acid, reagent grade.
6. Sodium phytate (hygroscopic), 99% purified, used for standards. Obtain a Certificate of Analysis or standardize as described below.

Solutions

Two systems have been tested and work equally satisfactorily. One system utilizes N-methyl piperazine·HNO_3 buffer with sodium nitrate as the gradient; the second system utilizes the N-methyl piperazine buffer with sodium chloride as the gradient. As a displacement anion, either nitrate or chloride ions have similar properties.[42]

1. 0.01 mol/L methyl piperazine·HNO_3 buffer (pH 4.0). Weigh 1.0 g/L of N-methyl piperazine into a small beaker. Wash into an appropriate graduate cylinder containing about 500 mL of HPLC-grade water (milliQ water is satisfactory). Fill to volume with HPLC-grade water. Stir for about 5 min with a magnetic stirrer. The initial pH of this buffer is about 10. This should be adjusted to pH 4 with either 1 mol/L nitric acid or 1 mol/L hydrochloric acid, depending upon which system is being utilized. Filter through 0.45-μm nylon filter, degas with helium at 25 mL/min or a vacuum degasser if available with the HPLC system. Store in a stoppered clear glass bottle at room temperature. This is a stable reagent.
2. 0.5 mol/L sodium nitrate in 0.01 mol/L methyl piperazine·HNO_3 buffer (pH 4.0). Weigh 42.5 g sodium nitrate, place into a 1-L graduate cylinder, make to volume with buffer. Alternatively, weigh the sodium nitrate and 1 g of N-methyl-piperazine and make to volume. Adjust to pH 4.0 with 1 mol/L nitric acid, filter through 0.45 μm nylon filter, degas as above. (With some HPLC systems it may be necessary to increase the sodium nitrate concentration to 0.6 mol/L or 51.0 g/L to effect separations within the operating framework.) The pK of N-methyl-piperazine is about 4.2–4.3. These solutions are colorless and stable.
3. Alternate: 0.7 mol/L sodium chloride in 0.01 mol/L methyl piperazine·HCl buffer (pH 4.0). Weigh 40.9 g sodium chloride, place into a 1-L graduate cylinder, make to volume with buffer adjusted with 1 mol/L HCl. Alternatively, weigh the sodium chloride and 1 g of N-methyl-piperazine and make to volume. Adjust to pH 4.0 with 1 mol/L hydrochloric acid, filter through 0.45 μm nylon filter, degas as above. The buffered solutions are prepared as above and adjusted to pH 4 with

1 mol/L HCl. The initial pH for the piperazine solutions will be 9 to 10.5. This solution is colorless and stable when stored in a stoppered glass bottle at room temperature.

4. Wade's reagent. Weigh 0.2 g (0.74 mmol) ferric chloride·6H$_2$O. Weigh 1.5 g (6.87 mmol) 5-sulfosalicylic acid (SSA). Combine into a 1-L graduate cylinder, make to volume with HPLC-grade water, adjust to pH 1.8 with 1 mol/L HNO$_3$ or HCl as appropriate, filter through 0.45-μm nylon filter, store in brown glass bottle. This is a light-sensitive reagent but is stable for several months in a stoppered brown glass bottle at room temperature. This combination provides a 9.2:1 molar ratio of SSA to Fe in the reagent solution. Wade's reagent, ferric chloride and sulfosalicylic acid, initially should have a pH of 2.5–3.0. This solution will be reddish-purple in color; that is the reaction between ferric iron and sulfosalicylic acid. It has an absorbance maximum of 500 nm. Sulfosalicylic acid appears to have a pK of about 2–2.2 that provides some buffering in that pH range.

Extracting Solutions

As noted earlier, three extracting solutions are equally effective in extracting phytate, phosphate, and inositol phosphates from several food samples.

1. Trichloroacetic acid (10%): Weigh 100 g of TCA, make to 1 L with HPLC grade water. Filter through 0.45-μm nylon filter, store in a stoppered clean glass bottle. This reagent is stable for an extended period of time when stored at room temperature.
2. 0.5 M HCl: Measure 41.8 mL of concentrated HCl and make to 1 L. Filter through 0.45-μm nylon filter and store in a stoppered clean glass bottle. This is a very stable reagent for an extended period of time when stored at room temperature.
3. 0.66 M HCl: Measure 54 mL of concentrated HCl and make to 1 L. Filter through 0.45-μm nylon filter, store in a stoppered clean glass bottle. This is a very stable reagent for an extended period of time when stored at room temperature.

Preparation of Standards

Label information of sodium phytate as purchased is not reliable for standard preparation. A "Certificate of Analysis" based on the lot number may be available from the supplier which contains more detailed and more accurate information on each lot of sodium phytate. This may be available for download via the Internet using the lot number as the reference or may be requested from the supplier. As with many techniques, the results of analyses for phytate are determined by the care in preparation and accuracy of the standards. Dodecasodium phytate (FW 923.8) as purchased is adequate for standards with some precautions. The molecular weight of undissociated phytic acid (MW 660) has classically been used in the calculation of phytate equivalent from phosphate content of purified, ashed sodium phytate. There has been no absolute agreement that the phytate should be expressed on the basis of the undissociated phytic acid equivalent or MW 648, which is the molecular weight of the totally dissociated anion that is the active species. It makes little difference as long as everyone is consistent in this usage. Tradition has been to use MW 660 in all calculations where the specific species is not apparent. The analysis varies slightly from lot to lot and thus must be recalculated from the "Certificate of Analysis," which provides precise information for each lot, or the phytate must be restandardized within the laboratory.

Phosphorus or phosphate is one entity that can be reanalyzed by most laboratories to update the sodium phytate for use as a standard. Thus, procedures for restandardization of phytate are included later in this chapter. Calcium is variable for different lots and must be corrected individually. Water is a critical variable that may change with different climates and, in some cases, with different seasons of the year. Sodium phytate has a tendency to be hygroscopic and therefore must be stored carefully to prevent water accumulation. This can always be corrected if needed by phosphate analysis. Therefore, the weight of sodium phytate as purchased made to

100 mL with HPLC grade water to provide 1 g of phytic acid/100 mL is not constant and must be determined by each laboratory for the lot of sodium phytate utilized.

To calculate the weight of dodecasodium phytate as purchased for your standard, utilize the percent phosphorus (g/100 g) from the "Certificate of Analysis." Divide this by 0.282 (fractional portion of phosphorus in phytic acid; MW 660) or the percentage of phytic acid based on phosphorus analysis. To obtain 1 g phytate per 100 mL, divide 1 g by the fractional portion of phytic acid to obtain the grams of that lot necessary to obtain that 1 g, and dilute to 100 mL with 0.5 N HCl to correct for acid effects.

This would be equivalent to 200 μg (303 nmol) phytate (MW 660)/20 μL injection and is the stock standard. Working standards are prepared by dilution of the stock standard, i.e., 1:4 = 50 μg (75.7 nmol); 1:8–25 μg (37.9 nmol); 1:10 = 20 μg (30 nmol); 1:25 = 8 μg (12.1 nmol); and 1:50 = 4 μg (6 nmol) per 20 μL injection.

For 5-μL injection, dilutions of stock standard would be 1:2 = 25 μg (37.85 nmol); 1:4 = 12.5 μg (18.925 nmol); 1:10 = 5.0 μg (7.5 nmol); 1:25 = 2.0 μg (3.025 nmol); and 1:50 = 1 μg (1.5 nmol). The 1:50 may be below the detection limit for some instruments.

Procedure

The prepared solutions are placed in their appropriate locations. The N-methyl piperazine may also be used as the wash solution for washing the injection needle of the autosampler. The piperazine buffer and gradient solutions are pumped with the gradient pump; Wade's reagent is pumped with the auxiliary pump. The piperazine buffer and Wade's reagent are pumped until stability is reflected on the detector and system pressures are stabilized. The instrument operates at relatively low pressures, but these pressures may be different for each analytical HPLC system. Several parameters should be monitored, i.e., pressures of both pumps, pH of the final eluent, flow rate of each pump, and total flow rate.

The principle of the method is to separate inorganic phosphate and the various inositol phosphates in the sample by eluting them from the column with the gradient of $NaNO_3$ or NaCl. The buffer or buffered gradient mixed with the Wade's reagent forms a stable baseline. When phosphate or inositol phosphates are eluted from the column, they form a more stable complex with ferric iron than does sulfosalicylic acid. Thus, they displace ferric iron from the colored complex, reducing the color produced by the complex. Ferric phytate is white and thus decreases the color produced by the ferric sulfosalicylate reaction. The decreased color is recorded as a decreased absorbance and is proportional to the concentration of phytate or inositol phosphates in the eluting sample. Negative peaks are an inherent part of this procedure but can be made positive by reversing the polarity of the recording instrument or inverting the peaks within the software of most instrument outputs. The mechanism for accomplishing this is otherwise individual for each of the software systems available.

Instrumentation Conditions

Equilibrate the system with 1 mL/min N-methyl piperazine buffer and 0.5 mL/min Wade's reagent until the absorbance changes only minimally. The following are typical operating conditions, but these may vary slightly for different systems:

A. Column — PL-SAX or equivalent strong anion exchange column.
B. Column temperature — ambient.
C. Gradient — 100% N-methyl piperazine buffer at baseline or zero time; 100% buffered salt (nitrate or chloride) at the end of the run (26 or 30 minutes).
D. Injector temperature — ambient.
E. Detector — Visible region, 500 nm.
F. Injection volume — 5 or 20 μL, depending on column diameter.

G. Total run time — 31 or 36 min, which sometimes varies with different HPLC systems and buffered salt concentrations.

H. Gradient time — 26 or 30 min, again dependent upon different HPLC systems and choice of buffered salt concentrations.

I. Flow rate — 1 mL/min for the baseline buffer and gradient buffer salt solutions. 0.5 mL/min Wade's reagent.

J. Pressures — 200–400 pounds per square inch (psi) or equivalent should be appropriate for starting or baseline pressures. When pressures increase above 1000–1200 psi, this should be an indication of a need to change filter frits or locate a precipitate plug in the system. Cautions are discussed below.

Extraction of Samples

Three extraction solutions were shown to be comparable for extracting samples. When tested on identical samples, 10% trichloroacetic acid, 0.5 mol/L HCl, or 0.66 mol/L HCl gave results that were not different statistically. Neither 3% TCA nor 5% TCA provided comparable results when used as extracting solutions. Recovery studies that add very water-soluble sodium phytate to a sample and consider the recovery of this as a measure of completeness of recovery from the matrix are not adequate as a measure of completeness of recovery from the matrix. Food matrices are too complex for this criterion to be meaningful.

Weigh approximately 1 g of sample (1.0000–1.2000 g is a good guide) and place 10 mL of one of the extracting solutions on the sample. Stir vigorously to be certain the sample is wet throughout. Place the samples on the appropriate device for gentle agitation. It is important that the samples be extracted by gentle agitation over a large surface area. This may be accomplished in several ways. A 50-mL polyethylene or polypropylene centrifuge tube with a screw cap may be satisfactory. It may be necessary to mix the tubes on a vortex before shaking and at about the midpoint, to assure that all of the sample is wet and to incorporate that which is clinging to the side of the tube into the extraction process. These tubes laid on their sides and taped to an orbital shaker or other mild shaking device should serve satisfactorily. A 125-mL Erlenmeyer flask will serve well, either on an orbital shaking platform, a dry Dubnoff shaking incubator, a radial arm shaker at low speed, or some other device that will roll or shake gently over the large surface at the bottom of the flask. Samples should be shaken for a minimum of 2 h but preferably 3 or more hours. Depending on circumstances, samples may be shaken overnight.

After extraction, the extract must be removed from the matrix. This can be accomplished in several ways. If the centrifuge tubes are used for extraction, they may be centrifuged using a clinical centrifuge at about 3500 rpm (~1800 g) for 20 minutes (a high-speed centrifuge is not necessary). At this point several secondary measures may be taken. First, the extracting solution may be removed from the top of the centrifuge tube with a Pasteur pipet, placed in a micro-centrifuge tube, and centrifuged a second time using a higher-speed centrifuge for 10 min. Transfer the supernatant with a Pasteur pipet directly to a HPLC vial. Second, the extractant from the first centrifugation may be placed into a 3-mL polyethylene syringe and forced through a 0.45-µm nylon filter directly into a HPLC vial. Third, if extraction was done in an Erlenmeyer flask, the sample may be filtered with gravity or vacuum through Whatman #1, 2, or equivalent filter paper. Then place some filtrate into a micro-centrifuge tube as above or force it through a 0.45-µm filter.

Precautions

Ferric phytate is insoluble in dilute acid and forms a precipitate in the system. This is effectively removed by the inline filter frit. The frits must be exchanged or cleaned frequently; otherwise, pressures may increase rapidly. These frits can be readily cleaned in one of several ways. The filter can be cleaned by pumping 0.2 mol/L sodium hydroxide through the reagent side only, then flushing thoroughly with water. The filter frits may be removed and replaced with clean filter frits. The plugged filter frits then can be collected and sonicated with dilute, mild detergent or, if necessary, with 30% nitric acid, rinsed by sonication with water, and recycled. Sometimes more than one procedure is needed.

When the phytate reaction occurs, the ideal window of reaction should occur between pH 1.5 and 2.5. For this reaction to be most stable, all solutions are adjusted to specific pH's of 4 for the buffered solutions and 1.8 for the Wade's reagent. This provides a final pH of 2.1–2.2 at most times. This is not the pH of maximum precipitation for ferric phytate, which is about 1, but provides a stable environment for the reaction to occur.

RESTANDARDIZATION OF SODIUM PHYTATE

Though sodium phytate as purchased is quite stable and free of most contaminating phosphate compounds, there may be occasions that necessitate the analysis and standardization for use as a standard, i.e., inability to obtain a "Certificate of Analysis," long-term storage, etc. It will be necessary to be able to analyze the inorganic phosphate in the presence of and without hydrolyzing any phytate. Total phosphate following an ashing procedure is also needed. This phosphate procedure is a modification of the Fiske–Subbarow[43] method. It has a long history, has stable reagents, and can be read from 640 to 720 nm with equal sensitivity.

Reagents

1. Sulfuric (sulphuric) acid (5 N). Dilute 70 mL of concentrated sulfuric acid to 500 mL. Stable reagent.
2. Ammonium molybdate reagent. Dissolve 12.5 g ammonium molybdate in 200 mL water. Transfer to a 500-mL volumetric flask, add 100 mL 5 N sulfuric acid, and dilute to volume with water. This is a stable reagent.
3. Sulfonic acid reagent (1-amino-2-naphthol-4-sulfonic acid). Dissolve 0.16 g 1-amino-2-naphthol-4-sulfonic acid, 1.92 g sodium sulfite, and 9.6 g sodium bisulfite in about 90 mL water. Heat to dissolve if necessary. Quantitatively transfer to 100-mL volumetric flask. Make to volume with water. Store in brown bottle or cover flask with brown paper or aluminum foil and refrigerate. Stable for at least 2 weeks.

Standard Phosphate Solution

Stock phosphate solution. Prepare a standard solution by weighing 0.1757 g of dried, dessicated, potassium dihydrogen phosphate (primary standard) per liter in a volumetric flask. Add 20 mL 5 N sulfuric acid and make to volume with water. This solution contains 40 mg P (as phosphate) per liter (40 µg/mL). Dilute as necessary to obtain other standard concentrations.

Procedure

This can be done in 25- or 50-mL volumetric flasks, provided the standard curve is determined in the same-sized flasks. Pipette blank (water), standard, or sample (in duplicate or triplicate) into an appropriate set of flasks. Add distilled water to about 10 or 20 mL, depending on flask size. Mix thoroughly. Add 2 mL molybdate reagent; mix well. Add 1 mL sulfonic acid reagent, dilute to volume, and mix well. Wait 15 min and read at 640 nm. The peak for this reaction is about 910 nm, but the slope is so gradual as to provide stability at 640 nm, which is within the capability of all spectrophotometers.

Total Phosphate

After measuring the inorganic phosphate, it is necessary to hydrolyze the phytate and measure the total phosphate. There are several important considerations necessary when wet-ashing samples for phosphate analysis. Phosphoric acid has several forms which boil at fairly low temperatures. According to the *Handbook of Chemistry and Physics*, hypophosphoric acid decomposes at 100°C, metaphosphoric acid sublimates, and orthophosphoric acid decomposes at temperatures less than 213°C. Various forms of phosphorus acids decompose or boil below 200°C. The importance of all this is that it is necessary to hydrolyze the phytate samples completely, the wet-ash must be at as low a temperature as possible, and the heating time should be the minimum required. Otherwise, variability may be encountered in phosphate content by any or all of the above.

Procedure

Pipette a measured aliquot of phytate solution to be standardized into a microkjeldahl flask or 25×200 mm digestion tubes. Add 0.5 mL concentrated sulfuric acid to each tube. Add 2 mL of 30% hydrogen peroxide to each tube. Add two boiling beads to each tube. Heat on a microkjeldahl digestion rack or block heater until only the sulfuric acid remains. If the digestion solution is clear, digestion is complete; in the event of any color or turbidity, cool to touch, add 1 mL 30% hydrogen peroxide, and continue heating as before. Continue the process until a clear solution results. Quantitatively transfer samples to appropriate volumetric flasks and continue color development and measurement as above.

Calculations

The calculation of phytate concentrations from the analyses begins with the understanding of the formula from the Beer–Lambert Law as follows:

$$\frac{\text{Concentration}_{\text{Standard}}}{\text{Absorbance (Response)}_{\text{Standard}}} = \frac{\text{Concentration}_{\text{Sample}}}{\text{Absorbance (Response)}_{\text{Sample}}}$$

$$\text{Sum [Concentration}_{\text{Standard}} / \text{Absorbance (Response)}_{\text{Standard}}] / n_{\text{Standards}} = \text{Mean K}$$

$$\text{Mean K} \times \text{R} \times \text{W} \times \text{M} = \text{mg phytate/g sample}$$

where

$\quad$ Mean K $\quad$ = mean of the concentrations (nmol)/response (area) for standards

$\quad R_{5 \text{ or } 20 \text{ mL}}$ $\quad$ = $\text{Response}_{\text{Sample}}$

$\quad W_{5 \text{ mL}}$ $\quad$ = 2000 ($20 \times 10 \times 10$ mL extractant/sample weight (g)) [corrects for volume and weight of sample] (5 mL $\times$ 20 = 0.1 mL) (0.1 mL $\times$ 10 = 1.0 mL) (1.0 mL $\times$ 10 mL extractant corrects for volume of extractant)

$\quad W_{20 \text{ mL}}$ $\quad$ = 500 ($5 \times 10 \times 10$ mL extractant)/sample weight (g) [corrects for volume and weight of sample] (20 mL $\times$ 5 = 0.1 mL), etc.

$\quad M_{5 \text{ or } 20 \text{ mL}}$ = 660 (MW)/10^6 [Corrects for nmol/g to mg/g]

$\qquad$ multiply mg/g phytate by 1000 = mg phytate/kg sample

$\qquad$ multiply mg/g phytate by 100/1000 = % phytate in sample

Molar Ratios

When calculating this ratio, it is important that the initial units of both components be the same (i.e., mg/kg, mg/100 g, g/kg, etc.):

$$\frac{\dfrac{\text{mg/kg phytate}}{660 \text{ (MW)}}}{\dfrac{\text{mg/kg zinc}}{65.4 \text{ (At wt)}}} = \text{Phytate:Zinc molar ratio}$$

When calculating [Ca][Phytate]/Zn molar ratio, which is more precise, it is necessary to convert all components to grams per kilogram and thus the appropriate definition of molar.

$$\frac{\dfrac{\text{g/kg phytate}}{660 \text{ (MW)}} \times \dfrac{\text{g/kg calcium}}{40.1 \text{ (At wt)}}}{\dfrac{\text{g/kg zinc}}{65.4 \text{ (At wt)}}} = [\text{Calcium}][\text{Phytate}]:[\text{Zinc}] \text{ molar ratio}$$

ACKNOWLEDGMENT

The HPLC method described above was developed in the laboratories and with the assistance and cooperation of Gerber Products Company, Fremont, Michigan, and its employees. This assistance is greatly appreciated.

REFERENCES

1. Oberleas, D., The determination of phytate and inositol phosphates, in *Methods of Biochemical Analysis*, vol. 20, Glick, D., Ed., Wiley, New York, 1971, 87.
2. Cosgrove, D. J., *Inositol Phosphates*, Elsevier, Amsterdam, 1980, 12.
3. Cheryan, M., Phytic acid interactions in food systems, *CRC Crit. Revs. Food Sci. Nutr.*, 1980, 297.
4. Maga, J. A., Phytate: its chemistry, occurrence, food interactions, nutritional significance, and methods of analysis, *J. Agri. Food Chem.*, 30, 1, 1982.
5. Oberleas, D., Phytate content in cereals and legumes and methods of determination, *Cereal Foods World*, 28, 352, 1983.
6. Oberleas, D. and Harland, B. F., Analytical methods for phytate, in *Phytic Acid: Chemistry and Applications*, Graf, E., Ed., Pilatus Press, Minneapolis, 1986, 77.
7. Wade, H. E. and Morgan, D. M., Fractionation of phosphates by paper ionophoresis and chromatography, *Biochem. J.*, 60, 264, 1955.
8. Sobolev, A. M. and Vyskrebentseva, E. I., The problem of identification of organic acid-soluble phosphorus compounds in plants by means of regulated paper chromatography, *Fiziol. Rastenii*, 6, 257, 1958.
9. Smith, D. H. and Clark, F. E., Chromatographic separations of inositol phosphorus compounds, *Soil Sci. Soc. Proc.*, 1952, 170.
10. Tomlinson, R. V. and Ballou, C. E., Myoinositol polyphosphate intermediates in the dephosphorylation of phytic acid by phytase, *Biochem.*, 1, 166, 1962.
11. Cosgrove, D. J., The isolation of *myo*inositol pentaphosphates from hydrolysates of phytic acid, *Biochem. J.*, 89, 172, 1963.
12. Cosgrove, D. J., The chemistry and biochemistry of inositol polyphosphates, *Rev. Pure Appl. Chem.*, 16, 209, 1966.
13. Cosgrove, D. J., Ion-exchange chromatography of inositol polyphosphates, *Ann. N.Y. Acad. Sci.*, 165, 677, 1969.
14. Cosgrove, D. J., Chemical nature of soil organic phosphorus. II. Characterization of the supposed DL *chiro*-inositol hexaphosphate component of soil phytate as D *chiro*-inositol hexaphosphate, *Soil Biol. Biochem.*, 1, 325, 1969.
15. Irving, G. C. J. and Cosgrove, D. J., Inositol phosphate phosphatases of microbiological origin. Inositol pentaphosphate products of *Aspergillus ficuum* phytases, *J. Bacteriol.*, 112, 434, 1972.

16. Cosgrove, D. J., Inositol phosphate phosphatases of microbiological origin. Inositol phosphate inter-mediates in the dephosphorylation of the hexaphosphates of *myo*-inositol, *scyllo*-inositol and D-*chiro*-inositol by a bacterial species (*Pseudomonas sp.*) phytase, *Aust. J. Biol. Sci.*, 23, 1207, 1970.

17. Cosgrove, D. J., Phosphorylation of epi-inositol and *muco*-inositol with phosphoric acid, *Carbohydrate Res.*, 40, 380, 1975.

18. Heubner, W. and Stadler, H., Uber eine Titration-methode zur Bestimmung des Phytins, *Biochem. Z.*, 64, 422, 1914.

19. Rather, J. B., Determination of phytin phosphorus in plant products, *J. Am. Chem. Soc.*, 39, 2506, 1917.

20. Averill, H. P. and King, C. G., The phytin content of foodstuffs, *J. Am. Chem. Soc.*, 48, 724, 1926.

21. Latta, M. and Eskin, M., A simple and rapid colorimetric method for phytate determination, *J. Agri. Food Chem.*, 28, 1313, 1980.

22. de Lange, D. J., Joubert, C. P., and du Peez, S. F. M., The determination of phytic acid and factors which influence its hydrolysis in bread, *Proc. Nutr. Soc. S. Africa*, 2, 69, 1961.

23. Wheeler, E. L. and Ferrel, R. E., A method for phytic acid determination in wheat and wheat fractions, *Cereal Chem.*, 48, 312, 1971.

24. Cilliers, J. L. and van Niekerk, P. J., LC determination of phytic acid in food by postcolumn colorimetric detection, *J. Agri. Food Chem.*, 34, 680, 1986.

25. Tangendjaja, B., Buckle, K. A., and Wootton, M., Analysis of phytic acid by high-performance liquid chromatography, *J. Chromat.*, 197, 274, 1980.

26. Bos, K. D., Verbeek, C., van Eeden, C. H. P., Slump, P., and Wolters, M. G. E., Improved determination of phytate by ion-exchange chromatography, *J. Agri. Food Chem.*, 39, 1770, 1991.

27. Oberleas, D., Dietary Factors Affecting Zinc Availability, Ph.D. dissertation, University of Missouri-Columbia, 1964.

28. Graf, E. and Dintzis, F. R., High-performance liquid chromatographic method for the determination of phytate, *Anal. Biochem.*, 119, 413, 1982.

29. Samotus, B. and Schwimmer, S., Phytic acid as a phosphorus reservoir in the developing potato tuber, *Nature*, 194, 578, 1962.

30. McCance, R. A. and Widdowson, E. M., Phytin in human nutrition. *Biochem. J.*, 29, 2694, 1935.

31. Young, L., The determination of phytic acid, *Biochem. J.*, 30, 252, 1936.

32. Harland, B. F. and Oberleas, D., A modified method for phytate analysis using an ion-exchange procedure: application to textured vegetable proteins, *Cereal Chem.*, 54, 827, 1977.

33. Camire, A. L. and Clydesdale, F. M., Analysis of phytic acid in foods by HPLC, *J. Food Sci.*, 47, 575, 1982.

34. Earley, E. B. and DeTurk, E. E., Time and rate of synthesis of phytin in corn grain during reproductive period, *J. Am. Soc. Agron.*, 36, 803, 1944.

35. Earley, E. B., Determining phytin phosphorus: stoichiometric relation of iron and phosphorus in ferric phytate, *Anal. Chem.*, 16, 389, 1944.

36. Haug, W. and Lantzsch, H-J., Sensitive method for rapid determination of phytate in cereals and cereal products, *J. Sci. Food Agri.*, 34, 1423, 1983.

37. Graf, E. and Dintzis, F. R., Determination of phytic acid in foods by high-performance liquid chro-matography, *J. Agri. Food Chem.*, 30, 1094, 1982.

38. Lee, K. and Abendroth, J. A., High performance liquid chromatographic determination of phytic acid in foods, *J. Food Sci.*, 48, 1344, 1983.

39. Fitchett, A. W. and Woodruff, A., Determination of polyvalent anions by ion chromatography, *Liq. Chromat. HPLC*, 1, 48, 1983.

40. Phillippy, B. Q. and Johnston, M. R., Determination of phytic acid in foods by ion chromatography with post-column derivatization, *J. Food Sci.*, 50, 541, 1985.

41. Rounds, M. A. and Nielsen, S. S., Anion-exchange method for determination of phytate in foods, *J. Chromat. A*, 653, 148, 1993.

42. Snyder, L. R. and Kirkland, J. J., *Introduction to Modern Liquid Chromatography*, 2nd ed., John Wiley, New York, 1979, 410.

43. Fiske, C. H. and Subbarow, Y., The colorimetric determination of phosphorus, *J. Biol. Chem.*, 66, 375, 1925.

Determination of the Saponin Content of Foods

David Oakenfull and John D. Potter

INTRODUCTION

There is currently much interest in the nutritional properties of "phytochemicals" — plant materials present at relatively low levels in foods but with significant biological activity.[1] Saponins are one such class of phytochemicals which are present in many fiber-rich foods, particularly legumes. Their presence is relevant to human nutrition because they have been shown to increase fecal excretion of bile acids in human[2,3] and animal studies.[4-6] In particular, yucca saponins[2] and saponin-rich alfalfa seeds[7] have been shown to lower plasma cholesterol in humans.

Saponins are a structurally diverse group of triterpene or steroid glycosides.[8,9] The molecules are amphiphilic, the triterpene or steroid part being hydrophobic and the sugar part hydrophilic. This gives saponins their characteristic surface activity, from which the name is derived. The structure of a typical saponin, one of those present in soybeans, is shown in Figure 3.8.1. Saponins have been identified in many hundreds of plant species, but only a few of these are used as food by humans (see Appendix, Table 9).

There appear to be two mechanisms by which saponins can affect cholesterol metabolism:

1. Some saponins, with particularly defined structural characteristics, form insoluble complexes with cholesterol (e.g., the well-known precipitation of cholesterol by digitonin). When this complexation process occurs in the gut, it inhibits the intestinal absorption of both endogenous and exogenous cholesterol.[10]
2. Saponins can interfere with the enterohepatic circulation of bile acids by forming mixed micelles. These can have molecular weights of several millions,[11] and the reabsorption of bile acids from the terminal ileum is effectively blocked.[12]

EXTRACTION PROCEDURE

The dried plant material is first extracted with acetone, chloroform, or hexane, preferably using a Soxhlet extractor, to remove lipids, pigments, etc. The residue is then further extracted with methanol, which removes the saponins, along with many other compounds, such as simple sugars, oligosaccharides, and flavonoids.

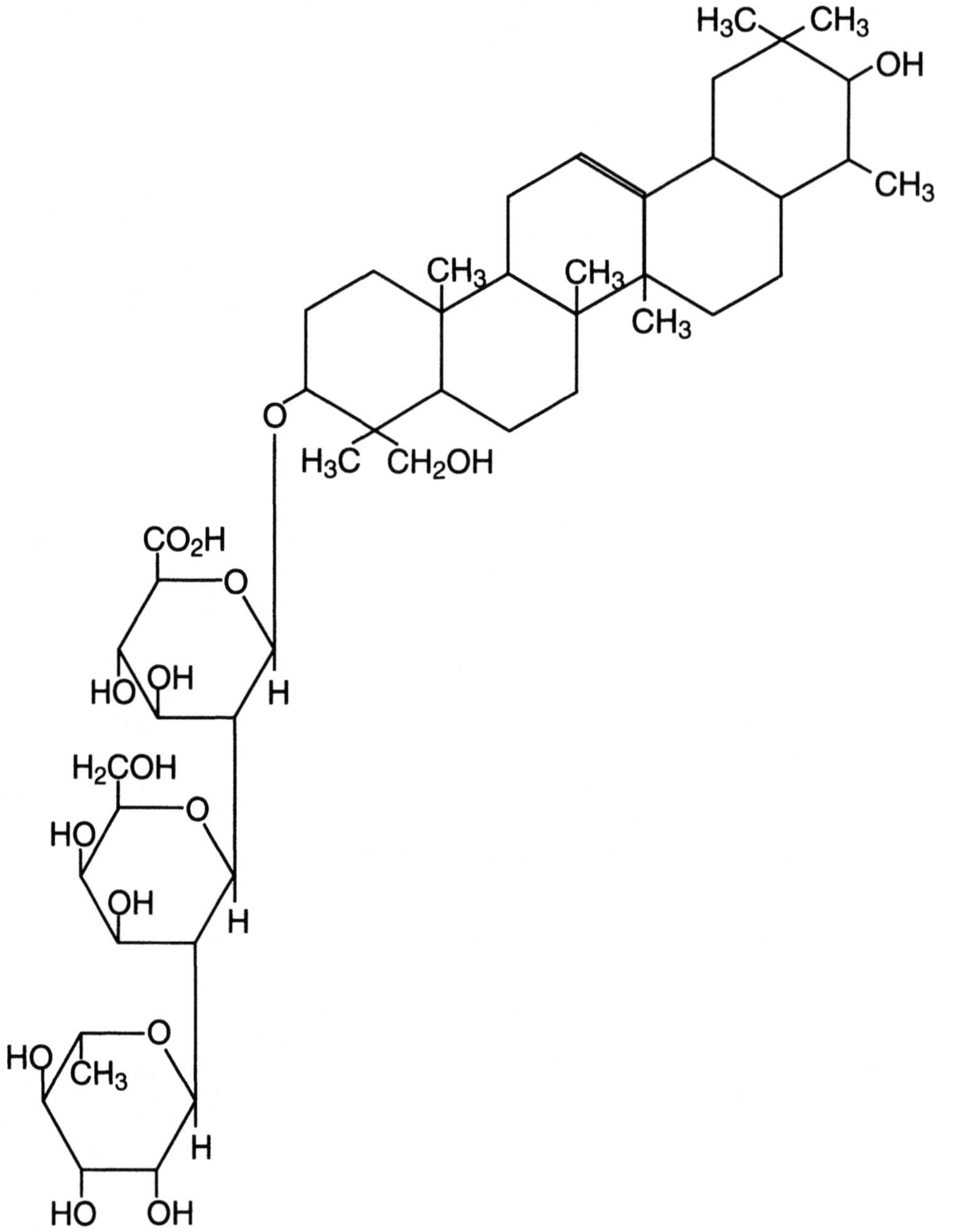

Figure 3.8.1 Structure of one of the saponins from soybeans.

METHODS OF ANALYSIS

Saponins have proved very difficult to assay, and many of the results in the literature are, at best, only approximations. For this reason, the majority of the values given in Table 3.8.1 of the Appendix are quoted as a range — there are often major discrepancies between results from different techniques and different laboratories. The difficulty is compounded by the fact that saponin content can vary considerably between different cultivars of the same plant species and can also depend on growing conditions. The major methods of analysis are thin-layer chromatography (TLC),[13,14] high-performance liquid chromatography (HPLC),[15,16] and gas chromatography with mass spectroscopy to identify the saponin (trimethylsilylated sapogenol) peaks (GC-MS).[17]

TLC

The essence of the technique is to spot a TLC plate with a crude saponin extract, develop the plate with a suitable solvent system, and use one of a number of methods for estimating the quantity of saponin on the plate. Suitable solvent systems are n-butanol–ethanol–concentrated ammonia (7:2:5) or chloroform–methanol–water (13:7:2). Spots can be visualized by spraying with 10% H_2SO_4 in ethanol or p-anisaldehyde–H_2SO_4–glacial acetic acid (1:2:100) and estimated by densitometry. The method is open to criticism in that spots may be wrongly identified as saponins or may be overlapped by other compounds (such as oligosaccharides). (However, techniques such as atomic bombardment mass spectrometry have been used to unequivocally identify the spots.[18])

HPLC

This technique has been used for the separation and analysis of both aglycones (the steroid or triterpene part of the molecule) and intact saponins. A rapid method for soybean saponins has been described[16] in which defatted soy flour is boiled under reflux with 1.5 M H_2SO_4 in dioxane–water (1:3). This hydrolyzes the saponins, and the sapogenins can then be extracted with ethyl acetate. HPLC is carried out with a commercial silica column, eluting with light petroleum–ethanol with a gradient technique. The saponin content can be estimated by assuming that the carbohydrate-to-sapogenin ratio is 1:1 (by weight).

Table 3.8.1 Plant Foods that Contain Significant Levels of Saponins and Their Estimated Saponin Content

David Oakenfull and John D. Potter

Plant	Saponin Content (g/kg dry weight)
Alfalfa sprouts (*Medicago sativa*)	80
Asparagus (*Asparagus officinalis*)	15
Broad bean (*Vicia faba*)	3.5
Chickpea (*Cicer arietinum*)	0.7–60
Green pea (*Pisum sativum*)	1.8–11
Kidney bean (*Phaseolus vulgaris*)	2–16
Lentil (*Lens culinaris*)	0.7–1.1
Mung bean (*Phaseolus mungo*)	0.5–6
Navy bean (*Phaseolus vulgaris*)	4.5–21
Oats (*Avena sativa*)	0.2–0.5
Peanut (*Arachis hypogaea*)	0.05–16
Quinoa (*Chenopodium quinoa*)	10–23
Sesame seed (*Sesamum indicum*)	3
Silver beet (*Beta vulgaris*)	58
Soy bean (*Glycine max*)	5.6–56
Spinach (*Spinacea oleracia*)	47
Sweet lupin (*Lupinus augustifolius*)	0.4–0.7

GC-MS

A method has been described in which the methanol saponin extract is evaporated to dryness and hydrolyzed by refluxing with dry HCl in methanol (5% v/v). The mixture is neutralized with ammonia and the sapogenols extracted with ethyl acetate. The dry sapogenols are derivatized by heating with bis(trimethylsilyl)trifluoroacetamide in pyridine prior to chromatography on a silica column. Quantitation is via an internal standard (cholesteryl *n*-decylate) and comparison with isolated, pure sapogenols. Peak identities are confirmed by mass spectroscopy.[18]

REFERENCES

1. Temple, N. J., Antioxidants and disease: more questions than answers, *Nutr. Res.*, 20, 449, 2000.
2. Bingham, R., Harris, D. H., and Laga, T., Yucca plant saponins in the treatment of hypertension and hypercholesterolemia, *J. Appl. Nutr.*, 30, 127, 1978.
3. Potter, J. D., Illman, R. J., Calvert, G. D., Oakenfull, D. G., and Topping, D. L., Soya saponins, plasma lipids, lipoproteins and fecal bile acids: a double-blind cross-over study, *Nutr. Rep. Int.*, 22, 521, 1980.
4. Malinow, M. R., McLaughlin, P., Kohler, G. O., and Livingston, A. L., Prevention of elevated cholesterolemia in monkeys by alfalfa saponins, *Steroids*, 29, 105, 1977.
5. Oakenfull, D. G., Fenwick, D. E., Topping, D. L., Illman, R. J., and Storer, G. B., Effects of saponins on bile acids and plasma lipids in the rat, *Br. J. Nutr.*, 42, 209, 1979.
6. Topping, D. L., Storer, G. B., Calvert, G. D., Illman, R. J., Oakenfull, D. G., and Weller, R. A., Effect of dietary saponins on fecal bile acids and neutral sterols, plasma lipids and lipoprotein turnover in the pig, *Am. J. Clin. Nutr.*, 33, 783, 1980.
7. Molgaard, J., von Schenk, H., and Olsson, A. G., Alfalfa seeds lower low density lipoprotein cholesterol and apoprotein B concentration in patients with type II hyperlipoproteinemia, *Atherosclerosis*, 65, 173, 1987.
8. Oakenfull, D. G. and Sidhu, G. S., Could saponins be a useful treatment for hypercholesterolaemia?, *Eur. J. Clin. Nutr.*, 65, 173, 1987.
9. Oakenfull, D. G. and Sidhu, G. S., Saponins, in *Toxicants of Plant Origin*, vol. 2, Cheeke, P., Ed., CRC Press, Boca Raton, FL, 1989.
10. Gestetner, B., Assa, Y., Henis, Y., Tencer, Y., Royman, M., Birk, Y., and Bondi, A., Interaction of lucerne saponins with sterols, *Biochim. Biophys. Acta*, 270, 181, 1972.
11. Oakenfull, D., Aggregation of saponins and bile acids in aqueous solution, *Aust. J. Chem.*, 39, 1671, 1986.
12. Oakenfull, D. G. and Sidhu, G. S., A physico-chemical explanation for the effects of dietary saponins on cholesterol and bile salt metabolism, *Nutr. Rep. Int.*, 27, 1253, 1983.
13. Fenwick, D. E. and Oakenfull, D. G., Saponin content of soya beans and some commercial soya products, *J. Sci. Food Agric.*, 32, 273, 1981.
14. Price, K. R., Curl, C. L., and Fenwick, G. R., The saponin content and sapogenol composition of the seed of thirteen varieties of legume, *J. Sci. Food Agric.*, 37, 115, 1986.
15. Kesselmeier, J. and Stack, D., High performance liquid chromatography analysis of steroidal saponins from *Avena sativa* L., *Z. Naturforsch.*, 36c, 1072, 1981.
16. Ireland, P. A. and Dziedzic, S. Z., High performance liquid chromatography on silica phase with evaporative light scattering detection, *J. Chromatogr.*, 361, 410, 1986.
17. Ng, K. G., Price, K. R., and Fenwick, G. R., A TLC method for the analysis of quinoa (*Chenopodium quinoa*) saponins, *Food Chem.*, 49, 311, 1994.
18. Ridout, C. L., Price, K. R., DuPont, M. S., Parker, M. L., and Fenwick, G. R., Quinoa saponins — analysis and preliminary investigations into the effects of reduction by processing, *J. Sci. Food Agric.*, 54, 165, 1991.

Physiological and Metabolic Effects of Dietary Fiber

CHAPTER **4.1**

Effect of Dietary Fiber on Protein Digestibility and Utilization

Daniel D. Gallaher and Barbara O. Schneeman

Determination and prediction of the quality of dietary protein has been a research interest almost since the beginning of nutrition as a science. For many years attention focused primarily on the evaluation of particular protein sources, either by chemical analysis or by biological assay using standardized diets. However, there is considerable interest in the influence on protein quality of dietary components other than protein. For example, the influence of digestible carbohydrates, particularly starch, has been studied extensively.[9] Dietary fiber, an indigestible carbohydrate, has also received considerable attention with regard to its effect on protein digestibility and utilization. This chapter is a collation of data from these studies.

Three pairs of tables are presented. For each pair, the first table contains information from studies using purified dietary fibers, with the second describing studies where fiber-rich sources were utilized. In all tables, information on diet composition, species studied, time period evaluated, and the method of fiber incorporation has been included to assist in evaluating the results of each study. The method of incorporation of the fiber or fiber source into the diet is of particular interest, since it influences the protein-to-calorie ratio of the diet. One of two methods is usually employed. The more common method is incorporation by substitution, in which the fiber is added to the diet at the expense of the digestible carbohydrate source. With the second method, called the dilution (or addition) method, the fiber is added to the basal or control diet, thus causing a dilution of all components of the diet.

With the substitution method, the protein content remains unchanged on a weight basis, but the protein-to-calorie ratio is increased. In contrast, with a fiber-diluted diet the protein-to-calorie ratio remains unchanged. As animals will normally consume diets to meet their energy needs,[31,32,37] incorporation of moderate amounts of fiber usually causes an increased food intake. Hence, with incorporation of fiber by substitution, animals will be consuming a greater proportion of their diet as protein than will animals fed a fiber-free or low-fiber diet. Animals fed a fiber-diluted diet, however, are likely to consume an equivalent amount of protein compared to control animals. In some studies, in which very high levels of fiber have been fed and/or weanling animals used, the animals have not been able to increase food intake sufficiently to meet their energy needs. This problem is a complicating factor in whether fiber is incorporated by substitution or dilution. The difference in the incorporation method becomes potentially significant when one considers that utilization of a protein varies with the amount of protein consumed.[26] This problem has been examined experimentally by Delorme et al.,[7] who showed that when rats were fed cellulose in the diet by the substitution method, the protein efficiency ratio (PER) decreased with increasing cellulose. However, when the diet was diluted with cellulose, the PER did not change, except at the very highest level of cellulose, where a slight decrease was noted. Thus, for experiments investigating the effect of dietary fiber on measures of protein utilization, it would appear that diet dilution is the better method of fiber incorporation.

The effect of purified dietary fibers on protein digestibility in animals and humans is presented in Table 4.1.1. In most cases, only apparent digestibility was determined. However, in those instances where both apparent and true digestibility were reported, the trend was similar for both. In most instances, purified fibers, regardless of type, reduced digestibility significantly in animals. Two carbohydrates with fiber-like properties, inulin and resistant starch, have also been shown to significantly reduce protein digestibility.[50, 53] This is consistent with several reports of increased protein in the small-intestinal contents when cellulose or wheat bran is fed.[34,35] The two human studies reported, however, showed no effect of purified fiber on digestibility.[38] Protein digestibility during consumption of fiber-rich sources is shown in Table 4.1.2. As with the purified fibers, the presence of fiber-rich sources in the diet led to significant decreases in both apparent and true digestibility in animals for all fibers for which statistics were reported. In contrast to the diets containing purified fibers, protein digestibility was lower in humans consuming the fiber-rich sources.

Fiber-rich sources usually contain significant quantities of protein which can influence the digestibility data, since part of this protein is indigestible.[13] This points out a potential difference in the source of fecal nitrogen between the purified fibers and the fiber-rich sources. For the purified fibers containing no protein (guar gum, usually considered a purified fiber, often contains a small amount of protein), the source of fecal protein must be from incomplete digestion of the dietary protein, the secreted digestive enzymes, sloughed mucosal cells, and microbial protein. In the case of fiber-rich sources, the protein associated with the fiber source will contribute to the fecal nitrogen. Thus, a low protein digestibility may be due, in part, to the presence of indigestible protein within the fiber source. Weber et al.[48] examined this possibility in cirrhotic subjects fed an animal or vegetable diet. They found that little fecal nitrogen was associated with the fecal fiber fraction, regardless of the diet. Large increases in fecal nitrogen with the vegetable diet were due to increases in the bacterial fraction and, to a lesser extent, the soluble fraction. Thus, at least for vegetable sources of fiber, fiber-associated protein appears to contribute little to fecal nitrogen.

Which attribute of dietary fiber is most responsible for the reduction in protein digestibility is unclear. Generally, the viscous and highly fermentable fibers, such as pectin and guar gum, reduce digestibility more than the nonviscous and relatively nonfermentable fibers such as cellulose on an equal weight basis. Fermentation could reduce protein digestibility by its action of promoting microbial growth, whereas viscosity could reduce digestibility by slowing protein digestion and absorption in the small intestine. Both these attributes could contribute to the effect, as they are not mutually exclusive. At this time, however, experiments feeding fiber sources that would allow the attribute most responsible for the reduced protein digestibility to be identified have not been published.

Most studies on fiber digestibility have been conducted in animals, usually rats. The question naturally arises as to how good animals are as a model for the effect of dietary fiber on protein digestibility. Bach Knudsen et al.[49] have examined this question directly by measuring protein digestibility in both humans and rats fed identical diets. They used diets containing either fruits and vegetables, a citrus fiber concentrate, or insoluble barley fiber as the fiber sources. Their results indicated that overall, apparent protein digestibilities were similar between the two species, and that the rank of the protein digestibilities of the different diets was the same for both rats and humans. Thus, rats would appear to be a very good model for humans in this context.

Table 4.1.1 Effect of Purified Dietary Fibers on Protein Digestibility

Fiber	Method of Incorporation[a]	Species Studied	Time on Diet[b] Adaptation → Balance (days)	Concentration in Diet Fiber (%)	Concentration in Diet Protein[c] (%)	Protein Digestibility Apparent (%)	Protein Digestibility True (%)	Ref.
Cellulose	Substitution	Rats, weanling ♂ and ♀	10	2.0	(10.0)	92.5 NR[d]		46
				7.0		92.0		
				12.0		90.0		
Cellulose	Substitution	Rats, weanling ♂	5 → 4	0.0	(12.0)	89.0 ± 4.7[e]NR		28
				10.0		86.0 ± 5.5		
				20.0		85.3 ± 6.9		
Cellulose	Substitution	Rats, weanling ♂	25 → 3	0.0	(8.5)	93.0 ± 1.0		19
				2.5		92.0 ± 0.7		
				5.0		90.4 ± 0.6		
				10.0		89.8 ± 1.1		
				20.0		81.6 ± 2.3		
						r = 0.851		
Cellulose	Substitution	Rats, ♂	4 to 56 → 5	0.0	(14.0)	89.7		50
				8.0		89.2		
Cellulose	Substitution	Rats, weanling ♂	25 → 3	0.0	(22.0)	94.9 ± 0.6		19
				2.5		96.1 ± 0.6		
				5.0		95.5 ± 0.8		
				10.0		92.6 ± 0.7		
				20.0		91.6 ± 0.5		
						r = −0.801		
Cellulose	Dilution	Rats, weanling ♂	21	0.0	(10.0)	92.3 ± 0.5	92.9 ± 0.5	36
				5.0	(9.5)	88.7 ± 0.6*	90.8 ± 0.8	
				10.0	(9.0)	86.4 ± 0.9*	89.2 ± 0.9*	
				20.0	(8.0)	81.9 ± 0.6*	86.2 ± 0.6*	
Cellulose	Substitution	Rats, weanling ♂	21 → 7	0.2	12.4	93.0 NR		7
				5.9	11.6	91.9		
Cellulose	Dilution	Rats, weanling ♂	21 → 7	0.1	10.4	89.3 NR		7
				4.9	9.9	90.3		
				8.9	10.0	85.9		
				16.2	8.6	85.8		
				27.5	8.3	74.7		
Cellulose	Substitution	Rats, ♂	4 → 5	5.2	9.3		100.0	2
				15.2			99.4	

Table 4.1.1 (Continued) Effect of Purified Dietary Fibers on Protein Digestibility

Fiber	Method of Incorporation[a]	Species Studied	Time on Diet[b] Adaptation → Balance (days)	Concentration in Diet Fiber (%)	Concentration in Diet Protein[c] (%)	Protein Digestibility Apparent (%)	Protein Digestibility True (%)	Ref.
Cellulose	Substitution	Mice, weanling ♂	28	5.0	(10.0)	86.7 ± 0.7		21
				10.0		82.2 ± 2.5		
				20.0		77.5 ± 3.9*		
Cellulose	Dilution	Dogs, ♀	14 → 5	0.0		37.8	90.8 ± 0.9	3
				2.9		29.5	88.8 ± 0.5	
				5.6		30.2	87.7 ± 1.0	
				8.3		28.5	87.0 ± 1.4	
							r = −0.59[f]	
Cellulose	Substitution	Rats, weanling ♂	35	0.0	10.0	92.8		12
				10.0	9.0	85.4*		
Cellulose	Dilution	Human, adult, ♀	20 → 30	9.5 g/d NDF[g] 23.5 g/d NDF	23.0	93.2 ± 0.8		38
Hemicellulose	Substitution	Mice, weanling ♂	28	5.0	(10.0)	74.4 ± 2.6		21
				10.0		67.0 ± 3.7*		
				20.0		62.0 ± 6.1*		
Xylan	Substitution	Rats, weanling ♂	35	0.0	10.0	92.8		12
				10.0	9.8	80.8		
Raffinose	Substitution	Rats, weanling ♂	35	0.0	10.0	92.8		12
				1.0	8.8	90.9		
Lignin	Substitution	Mice, weanling ♂	28	5.0	(10.0)	74.4 ± 2.6		21
				10.0		67.0 ± 3.7*		
				20.0		62.0 ± 6.1*		
Lignin	Dilution	Rats, weanling ♂	21	0.0	(10.0)	92.3 ± 0.5	92.9 ± 0.5	36
				3.0	(9.7)	89.5 ± 0.7*	90.6 ± 0.8*	
				6.0	(9.4)	84.8 ± 0.4*	87.4 ± 0.5*	
Acid detergent fiber	Substitution	Rats, ♂ and ♀	7 → 10	0.0	16.0	90.9 ± 0.8		14
				5.0		87.8 ± 1.6*	83.6 ± 2.1*	
				10.0			82.6 ± 1.3*	
				15.0				
Pectin	Substitution	Rats, weanling ♂ and ♀	10	0.0	(10.0)	92.5	NR	17
				5.0[h]		85.5		
				10.0[h]		79.5		
				10.0[i]		79.0		

Fiber	Method	Animal	Age	Level	Detail	Value	Value	Ref
Pectin	Substitution	Rats, weanling ♂	25 → 3	0.0	(8.5)	93.3 ± 0.5		19
				2.5		88.3 ± 1.4		
				5.0		88.7 ± 0.6		
				7.5		86.0 ± 0.8		
				10.0		85.1 ± 21		
						r = −0.78^f		
Pectin	Substitution	Rats, weanling ♂	25 → 3	0.0	(22.0)	95.4 ± 0.1		19
				2.5		94.8 ± 0.5		
				5.0		94.6 ± 0.8		
				7.5		92.3 ± 1.5		
				10.0		91.5 ± 0.8		
						r = −0.68^f		
Pectin	Dilution	Rats, weanling ♂	21	0.0	(10.0)	92.3 ± 0.5	92.9 ± 0.5	36
				5.0	(9.5)	86.3 ± 0.2*	88.9 ± 0.3*	
				10.0	(9.0)	83.4 ± 0.4*	88.4 ± 0.5*	
				20.0	(8.0)	79.1 ± 1.0*	86.9 ± 0.9*	
Pectin	Substitution	Rats, weanling ♂	3 → 7	0.0	(10.0)	92.0 ± 0.3		1
				10.0	(HMW,HDE)^j	79.4 ± 2.2*		
				10.0	(HMW,LDE)	87.4 ± 0.06*		
				10.0	(LMW,HDE)	81.6 ± 1.0*		
				10.0	(LMW,LDE)	87.4 ± 0.6*		
Pectin	Substitution	Rats, ♂	4 → 5	0.0	(10.0)	92.8 ± 1.2	101.8 ± 1.2	30
				9.3	(HDE)	77.7 ± 1.0*	86.9 ± 1.0*	
				9.4	(LDE)	81.9 ± 1.0*	91.1 ± 1.0*	
Pectin	Substitution	Rats, weanling ♂	35	0.0		92.8		12
				10.0	10.0	78.2*		
Pectin	Substitution	Rats, ♂	4 to 56 → 5	0.0	(14.0)	89.7		50
				8.0		84.5*		
Guar gum	Dilution	Rats, weanling ♂	21	0.0	(10.0)	92.3 ± 0.5	92.9 ± 0.5	36
				5.0	(9.5)	81.4 ± 0.8*	83.9 ± 0.8*	
				10.0	(9.0)	79.9 ± 0.9*	84.5 ± 1.1*	
				20.0	(8.0)	63.3 ± 1.3*	70.8 ± 1.3*	
Guar gum	Substitution	Rats, ♂	4 → 5	0.0	10.0	92.8 ± 1.2	101.8 ± 1.2	30
				10.0		78.3 ± 2.3*	87.2 ± 5.1*	
Guar gum	Substitution	Rats, weanling ♂	3 → 8	0.0	8.0	87.8 ± 0.5		16
				10.0		78.0 ± 0.4*		
Guar gum	Dilution	Rats, weanling ♂	21	0.0	9.4	89.4 ± 0.4		15
				4.8	9.4	82.3 ± 0.3*		
				0.0	4.7	80.0 ± 1.3		
				4.8	4.7	70.4 ± 1.4*		

Table 4.1.1 (Continued) Effect of Purified Dietary Fibers on Protein Digestibility

Fiber	Method of Incorporation[a]	Species Studied	Time on Diet[b] Adaptation → Balance (days)	Concentration in Diet		Protein Digestibility		Ref.
				Fiber (%)	Protein[c] (%)	Apparent (%)	True (%)	
Guar gum	Substitution	Rats, ♂	4 to 56 → 5	0.0 8.0	(14.0)	89.7 83.8*		50
Guar gum	Dilution	Dogs, ♂ & ♀	21 → 7	0 7	(24.5) (23.0)	90.9 ± 1.2 85.6 ± 3.3*		53
Agar	Substitution	Rats, weanling ♂	3 → 8	0.0 10.0	8.0	87.8 ± 0.5 79.5 ± 0.2*		16
Alginate, Na	Substitution	Rats, weanling ♂	3 → 8	0.0 10.0	10.0	87.7 ± 0.5 81.0 ± 0.2*		16
Alginate, Na	Substitution	Rats, weanling ♂ and ♀	10	0.0 10.0	(10.0)	92.5 NR 88.5		46
Carrageenan	Substitution	Rats, weanling ♂	3 → 8	0.0 10.0	8.0	87.8 ± 0.5 82.6 ± 0.6*		16
Carob bean gum	Substitution	Rats, weanling ♂	3 → 8	0.0 10.0	8.0	87.8 ± 0.5 75.0 ± 0.8*		16
Ispaghula husk (Isogel)	Dilution	Humans, adult ♂ and ♀	14 → 5	0 g (19.7 g)[k] 25 g (43.5 g)[k]	Not stated	88.5 NR 87.3		33
Inulin	Dilution	Dogs, ♂ & ♀	21 → 7	0 7	(24.5) (23.6)	90.9 ± 1.2 88.3 ± 1.5*		53
Resistant starch	Substitution	Rats, ♂	4 to 56 → 5	0.0 8.0	(14.0)	89.7 85.6*		50

Mixed (oligofructose & sugar beet fiber, 4:1)	Substitution	Dogs, ♂	35 → 7	0 5 10	65 g/1000 kcal 66.9 g/1000 kcal 68.8 g/1000 kcal	87.8 ± 0.5 86.3 ± 0.5 83.8 ± 1.0*	52
Mixed (cellulose, pectin, xylan, 32.5%; raffinose; 2.4%)	Substitution	Rats, weanling ♂	35	0.0 10.2	10.0 9.6	92.8 82.2*	12

Note: An asterisk indicates that the value is significantly different from fiber-free or low fiber control group ($p < 0.05$).

a Indicates method by which fiber or fiber source was incorporated into the diet. Substitution signifies addition to the diet at the expense of the digestible carbohydrate source. Dilution signifies addition to the diet, resulting in a whole diet dilution. In the case of dilution, the fiber or fiber source concentration in the diet indicates the actual concentration of fiber in the diet, not the percentage of fiber added to the diet. See text for further explanation.

b Indicates time of the experimental diet. Where two values appear separated by an arrow, the first value is the time allowed for adaptation to the experimental diet. The value after the arrow, or where only one value is present, indicates the length of time for which sample collections were made.

c Values in parentheses indicate concentration of protein sources (usually casein) in diet, as the actual crude protein concentration was not reported, otherwise reported as grams per day or grams nitrogen (N) per day.

d NR, no statistics reported.

e Mean ± SEM.

f Correlation between the percentage of fiber in the diet and the apparent protein digestibility. The correlation is statistically significant.

g NDF, neutral detergent fiber.

h Slow setting, 55% esterified.

i Fast setting, 65% esterified.

j MW, molecular weight; DE, degree of esterification; H, high; L, low.

k Total dietary fiber.

Table 4.1.2　Effect of Fiber-Rich Sources on Protein Digestibility

Fiber	Method of Incorporation[a]	Species Studied	Time on Diet[b] Adaptation → Balance (days)	Concentration in Diet		Protein Digestibility		Ref.
				Fiber (%)	Protein[c] (%)	Apparent (%)	True (%)	
Wheat bran	Substitution	Rats, ♂	4 → 5	0.0	(10.0)	92.8 ± 1.2[d]	101.8 ± 1.2	30
				10.0		87.4 ± 1.2*	96.2 ± 1.3*	
Wheat bran	Dilution	Rats, weanling ♂	21	0.0	(10.0)	92.3 ± 0.5	92.9 ± 0.5	36
				5.0	(9.5)	89.0 ± 0.4*	89.9 ± 0.5	
				10.0	(9.0)	86.3 ± 0.4*	87.9 ± 0.4*	
				20.0	(8.0)	77.0 ± 1.0*	77.7 ± 0.8*	
Wheat bran	Substitution	Rats, weanling ♂	35	0.0	10.0	92.8		12
				16.8	12.5	83.0*		
Wheat bran	Dilution	Humans, adult ♂	18 → 4	0 (33.0 g/d)[e]	15.4 g N/d	89.7 ± 0.6		11
				12 g (53.5 g/d)	16.4 g N/d	87.6 ± 0.5*		
Wheat bran	Substitution	Rats, ♂	9 → 5	0(4.3)[h]	9.8		97.9	8
				5.2[i]			97.2	
				6.1			96.3	
				7.9			95.2*	
				11.6			92.6*	
Wheat bran	Dilution	Pigs, ♂	20 → 10	0.0	16.9	97.01		42
				6.9[e]	16.3	93.4		
				12.8	16.3	91.8		
				18.0	15.6	88.5		
				22.4	15.6	78.9		
Wheat bran	Substitution	Pigs, ♂	7 → 7	1.21	(8.13)	91.3		55
				6.38	(8.90)	85.8*		
Wheat bran	Substitution	Chickens, ♂	7	4.5	(15.7)	67		54
				13.2	(17.1)	61*		
				20.3	(18.4)	57*		
Corn bran	Substitution	Rats, weanling ♂	35	0.0	10.0	92.8		12
				16.8	12.5	83.0*		
Oat bran	Dilution	Humans, adult ♂	14	0 (3.8 g/d)[e]	10.7 g N/d	91 ± 3 NR[f]		4
				45 g (12.0 g/d)	10.5 g N/d	85 ± 4		
Oat bran	Substitution	Chickens, ♂	7	4.5	(15.7)	67		54
				9.1	(18.9)	64*		
				12.7	(21.1)	55*		

Fiber	Method	Species	Level	Fiber	10.6 g N/d			Ref.
Sorghum meal	Substitution	Humans, adult ♂	5 → 6	3.3e 4.8 5.4		65.4 ± 1.8 60.5 ± 2.1* 56.9 ± 2.3*		5
Pea fiber	Substitution	Chickens, ♂	7	4.5 14.9 25.1	(15.7) (15.3) (16.0)	63 60* 55*		54
Barley fiber, insoluble	Substitution	Humans, adult ♀	14 → 7	5.4 8.7 9.2	(16.4) (15.9) (11.6)	87.0 86.2 79.9NR		49
Barley hulls	Substitution	Rats, ♂	4 → 5	0.0 10.0	9.3	100.0 97.3*		2
Barley fiber, insoluble	Substitution	Rats, ♂	17 → 5	5.4 8.7 9.2	(16.4) (15.9) (11.6)	91.7 88.5 87.0NR		49
Barley husk	Substitution	Rats, ♂	4 → 5	0.0 7.7e	9.7 12.8		87.8 86.9*	10
Barley husk	Substitution	Rats, ♂	9 → 5	0(4.3)h 5.1i 6.0 7.9 11.7	9.8 9.7 9.7		97.9 98.4 96.7 96.1* 94.9*	8
Maize hulls	Dilution	Pigs, ♂	20 → 10	0.0 7.4e 14.7 21.7 23.6	16.9 15.6 14.4 13.8 12.5	97.0 94.7 91.3 88.0 83.7		42
Oat hulls	Dilution	Pigs, ♂	20 → 10	0.0 7.4e 14.7 21.8 28.7	16.9 15.6 14.4 13.1 11.9	97.0i 95.5 94.1 92.6 90.7		42
Soybean hulls	Dilution	Pigs, ♂	20 → 10	0.0 7.3e 14.1 20.6 26.6	16.9 14.4 15.6 15.0 14.4	97.0i 93.0 88.6 82.9 80.3		42
Soybean hulls	Substitution	Rats, ♂	16	0 12	13 14	98 92*		47

Table 4.1.2 (Continued) Effect of Fiber-Rich Sources on Protein Digestibility

Fiber	Method of Incorporation[a]	Species Studied	Time on Diet[b] Adaptation → Balance (days)	Concentration in Diet		Protein Digestibility		Ref.
				Fiber (%)	Protein[c] (%)	Apparent (%)	True (%)	
Soybean hulls	Substitution	Dogs, ♂ & ♀	10 → 4	3.05	93.4	84.3		51
				4.09	80.4	81.4		
				6.03	83.4	82.7		
				7.32	93.9	83.2		
Lupin hulls	Dilution	Pigs, ♂	20 → 10	0.0	16.9	97.0[i]		42
				7.41	15.6	91.9		
				14.5	14.4	90.7		
				21.6	13.1	86.0		
				28.5	12.5	81.4		
Pea hulls	Dilution	Pigs, ♂	20 → 10	0.0	16.9	97.0[i]		42
				7.21	15.6	89.6		
				13.8	14.4	81.7		
				19.8	13.1	74.8		
				25.4	12.5	65.3		
Canola hulls	Substitution	Rats, ♂	16	0.0	13	98		47
				12	15	87*		
Bean cell wall	Substitution	Rats, weanling ♂	35	0.0	10.0	92.8		12
				10.0	11.8	85.8*		
Soybean cell wall	Substitution	Rats, ♂	16	0.0	13	98		47
				12	14	90*		
Soy polysaccharide	Formulated[h]	Humans, ♂ a&nd ♀	3 → 4–5	0.0 g/d	13.1 g/d	92.2 ± 2.9		18
				8.8 g/d	14.3 g/d	90.0 ± 1.6		
Canola cell wall	Substitution	Rats, ♂	16	0.0	13	98		47
				12	13	90*		
Sugar beet fiber	Substitution	Rats, ♂	4 → 5	0.0	(10.0)	92.8 ± 1.2	101.8 ± 2.6	30
				10.0		84.6 ± 0.8*	92.5 ± 0.8*	
				10.0[g]		83.0 ± 1.5	92.0 ± 1.5*	
Sugar beet fiber	Dilution	Dogs, ♂ & ♀	21 → 7	0	(24.5)	90.9 ± 1.2		53
				7	(23.3)	88.2 ± 1.6*		

Food source	Type	Subject	Sex	Period	Fiber intake	N/protein intake	Digestibility	Ref.
Brown rice	Substitution	Humans, adult	♂	1 → 14	5.7 g/dᵉ	4.74 g N/d	68.0 ± 3.5	27
					13.9 g/dᵉ	4.65 g N/d	48.4 ± 3.8*	57
Barley, wheat, pea fiber, and pectin	Substitution	Rats, ♂		4	5.6	(15.5)	86.1	
					25.7	(17.2)	72.7*	
Fruits, vegetables, and whole meal bran	Unclear	Human, ♂		2 → 7	6.2 g/d	13.1 g N/d	92.1 ± 0.6NR	40
					16.2 g/d	13.9 g N/d	90.8 ± 0.5	
					31.9 g/d	14.7 g N/d	85.2 ± 0.5	
Fruits and vegetables	Unclear	Humans, adult	♂	19 → 7	3.6 g/dᵉ	93.0 g/d	90.4 ± 0.9	22
					20.0 g/d	96.0 g/d	81.1 ± 1.1*	
Fruits and vegetables	Unclear	Humans, adult	♂	14 → 7	1.9 g/d	13.6 N/d	89.9 ± 0.5	23
					10.0 g/d	14.1 g N/d	86.9 ± 0.7*	
					19.4 g/d	13.8 g N/d	83.5 ± 0.8*	
					25.6 g/d	13.9 g N/d	81.2 ± 1.1*	
Fruits and vegetables	Substitution	Humans, adult	♂	21 → 7	17.8 g/d	15.8 g N/d	90 ± 2	25
					41.0 g/d	16.5 g N/d	84 ± 4*	
Fruits and vegetables	Substitution	Human, adult	♀	14 → 7	7.3	(19.3)	90.0	49
					14.6	(20.3)	84.1	
Fruits and vegetables	Substitution	Rats, ♂		17 → 5	7.3	(19.3)	91.5	49
					14.6	(20.3)	85.8	
Konjac and seaweed	Substitution	Humans, adult	♀	5	0.0	26 g/d	81.2	20
					18 g/dᵉ	27 g/d	55.5*	
"Guatemalan" diet	Dilution	Humans, adult	♂	14	3.8 g/d	10.7 g N/d	91 ± 3 NR	4
					93.0 g/d	10.8 g N/d	69 ± 2	

Note: An asterisk indicates that the value is significantly different from fiber-free or low-fiber control group ($p < 0.05$).

a See footnote a of Table 4.1.1.
b See footnote b of Table 4.1.1.
c See footnote c of Table 4.1.1.
d Mean ± SEM.
e Neutral detergent fiber.
f NR, no statistics reported.
g Treated with hot water to increase the solubility of pectin.
h Enteral formulas.
i Total dietary fiber.
j Statistically significant linear decrease ($p < 0.001$) with increased NDF intake.

Tables 4.1.3 and 4.1.4 show the effect of fibers on nitrogen excretion and on nitrogen balance for the purified and fiber-rich sources. It is apparent from the data that fiber consumption causes a shift in the pattern of nitrogen excretion. Fecal nitrogen increases are often accompanied by a decrease in urinary nitrogen. This occurred with all types of fibers and fiber sources. However, in most instances the decrease in urinary nitrogen did not fully compensate for the increase in fecal nitrogen, such that nitrogen balance was often significantly reduced, although in all cases it remained positive.

The effect of dietary fibers on several measures of protein utilization is found in the last two tables (Tables 4.1.5 and 4.1.6). The most common measure of protein utilization is the protein efficiency ratio, undoubtedly due to its ease of determination. It should be understood, however, that this is not the same PER as described by the AOAC, since the cellulose concentrations differed from 1% and the protein concentrations were not always in the 9.5 to 10.5% range. However, the term is retained, since the PER is calculated in the same way (body weight gain per protein consumed). Given the decrease in protein digestibility and the consequent increase in fecal nitrogen, one might expect a decrease in protein utilization parameters that have a digestibility component, such as PER and net protein utilization (NPU), and an increase in parameters measuring the utilization of absorbed protein, such as biological value (BV). However, the results from protein utilization studies are quite variable. For example, in rats the PER of diets containing 10 to 12% cellulose are either significantly higher,[12] lower,[7] or unchanged,[38,47] than in fiber-free controls. The fiber with the most consistent effect on PER is pectin. A level of 10% or greater in the diet almost invariably led to a significant reduction in this measure of protein utilization. Interestingly, two other soluble fibers showed divergent effects on the PER. Guar gum at 10% of the diet led to a significant reduction in PER,[36] whereas alginate did not.[46] Few studies have investigated the effect of fibers on NPU and, consequently, no trends can be discerned regarding the effect of fibers on NPU. Although a large number of studies have reported the BV of fiber-containing diets, the results are too inconsistent to make any meaningful statements about the effect of fibers as a whole. Unfortunately, because of differences in the protein and/or fiber concentrations of the diets, as well as the method of fiber incorporation into the diet, comparisons between studies using the same fiber type are often not possible.

From the available studies it is clear that dietary fiber and fiber-rich foods reduce protein digestibility, often in an approximately linear fashion. However, it remains to be established whether dietary fiber has a detrimental effect on protein utilization.

This review covers the published literature through November 2000.

Table 4.1.3 Effect of Purified Dietary Fibers on Nitrogen Excretion and Balance

Fiber	Method of Incorporation[a]	Species Studied	Time on Diet[b] Adaptation → Balance (days)	Fiber in Diet	Nitrogen Intake (g/day)	Nitrogen Excretion		Nitrogen Balance (mg/day)	Ref.
						Fecal (mg/day)	Urinary (mg/day)		
Cellulose	Substitution	Rats, weanling ♂	5 → 4	0.0 10.0 20.0	0.121 0.132 0.132	22.9±3.2 NR[d] 20.2±2.9 19.8±3.1	10.4±1.4 NR 11.1±1.5 12.7±1.6	40.0±4.6 NR 45.1±5.6 51.3±6.8	18
Cellulose	Dilution	Rats, weanling ♂	21	0.0 5.0 10.0 20.0	0.289 0.276 0.266 0.264	22.0(6)[e] 31.0*(10*) 36.0*(12*) 47.0*(16*)			36
Celulose[f]	Dilution	Rats, ♂	35 → 7	0.0 2.0 g/d	0.188	16.0±2.4 NR 25.5±5.0	163.4±8.3 NR 249.4±4.3	8.2 NR 12.7	44
Cellulose[g]	Substitution	Rats, ♂	21 → 7	0.0 2.1	0.289 0.287	18.0 17.0	9.60 106.0	181.0 165.0	29
Cellulose[h]	Substitution	Rats, ♂	21 → 7	0.0 2.1	0.319 0.316	20.0 21.0	139.0 114.0*	154.0 186.0*	29
Cellulose	Substitution	Mice, weanling ♂	28	5.0 10.0 20.0	0.080 0.070 0.070	10.0±1 10.0±1 20.0±2	10.0±3 10.0±2 10.0±3	50.0±7 50.0±9 50.0±10	21
Cellulose	Substitution	Rats, growing ♂ and ♀	30 → 1	0.0 15.0	0.256	133.0±30 131.0±12			17
Cellulose	Dilution	Monkeys, ♂	7 → 7	1.0 g/d 7.0 g/d 16.0 g/d 20.0 g/d		250 200 225 275			41
Cellulose	Dilution	Humans, adult, ♀	3 → 4	0 (6.8 g/d)[i] 14.2 g/d (21.0 g/d)	7.910	970 1140*	5840 5950	1100 820*	24
Cellulose	Dilution	Humans, adult, ♂ and ♀	3 → 7	0 (6.8 g/d)[i] 14.2 g/d (21.0 g/d)	7.880	910 1170*	5750 5740	1220 970*	24

Table 4.1.3 (Continued) Effect of Purified Dietary Fibers on Nitrogen Excretion and Balance

Fiber	Method of Incorporation[a]	Species Studied	Time on Diet[b] Adaptation → Balance (days)	Fiber in Diet	Nitrogen Intake (g/day)	Nitrogen Excretion Fecal (mg/day)	Nitrogen Excretion Urinary (mg/day)	Nitrogen Balance (mg/day)	Ref.
Cellulose	Dilution	Humans, adolescent ♂	3 → 4	0	7.850	860	5080	1910	24
				(6.8 g/d)[i]					
				14.2 g/d		920	5570	1360*	
				(21.0 g/d)					
Hemicellulose	Substitution	Mice, weanling ♂	28	5.0	0.060	20.0 ± 4	10.0 ± 4	30.0 ± 4	21
				10.0	0.070	20.0 ± 4*	10.0 ± 4	40.0 ± 6	
				20.0	0.060	20.0 ± 5*	10.0 ± 5	30.0 ± 6	
Hemicellulose	Dilution	Humans, adult ♀	3 → 4	0	7.910	970	5840	1100	24
				(6.8 g/d)[i]					
				14.2 g/d		1180*	5990	740*	
				(21. g/d)					
Hemicellulose	Dilution	Humans, adult ♂ and ♀	3 → 7	0	7.880	910	5750	1220	24
				(6.8 g/d)[i]					
				14.2 g/d		1290*	5730	860*	
				(21.0 g/d)					
Hemicellulose	Dilution	Humans, adolescent ♂	3 → 4	0	7.850	860	5080	1910	24
				(6.8 g/d)[i]					
				14.2 g/d		1110*	5730	1380*	
				(21.0 g/d)					
Lignin	Dilution	Rats, weanling ♂	21	0.0	0.289	22.0(6)[e]			36
				3.0	0.275	29.0(10*)			
				6.0	0.264	40.0*(14)			
Lignin	Substitution	Mice, weanling ♂	28	5.0	0.070	10.0 ± 3	10.0 ± 5	40.0 ± 15	21
				10.0	0.070	10.0 ± 2	20.0 ± 6	40.0 ± 9	
				20.0	0.050	10.0 ± 4	20.0 ± 7	20.0 ± 8*	
Neutral detergent fiber (wheat bran)[g]	Substitution	Rats, ♂	21 → 7	0.0	0.289	18.0	96.0	181.0	29
				2.1	0.297	26.0*	80.0	187.0	

Neutral detergent fiber (wheat bran)[h]	Substitution	Rats, ♂	21 → 7	0.0 2.1	0.319 0.332	20.0 34.0*	139.0 118.0*	154.0 172.0	29
Acid detergent fiber (wheat bran)[h]	Substitution	Rats, ♂	21 → 7	0.0 2.1	0.289 0.289	18.0 22.0*	96.0 90.0	181.0 182.0	29
Acid detergent fiber (wheat bran)[h]	Substitution	Rats, ♂	21 → 7	0.0 2.1	0.319 0.321	20.0 25.0	13.9 122.0*	154.0 174.0*	29
Pectin	Substitution	Rats, ♂	4 → 5	0.0 9.3 (LDE)[j] 9.4 (HDE)		10.5 23.7* 30.0*			30
Pectin[g]	Substitution	Rats, ♂	21 → 7	0.0 2.1	0.289 0.288	18.0 24.0*	96.0 97.0	181.0 182.0	29
Pectin[h]	Substitution	Rats, ♂	21 → 7	0.0 2.1	0.319 0.316	20.0 25.0	139.0 132.0	154.0 159.0	29
Pectin[h]	Substitution	Rats, ♂	21 → 7	0.0 2.1	0.319 0.316	20.0 25.0	139.0 132.0	154.0 159.0	29
Pectin	Dilution	Humans, adult, ♂ and ♀	3 → 4	0 (6.8 g/d)[i] 14.2 g/d (21.0 g/d)	7.910	970.0 1060.0	5840.0 5510.0	1100.0 1090.0	24
Pectin	Dilution	Humans, adult, ♂ and ♀	3 → 7	0 (6.8 g/d)[i] 14.2 g/d (21.0 g/d)	7.880	910 1060	5750 5510	1220 1310	24
Pectin	Dilution	Humans, adolescent, ♂	3 → 4	0 (6.8 g/d)[i] 14.2 g/d (21.0 g/d)	7.850	860 1010	5080 5010*	1910 1830	24
Pectin	Dilution	Monkeys, ♂	7 → 7	1.0 g/d 7.0 g/d 13.0 g/d 20.0 g/d		190 250 210 230			41
Pectin	Dilution	Rats, weanling, ♂	21	0.0 5.0 10.0 20.0	0.289 0.241* 0.191* 0.146*	22.0(6)[e] 33.0*(11*) 31.0*(15*) 30.0*(19*)			36

Table 4.1.3 (Continued)   Effect of Purified Dietary Fibers on Nitrogen Excretion and Balance

Fiber	Method of Incorporation[a]	Species Studied	Time on Diet[b] Adaptation → Balance (days)	Fiber in Diet	Nitrogen Intake (g/day)	Nitrogen Excretion Fecal (mg/day)	Nitrogen Excretion Urinary (mg/day)	Nitrogen Balance (mg/day)	Ref.
Guar gum	Substitution	Rats, weanling, ♂	3 → 8	0.0	0.142	17.3 ± 0.6	58.9 ± 1.6	66.0[k]	16
				10.0	0.152	33.5 ± 1.0*	43.8 ± 1.3*	75.0	
Guar gum[l]	Dilution	Rats, ♂		0.0	0.335	6.0	92.0	234.0	45
				5.0	0.311	18.0*	56.0	228.0	
Guar gum	Dilution	Rats, weanling, ♂	8		Casein				15
				0.0	0.234	24.5	152.3	57.2[k]	
				5.0	0.237	42.0	129.5*	65.6	
					Egg albumin				
				0.0	0.109	21.8	69.4	17.7	
				5.0	0.114	33.8*	57.6*	22.5	
Guar gum	Substitution	Rats, ♂	4 → 5	0.0		10.5			30
				5.0		26.8*			
				10.0					
Guar gum	Dilution	Rats, weanling, ♂	21	0.0	0.289	22.0(6)[e]			36
				5.0	0.259	48.0*(12*)			
				10.0	0.217	44.0*(17*)			
				20.0	0.168	61.0*(20*)			
Carrageenan	Substitution	Rats, ♂ and ♀	148	0.0			55.0 ± 4.8%[m]		17
				2.0			49.0 ± 3.0%		
				5.0			53.0 ± 2.9%		
				10.0			52.0 ± 3.0%		
				15.0			44.0 ± 3.0%		
				20.0			43.0 ± 4.2%		

Carrageenan	Substitution	Rats, weanling, ♂	3 → 8	0.0 10.0	0.142 0.138	17.3 ± 0.6 24.8 ± 0.5*	58.9 ± 1.6 61.9 ± 0.6*	66.0* 51.0	16
Carob bean gum	Substitution	Rats, weanling, ♂	3 → 8	0.0 10.0	0.142 0.154	17.3 ± 0.6 38.4 ± 1.4*	58.9 ± 1.6 49.5 ± 1.3*	66.0k 66.0	16
Na-alginate	Substitution	Rats, weanling, ♂	3 → 8	0.0 10.0	0.142 0.149	17.3 ± 0.6 28.2 ± 1.0*	58.9 ± 1.6 51.4 ± 1.9*	66.0k 70.0	16
Algar	Substitution	Rats, weanling, ♂	3 → 8	0.0 10.0	0.142 0.134	17.3 ± 0.6 27.5 ± 1.6*	58.9 ± 1.6 61.2 ± 1.8	66.0 45.0	16
Vegetable	Substitution	Humans, adult	3 → 6	0.15 g/kg 0.67 g/kg	118.2 mg/kg 124.8 mg/kg	11.7 ± 1.7 mg/kg 27.6 ± 4.7* mg/kg	106.0 ± 6.5 mg/kg 85.3 ± 4.1* mg/kg	−3.4 ± 4.1 mg/kg 6.4 ± 6.5 mg/kg	48

Note: An asterisk indicates that these values are significantly different from the fiber-free or low-fiber control group ($p < 0.05$).

a   See footnote a in Table 4.1.1.
b   See footnote b in Table 4.1.1.
c   Mean ± SEM.
d   Nr, no statistics reported.
e   Endogenous fecal nitrogen, uncorrected for nitrogen content of nonprotein diet.
f   Rats were made obese, then fed an energy-restricted regime with or without cellulose.
g   Metabolizable energy of diet was 57 kcal/day.
h   Metabolizable energy of diet was 67 kcal/day.
i   Total dietary fiber intake.
j   De, degree of esterification; L, low; H, high.
k   Calculated from intake and excretion means.
l   Data chosen from 1.2% dietary arginine groups. Nitrogen intake and balance calculated from data presented in article.
m   Values are mean ± SEM for nitrogen excreted per day as a percentage of ingested nitrogen.

Table 4.1.4   Effect of Fiber-Rich Sources on Nitrogen Excretion and Balance

Fiber	Method of Incorporation[a]	Species Studied	Time on Diet[b] Adaptation → Balance (days)	Fiber in Diet	Nitrogen Intake (g/day)	Nitrogen Excretion Fecal (mg/day)	Urinary (mg/day)	Nitrogen Balance (mg/day)	Ref.
Wheat bran	Substitution	Rats, ♂	4 → 5	0.0% / 10.0%		10.5 / 19.7			30
Wheat bran	Substitution	Rats, ♂	28 → 7	0.0% / 2.0%	0.289 / 0.287	18.0 / 26.0*	96.0 / 80.0	181.0 / 185.0	29
Wheat bran	Dilution	Rats, ♂	3 → 15	0.0% / 5.0%	0.335 / 0.322	6.0 / 12.0*	92.0 / 87.0*	237.0[c] / 223.0	45
Wheat bran (largely)	Dilution	Humans, adult	18 → 4	0.0% / 12.0%			6300		11
Wheat bran	Substitution	Humans, adult, ♂ and ♀	4–5 → 7	0.0 / 5.0 g	18.2 ± 0.8[d] / 19.1 ± 0.9	1150 ± 210 NR[e] / 1650 ± 220	8200*		39
Wheat bran	Not stated	Humans	14 → 7	0.0 / 18.0 g		1400 NR / 2000			43
Wheat fiber[f]	Substitution	Humans, ♂	21	0 / (21.8 g/d)[g] / 31 g/d / (53.2 g/d)	21.9 / 26.9	1400 ± 300 / 2490 ± 100*			6
Sorghum fiber	Substitution	Humans	5 → 6	3.3%[h] / 4.8% / 5.4%	10.6 / 10.6 / 10.6	4020 ± 270 / 4139 ± 240 / 4730 ± 390	5500 ± 360 / 4830 ± 200 / 4960 ± 270	2020 ± 230 / 1470 ± 210* / 1110 ± 310*	5
Oat bran[i]	Substitution	Humans, ♂	14	3.8 g/d / 12.0 g/d	10.7 ± 0.9 / 10.5 ± 0.8	1000 ± 320 NR / 1610 ± 560	8390 ± 420 NR / 8160 ± 280	800 ± 440* NR / 260 ± 320	4
Sugar beet fiber	Substitution	Rats, ♂	4 → 5	0.0% / 10.0%	10.5 / 26.2*				30
Locust bean gum	Dilution	Monkeys, ♂	7 → 7	1.0 g/d / 15.0 g/d[l]	260 / 280				41

Food source	Method	Species	n	Fiber					Ref.
Slippery elm	Dilution	Monkeys, ♂	7 → 7	1.0 g/d 20.0 g/d[l]	190 390				41
Rice hulls	Dilution	Monkeys, ♂	7 → 7	1.0 g/d 16.0 g/d[l]		200 335			41
Oat straw	Dilution	Monkeys, ♂	7 → 7	1.0 g/d 15.0 g/d[l]		200 385			41
Soy husks	Dilution	Monkeys, ♂	7 → 7	1.0 g/d 20.0 g/d[l]		205 470			41
Psyllium seed	Dilution	Monkeys, ♂	7 → 7	1.0 g/d 18.0 g/d[l]		335 320			41
Fruits and vegetables	Substitution (?)	Humans, ♂	19 → 7	3.6 g/d[i] 20.0 g/d	14.9 15.4	1350 2480	11450 10810	1090 740	22
Fruits and vegetables	Substitution	Humans, ♂	14 → 7	1.9 g/d[j] 10.1 g/d 19.4 g/d 25.6 g/d	13.6 14.1 13.8 13.9			1380 ± 80 1840 ± 120* 2280 ± 140* 2600 ± 180*	23
Cabbage	Not stated	Humans	4 → 7	0.0 g/d 18.3 g/d		1400 2100			43
Vegetables	Substitution	Humans, adult (cirrhotic)	3 → 6	12.5 g/d 55.6 g/d	9.8 10.4	955 2291*	8798 7080*	−282 531	48
Brown rice	Substitution	Humans, adult ♂	1 → 15	5.7 g/d[j] 13.9 g/d	4.74 ± 0.65 4.65 ± 0.64	1500 ± 140 2410 ± 430	3950 ± 390 3330 ± 510	−710 ± 290 −1090 ± 330	27

Note: A single asterisk indicates that the value is significantly different from the fiber-free or low-fiber control group ($p < 0.05$).

a See footnote a in Table 4.1.1.
b See footnote b in Table 4.1.1.
c Calculated from intake and excretion means.
d Mean ± SEM.
e NR, no statistics reported.
f High protein diets.
g Total dietary fiber.
h Crude fiber.
i Data from untoasted oat bran group study.
j Neutral detergent fiber.
k Corrected balance, with one subject omitted.
l Highest level fed.

Table 4.1.5 Effect of Purified Dietary Fibers on Measures of Protein Utilization

Fiber	Method of Incorporation[a]	Species Studied	Concentration in Diet Fiber (%)	Concentration in Diet Protein[b] (%)	Measures of Protein Utilization[c] PER	Measures of Protein Utilization[c] NPU	Measures of Protein Utilization[c] BV	Ref.
Cellulose	Substitution	Rats	0.0	7.6			76.0	19
			2.5	(8.5)			78.0	
			5.0				76.0	
			10.0				79.0	
			20.0				76.0	
			0.0	19.7			64.0	
			2.5	(22.0)			72.0	
			5.0				61.0	
			10.0				65.0	
			20.0				69.0	
Cellulose	Substitution	Rats	0.0	9.98	2.89(2.50)[d]			12
			10.0	8.98	3.94*(3.41)			
Cellulose	Substitution	Rats	0.0	10.0		79.1 ± 4.6[e] NR[f]	60.4 ± 3.6 NR	28
			10.0	(12.0)		80.2 ± 5.3	57.8 ± 3.1	
			20.0			78.1 ± 4.2	63.4 ± 3.8	
			0.0	9.5% of calories		83.7 ± 6.1	64.7 ± 5.0	
			10.0	(12.0)		84.9 ± 5.7	58.9 ± 4.3	
			20.0			80.7 ± 5.6	59.3 ± 4.0	
Cellulose	Substitution	Rats	0.0	12.38	2.24 ± 0.21			7
			5.0	11.61	2.29 ± 0.10			
			10.0	11.89	2.06 ± 0.05*			
			20.0	12.05	2.06 ± 0.12*			
			40.0	11.82	1.98 ± 0.06*			
	Dilution		0.0	10.38	2.70 ± 0.24			
			5.0	9.94	2.72 ± 0.12			
			10.0	9.95	2.57 ± 0.11			
			20.0	8.58	2.82 ± 0.22			
			40.0	8.25	2.36 ± 0.19*			
Cellulose	Substitution	Rats	0.0	(10.0)	3.2 ± 0.2			46
			5.0		3.3 ± 0.1			
			10.0		2.8 ± 0.7			
Cellulose	Substitution	Mice	5.0	10.0	1.7 ± 0.2			21
			10.0	(10.0)	1.7 ± 0.5			
			20.0		1.4 ± 0.3			

Fiber	Method	Animal	Fiber level (%)	Dietary protein level	Value 1	Value 2	Reference
Cellulose	Dilution	Rats	0.0	10.0	3.98 ± 0.14⁹(87)ʰ	4.31 ± 0.15ʲ (4.28 ± 0.14)ʲ	36
			5.0		3.90 ± 0.21 (85)	4.40 ± 0.29 (4.30 ± 0.28)	
			10.0		3.71 ± 0.37 (81)	4.30 ± 0.50 (4.16 ± 0.47)	
			20.0		3.79 ± 0.20 (83)	4.63 ± 0.19* (4.40 ± 0.19)	
Cellulose	Substitution	Rats	0.0*	12.78 (2.044% N)	2.89	75.4	29
			2.1		2.95	70.2	
			0.0ᶠ		1.86	63.9	
			2.1		1.98*	74.4*	
Cellulose	Substitution	Rats	5.2	9.38 (1.5% N)	3.00	95.7	2
			15.2		2.99	93.3*	
Cellulose	Substitution	Rats, ♂	0.0	13		87.4	47
			12	13		87.7	
Xylan	Substitution	Rats	0.0	9.98	2.89 (2.50)ᶜ		
			10.0	9.75	3.79*(3.28)		
Hemicellulose	Substitution	Mice	5.0	10.0	1.1 ± 0.3		
			10.0	(10.0)	2.3 ± 0.5*		
			20.0		1.9 ± 0.7		
Lignin	Substitution	Mice	5.0	10.0	1.2 ± 0.6		21
			10.0	(10.0)	2.3 ± 0.4		
			20.0		1.0 ± 0.9		
Lignin	Dilution	Rats	0.0	10.0	3.98 ± 0.14⁹(87)ʰ	4.31 ± 0.15ʲ (4.28 ± 0.14)ʲ	36
			3.0		3.48 ± 0.22 (76)	3.89 ± 0.20 (3.83 ± 0.20)	
			6.0		3.05 ± 0.20 (67)	3.60 ± 0.24 (3.49 ± 0.23)	
Neutral detergent fiber (wheat bran)	Substitution	Rats	0.0*	12.78 (2.044% N)	2.89	75.4	29
			2.1		2.91	78.0	
			0.0ᶠ		1.86	63.9	
			2.1		1.96*	71.3*	
Acid detergent fiber (wheat bran)	Substitution	Rats	0.0*	12.78 (2.044% N)	2.89	75.4	29
			2.1		2.91	77.7	
			0.0ᶠ		1.86	63.9	
			2.1		1.99*	70.7*	

Table 4.1.5 (Continued) Effect of Purified Dietary Fibers on Measures of Protein Utilization

Table 4.1.5 (Continued) Effect of Purified Dietary Fibers on Measures of Protein Utilization

Fiber	Method of Incorporation[a]	Species Studied	Concentration in Diet		Measures of Protein Utilization[c]			Ref.
			Fiber (%)	Protein[b] (%)	PER	NPU	BV	
Pectin	Substitution	Rats	0.0	7.6			75.0	19
			2.5	(8.5)			83.0	
			5.0				78.0	
			10.0				76.0	
			20.0				72.0	
			0.0	19.7			66.0	
			2.5	(22.0)			66.0	
			5.0				63.0	
			10.0				64.0	
			20.0				63.0	
Pectin	Substitution	Rats	0.0	10.0	3.2 ± 0.2			46
			5.0[i]		3.6 ± 0.5			
			10.0[i]		2.8 ± 0.3			
			10.0[i]		2.3 ± 0.3*			
Pectin	Substitution	Rats	0.0	9.98	2.89 (2.50)[d]			12
			10.0[i]	9.95	2.21* (1.91)			
Pectin	Substitution	Rats	0.0	(10.0)		64.3 ± 8.0	67.9 ± 8.9	1
			10.0 (HDE, HMW)[m]			60.0 ± 11.5	76.4 ± 18.1	
			10.0 (LDE, HMW)			71.3 ± 5.2*	81.6 ± 5.5*	
			10.0 (HDE, LMW)			67.4 ± 5.3	82.7 ± 7.0*	
			10.0 (LDE, LMW)			74.5 ± 6.4*	85.4 ± 8.0*	
Pectin	Substitution	Rats	0.0	12.78	2.89		75.4	29
			2.1	(2.044% N)	2.96		78.2	
			0.0		1.86		63.9	
			2.1		2.11*		66.4	
Pectin	Dilution	Rats	0.0	(10.0)	3.98 ± 0.14[g](87)[h]		4.31 ± 0.15[j] (4.28 ± 0.14)[j]	36
			5.0		3.05 ± 0.33*(66)		3.54 ± 0.04* (3.44 ± 0.38)*	
			10.0		3.00 ± 0.42*(65)		3.59 ± 0.47* (3.39 ± 0.47)*	
			20.0		1.83 ± 0.31*(40)		2.32 ± 0.40* (2.11 ± 0.37)*	

Pectin	Substitution	Rats	0.0		82.9 ± 4.4	(10.0)	30
			9.3 (HDE)[m]		81.6 ± 3.1		
			9.4 (LDE)		79.9 ± 5.0		
Guar gum	Substitution	Rats	0.0		82.9 ± 4.4	(10.0)	30
					84.3 ± 3.1		
Guar gum	Dilution	Rats	0.0	3.98 ± 0.149(87)[h]	4.31 ± 0.15[j]	(10.0)	36
					(4.28 ± 0.14)[j]		
			5.0	3.65 ± 0.38(79)	4.48 ± 0.35		
					(4.35 ± 0.32)		
			10.0	3.45 ± 0.18*(76)	4.33 ± 0.30		
					(4.00 ± 0.30)		
			20.0	2.24 ± 0.32*(47)	3.57 ± 0.64*		
					(3.19 ± 0.56)*		
Algin	Substitution	Rats	0.0	3.2 ± 0.2		(10.0)	46
			10.0	2.9 ± 0.4			

Note: An asterisk indicates that the value is significantly different from the fiber-free or low-fiber control group ($p < 0.05$).

[a] See footnote a of Table 4.1.1.
[b] Values in parentheses are the concentrations of the protein source (usually casein) or the percentage of nitrogen (where so indicated) in the diet.
[c] PER, protein efficiency ratio; NPU, net protein utilization; BV, biological value.
[d] PER, corrected for fiber-free group = 2.50.
[e] Mean ± SD.
[f] NR, no statistics reported.
[g] Net protein ratio (NPR).
[h] Relative net protein ratio (RNPR).
[i] NPR ÷ apparent digestibility (NPR/AD).
[j] NPR ÷ true digestibility (NPR/TD).
[k] Metabolizable energy of diet was 57 kcal/day.
[l] Metabolizable energy of diet was 67 kcal/day.
[m] DE, degree of esterification; MW, molecular weight; L, low; H, high.

Table 4.1.6 Effect of Fiber-Rich Sources on Measures of Protein Utilization

Fiber	Method of Incorporation[a]	Species Studied	Concentration in Diet		Measures of Protein Utilization[c]			Ref.
			Fiber (%)	Protein[b] (%)	PER	NPU	BV	
Wheat bran	Substitution	Rats	0.0	9.98	2.87 (2.50)[d]			12
			10.0	12.50	3.02 (2.61)			
Wheat bran	Substitution	Rats	0.0	(10.0)			82.9 ± 4.4	24
			10.0				77.1 ± 5.1	
Wheat bran	Dilution	Rats	0.0	(10.0)	2.98 ± 0.14[e,f](87)[g]		4.31 ± 0.15[h] (4.28 ± 0.14)[j]	36
			5.0		3.22 ± 0.22*(70)		3.61 ± 0.26* (3.57 ± 0.26*)	
			10.0		2.92 ± 0.18*(64)		3.38 ± 0.22* (3.33 ± 0.22*)	
			20.0		2.52 ± 0.12*(55)		3.28 ± 0.17* (3.16 ± 0.16*)	
Wheat bran	Substitution	Rats	0.0[i]	12.78	2.89		75.4	29
			5.0	(2.044% N)	3.03*		80.1	
			0.0[k]		1.86		63.9	
			5.0		2.07*		69.5*	
Wheat bran	Substitution	Rats, ♂	0(4.3)[n]	9.8		82.6	84.3	8
			5.2[l]	9.8		83.3	85.8	
			6.1[l]	9.8		83.3	86.5	
			7.9[l]	9.8		83.4	88.3*	
			11.6[l]	10.0		83.3	90.1	
Corn bran	Substitution	Rats	0.0	9.98	2.89 (2.50)[d]			12
			10.0	10.59	3.26 (2.82)			
Barley hulls	Substitution	Rats	0.0	9.38		87.4	95.7	2
			10.0	(1.5% N)		87.5	94.2*	

Barley husk	Substitution	Rats, ♂	0(4.3)[n]	9.8		82.6	84.3	8
			5.1[i]	9.7		80.7	83.5	
			6.0[i]	9.7		80.7*	83.5	
			7.9[i]	9.8		80.1*	83.4	
			11.7[i]	9.8		79.5*	83.7	
Barley husk	Substitution	Rats, ♂	0.0	9.7		68.0	77.4	10
			7.7[o]	12.8		67.9	78.1	
Sugar beet fiber	Substitution	Rats	0.0	(10.0)			92.9 ± 4.4	24
			10.0(7.67)[l]				75.2 ± 3.3*	
			10.0[m](7.43)				74.4 ± 4.3*	
Bran cell wall fiber	Substitution	Rats	0.0	9.98	2.89 (2.50)[d]			10
			10.0	11.78	2.97 (2.57)			

Note: An asterisk indicates that the value is significantly different from the fiber-free or low-fiber control group ($p < 0.05$).

a See footnote a in Table 4.1.1.
b See footnote b in Table 4.1.1.
c See footnote c in Table 4.1.1.
d PER, corrected for fiber-free group = 2.50.
e Mean ± SD.
f Net protein ratio (NPR).
g Relative net protein ratio (RNPR).
h NPR ÷ apparent digestibility (NPR/AD).
i NPR ÷ true digestibility (NPR/TD).
j Metabolizable energy of diet was 57 kcal/day.
k Metabolizable energy of diet was 67 kcal/day.
l Total dietary fiber.
m Treated with hot water to increase the solubility of pectin.
n Cellulose content of 0% fiber diet.
o Neutral detergent fiber.

REFERENCES

1. Atallah, M. T. and Melnik, T. A., Effect of pectin structure on protein utilization by growing rats, *J. Nutr.*, 112, 2027, 1982.
2. Beames, R. M. and Eggum, B. O., The effect of type of and level of protein fiber and starch on nitrogen excretion patterns in rats, *Br. J. Nutr.*, 46, 301, 1981.
3. Burrows, C. F., Kronfeld, D. S., Banta, C. A., and Merritt, A. M., Effects of fiber on digestibility and transit time in dogs, *J. Nutr.*, 112, 1726, 1982.
4. Galloway, D. H. and Kretsch, M. J., Protein and energy utilization in men given a rural Guatemalan diet and egg formulas with and without added oat bran, *Am. J. Clin. Nutr.*, 31, 1118, 1978.
5. Corms, A. and Delpeuch, F., Effect of fiber in sorghum on nitrogen digestibility, *Am. J. Clin. Nutr.*, 34, 2454, 1981.
6. Cummings, J. H., Hill, M. L, Bone, E. S., Branch, W. J., and Jenkins, D. J. A., The effect of meat protein and dietary fiber on colonic function and metabolism. II. Bacterial metabolites in feces and urine, *Am. J. Clin. Nutr.*, 32, 2094, 1979.
7. Delorme, C. B., Wojcik, J., and Gordon, C., Method of addition of cellulose to experimental diets and its effect on rat growth and protein utilization, *J. Nutr.*, 111, 1522, 1981.
8. Donangelo, C. M. and Eggum, B. O., Comparative effects of wheat bran and barley husk on nutrient utilization in rats, *Br. J. Nutr.*, 54, 741, 1985.
9. Dreher, M. L., Dreher, C. J., and Berry, J. W., Starch digestibility of foods: a nutritional perspective, *CRC Crit. Rev. Food Sci. Nutr.*, 20, 47, 1984.
10. Eggum, B. O., Beames, R. M., Wolstrup, J., and Bach Knudsen, K. E., The effect of protein quality and fibre level in the diet and microbial activity in the digestive tract on protein utilization and energy digestibility in rats, *Br. J. Nutr.*, 51, 305, 1984.
11. Farrell, D. J., Girle, L., and Arthur, J., Effects of dietary fiber on the apparent digestibility of major food components and on blood lipids in men, *Aust. J. Exp. Biol. Med. Sci.*, 56, 469, 1978.
12. Fleming, S. E. and Lee, B., Growth performance and intestinal transit time of rats fed purified and natural dietary fibers, *J. Nutr.*, 113, 592, 1983.
13. Food and Agriculture Organization, Amino Acid Content of Foods and Biological Data on Protein, Nutritional Studies No. 24, FAO, Rome, 1970.
14. Garrison, M. V., Rein, R. L., Fawley, P., and Breidenstein, C. P., Comparative digestibility of acid detergent fiber by laboratory albino and wild Polynesian rats, *J. Nutr.*, 108, 191, 1978.
15. Harmuth-Hoene, A. E., Jakubick, V., and Schelenz, R., Der einfluss von guarmehl in der nahrung auf die stickstoffbilanz, den proteinstoff-wechsel und die transitzeit der nahrung in ratten, *Nutr. Metab.*, 22, 32, 1978.
16. Harmuth-Hoene, A. E. and Schwerdtfeger, E., Effect of indigestible polysaccharides on protein digestibility and nitrogen retention in growing rates, *Nutr. Metab.*, 23, 399, 1979.
17. Hawkins, W. W. and Yaphe, W., Carrageenan as a dietary constituent for the rat: faecal excretion, nitrogen absorption and growth, *Can. J. Biochem.*, 43, 479, 1965.
18. Heymsfield, S. B., Roongspisuthipong, C., Evert, M., Casper, K., Heller, P., and Akrabawi, S. S., Fiber supplementation of enteral formulas: effects on the bioavailability of major nutrients and gastrointestinal tolerance, *J. Parenter. Enteral. Nutr.*, 12, 265, 1988.
19. Hove, E. L. and King, S., Effects of pectin and cellulose on growth, feed efficiency and protein utilization, and their contribution to energy requirement and cecal VFA in rats, *J. Nutr.*, 109, 1274, 1979.
20. Kaneko, K., Nishida, K., Yatsuda, J., Osa, S., and Koike, G., Effect of fiber on protein, fat and calcium digestibilities and fecal cholesterol excretion, *J. Nutr. Sci. Vitaminol.*, 32, 317, 1986.
21. Keim, K. and Kies, C., Effects of dietary fiber on nutritional status of weanling mice, *Cereal Chem.*, 56, 73, 1979.
22. Kelsay, J. L., Behail, K. M., and Prather, E. S., Effect of fiber from fruits and vegetables on metabolic responses of human subjects. I. Bowel transit time, number of defecations, fecal weight, urinary excretions of energy and nitrogen and apparent digestibilities of energy, nitrogen and fat, *Am. J. Clin. Nutr.*, 31, 1149, 1978.
23. Kelsay, J. L., Clark, W. M., Herbst, B. J., and Prather, E. S., Nutrient utilization by human subjects consuming fruits and vegetables as sources of fiber, *J. Agric. Food Chem.*, 29, 461, 1981.
24. Kies, C. and Fox, H. M., Fiber and protein nutritional status, *Cereal Foods World*, 23, 249, 1978.

25. Miles, C. W., Kelsay, J. L., and Wong, N. P., Effect of dietary fiber on the metabolizable energy of human diets, *J. Nutr.*, 118, 1075, 1988.
26. Miller, D. S. and Payne, P. R., Problems in the prediction of protein values of diets. The influence of protein concentration, *Br. J. Nutr.*, 15, 11, 1961.
27. Miyoshi, H., Okuda, T., Okuda, K., and Koishi, K., Effects of brown rice on apparent digestibility and balance of nutrients in young mean on low protein diets, *J. Nutr. Sci. Vitaminol.*, 33, 207, 1987.
28. Narayana Rao, M. and Sunderavalli, O. E., Extraneous cellulose: effect on protein utilization, *J. Am. Dietet. Assoc.*, 57, 517, 1970.
29. Nomani, M. Z., Fashandi, E. F., Davis, G. K., and Bradac, C. J., Influence of dietary fiber on the growth and protein metabolism of the rat, *J. Food Sci.*, 44, 745, 1979.
30. Nyman, M. and Asp, N-G., Fermentation of dietary fiber components in the rat intestinal tract, *Br. J. Nutr.*, 47, 357, 1982.
31. Peterson, A. D. and Baumgardt, B. R., Food and energy intake of rats fed diets varying in energy concentration and density, *J. Nutr.*, 101, 1059, 1971.
32. Peterson, A. D. and Baumgardt, B. R., Influence of level of energy demand on the ability of rats to compensate for diet dilution, *J. Nutr.*, 101, 1069, 1971.
33. Prynne, C. J. and Southgate, D. A. T., The effects of a supplement of dietary fiber on fecal excretion by human subjects, *Br. J. Nutr.*, 41, 495, 1979.
34. Schneeman, B. O. and Gallaher, D., Changes in small intestinal digestive enzyme activity and bile acids with dietary cellulose in rats, *J. Nutr.*, 110, 584, 1980.
35. Schneeman, B. O., Richter, B. D., and Jacobs, L. R., Response to dietary wheat bran in the exocrine pancreas and intestine of rats, *J. Nutr.*, 112, 283, 1982.
36. Shah, N., Attallah, M. T., Mahoney, R. R., and Pellett, P. L., Effect of dietary fiber components on fecal nitrogen excretion and protein utilization in growing rats, *J. Nutr.*, 112, 658, 1982.
37. Sibbald, I. R., Berg, R. T., and Bowland, J. P., Digestible energy in relation to food intake and nitrogen retention in the weanling rat, *J. Nutr.*, 59, 385, 1956.
38. Slavin, J. L. and Marlett, J. A., Effect of refined cellulose on apparent energy, fat and nitrogen digestibilities, *J. Nutr.*, 110, 2020, 1980.
39. Southgate, D. A. T., Branch, W. J., Hill, M. J., Draser, B. S., Welters, R. L., Davies, P. S., and Baird, I. M., Metabolic responses to dietary supplements of bran, *Metabolism*, 25, 1129, 1976.
40. Southgate, D. A. T. and Durnin, J. V., Calorie conversion factors. An experimental reassessment of the factors used in the calculation of the energy value of human diets, *Br. J. Nutr.*, 24, 517, 1970.
41. Spiller, G. A., Effect of graded dietary levels of plant fibers on fecal output in pig-tailed monkeys, *Nutr. Rep. Int.*, 23, 313, 1981.
42. Stanogias, G. and Pearce, G. R., The digestion of fibre by pigs. I. The effects of amount and type of fibre on apparent digestibility, nitrogen balance and rate of passage, *Br. J. Nutr.*, 53, 513, 1985.
43. Stephen, A. M. and Cummings, J. H., The influence of dietary fiber on fecal nitrogen excretion in man, *Proc. Nutr. Soc.*, 38, 141A, 1979.
44. Sundaravalli, O. E., Shurpalekar, K. S., and Narayana Rao, M., Inclusion of cellulose in calorie-restricted diets, *J. Am. Dietet. Assoc.*, 62, 41, 1973.
45. Ulnan, E. A. and Fisher, H., Arginine utilization of young rats fed diets with simple versus complex carbohydrates, *J. Nutr.*, 113, 131, 1983.
46. Viola, S., Zimmerman, G., and Mokady, S., Effect of pectin and algin upon protein utilization, digestibility of nutrients and energy in young rats, *Nutr. Rep. Int.*, 1, 367, 1970.
47. Ward, A. T. and Reichert, R. D., Comparison of the effect of cell wall and hull fiber from canola and soybean on the bioavailability for rats of minerals, protein and lipid, *J. Nutr.*, 116, 233, 1986.
48. Weber, F. L., Minco, D., Fresard, K. M., and Banwell, J. G., Effects of vegetable diets on nitrogen metabolism in cirrhotic subjects, *Gastroenterology*, 89, 538, 1985.
49. Bach Knudsen, K. E., Wisker, E., Daniel, M., Feldheim, W., and Eggum, B. O., Digestibility of energy, protein, fat and non-starch polysaccharides in mixed diets: comparative studies between man and the rat, *Br. J. Nutr.*, 71, 471, 1994.
50. Brunsgaard, G., Bach Knudsen, K. E., and Eggum, B. O., The influence of the period of adaptation on the digestibility of diets containing different types of indigestible polysaccharides in rats, *Br. J. Nutr.*, 74, 833, 1995.

51. Cole, J. T., Fahey, G. C., Jr., Merchen, N. R., Patil, A. R., Murray, S. M., Hussein, H. S., and Brent, J. L., Jr., Soybean hulls as a dietary fiber source in dogs, *J. Anim. Sci.*, 77, 917, 1999.

52. Diez, M., Hornick, J.-L., Baldwin, P., and Istasse, L., Influence of a blend of fructo-oligosaccharides and sugar beet fiber on nutrient digestibility and plasma metabolite concentrations in healthy Beagles, *Am. J. Vet. Res.*, 58, 1238, 1997.

53. Diez, M., Hornick, J. L., Baldwin, P., Van Eenaeme, C., and Istasse, L., The influence of sugar-beet fibre, guar gum and inulin on nutrient digestibility, water consumption and plasma metabolites in healthy Beagle dogs, *Res. Vet. Sci.*, 64, 91, 1998.

54. Jørgensen, H., Zhao, X.-Q., Bach Knudsen, K. E., and Eggum, B. O., The influence of dietary fibre source and level on the development of the gastrointestinal tract, digestibility and energy metabolism in broiler chickens, *Br. J. Nutr.*, 75, 379, 1996.

55. Leenaars, M. and Moughan, P. J., The apparent digestibility of energy, nitrogen, and fibre and the biological value of protein in low- and high-fibre wheat breads, *Plant Foods Human Nutr.*, 44, 187, 1993.

56. Pettersson, D. and Razdan, A., Effects of increasing levels of sugar-beet pulp in broiler chicken diets on nutrient digestion and serum lipids, *Br. J. Nutr.*, 70, 127, 1993.

57. Zhao, X., Jorgensen, H., and Eggum, B. O., The influence of dietary fibre on body composition, visceral organ weight, digestibility and energy balance in rats housed in different thermal environments, *Br. J. Nutr.*, 73, 687, 1995.

Effects of Dietary Fiber and Phytate on the Homeostasis and Bioavailability of Minerals

Barbara F. Harland and Donald Oberleas

Phytate is found in all plant seeds (both cereals and legumes), many roots and tubers, and in fruits. Dietary fiber is also derived from many of these same plants as a part of the stems, stalks, and leaves that support the growing plant. Phytate is a distinct, identifiable, and quantifiable compound, but it is frequently considered a component of dietary fiber — particularly in cereal bran. Other components of dietary fiber such as cellulose, hemicellulose, pectin, gums, and lignin have properties generally associated with fiber or roughage.

In order to understand the effects of these various components of dietary fiber, it is important to understand the physical and chemical properties of these various constituents that make up dietary fiber. The two major components are the water-insoluble cellulose, lignin, and some hemicelluloses and the water-soluble pectin, gums, and other hemicelluloses. With the exception of lignin, these all consist of polysaccharides or poly-alcohols. Pectin and gums hydrate and imbibe water and thus tend to provide bulk and lubrication to the GI tract; the cellulose and lignin provide bulk without hydration. The hydroxyl groups are weak binding and complexing sites and thus, with the exception of adsorption of the minerals on the large cellulose structure, fibers do not have sufficient binding characteristics to significantly alter the balance of any minerals.

Phytate, on the other hand, has strongly electrovalent phosphate acid groups that have stronger binding and complexing properties. Also, for this relatively small molecule there is a large capacity for the complexation of essential divalent cations. There is also good evidence that calcium, magnesium, and zinc are recycled through the pancreas.[1] This should make these essential divalent mineral elements more vulnerable to complexation. Though fiber would pass through this same region of the GI tract, the greater compleximetric strength of phytate toward cations would favor phytate as having the greater effect on the homeostasis of these minerals. The special exception to this may be iron, which has special complexing properties with phytate.[2]

All people who consume a well-balanced diet also consume a diet containing phytate.[3] Therefore, phytate is a component of most human diets throughout the world. Whereas phytate and inositol phosphates cannot be absorbed,[4] phytate's hydrolysis products, both phosphate and inositol, are absorbable. Independent of phosphate esters, inositol is absorbable and is metabolized as glucose. Thus, if dietary phytate is to exhibit some effect, that effect must be limited to the gastrointestinal tract.

The other characteristic chemical property of phytate is that it dissociates to a very large anion in acid solution and has a capability for complexing heavy metals. This complexation effect may be positive, as in the case of non-essential metals such as cadmium and lead, or negative, as in the case of essential metal elements such as calcium, iron, and zinc, and to a lesser extent copper, magnesium, manganese, and others. Only calcium, iron, and zinc have been studied in detail. Several *in vitro* studies have been carried out that have helped to clarify the complexing characteristics with various mineral elements.[5] More recent studies of several divalent cations *in vitro* demonstrated a reciprocal relationship between the atomic weights and the relative strengths of the phytate–cation complexes (Figure 4.2.1).[6]

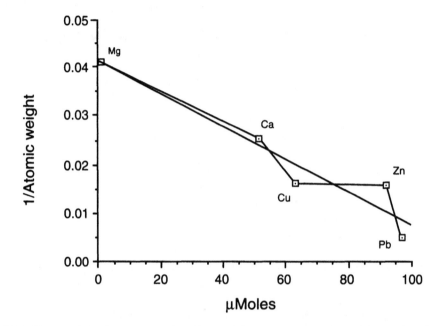

Figure 4.2.1 The correlation between atomic weight and the concentration of precipitates of each cation at a phytate-to-cation molar ratio of 1:2 at pH 6.0. The correlation equation is atomic weight $(Y) = 0.0412 - 0.0034X$ (μmoles precipitated), $r^2 = 0.92$. (*Source:* Oberleas, D. and Chan, H.-C., *Trace Elem. Elec.*, 14, 173, 1997. With permission.)

ZINC HOMEOSTASIS

Zinc deficiency was first described in rats by Todd et al.[7] This was accomplished with a diet that was chemically depleted of zinc. So little zinc was required to meet the needs of the animals, it was thought that zinc deficiency was not possible with natural foodstuffs. Yet zinc deficiency, with apparent adequate dietary zinc but containing plant seed protein, was reported by Tucker and Salmon.[8] Phytate was not implicated in zinc deficiency until O'Dell and Savage[9] demonstrated that, with chickens, phytic acid added to a casein-based (animal protein) diet produced the same deficiency symptoms as a soybean-based (plant seed protein) diet. This was repeated in several species including rainbow trout,[10] Japanese quail,[11] rats,[5] pigs,[12] dogs,[13] and humans.[14] These observations established a definite relationship between phytate and zinc homeostasis.

Most investigators continued to believe that the major effect of phytate was on the absorption of dietary zinc. The word "bioavailability" was coined in the early 1970s to describe this phenomenon. *In vitro* studies have also shown that zinc complexes strongly with phytate at pH 6.[5] This pH is ideal for maximum complexation and is also the approximate pH of the duodenum.

Investigators have ignored the secretion of zinc via the pancreatic fluid in quantities as much as four times that likely to be consumed in foods each day.[15-17] Evidence in other species has continued to be developed.[18-20] Zinc is the only essential divalent trace element cation that is secreted via the pancreas. It is also obvious that much of this secreted zinc must be reabsorbed in order for zinc homeostasis to be sustained. With dietary zinc representing only 20 to 25% of the duodenal pool, it was possible to measure relative absorption of dietary zinc utilizing radioactive ^{65}zinc. However, any result must be assigned to the total duodenal zinc pool to become of any value. This parameter is more difficult to measure and has as yet to be adequately determined in humans.[21] Computer models developed to study human fluxes have either avoided or ignored this fact.[22-25]

Only recently were efforts made to understand the pancreatic pool and its importance in the maintenance of zinc homeostasis. This was done using a rat model in which the endogenous pool was labeled with radioactive ^{65}zinc (Oberleas[20]). Some of the rats were fed a phytate-containing diet using soybean protein as the native phytate source. An equal number of animals were fed a non-phytate-containing animal protein diet. Simply measuring the differential of fecal zinc excretion and comparing the ratio of radioactive excretion indicates that the major effect of phytate is not on the dietary pool, but rather on the duodenal pool. Thus, the effect is not dietary zinc bioavailability but zinc homeostasis. The results of these studies are shown in Figure 4.2.2. This clearly shows that the effect of phytate on endogenous zinc is two to four times the effect on dietary zinc. From these results a theoretical model was developed. This theoretical model is represented in Figure 4.2.3.[20] This model has been confirmed also in rats, as shown in Figure 4.2.4.[26]

Little effort has been made to study this zinc pool, and most investigators utilize experimental diets in animal studies that contain dehydrated ovalbumin, again an animal protein deficient in zinc. No population group in the world consumes such a diet; therefore, a practical relationship of this type of diet to any culture or world population is nonexistent.

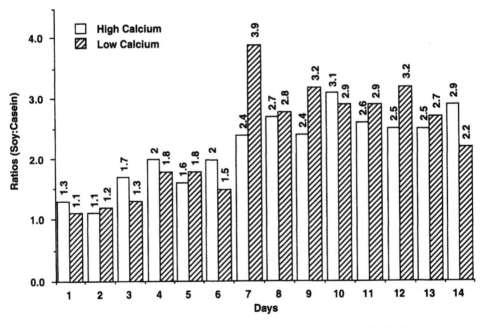

Figure 4.2.2 Ratios of ^{65}zinc excreted following intraperitoneal injection as affected by isolated soybean–casein diets and dietary calcium levels. (*Source:* Oberleas, D., *J. Inorg. Biochem.*, 62, 231, 1996. With permission.)

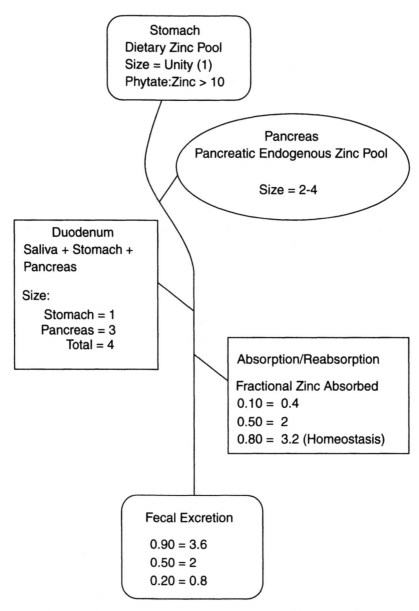

Figure 4.2.3 A mathematical model for zinc homeostasis. This model assumes a daily dietary intake expressed as unity, and all other values are relative to the dietary intake. (*Source:* Oberleas, D., *J. Inorg. Biochem.*, 62, 231, 1996. With permission.)

MAGNESIUM BIOAVAILABILITY

In humans, magnesium is absorbed in both the jejunum and the ileum. Magnesium is secreted into the GI tract related to the flux of water,[1] with absorption dependent upon the movement of water. The concentrations of secretory fluids in decreasing order are bile, 0.70 mmol/L; gastric fluid, 0.50 mmol/L; saliva, 0.15 mmol/L; and pancreatic fluid, 0.05 mmol/L. Secreted magnesium appears to be almost completely reabsorbed. The efficiency of absorption ranges from 21 to 70%. Some factors which influence magnesium absorption include dietary intake, intestinal transit time, rate of water absorption, dietary calcium and phosphate, source of magnesium, and age. The kidney

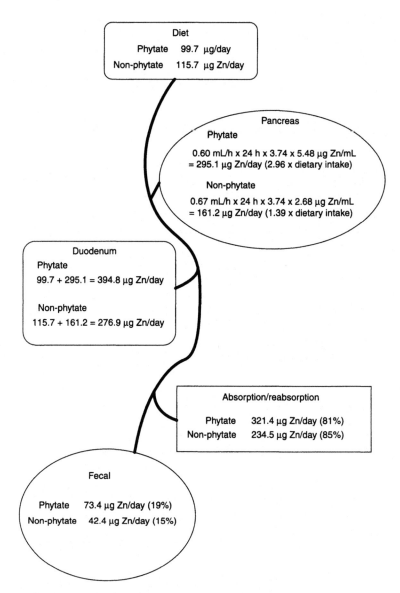

Figure 4.2.4 Confirmation of zinc homeostasis with the rat as the experimental model. (*Source:* Oberleas, D. and Kwun, I. S., in *Metal Ions in Biology and Medicine*, vol. 5, Collery, P., Bratter, P., Negretti de Bratter, V., Khassanova, L., and Etienne, J. C., Eds., John Libbey Eurotext, Paris, 1998, 140. With permission.)

is the primary site for magnesium reabsorption and regulation of homeostasis, where it may be influenced by water reabsorption and parathormone. Considerable magnesium excretion may occur via sweat loss.

Much of the fecal magnesium appears to be unabsorbed dietary magnesium. Ten to 30% of plant cell magnesium is associated with chlorophyll. Nothing is known about the bioavailability of chlorophyll magnesium, which could be a major contributor to the fiber effect. Several reports of decreased magnesium absorption with human subjects have been reported using cellulose as the fiber source,[27–31] and Kelsay et al.[32] used pectin as the fiber source. Drews et al.[33] reported no effect with adolescent male subjects, utilizing either cellulose or pectin.

With phytate, magnesium alone does not complex well,[6] but magnesium serves well as a tertiary synergistic cation. Several studies with a rat model reported an adverse effect of dietary phytate on magnesium absorption.[34–37] Two studies with human subjects reported a negative effect of dietary phytate on magnesium absorption.[38,39]

CALCIUM BIOAVAILABILITY

Calcium is normally the divalent mineral cation in greatest concentration in the diet. Calcium absorption occurs from all segments of the small intestine, particularly the proximal colon.[40] Calcium is also secreted into the duodenum at 30 to 40% of the dietary concentration.[1] Calcium absorption is enhanced by lysine, arginine, fructose, glucose, lactose, and xylose.[41] Phytate, fiber, and oxalate decrease the absorption of calcium by forming complexes, and some adsorption occurs in the case of fiber. Calcium does not complex as tightly with phytate as does copper or zinc, but by virtue of its dietary concentration it is usually, but erroneously, given responsibility for the synergistic secondary cation effect observed in practical animal experiments.[6,9] Truly, the synergism works both ways and, thus, that affected by other dietary divalent cations makes calcium vulnerable to phytate complexation and subsequent decreased absorption. There are many accessory dietary factors that need to be evaluated to determine the net effect of phytate on calcium absorption and bioavailability. It is difficult to arrive at a uniform conclusion because most experiments used diets containing both phytate and dietary fiber,[33,38,39,42,43] and, under these circumstances, differentiating between a phytate effect and a fiber effect is most difficult.

Again, a true effect of fiber is difficult to ascertain. The adsorption of an insoluble calcium salt onto a fiber matrix without the demonstration of a chemical complex formation is not an effect of fiber in reducing the absorption of that mineral. An insoluble calcium salt that coincidentally adsorbs upon a fiber matrix without chemical reaction with some fiber component would not have been absorbed if the diet were devoid of fiber. This is one reason for the variety of results that make simple conclusions questionable.[33,44]

An important characteristic of dietary fiber or dietary fiber adjuncts in our diets is that they are fully or partially fermented in the large intestine where the lower pH fosters this activity. Soluble oligosaccharides such as inulin and fructooligosaccharides have been shown to enhance calcium and magnesium absorption quantifiable by increased femoral bone volume and mineral concentrations in rats.[45] In another study, Bird et al.[46] showed decreased large bowel calcium concentrations in pigs fed brown rice compared with boiled white rice, showing significantly greater calcium absorption from all sections of the lower bowel.

COPPER BIOAVAILABILITY

In most species, dietary copper is poorly absorbed.[47] The extent of absorption is influenced by the amount and chemical form of the copper ingested, by the dietary level of other metal ions, and by organic substances that may include both dietary fiber and phytate. In adults, copper is absorbed from the stomach and all portions of the small intestine with decreasing efficiency in descending order.[48–51] Copper is absorbed in the cupric state and is more easily oxidized and/or reduced than is iron. Thus, those substances that tend to favor the absorption of iron by reducing ferric iron to ferrous can have a devastating effect on copper absorption. Ascorbic acid is renowned in this regard,[52–54] and fructose or fructose-containing sugars, i.e., sucrose, have been shown to alter copper absorption.[55]

The normal site of excretion of copper is via the bile. The excretory products are very stable complexes which are not susceptible to being reabsorbed or altered by dietary fiber or phytate. Thus, any effect of fiber or phytate on copper in the GI tract must be on dietary copper. There is little agreement on fiber having an effect on copper bioavailability, but it could contribute to the synergistic co-precipitation of calcium, lead, magnesium, and zinc by phytate in the GI tract.[6]

Very little interest has been shown regarding the effect of phytate or fiber directly on copper absorption or bioavailability. Davis et al.[56] reported that an isolated soybean protein diet fed to chickens decreased the bioavailability of copper. This was later confirmed by Davies and Nightingale using a rat model.[37] Human studies indicating an effect of phytate on copper absorption have been reported by Moser et al.[57] Without further information on details of the diets used in these studies, investigators must withhold definitive conclusions.

IRON BIOAVAILABILITY

Several studies have indicated that phytate in the diet decreases the iron balances in human subjects.[38,58–64] Some animal studies have also confirmed the effect of phytate on iron absorption to a greater[37] or lesser[65–67] extent. Iron absorption is dependent upon several factors, including the size of iron stores and particularly the extent of stores in enterocytes, which are the sites of regulation of iron absorption. There are two chemical forms of dietary iron: heme and non-heme. Heme iron is present in hemoglobin from blood and myoglobin from muscle meat. Heme iron, by the presence of the heme complex, is non-ionic and is absorbed intact and thus protected from the possible complexation by phytate. Heme represents approximately 10 to 15% of the total iron intake within the developed world.[67]

Non-heme iron is also found in two forms: ferrous and ferric iron. Though the chemical difference is one electron, this makes for considerable chemical and physiological difference, including its reaction with phytate. Non-heme iron constitutes the remaining 85 to 90% of dietary iron in the developed world and maybe more in the developing countries. The most active site of iron absorption is the duodenum and upper jejunum. However, the effect of phytate on iron absorption may have already occurred in the stomach. Ferric ion was declared the only ion that would complex with phytate in dilute acid conditions and thus was the basis for the first and many subsequent analytical methods for phytate.[68] More recently, *in vitro* studies have been made of the complexation between phytate and ferric and ferrous ions independently. It is this chemistry of ferric ions with phytate that describes the mechanism for the alteration of ferric iron availability. Thus, the resultant complexation does not occur in the duodenum as with most cations but in the stomach, where the acid conditions dissociate phytate from its various dietary complexes and provide the ideal environment for complexation with ferric iron. Interestingly, ferrous iron, though not quite as insoluble as ferric iron, starts precipitating at about pH 2, which also gives it some advantage over other essential cations for complexation, and thus, vulnerability toward reduced iron bioavailability. The other important characteristic of both ferric and ferrous complexes is that they remain fairly stable through pH 7. This is shown in Figure 4.2.5. Since there is no recycling of iron via the duodenum or bile, the only logical mechanism is that iron merely gets first chance to complex and, whereas other cation complexes are soluble in dilute acid, ferric and ferrous irons form very stable, insoluble complexes.

MANGANESE BIOAVAILABILITY

Manganese may be found in several valence states from +1 to +7, with Mn^{+2} being the most stable. Absorption has been reported as low as 1%[69] to as high as 40%[70] using rat models. The dietary factors which affect the absorption and distribution of manganese have not been clearly identified. Only Davies and Nightingale[37] have reported an effect of phytate on the absorption of manganese, also in a rat model. The main route of manganese excretion is via the bile.[71] The homeostatic regulation of manganese in the body appears to be effected by a very efficient excretory process.[72] Much of the excreted manganese may be reabsorbed in a hormonally regulated pattern.

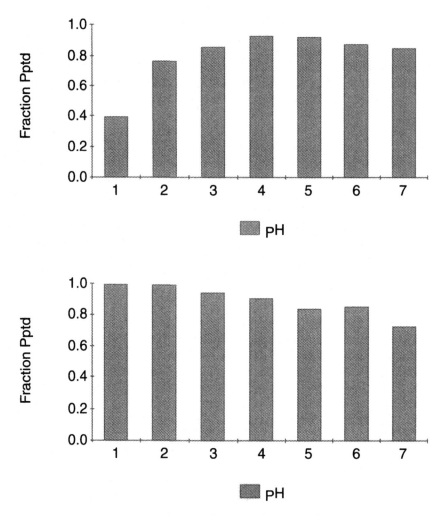

Figure 4.2.5 Chemical precipitation of ferrous (top) and ferric (bottom) ions at various pHs at a 2:1 molar ratio of cations to phytate. (*Source:* Oberleas, D., in *Metal Ions in Biology and Medicine*, vol. 6, Centano, J. A., Collery, P., Vernet, G., Finkelman, R. B., Gibb, H., and Etienne, J. C., Eds., John Libbey Eurotext, Paris, 2000, 558. With permission.)

At this time it is difficult to ascertain whether either phytate or dietary fiber could have a significant effect on manganese homeostasis.

PHOSPHORUS BIOAVAILABILITY

Phytate is rich in phosphate, but its non-availability to monogastric species was first shown by Common[73] with young chicks as the model. This has been confirmed many times in several monogastric species reviewed by Nelson[74] and more recently by Soares.[75] Since phosphorus is absorbed as orthophosphate, the conclusion was that chicks did not have the inherent ability to hydrolyze phytate. This same conclusion has been shown for rats,[76] pigs,[77] and recently with dogs by Schoenherr et al.[4] This is a fair conclusion for humans, also.[38,78]

This lack of bioavailability of phosphorus from phytate means that much of the dietary phosphorus is excreted in the feces. Phosphorus from phosphorus-rich chicken and pig manure has created another international problem of phosphorus pollution when applied to cropland as fertilizer in the Netherlands, Germany, and Taiwan and in the U.S. (North Carolina, Maryland, Delaware, Virginia, and Arkansas), where chicken and pig production is high and the land available for spreading the manure is limited. This has led to the development of microbial phytase products that, when added to animal diets, are effective in improving the utilization of phytate phosphorus in both pigs and poultry.[79,80] Incorporating phytase into animal feeds can improve phytate phosphorus bioavailability by 40 to 50%. An added benefit from phytase is an enhancement of the bioavailability of copper, zinc, and other divalent trace minerals.[81]

The effect of fiber (cellulose) on phosphorus bioavailability is less distinctive. Only Godara et al.[82] reported some decrease in phosphorus absorption, whereas others indicated no differences.[32,43] Here again, the effect may be related to the relative solubility of the phosphate salts contained in the diet and the greater or lesser degree of adsorption of these salts on the dietary fiber components.

SUMMARY

It is well established that phytate, with its strong complexing bonds, is capable of combining with essential divalent cations, decreasing their absorption or, in the case of zinc and possibly magnesium, their reabsorption and thus homeostasis. The environmental conditions, such as the pH of the GI tract (acidic in the stomach for iron and about pH 6 in the duodenum and upper jejunum), combined with the secretion of calcium, magnesium, and particularly zinc, create realistic metabolic deficits. With respect to dietary fiber, the case is not as well defined. The fibers provide bulk, and pectin and gums provide osmotic potential. However, these compounds have weak binding characteristics, and thus much of their effect is limited to the adsorption of the mineral elements. Adsorption has a less reliable and less effective impact on the mineral elements and, coupled with several dietary variables, produces outcomes that are less conclusive.

REFERENCES

1. Cragle, R. G., Dynamics of mineral elements in the digestive tract of ruminants, *Fed. Proc.*, 32, 1910, 1973.
2. Oberleas, D., Ferrous and ferric ions with phytate *in vitro, Metal Ions in Biology and Medicine*, vol. 6, Centano, J. A., Collery, P., Vernet, G., Finkelman, R. B., Gibb, H., and Etienne, J. C., Eds., John Libbey Eurotext, Paris, 558, 2000.
3. Harland, B. F. and Morris, E. R., Fibre and mineral absorption, in *Fibre Perspectives*, vol. 1, Leeds, A. R., Ed., John Libby and Sons, London, 1985, 72.
4. Schoenherr, W., Davidson, S., Stephens, L., Grieti, J., Wedekind, K., and Harmon, D., Digestion and absorption of phytate in mature dogs, *FASEB J.*, 14, 160.10, 2000.
5. Oberleas, D., Muhrer, M. E., and O'Dell, B. L., Dietary metal-complexing agents and zinc availability in the rat, *J. Nutr.*, 90, 56, 1966.
6. Oberleas, D. and Chan, H.-C., Cation complexation by phytate, *Trace Elem. Elec.*, 14, 173, 1997.
7. Todd, W. R., Elvehjem, C. A., and Hart, E. B., Zinc in the nutrition of the rat, *J. Biol. Chem.*, 107, 146, 1934.
8. Tucker, H. F. and Salmon, W. D., Parakeratosis or zinc deficiency disease in the pig, *Proc. Soc. Exptl. Biol. Med.*, 88, 613, 1955.
9. O'Dell, B. L. and Savage, J. E., Effect of phytic acid on zinc availability, *Proc. Soc. Exp. Biol. Med.*, 103, 304, 1960.
10. Ketola, H. G., Influence of dietary zinc on cataracts in rainbow trout (*Salmo gairdneri*), *J. Nutr.*, 109, 965, 1979.
11. Fox, M. R. S. and Harrison, B. N., Use of Japanese quail for the study of zinc deficiency, *Proc. Soc. Exp. Biol. Med.*, 116, 256, 1964.

12. Oberleas, D., Muhrer, M. E., and O'Dell, B. L., Effects of phytic acid on zinc availability and parakeratosis in swine, *J. Anim. Sci.*, 21, 57, 1962.

13. Robertson, B. T. and Burns, M. J., Zinc metabolism and the zinc deficiency syndrome in the dog, *Am. J. Vet. Res.*, 24, 997, 1963.

14. Prasad, A. S., Halsted, J. A., and Nadimi, M., Syndrome of iron deficiency anemia, hepatosplenomegaly, hypogonadism, dwarfism and geophagia, *Am. J. Med.*, 31, 532, 1961.

15. Montgomery, M. S., Sheline, G. E., and Chaikoff, I. L., The elimination of administered zinc in pancreatic juice, duodenal juice and bile of the dog as measured by its radioactive isotope ^{65}Zn, *J. Exp. Med.*, 78, 151, 1943.

16. Birnstingl, M., Stone, B., and Richards, V., Excretion of radioactive zinc (Zn-65) in bile, pancreatic and duodenal secretions of the dog, *Am. J. Physiol.*, 186, 377, 1956.

17. Cotzias, G. C., Borg, D. C., and Selleck, B., Specificity of zinc pathway through the body: turnover of 65-Zn in, the mouse, *Am. J. Physiol.*, 202, 359, 1962.

18. Pekas, J. C., Zinc-65 metabolism: gastrointestinal secretion by the pig, *Am. J. Physiol.*, 211, 407, 1966.

19. Schneeman, B. O., Lonnerdal, C. L., and Hurley, L. S., Zinc and copper in rat bile and pancreatic fluid: effects of surgery, *J. Nutr.*, 113, 1165, 1983.

20. Oberleas, D., Mechanism of zinc homeostasis, *J. Inorg. Biochem.*, 62, 231, 1996.

21. Oberleas, D., In search of a human model for zinc homeostasis, in *Proceedings of the 2nd International Symposium on Trace Elements in Human: New Perspectives*, Ermidou-Pollet, S. and Pollet, S., Eds., G. Morogianni, Athens, Greece, 2000, 651–659.

22. Aamodt, R. L., Rumble, W. F., and Henkin, R. I., Zinc absorption in humans, in *Nutritional Bioavailability of Zinc*, Inglett, G.E., Ed., American Chemical Society, Washington, D.C., 1983, 61.

23. Wastney, M. E. and Henkin, R. I., Development and application of a model for zinc metabolism in humans, *Prog. Food Nutr. Sci.*, 12, 243, 1988.

24. Lowe, N. M., Shames, D. M., Woodhouse, L. R., Matel, J. S., Roehl, R., Saccomani, M. P., Toffolo, G., Cobelli, C., and King, J., A compartmental model of zinc metabolism in healthy women using oral and intravenous stable isotope tracers, *Am. J. Clin. Nutr.*, 65, 1810, 1997.

25. Lowe, N. M., Woodhouse, L. R. Matel, J. S., and King, J. C., Comparison of estimates of zinc absorption in humans by using 4 stable isotopic tracer methods and compartmental analysis, *Am. J. Clin. Nutr.*, 71, 523, 2000.

26. Oberleas, D. and Kwun, I. S., Confirmation of the mechanism of zinc homeostasis, *Metal Ions in Biology and Medicine*, vol. 5, Collery, P., Bratter, P., Negretti de Bratter, V., Khassanova, L., and Etienne, J. C., Eds., John Libbey Eurotext, Paris, 140, 1998.

27. Ismail-Beigi, F., Reinhold, J. G., Faraji, B., and Abadi, P., Effects of cellulose added to diets of low and high fiber content upon metabolism of calcium, magnesium, zinc and phosphorus, by man, *J. Nutr.*, 107, 510, 1977.

28. Slavin, J. L., Marlett, M. S., and Marlett, J. A., Influence of refined cellulose on human bowel function and calcium and magnesium balances, *Am. J. Clin. Nutr.*, 33, 1932, 1980.

29. McHale, M., Kies, C., and Fox, H. M., Calcium and magnesium nutritional status of adolescent humans fed cellulose or hemicellulose supplements, *J. Food Sci.*, 44, 1412, 1979.

30. Revusova, V., Sodium cellulose phosphate-induced increment in urinary calcium/magnesium ratio, *Eur. Urol.*, 1, 294, 1975.

31. Parfitt, A. M., Effect of cellulose phosphate on calcium and magnesium homeostasis: studies in normal subjects and patients with latent hypoparathyroidism, *Clin. Sci. Mol. Med.*, 49, 83, 1975.

32. Kelsay, J. L., Behall, K. M., and Prather, E. S., Effect of fiber from fruits and vegetables on metabolic responses of human subjects, *Am. J. Clin. Nutr.*, 32, 1876, 1979.

33. Drews, L. M., Kies, C., and Fox, H. M., Effects of dietary fiber on copper, zinc and magnesium utilization in adolescent boys, *Am. J. Clin. Nutr.*, 32, 1893, 1979.

34. Roberts, A. H. and Yudkin, J., Dietary phytate as a possible cause of magnesium deficiency, *Nature*, 185, 823, 1960.

35. Seelig, M. S., Requirement of magnesium by the normal adult, *Am. J. Clin. Nutr.*, 14, 342, 1964.

36. Likuski, H. J. A. and Forbes, R. M., Mineral utilization in the rat. IV. Effects of calcium and phytic acid on the utilization of dietary zinc, *J. Nutr.*, 85, 230, 1965.

37. Davies, N. T. and Nightingale, R., The effects of phytate on intestinal absorption and secretion of zinc, and whole-body retention of zinc, copper, iron and manganese in rats, *Br. J. Nutr.*, 34, 243, 1975.

38. McCance, R. A. and Widdowson, E. M., Mineral metabolism of healthy adults on white and brown bread dietaries, *J. Physiol.*, 101, 44, 1942.

39. Reinhold, J. G., Faraji, B., Abadi, P., and Ismail-Beigi, F., Decreased absorption of calcium, magnesium, zinc and phosphorus by humans due to increased fiber and phosphorus consumption as wheat bread, *J. Nutr.*, 106, 493, 1976.

40. Bronner, F., Dynamics and function of calcium, in *Mineral Metabolism: An Advanced Treatise.* 1st ed., vol. IIA, Comar, C. L. and Bronner, F., Eds., Academic Press, New York, 1964, 341.

41. Weiser, M. M., Calcium, in *Absorption and Malabsorption of Mineral Nutrients*, 1st ed., Solomons, N. W. and Rosenberg, I. H., Eds., Alan R. Liss, New York, 1984, 39.

42. Walker, A. R. P., Fox, F. W., and Irving, J. R., The effect of bread rich in phytate phosphorus on the metabolism of certain mineral salts, with special reference to calcium, *Biochem. J.*, 42, 452, 1948.

43. Sandberg, A.-S., Hasselblad, C., and Hasselblad, K., The effect of wheat bran on the absorption of minerals in the small intestine, *J. Nutr.*, 48, 185, 1982.

44. Aro, A., Usiteyra, M., Korhonen, T., and Sitonen, O., Dietary fiber and calcium excretion in diabetes, *Br. Med. J.*, 281, 831, 1980.

45. Takahara, S., Morohashi, T., Sano, T., Ohta, A., Yamada, S., and Sasa, R., Fructooligosaccharide consumption enhances femoral bone volume and mineral concentrations in rats, *J. Nutr.*, 130, 1792, 2000.

46. Bird, A. R., Hayakawa, T., Marsono, Y., Gooden, J. M., Record, I. R., Correll, R. L., and Topping, D. L., Coarse brown rice increases fecal and large bowel short-chain fatty acids and starch but lowers calcium in the large bowel of pigs, *J. Nutr.*, 130, 1780, 2000.

47. Schultze, M. O., Elvehjem, C. A., and Hart, E. B., Further studies on the availability of copper from various sources as a supplement to iron in hemoglobin formation, *J. Biol. Chem.*, 115, 453, 1936.

48. Owen, C. A., Jr., Absorption and excretion of ^{64}Cu-labeled copper by the rat, *Am. J. Physiol.*, 207, 1203, 1964.

49. Starcher, B. C., Studies on the mechanism of copper absorption in the chick, *J. Nutr.*, 97, 321, 1969.

50. Van Campen, D. R. and Mitchell, E. A., Absorption of Cu^{64}, Zn^{65}, Mo^{99}, and Fe^{59} from ligated segments of the rat gastrointestinal tract, *J. Nutr.*, 86, 120, 1965.

51. Bremner, I., Absorption, transport, and distribution of copper, *Biological Roles of Copper*, Ciba Foundation Symposium 79, Amsterdam, Excerpta Medica, 1980, 23.

52. Carlton, W. W. and Henderson, W., Studies in chickens fed a copper-deficient diet supplemented with ascorbic acid, reserpine, and diethylstilbesterol, *J. Nutr.*, 85, 67, 1965.

53. Hill, C. H. and Starcher, B., Effect of reducing agents on copper deficiency in the chick, *J. Nutr.*, 87, 271, 1965.

54. Hunt, C. E. and Carlton, W. W., Cardiovascular lesions associated with experimental copper deficiency in the rabbit, *J. Nutr.*, 87, 385, 1965.

55. Fields, M., Ferretti, R. J., Reiser, S., and Smith, J. C., Jr., The severity of copper deficiency in rats is determined by the type of dietary carbohydrate, *Proc. Soc. Exp. Biol. Med.*, 175, 530, 1984.

56. Davis, P. N., Norris, L. C., and Kratzer, F. H., Interference of soybean proteins with the utilization of trace minerals, *J. Nutr.*, 77, 217, 1962.

57. Moser, P. B., Reynolds, R. D., Acharya, S., Howard, M. P., Andon, M. B., and Lewis, S. A., Copper, iron, zinc, and selenium dietary intake and status of Nepalese lactating women and their breast-fed infants, *Am. J. Clin. Nutr.*, 47, 729, 1988.

58. McCance, R. A., Edgecombe, C. N., and Widdowson, E. M., Phytic acid and iron absorption, *Lancet*, II, 126, 1943.

59. Sharpe, L. M., Peacock, W. C., Cooke, R., Harris, R. S., Lockhart, H., Yee, H., and Nightingale, G., The effect of phytate and other food factors on iron absorption, *J. Nutr.*, 41, 433, 1950.

60. Turnbull, A., Cleton, F., and Finch, C. A., Iron absorption. VI. Absorption of hemoglobin iron, *J. Clin. Invest.*, 41, 1897, 1962.

61. Simpson, K. M., Eugene, B. S., and Cook, R. M. D., The inhibitory effect of bran on iron absorption in man, *Am. J. Clin. Nutr.*, 34, 1469, 1981.

62. Gillooly, M., Bothwell, T. H., Torrance, J. D., WacPhail, A. P., Derman, D. P., Bezwoda, W. R., Mills, W., and Charlton, R. W., The effects of organic acids, phytates and polyphenols on the absorption of iron from vegetables, *Br. J. Nutr.*, 49, 331, 1983.

63. Hallberg, L., Rossander, L., and Skanberg, A. B., Phytates and the inhibitory effect of bran on iron absorption in man, *Am. J. Clin. Nutr.*, 45, 988, 1987.

64. Hallberg, L., Brune, M., and Rossander, L., Iron absorption in man: Ascorbic acid and dose-dependent inhibition by phytate, *Am. J. Clin. Nutr.*, 49, 140, 1989.

65. Fuhr, I. and Steenbock, H., Effect of dietary calcium, phosphorus, and vitamin D on the utilization of iron. I. Effect of phytic acid on the availability of iron, *J. Biol. Chem.*, 147, 59, 1943.

66. Cowan, J. W., Esfahani, M., Salji, J. P., and Azzam, S. A., Effect of phytate on iron absorption in the rat, *J. Nutr.*, 90, 423, 1966.

67. Ranhotra, G. S., Loewe, R. J., and Puyat, L. V., Effect of dietary phytic acid on the availability of iron and phosphorus, *Cereal Chem.*, 51, 323, 1974.

67. Hallberg, L., Bioavailability of dietary iron in man, *Ann. Rev. Nutr.*, 1, 123, 1981.

68. Heubner, W. and Stadler, H., Uber eine Titration-methode zur Bestimmung des Phytins, *Biochem. Z.*, 64, 422, 1914.

69. Greenburg, D. M., Copp, B. D., and Cutherbertson, E. M., The distribution and excretion, particularly by way of the bile, of iron, cobalt, and manganese, *J. Biol. Chem.*, 147, 749, 1943.

70. Lee, D. Y. and Johnson, P. E., Factors affecting absorption and excretion of ^{54}Mn in rats, *J. Nutr.*, 118, 1509, 1988.

71. Bertinchamps, A. J., Miller, S. T., and Cotzias, G. C., Interdependence of routes excreting manganese, *Am. J. Physiol.*, 211, 217, 1966.

72. Howes, A. D. and Dyer, I. A., Diet and supplemental mineral effects on manganese metabolism in newborn calves, *J. Anim. Sci.*, 32, 141, 1971.

73. Common, R. H., Phytic acid and mineral metabolism in poultry, *Nature*, 143, 379, 1939.

74. Nelson, T. S., Utilization of phytate phosphorus by poultry: a review, *Poult. Sci.*, 46, 862, 1967.

75. Soares, J. H., Phosphorus bioavailability, in *Bioavailability of Nutrients for Animals*, 1st ed., Ammerman, C. B., Baker, D. H., and Lewis, A. J., Eds., Academic Press, New York, 1995, 257.

76. Oberleas, D., Dietary Factors Affecting Zinc Availability, Ph.D. dissertation, University of Missouri-Columbia, 1964.

77. Kornegay, E. T. and Thomas, H. R., Phosphorus in swine. II. Influence of dietary calcium and phosphorus levels and growth rate on serum minerals, soundness scores and bone development in barrows, gilts and boars, *J. Anim. Sci.*, 52, 1049, 1981.

78. Reinhold, J. G., Lahimgarzadeh, A., Nasr, K., and Hedayati, H., Effects of purified phytate and phytate-rich bread upon metabolism of zinc, calcium, phosphorus and nitrogen in man, *Lancet*, 1, 283, 1973.

79. Cromwell, G. L., Stahly, T. S., Coffey, R. D., Monegue, H. J., and Randolph, J. H., Efficacy of phytase in improving the bioavailability of phosphorus in soybean meal and corn-soybean meal diets for pigs, *J. Anim. Sci.*, 71, 1831, 1993.

80. Cromwell, G. L., Coffey, R. D., Parker, G. R., Monegue, H. J., and Randolph, J. H., Efficacy of a recombinant-derived phytase in improving the bioavailability of phosphous in corn-soybean meal diets for pigs, *J. Anim. Sci.*, 73, 2000, 1995.

81. Pallauf, V. J., Hohler, D., and Rimbach, G., Effect of microbial phytase supplementation to a maize-soya diet on the apparent absorption of Mg, Fe, Cu, Mn, and Zn and parameters of Zn status in piglets, *J. Anim. Physiol. Anim. Nutr.*, 68, 1, 1992.

82. Godara, R., Kaur, A. P., and Bhat, C. M., Effect of cellulose incorporation in a low fiber diet on fecal excretion and serum levels of calcium, phosphorus and iron in adolescent girls, *Am. J. Clin. Nutr.*, 34, 1083, 1981.

Effects of Dietary Fiber on Vitamin Metabolism

Heinrich Kasper

ABSORPTION OF VITAMINS

Fat-Soluble Vitamins

Starting from the fact that fecal fat excretion is increased after a high-fiber diet, the question arises whether dietary fiber substances (DF) affect ingested fat-soluble vitamins being utilized in the GI tract. The exact mechanism by which the intake of DF induces fecal fat excretion is not known. Interactions between DF and bile salts or the formation of micelles are discussed, as is the impaired activity of intestinal enzymes. DF binds components of mixed micelles, such as bile salts, fatty acids, monolene, phospholipids, etc., and may therefore impair fat absorption in the upper jejunum.[1] Reduced lymphatic absorption of both cholesterol and triglycerides in rats receiving pectin, alfalfa, and cellulose also supports this hypothesis.[2] Reports on the way different DFs influence pancreatic enzyme activity, especially lipase activity, are contradictory.[3–6] Due to the close relationship between the absorption of triglycerides and fat-soluble vitamins, disorders of fat absorption are invariably always associated with a disorder of the absorption of fat-soluble vitamins. Esters of fat-soluble vitamins, dissolved in nutritional fat, are hydrolyzed in the intestinal lumen by pancreatic carboxylic ester hydrolases.[7,8] Hydrolysis takes place in the intestinal lumen during solubilization of the vitamin esters in the mixed micelles.[9] Across the unstirred water layer the fat-soluble nutrients have to be moved toward the cell membrane in the form of mixed micelles.

Vitamin A and Carotene

Experiments on Test Animals

Experiments on rats have shown that there is no decrease in vitamin A accumulation in the liver when vitamin A or carotene and 3% of pectin are added to the feed, whereas the same amount of pectin has a hypocholesterinemic effect when cholesterin is added to the diet.[10] Due to the different concentrations of vitamin A and cholesterin when pectin is administered, the authors believe that this DF substance does not affect the common steps of vitamin A and cholesterin absorption. Even the addition of 5 or 10% of microcrystalline cellulose had no effects on the postprandial serum vitamin A concentrations in rats when radioactively labeled vitamin A was administered orally.[11] Under these experimental conditions there were no indications of DF influencing vitamin A or carotene absorption. Polish investigators[12] have shown that DF, according to individual test conditions, can have a positive as well as a negative effect on vitamin A absorption. Increased vitamin A absorption in rats, indicated by accumulation in the liver and plasma concentration, was found when the daily vitamin A intake with feed was 30 or 90 IU and 10% methylcellulose, agar, pectin, or wheat bran was added to the feed. With the vitamin A dose increased to 300 IU/day, the same amount of DF had a negative effect on vitamin A absorption.

Experiments on Man

Among the fat-soluble vitamins, vitamin A has been the most extensively studied in man. Mahle and Patton[13] reported that subsequent to 8 g of a hydrophilic mucilloid laxative extracted from psyllium being administered daily, neither the fecal excretion of vitamin A and carotene was increased nor were plasma vitamin A and carotene concentrations affected by long-term intake of hyrophilic mucilloid. In contrast to this, Kelsay et al.,[14] using other experimental conditions, reported that carotene excretion after a high-fiber diet was approximately double that of a low-fiber diet. In healthy subjects, a mixed diet containing fiber from fruits and vegetables was compared with the same diet, in which fruit and vegetable juices replaced the fruits and vegetables. Carotene was added to the low-fiber diet to make the two diets as equivalent as possible in all respects except fiber.

Besides fat intake and the efficiency of extraction from the food matrix, the amount and type of dietary fiber in the diet seem to determine carotenoid bioavailability (Parker 1997, Rock 1997, Williams et al., 1998). Because detailed information on the effect of different kinds of dietary fiber on carotenoid absorption in humans is lacking, the effects of different kinds of dietary fiber on the absorption of carotenoids were investigated. Six healthy young women received an antioxidant mixture consisting of β-carotene, lycopene, lutein, and canthaxanthin together with a standard meal. The meal did not contain additional dietary fiber or was enriched with pectin, guar, alginate, cellulose or wheat bran (0.15 g · kg body weight^{-1}). The increases in plasma carotenoid concentrations were followed over 24 h, and the areas-under-curves (AUC_{24h}) were calculated. The mean AUC_{24h} of β-carotene was significantly ($P < 0.05$) reduced by the water-soluble fibers pectin, guar, and alginate with a mean decrease of 33–43%. All tested fibers significantly reduced the AUC_{24h} of lycopene and lutein by 40–74% ($P < 0.05$). The dietary fiber effect on the AUC_{24h} of canthaxanthin was almost significant ($P = 0.059$). It is concluded that the biovailability of β-carotene, lycopene, and lutein given within a mixed supplement is markedly reduced by different kinds of dietary fiber.[58]

Wheat bran, pectin, carob seed flour, microcrystalline cellulose, and guar, administered together with a formula diet, had no negative effect on a vitamin A tolerance test in healthy subjects. Compared with the area under the postprandial serum concentration curve, there was an increase in vitamin A absorption subsequent to the above-mentioned DF being administered.[15] Barnard and Heaton[16] stress the point that in healthy subjects cholestyramine added to a test meal reduced vitamin A absorption, whereas lignin had no significant effect. In patients suffering from steatorrhea in the course of an excretory pancreatic insufficiency in chronic pancreatitis (mean daily fecal fat excretion 38 g), the additional ingestion of 10 g pectin together with a standard meal had no effect on the serum vitamin A concentrations when 300,000 IU vitamin A palmitate were added to the meal.[17]

Single tests are inappropriate to determine whether or not long-term administration of large amounts of DF leads to the concentration of an essential serum nutrient or impairment of the supply required. The three well-known long-term studies on man on serum vitamin A concentrations subsequent to increased ingestion of DF come to different conclusions. During an experiment on 68 patients receiving two tablespoons of bran per day over a period of at least 6 months, it was found that serum vitamin A concentrations were higher compared to the initial figures,[18] whereas in another experiment on 4 subjects after the daily intake of 15 g apple pectin or 30 g wheat bran over a period of 50 days, a decrease in vitamin A concentrations was found, while serum carotene concentrations remained unchanged.[16] Wahal and co-workers[19] tested the effect of wheat bran on serum vitamin A levels in healthy subjects during a 6-week trial. The addition of wheat bran to a standard diet with 20,000 units of vitamin A significantly lowered serum vitamin A levels within 1 week, and this trend continued over 3 weeks. They suggest that bran in the wheat flour which forms the staple diet in some parts of India may contribute towards the vitamin A deficiency state commonly observed in this country.

Vitamin D

Experiments on Test Animals

Investigations on chickens revealed that carboxymethylcellulose, pectin, and guar led to decreased fat and nitrogen utilization and, if given with diets marginally deficient in vitamin D_3, led to the development of rickets. These findings indicate that the above-mentioned carbohydrates have a negative effect on vitamin D_3 absorption.[20]

Experiments on Man

Several findings indicate that a high intake of fiber from unleavened whole meal wheat flat bread is responsible for rickets occurring in population groups in Asia. The significance of the rich phytate concentration and the role of wheat fiber, especially its lignin component, are currently being discussed. Lignin combines with bile acids and increases their excretion. The authors postulate that vitamin D probably becomes attached to the fiber/bile acid complex and is transported unabsorbed through the gut.[21] Serum or urinary calcium and phosphate concentrations and the serum alkaline phosphatase concentrations, obtained during investigations on children treated with bran for constipation, indicate that under this therapy vitamin D–deficiency rickets may develop.[22] Experimental high-fiber diets have been reported to reduce plasma half-life of 25 (OH) D.[23] This finding, in combination with a low vitamin D intake and bioavailability, may explain the high incidence of rickets and low plasma 25 (OH) D concentrations in some population groups and in infants on macrobiotic diets.[24,25]

Vitamin E

Experiments on Test Animals

There have been several fiber and vitamin E studies conducted on rats. From these studies it appears that intakes of pectin decrease vitamin E bioavailability, but fiber-containing breads or cereals have only transient or no effects.[26–28]

Experiments in Man

The glucomannan konjac mannan has a lowering effect on vitamin E absorption in healthy volunteers and in diabetic patients. This could be demonstrated with the vitamin E tolerance test when the glucomannan was added to the test meal.[29]

Riedl et al.[58] found that a meal enriched with pectin, guar, alginate, cellulose, or wheat bran (0.15 g · kg body weight) did not affect the plasma response curves of α-tocopherol.

Vitamin K

It is uncertain whether there are relations between vitamin K metabolism and ingestion of dietary fiber. Investigations on the influence of DF on vitamin K absorption and serum vitamin K concentration are not available. The prothrombin and thromboplastin times of diabetics who were treated with a high-fiber diet (25 to 35 g dietary fiber per 1000 kcal) for an average of 21 months remained unchanged. This indicates that the high-fiber diet does not impair vitamin K absorption.[30]

From the fact that the concentration of coagulation factors is changed if the fat and dietary fiber content of the diet is altered, it must be inferred that coagulation factors are not sufficiently reliable parameters for judging vitamin K absorption.[31]

Water-Soluble Vitamins

The underlying mechanisms of water-soluble vitamins being absorbed are more complex and less uniform than those of the fat-soluble vitamins. Some water-soluble vitamins, such as folic acid, must be transformed in the intestinal lumen prior to absorption.

Thiamin (Vitamin B1), Pantothenic Acid, Biotin

No data published.

Riboflavin (Vitamin B₂)

The influence of high- and low-fiber diets on urinary riboflavin excretion was examined in healthy subjects. Compared to a control group receiving a low-fiber diet, coarse and fine bran, cellulose, and cabbage increased urinary excretion for 8 h when 15 mg riboflavin-5′-phosphate were administered orally with breakfast. The authors concluded that dietary fiber accelerates GI riboflavin absorption.[32] In another study the impact of psyllium gum, wheat bran, and a combination of the two on the absorption of pharmacological doses of riboflavin (30 mg) was examined with a riboflavin load test. Fractional urine collections were made for 24 h. No effect of wheat bran on riboflavin absorption was detected, but psyllium gum reduced the 24-h apparent absorption of riboflavin from 31.8 to 25.4%.[33]

Pyridoxine (Vitamin B₆)

Experiments on Test Animals

A number of experiments on animals and man using natural and purified forms of dietary fiber suggest that dietary fiber has little effect on the bioavailability of vitamin B_6 in foods.[34] Bioassays on rats and chickens receiving cellulose, pectin, wheat bran, and mixtures of cellulose, pectin, and lignin indicated no inhibitory effect of these test materials on the bioavailability of pyridoxine.[35]

Experiments on Man

In man receiving 15 mg pectin daily, there was no negative effect on plasma pyridoxal-5′-phosphate concentration and urinary 4-pyridoxic-acid excretion. This indicates that dietary pectin supplementation has no effect on the utilization of dietary vitamin B_6.[36] There were no uniform results in experiments on the bioavailability of vitamin B_6 in bread containing varying amounts of wheat bran. Whereas some investigators[37] found similar plasma pyridoxal-5′-phosphate concentrations in man after the intake of white and whole wheat breads, others reported significantly higher fecal B_6 excretion with whole grain bread than with white bread. The plasma vitamin B_6 concentrations were slightly lower subsequent to whole grain bread being ingested.[37] It appears that the significantly higher consumption of dietary fiber by vegetarians has no adverse effect on the availability or metabolism of vitamin B_6.[38,39]

Nicotinic Acid (Niacin, Vitamin PP)

Sina et al.[11] studied the influence of microcrystalline cellulose on the absorption of radioactively labeled nicotinic acid in rats. Serum activity was measured subsequent to the labeled vitamin being administered orally with or without the addition of 5 or 10 g microcrystalline cellulose to the feed. Serum radioactivity was significantly higher when microcrystalline cellulose was added.

Folic Acid

According to the experiments of Luther et al.,[40] DF can bind pteroylmonoglutamates but not polyglutamates. This would suggest that naturally occurring dietary polyglutamates could be split by the normal intestinal conjugase activity, but the product might be bound in the presence of DF. Despite the fact that insoluble dietary residue of various foods was used in this study, other investigators[41] incubated folic acid with defined DF (cellulose, pectin, lignin, sodium alginate, and wheat bran) without observing an absorptive effect. No effects of these DF on plasma or hepatic folate concentrations could be demonstrated in feeding experiments on chickens. Two 6-month studies on patients with diverticulosis, constipation, and irritable colon yielded opposite results. In the patients of one study receiving 3 teaspoons of wheat bran daily, serum folic acid concentration was significantly decreased.[42] In the patients of the other study, administered 10 to 40 g wheat bran daily, there was a significantly higher average folic acid concentration at the end of the observation period than there was at the beginning.[17] These fluctuations of serum folic acid concentrations are probably due to different eating habits during the various seasons rather than to the ingestion of wheat bran. Results were negative when folic acid monoglutamate was incubated with high-fiber bread like that consumed in Iran. Experiments on healthy subjects showed that there is no change in folate absorption between the low-fiber and the high-fiber bread meals.[43] After a 21-month treatment of diabetics with a high-fiber diet, serum folic acid levels were normal.[30] The results of the investigation show that supply of folic acid requirements is not impaired if a mixed high-fiber diet is administered like the one recommended for prophylaxis and therapy of metabolic and GI disorders. Since, however, there are indications that conventional nutrition in Western industrialized countries does not invariably meet folic acid requirements,[44] it cannot be denied that ingestion of bran or isolated DF leads to folic acid requirements being impaired.

As studies on healthy subjects show, maximum postprandial serum folic acid concentrations were obtained subsequent to 200-mg folic acid monoglutamate being ingested together with a standardized test meal. The above-mentioned concentrations were obtained 1 to 2 h later than in the control experiment when 5 g guar, 10 g pectin, or 20 g wheat bran were added to the test meal. The areas under the folic acid concentration curves show that total absorption was significantly decreased up to 7 h after the intake when guar and bran were added to the test meal.[17] Keagy and co-workers[45] have examined the effect of wheat bran or California small white beans in the diet on absorption of monoglutamyl (PteGlu) and heptaglutamyl folic acid (PteGlu7) in healthy men. Relative folate absorption was determined by measuring 24-h urinary folate excretion and serum folate levels at 0, 1, and 2 h after ingestion of a formula meal containing 1.13 μmol PteGlu or PteGlu7 (500 μg PteGlu equivalent). Addition of 30 g wheat bran accelerated PteGlu absorption, whereas PteGlu7 absorption was not significantly affected by either food. Effects of the two foods were qualitatively different. Wheat bran increased the absorption of PteGlu relative to PteGlu7, whereas beans minimized the difference between PteGlu and PteGlu 7 serum areas.

Cobalamin (Vitamin B$_{12}$)

Experiments on Test Animals

Cullen and Oace[46] have examined the effects of cellulose or pectin supplements upon vitamin B$_{12}$ metabolism in rats. The experiments demonstrated that the addition of either 20 to 50% cellulose or 5 to 20% pectin to the semipurified B$_{12}$-deficient diet enhanced the depletion of body stores of vitamin B$_{12}$. The authors suggest that both fibers interfere with the recovery of biliary vitamin B$_{12}$ by binding to a residue that is little metabolized until it passes the ileum reabsorption site. Urinary methylmalonic acid excretion was also measured and used as a parameter of vitamin B$_{12}$ deficiency. Compared to the control group, urinary excretion increased significantly subsequent to cellulose and pectin being ingested. However, this occurred much earlier and to a greater extent with pectin than with cellulose. The reason for this is not known. The authors postulate that there may be greater production of propionate during the bacterial decomposition of pectin. In B$_{12}$ deficiencies, methylmalonic acid is produced from propionic acid in the liver. Another explanation would be a change in the intestinal flora, with a resulting increase in B$_{12}$ consumption.

Experiments on Man

The influence of DF on vitamin B$_{12}$ has not been studied systematically hitherto. It is only known that there is no change in serum vitamin B$_{12}$ concentrations in patients with diverticulosis on 6-month wheat bran therapy.[42] The serum vitamin B$_{12}$ concentration of diabetics 21 months subsequent to a high-fiber diet being administered was also in the normal range.[30] In healthy volunteers and in diabetic patients, vitamin B$_{12}$ absorption was not affected when the glucomannan konjac mannan was added to a test meal.[29]

Ascorbic Acid (Vitamin C)

With 100 mg ascorbic acid being administered daily to healthy subjects, a significant increase in urinary excretion of the vitamin was observed when 14 g hemicellulose was added to the diet. Cellulose and pectin had no effect on urinary ascorbic acid concentration.[47] Postprandial serum concentrations were not measured. Contrary to all expectations, these findings might indicate an increase in intestinal ascorbic acid absorption. Preliminary results of other investigators confirm these findings. They were able to show that 5 g pectin as well as 10 g wheat bran increase serum vitamin C concentration and urinary excretion significantly when they are ingested together with a formula diet containing 400 mg ascorbic acid.[48]

ENTERAL VITAMIN SYNTHESIS

Due to the findings of a large number of experiments on animals, it could be definitely demonstrated that those carbohydrates which are hard to digest stimulate the intestinal synthesis of B vitamins and vitamin K. There have been various studies, especially on raw potato starch, inositol, mannitol, sorbitol, pectin, and cellulose. Since the colon is the site of vitamin synthesis, vitamins synthesized in the intestine can probably contribute to the supply of what is required only when coprophagy takes place.[49] For example, rats resist dietary vitamin K deficiency by eating their own feces. Prevention of coprophagy in these animals leads to vitamin K deficiency after a short time.[50] There are findings, however, which indicate that vitamin K requirements even in man are met to a large extent by the intestinal flora.[51] It is not known whether during possible absorption of internally synthesized vitamin K the content of nutritional DF in man determines the amount of synthesized, and hence absorbed, vitamin K.

Since the human small intestine often harbors considerable microflora,[52] and a free intrinsic factor is often present in the lumen of the small intestine,[53] there has been speculation that vitamin B_{12} synthesized by the small intestinal flora contributes to vitamin B_{12} requirements being met. This might account for the absence of vitamin B_{12} deficiency in some groups of vegetarians.[54] It is not known to what extent bacterial vitamins synthesize in man's small intestine and thus, the requirement in vitamin B_{12} being met can be influenced by those carbohydrates being ingested which are difficult to absorb.

REFERENCES

1. Vahouny, G. V., Tombes, R., Cassidy, M. M., Kritchevsky, D., and Gallo, L. L., Dietary fibers. VI. Binding of fatty acids and monolein from mixed micelles containing bile salts and lecithin, *Proc. Soc. Exp. Biol. Med.*, 166, 12, 1981.
2. Vahouny, G. V., Roy, R., Gallo, L. L., Story, J. A., and Cassidy, M. M., Dietary fibers. III. Effects of chronic intake on cholesterol absorption and metabolism in the rat, *Am. J. Clin. Nutr.*, 33, 2182, 1980.
3. Dutta, S. K., Bustin, M., and Rubin, J., Effect of dietary fiber on pancreatic enzymes and fat malabsorption in pancreatic insufficiency, *Gastroenterology*, 80A, 1939, 1981.
4. Dunaif, G. and Schneeman, B. O., Effects of several sources of dietary fiber on human pancreatic enzymes activity in vitro, *Fed. Proc. Fed. Am. Soc. Exp. Biol.*, 40A, 3500, 1981.
5. Schneeman, B. O. and Gallaher, D., Loss of lipase activity with fiber treatment, *Fed. Proc. Fed. Am. Soc. Exp. Biol.*, 37, 849A, 1978.
6. Sommer, H. and Kasper, H., The effect of dietary fiber on the pancreatic excretory function, *Hepatogastroenterology*, 27, 477, 1980.
7. Lombardo, D. and Guy, O., Studies on the substrate specificity of a carboxyl esterhydrolase from human pancreatic juice. II. Action of cholesterol esters and lipid-soluble vitamin esters, *Biochim. Biophys. Acta*, 611, 147, 1980.
8. Mathias, P. M., Harries, J. T., Peters, T. J., and Muller, D. P. R., Studies on the in vivo absorption of micellar solutions of tocopherol and tocopheryl acetate in the rat, *J. Lipid Res.*, 22, 829, 1981.
9. Friedman, H. I. and Nylund, B., Intestinal fat digestion, absorption, and transport, *Am. J. Clin. Nutr.*, 33, 1108, 1980.
10. Phillips, W. E. J. and Brien, R. L., Effect of pectin, a hypocholesterolemic polysaccharide, on vitamin A utilization in rat, *J. Nutr.*, 100., 289, 1970.
11. Sina, P. A., Provenghi, R. R., and Cantone, A., Dietary cellulose and intestinal absorption of nutrients in rats, *Biochem. Exp. Biol.*, 12, 321, 1976.
12. Gronowska-Senger, A., Chudy, D., and Smaczny, E., Poziom blonnika w diecie a wykorzystanie witaminy. A przez organizm, *Roczn, Pzh.*, 30, 553, 1979.
13. Mahle, A. E. and Patton, H. M., Carotene and vitamin E metabolism in man: the excretion and plasma level as influenced by orally administered mineral oil and a hydrophilic mucilloid, *Gastroenterology*, 9, 44, 1947.
14. Kelsay, J. L., Behall, K. M., and Prather, E. S., Effect of fiber from fruits and vegetables on calcium, magnesium, iron, silicon and vitamin A balances of human subjects, *Fed. Proc. Fed. Am. Soc. Exp. Biol.*, 37, 755, 1978.
15. Kasper, H., Rabast, U., Fassl, H., and Fehle, F., The effect of dietary fiber on the postprandial serum vitamin A concentration in man, *Am. J. Clin. Nutr.*, 32, 1847, 1979.
16. Barnard, D. L. and Heaton, K. W., Bile acids and vitamin A absorption in man: the effects of two bile acid-binding agents, cholestyramine and lignin, *Gut*, 14, 316, 1973.
17. Kasper, H. and Schrezenmeir, J., unpublished data.
18. Rattan, J., Levin, N. E., Graff, N., Weizer, T., and Gilat, N., A high-fiber diet does not cause mineral and nutrient deficiencies, *J. Clin. Gastroenterol.*, 3. 389, 1981.
19. Wahal, P. K., Singh, R., Kishore, B., Prakash, V., Maheshwari, B. B., Gujral, V. K., and Jain, B. B., Effect of high fibre intake on serum vitamin A levels, *J. Assoc. Physicians India*, 34, 269, 1986.
20. Kratzer, F. H., Rajaguru, R. W., and Vohra, P., The effect of polysaccharides on energy utilization, nitrogen retention and fat absorption in chickens, *Poultry Sci.*, 46, 1489, 1967.

21. Reinhold, J. G., Rickets in Asian immigrants, *Lancet*, 2, 1132, 1976.
22. Zoppi, G., Gobio-Casali, L., Deganello, A., Astolfi, R., Saccomani, F., and Cecchettin, M., Potential complications in the use of wheat bran of constipation in infancy, *J. Pediatr. Gastroenterol. Nutr.*, 1, 91, 1982.
23. Batchelor, A. J. and Compston, J., Reduced plasma half-life of radio-labelled 25-hydroxyvitamin D_3 in subjects receiving a high-fibre diet, *Br. J. Nutr.*, 49, 213, 1983.
24. Dagnelie, P. C., Vergote, F. J. V. R. A., van Staveren, W. A., van den Berg, H., Dingjan, P. G., and Hautvast, J. G.A.J., High prevalence of rickets in infants on macrobiotic diets, *Am. J. Clin. Nutr.*, 51, 202, 1990.
25. Gibson. R. S., Bindra, G. S., Nizan, P., and Draper, H. H., The vitamin D status of East Indian Punjabi immigrants to Canada, *Brit. J. Nutr.*, 58, 23, 1987.
26. deLumen, B. O., Lubin, B., Chiu, D., Reyes, P., and Omaye, S. T., Bioavailability of vitamin E in rats fed diets containing pectin, *Nutr. Res.*, 2, 73, 1982.
27. Omaye, S. T. and Chow, F. I., Effect of hard red spring wheat bran on the bioavailability of lipid-voluble vitamins and growth of rats fed for 56 days, *J. Food Sci.*, 49, 504, 1984.
28. Schaus, E. E., deLumen, B. O., Chow, F. I., Reyes, P., and Omaye, S. T., Bioavailability of vitamin B in rats fed graded levels of pectin, *J. Nutr.*, 115, 263, 1985.
29. Doi, K., Matsuura, M., Kawara, A., Tanaka, T., and Baba, S., Influence of dietary fiber (konjac mannan) on absorption of vitamin B_{12} and vitamin E., *Tohoku J. Exp. Med.*, 141 (Suppl.), 677, 1983.
30. Anderson, J. W., Ferguson, S. K., et al., Mineral and vitamin status on high-fiber diets: long-term studies of diabetic patients, *Diabetes Care*, 3, 38, 1980.
31. Simpson, H. C. R. and Mann, J. I., Effect of high-fibre diet on haemostatic variables in diabetes, *Br. Med. J.*, 1, 1608, 1982.
32. Roe, D. A., Wrick, K., McLain, D., and van Soest, P., Effects of dietary fiber sources on riboflavin absorption, *Fed. Proc. Fed. Am. Soc. Exp. Biol.*, 3, 756, 1978.
33. Roe, D. A., Kalkwarf, H., and Stevens, J., Effect of fiber supplements on the apparent absorption of pharmacological doses of riboflavin, *J. Am. Dietetic Assoc.*, 88, 210, 1988.
34. Gregory, J. F. and Kirk, J. R., The bioavailability of vitamin B_6 in foods, *Nutr. Rev.*, 39, 1, 1981.
35. Nguyen, L. B., Gregory, J. F., and Damron, B. L., Effects of selected polysaccharides on the bioavailability of pyridoxine in rat and chickens, *J. Nutr.*, 111, 1403, 1981.
36. Miller, L. T., Schultz, T. D., and Leklem, J. E., Influence of citrus pectin on the bioavailability of vitamin B_6 in man, *Fed. Proc. Fed. Am. Soc. Exp. Biol.*, 39, 797, 1980.
37. Leklem, J. E., Miller, L. T., Perera, A. D., and Peffer, D. E., Bioavailability of vitamin B_6 from wheat bread in humans, *J. Nutr.*, 110, 1819, 1980.
38. Shultz, T. D. and Leklem, J. E., Vitamin B_6 status and bioavailability in vegetarian women, *Am. J. Clin. Nutr.*, 46, 447, 1987.
39. Lowik, M. R. H., Schrijver, J., van den Berg, H., Hulshof, K. F. A. M., Wedel, M., and Ockhuizen, T., Effect of dietary fiber on the vitamin B_6 status among vegetarian and nonvegetarian elderly (Dutch Nutrition Surveillance System), *J. Am. Coll. Nutr.*, 9, 241, 1990.
40. Luther, L., Santini, R., Brewster, C., Perez-Santiago, E., and Butterworth, C. E., Folate binding by insoluble components of American and Puerto Rican diets, *Ala. J. Med. Sci.*, 2, 389, 1965.
41. Ristow, K. A., Gregory, J. F., and Damron, B. L., The effect of dietary fiber on folic acid bioavailability, *Fed. Proc. Fed. Am. Soc. Exp. Biol.*, 40, 854, 1981.
42. Brodribb, A. J. M. and Humphreys, D. M., Metabolic effect of bran in patients with diverticular disease, *Br. Med. J.*, 1, 424, 1976.
43. Russell, R. M., Ismail-Beig, F., and Reinhold, J. G., Folate content of Iranian breads and the effect of their fiber content on the intestinal absorption of folic acid, *Am. J. Clin. Nutr.*, 29, 799, 1976.
44. Pietrzik, K., Urban, G., and Hötzel, D., Biochemische und haematologische Ma β stäbe zur Beurteilung des Folatstatus beim Menschen, *Int. Z. Vit. Ern. Forsch.*, 48, 391, 1978.
45. Keagy, P. M., Shane, B., and Oace, S. M., Folate bioavailability in humans: effects of wheat bran and beans, *Am. J. Clin. Nutr.*, 47, 80, 1988.
46. Cullen, R. W. and Oace, S. M., Methylmalonic acid and vitamin B_{12} excretion of rats consuming diets varying in cellulose and pectin, *J. Nutr.*, 108, 640, 1978.
47. Keltz, F. R., Kies, C., and Fox, H. M., Urinary ascorbic acid excretion in the human as affected by dietary fiber and zinc, *Am. J. Clin. Nutr.*, 31, 1167, 1978.

48. Kasper, H., Der Einfluss von Ballastoffen auf die Ausnutzung von Nährstoffen und Pharmaka, in *Pflanzenfasern-Ballastoffe in der menschlichen Ernährungs* Rottka, H., Ed., G. Thieme-Verlag, Stuttgart, 1980.

49. Hötzel, D. and Barnes, R. H., Contributions of the intestinal microflora to the nutrition of the host, *Vit. Horm.*, 24, 115, 1966.

50. Barnes, R. H., Kwong, E., and Fiala, G., Effects of the prevention of coprophagy in the rat, *J. Nutr.*, 68, 603, 1959.

51. Editorial: Intestinal microflora, injury and vitamin K deficiency, *Nutr. Rev.*, 38, 341, 1980.

52. Bhat, P., Shantakumarie, S., Rajan, D., Mathan, H. I., and Kapadia, C. R., Bacterial flora of the gastrointestinal tract in Southern Indian control subjects and patients with tropical sprue, *Gastroenterology*, 62, 11, 1972.

53. Kapadia, C. R., Mathan, V. J., and Bauer, S. J., Free intrinsic factor in the small intestine in man, *Gastroenterology*, 70, 70, 1976.

54. Albert, M. J., Mathan, V. J., and Baker, S. J., Vitamin B_{12} synthesis by human small intestinal bacteria, *Nature*, 283, 781, 1980.

55. Parker, R. S., Biovailability of carotenoids, *Eur. J. Clin. Nutr.*, 51, Suppl. 1, S86, 1997.

56. Rock, C. L., Carotenoids: biology and treatment, *Pharmacol. Ther.*, 75, 185, 1997.

57. Williams, A. W., Boileau, T. W. M., and Erdman, J. W., Factors influencing the uptake and absorption of carotenoids, *Proc. Soc. Exp. Biol. Med.*, 218, 106, 1998.

58. Riedl, J., Linseisen, J., Hoffmann, J., and Wolfram, G., Some dietary fibers reduce the absorption of carotenoids in women, *J. Nutr.*, 129, 2170, 1999.

The Effect of Dietary Fiber on Fecal Weight and Composition

John H. Cummings

HISTORICAL INTRODUCTION

Present-day interest in fiber stems from the middle of the nineteenth century when the preoccupation of the Victorians with their bowel habits led many physicians to declaim the virtues of bran. John Burne,[1] writing in 1840 in *A Treatise on the Causes and Consequences of Habitual Constipation*, recommends that "coarse brown and bran bread is very efficacious, the bran acting as a salutory stimulus to the peristaltic action of the intestines." There was little need to convince Burne and his generation that bran stimulated colonic movement and increased fecal output. Nevertheless, each generation of medical scientists seems to have to rediscover this fact for itself, and medical and nutritional literature in the 1970s contained many papers in which little else but the laxative properties of bran were reported.

By 1909, Sir Arthur Hertz (later Sir Arthur Hurst)[2] was writing, "One of the most valuable foods for constipation in whole-meal bread ... white bread, which is made of the endosperm alone and those varieties of brown bread, such as Hovis, which are made from the endosperm and germ, contain only about one-fifth of the cellulose present in whole-meal bread. It is clear, therefore, that the substitution of whole-meal bread for white bread is a very important part of the dietetic treatment of constipation." Thus, 75 years ago fiber was being singled out as the principal component of bran responsible for its colonic effects.

In 1936, Dimock,[3] in his M.D. thesis for the University of Cambridge entitled "Treatment of Habitual Constipation by the Bran Method," was able to review over 50 papers reporting clinical, biochemical, radiological, and physiological studies of the use of fiber in constipation. He discussed various current ideas about the way bran produces its laxative effect, such as the presence of undigestible fiber, its content of vitamin B, phytin, hemicellulose, inorganic salts, and the production of volatile fatty acids from decomposition of cellulose and hemicellulose. As a result of his own observations, he concluded, "My view is that bran exerts a mechanical laxative action due to its fibre content. The fibre mixes intimately with the food residues in the colon, even when bran is taken only once a day. I believe that by so doing, it not only retains moisture itself but enables the other residues in the colon to resist dehydration."

The 1930s were a time of vigorous investigation of the laxative properties of dietary fiber. Purified forms of fiber such as ispaghula, various celluloses, agar, karaya, sterculia, and psyllium were all in common use and were a focus of some interesting studies on their mechanism of action. It was widely believed at the time that fiber acted by virtue of its capacity to absorb and retain water in the gut.[4-8] However, the work by Williams and Olmsted,[9] which involved careful metabolic balance studies and fecal analysis of subjects ingesting various fibers prepared from peas, carrots, cabbage, corn bran, wheat bran, etc., concluded that "contrary to the accepted belief, the effectiveness of indigestible residues is not due primarily to the mechanical stimulus of distention but rather to chemical stimuli which arise from the destruction of hemicelluloses and cellulose by the intestinal bacterial flora. One of these stimulating products is the lower volatile fatty acids." These studies contradicted the experimental data of others and questioned the whole basis of then currently accepted beliefs about fiber. Surprisingly, perhaps because of the international conflict which involved many nations at that time, there followed an apparently complete loss of interest in the subject and no significant developments were reported for the next 30 years.

Attention to the effect of dietary fiber on bowel habit returned around 1970, not because of any new insights into the problem of constipation but as a result of epidemiological observations relating bowel habit to disease by Burkitt[10-14] and studies by Painter on the etiology and treatment of diverticular disease.[15-17] In his paper on the etiology of large bowel cancer in 1971, Burkitt suggests that fiber affects bowel function by speeding up transit time, diluting gut contents, and favorably influencing the microbial flora. At the same time, Painter was concluding a series of studies in the U.K. which he interpreted as showing that diverticular disease of the large intestine was due to lack of bulk in colonic contents. He surmised from these studies that propulsion of intestinal contents was more difficult if they were dry, inspissated, and of small volume, thus requiring increased intraluminal pressures. He then went on to show that, contrary to current medical opinion, diverticular disease could be satisfactorily treated by increasing the amount of dietary fiber in the form of wheat bran. These studies stimulated new research into the mode of action of fiber in the colon. Since then, much of the early work on fiber has inevitably been repeated and many papers do little if anything to advance our knowledge or understanding of the mode of action of dietary fiber in the colon. However, as a result of better chemical techniques and advancing knowledge of colonic physiology, new concepts have emerged with regard to the mode of action of fiber in the colon and its role in determining colonic function.

Table 4.4.1 Average Increase in Fecal Output per Gram Fiber Fed

Source	Increase g/g Fiber ± SEM	No. of Studies (see Tables 2-15)	Comments
Wheat	5.4 (0.7)	41	Mainly bran. Raw 7.2; cooked 4.9 ($p < 0.05$)
Fruit and vegetables	4.7 (0.7)	28	Carrot, peas, cabbage, apple, potato, banana, prunes, and mixed sources
Gums and mucilages	3.7 (0.5)	27	Psyllium/ispaghula, 4.0 (N = 14). Other: traga canth, xanthan, sterculia, bassara, xylan, agar, gum arabic, 4.0 (N = 9.0)
Cellulose	3.5 (0.8)	7	Also carboxymethylcellulose, 4.9 (N = 3); methylcellulose, 8.9 (N = 4)
Oats	3.4 (1.1)	4	Oat bran or oats
Corn	3.3 (0.3)	5	Corn meal or bran
Legumes	2.2 (0.3)	17	Soya products, 2.5 (N =11)
Pectin	1.2 (0.3)	11	Degree of methoxylation not important

MODERN STUDIES

Table 4.4.1 is a summary of the result of nearly 100 studies of the effect of the dietary fiber on bowel habit and fecal composition published between 1932 and 1984 and given in detail in Tables 4.4.2 to 4.4.9. All sources of fiber lead to an increase in fecal output and therefore in the components which make up feces such as fat, nitrogen, water, minerals, and trace elements. What is clear from Table 4.4.1, however, is that not all fibers are equal in this respect, pectin for example giving an increase of about 1.3 g of stool per gram of fiber fed while pure cellulose has an effect more than double (3.0 g/g fiber fed), and fruit, vegetables, and bran as sources of fiber being yet more effective (4.9 and 5.7 g/g, respectively).

The reasons for these differences relate to the physicochemical properties of dietary fiber. Two factors, particle size and chemical composition of individual fiber polysaccharides, have already emerged from experimental studies as specifically affecting the mode of action of dietary fiber. Table 4.4.10 summarizes studies of the effect of particle size on the efficacy of wheat bran in altering colonic function. In general, these show that if exactly the same source of fiber is fed at two different particle sizes, the greater particle size preparation will produce larger changes in stool output. The reason for this is thought to relate to the extent and rate of breakdown of dietary fiber in the large intestine. Large particles are more slowly degraded and so are more likely to survive passage through the gut. In so doing they are able to exert a physical effect on colonic function by providing both bulk to gut contents and a surface for the bacteria which allows for their more efficient metabolism.

Chemical analysis of dietary fiber sources also shows a relation to fecal bulking properties. The more pentose sugars present in the dietary fiber polymers, the greater the increase in stool weight (other factors being equal).[18] This association is an intriguing one and one which is at the present time unexplained. It was initially felt that the response to pentose-containing polysaccharides was simply a reflection of the water-holding capacity of a particular fiber. However, both pentose- and hexose-containing polysaccharides hold water and further research has cast doubt on the water-holding hypothesis[19] as the sole explanation for the action of fiber, although its water-holding properties are still an important component of the explanation of its role in altering gut function.[20–25]

The most telling argument against the water-holding hypothesis is that virtually all fiber is broken down in the gut. Fiber digestion in man has been reported in the literature on many occasions in the past century. Despite this, the popular view has persisted that it is not degraded, although there is now ample evidence to the contrary.[26,27] For example, when fiber in mixed diets is fed to healthy subjects, 70 to 80% of it disappears during passage through the gut.[28] The cellulosic fraction tends to survive digestion better than the noncellulosic polysaccharides, and fiber from cereals survives better than that from fruit and vegetables. When the digestion of cabbage and bran fiber was compared in healthy subjects taking equal doses of each material, only 10% of the cabbage fiber could be recovered in feces, while 60% of bran fiber was excreted.[25]

Since fiber is extensively degraded, it is not surprising that its water-holding capacity alone is insufficient to explain its physiological effects in the colon. Another mechanism has to be sought whereby fiber can alter colonic metabolism. Williams and Olmsted[9,29] were probably the first to recognize the significance of the extensive breakdown of fiber in the human gut. They suggested that the fecal bulking by fiber could be accounted for by the stimulatory effect on colonic smooth muscle of the major end products of fiber breakdown, the short chain, or volatile fatty acids. Today, however, short-chain fatty acids are known to be rapidly absorbed from the human colon and are thought not to control laxation in man.[30] Because of this, little has been learned from the study of their fecal excretion and, therefore, data from the few studies where they have been measured are not included in the accompanying tables.

A component of normal stools that has been neglected in studies of fiber for many years is the microflora. Bacteria are about 80% water and, therefore, a potentially important component of stools. Because of their ability to resist dehydration, bacteria are more likely to retain their water against the absorptive forces of the colonic mucosa than are the cellular skeletons of plant material that remain after cooking of food and its subsequent passage through the gut. Stephen and colleagues[31] developed a method for fractionating human feces which allows the contribution from microbial material to be estimated. Using this technique, it can be shown that bacteria compose up to half of the fecal solids in subjects eating typical Western diets. Bacteria are therefore probably an underestimated component of human feces, and their role in changes in fecal composition is important. In Tables 4.4.2 to 4.4.9, it will be seen that fiber almost always brings about an increase in fecal nitrogen excretion. Studies in both man[32] and animals[33-34] have shown that this N is most likely to be bacterial N which increases as the result of microbial growth in the colon through fermentation of fiber. An increase in lipid excretion may, in part, also be explained this way.

MECHANISM OF ACTION OF DIETARY FIBER

The way in which dietary fiber affects bowel habit cannot be explained on the basis of one simple hypothesis. There are probably at least four distinct effects of fiber by which it brings about an increase in stool weight. First, plant cell walls which resist breakdown by the microflora, e.g., because of lignification as in bran, are able to exert a physical effect on intestinal bulk by retaining water within their cellular structure. Increasing bulk stimulates colonic movement. Second, most forms of dietary fiber are extensively degraded by the microflora. The result of this is to stimulate microbial growth and a greater excretion of microbial products in feces. This again contributes to the change in fecal mass. Third, substances which increase bulk in the large intestine often speed up the rate of passage through the bowel. As transit time falls, the efficiency with which the bacterica grows improves. Shortened transit time also leads to reduced water absorption by the colon and therefore wetter stools. Fourth, dietary fiber is an important source of gas in the colon since the gases H_2, CH_4, and CO_2 are some of the principal end products of fermentation. Gas trapped within gut contents again adds to their bulk. These mechanisms together combine to increase stool weight.

Many workers who have studied the effect of dietary fiber on bowel function have noted the wide range in response among individuals. Table 4.4.11 summarizes studies of dietary fiber in subjects with diverticular disease of the colon. In general, it would appear that in response to bran, these patients exhibit only about 50% of the response seen in healthy subjects. Whether this is the result or cause of the diverticular disease cannot be said but is worth further study.

Although the literature on dietary fiber and bowel habit contains much that is repetitious, in a small number of papers evenly distributed over the years, experiments are described which demonstrate new aspects of large bowel physiology hitherto unrecognized. The advent of better carbohydrate chemistry, microbiological techniques, and noninvasive methods of studying colonic function has allowed investigators in recent years to show that dietary fiber has, through its breakdown in the large intestine by the microflora, an important role in maintaining normal digestive function as it does in the ruminant and other hind gut fermenting species.

NOTES TO TABLES

Selection of Papers

These tables summarize essential experimental details from a selection of reports of the effect of dietary fiber, in many forms, on bowel function, fecal weight, and composition published during the past 55 years. It is not a comprehensive survey since such a report would have been very extensive and have contained probably little more useful information than the present one. Studies have been selected for inclusion provided they were conducted on man, were reported as full papers in the English language, and contained numerical data on changes in large bowel function, particularly fecal output and composition. Many early studies from the period 1920 to 1950[35-52] have not been included because they report only qualitative data, percent changes, or results that are otherwise difficult to convert to tabular form. Nevertheless, some of these studies are detailed and thoughtful and well worth consulting .

The series of papers by Fantus and colleagues in 1940 to 1942,[37,40,41] together with the classic work of Williams and Olmsted,[9,29,53-56] that of Cowgill and associates,[58,59] and the Comprehensive studies of Tainter et al.[7,8,60,61] on the mode of action of bulk laxatives, laid the foundation for much of present-day thinking about dietary fiber. Unfortunately, only a minority of modern researchers seem to have read or taken note of these early studies. If these studies had received greater attention, much that is mundane and repetitious in current nutritional research would have been obviated.

A great deal that is written about fiber and bowel habit concerns constipation. The majority of these papers, however, are worthless, being reports of uncontrolled studies which usually show a beneficial effect of bran or other bulk laxatives. They have not been included in this survey unless they contain clear data on the role of fiber. In general, studies of young children have also been excluded, as have those where data are based on a single stool or only 1 day of fecal collection.

Most studies reported are within-subject crossover type design where each person takes both test and control diets. To say that they are solely experiments to determine the effect of dietary fiber on bowel function is an overstatement, however, since many investigators have used fiber sources such as bran or foods which contain other nutrients. Nevertheless, there are problems in interpreting information and extrapolating foods that are normally eaten when dealing with studies where purified materials, such as cellulose, are used.[62] Thus, both types of experiments, whole foods and purified materials, are needed to give a full understanding of the effects of fiber. The problem of the purity of fiber sources has been recognized for many years and early studies of bran, such as those reported by Dimock,[3] discuss at length the potential of various components of bran to induce laxation. The answers to some of the questions Dimock posed have not yet been found or even looked for.

Finally, the age-old question "what is fiber" constantly appears when reading the literature. The word "fiber" is used in many different contexts in the papers reported here and clearly means different things to different investigators. All definitions and concepts are included in the tables. Some guide as to the meaning of the word in individual studies is given by an indication of the chemical methods used in the study to measure fiber intake in the experimental subjects.

TABLES 4.4.2 TO 4.4.11

An asterisk in all columns means that the value is significantly different from basal (or other appropriate) control diet.

Column 1: Literature Sources, Diet, Fiber Source

The principal *literature sources* for the data given in the table are recorded in column 1. In recent years the practice has developed in which authors publish the results of a single complete study in several parts, possibly in different journals. Alternatively, and to be decried, is the repeated publication of the same data in several journals. Small alterations may be made to numbers of subjects or details and the work republished. All this conspires to crowd the literature with irrelevant and superfluous information while apparently enhancing the reputation of the authors for industry, science, and original thought. As a means of guiding the reader through this morass, all citations to a single experiment are recorded in this column, insofar as they can be identified.

Diets are either "controlled" or *ad lib*. Controlled diets are where the food is cooked and prepared for the subjects by the investigators and provides a constant background against which to judge the effect of fiber. These are sometimes referred to as "metabolic studies." Commendably, many studies are now carried out in this way. *Ad lib* diets are self-selected by the subjects.

Fiber sources are described as in the paper.

Column 2: Total Number of Subjects in Study, Sex, and Age

The number of subjects of each sex (M = male, F = female) who took part in the whole study or part of the study are recorded together with the range of ages. A dash indicates that no data are available.

Column 3: Study Period

Study period describes the diet and/or fiber source relevant to the data given on that line. Basal = control diet against which fiber supplements were compared.

Column 4: Fiber Intake (g/day) and Fiber Method

Many authors have attempted to measure fiber intake using one of a number of methods (see below). Where no method is given in the paper, an attempt has been made to calculate dietary fiber intakes using currently available food tables or analytical information. If errors have been committed or wrong assumptions have been made by me in doing this, I apologize in advance to the investigators concerned.

    I. Crude fiber [63-64]
    II. Williams and Olmsted 1935[56]
    III. Southgate[65-70]
    IV. Paul and Southgate[71]
    V. Van Soest and modifications [72-76]
    VI. Crampton and Maynard[77]
    VII. O'Shea, Ribiero, and Moran[78]
    VIII. McCance, Widdowson, and Shackleton[79]
    IX. Katan and von de Bovenkamp[80]
    X. Englyst[81-82]
    XI. Schweizer[83-84]
    XII. Angus, Sutherland, and Farrell [85]

Column 5: Days on Diet

This information appears as in the paper. Where this was varied, a range is given. (No figure is given for *ad lib* diets since it is assumed to be the subject's usual diet.)

Column 6: Fecal Collection Period (Days)

This is the number of days of fecal collection pooled for analysis. It is the *minimum* included since investigators have used, on occasion, averages of several collection periods for the data.

Column 7: Number of Subjects Collecting Feces

This number may be less than the total number participating in the study either because the subjects were split into groups or some did not collect feces. It is the number which has been used to calculate standard errors in other columns.

Column 8: Fecal Weight (g/day)

Average value (± 1 SE of the mean). Some of these figures are derived by calculation on the basis of data in the original papers. Any errors are therefore not the fault of the original authors, and investigators seeking to follow up these studies should consult the publications themselves. Where data are given in the paper for several periods on the same diet, the information relating to the *final* period has been used in this table.

Column 9: Percent Moisture

If not given in the original paper, this has been calculated as:

$$\frac{\text{total fecal weight g/day} - \text{fecal solids g/day}}{\text{total stool weight g/day}} \times 100$$

Column 10: Fecal Solids (g/day)

As given in the paper or calculated from data related to percent moisture of feces (± 1 SE of the mean).

Column 11: Apparent Increase in Fecal Weight Per Gram Dietary Fiber Fed

Calculated as:

$$\frac{\text{fecal output with fiber source g/day} - \text{basal fecal output g/day}}{\text{g fiber fed per day}}$$

Gram of fiber fed per day is always "dietary fiber" as defined in 1972 and 1976.[86-87] Where dietary fiber data are not given in the paper, these have been calculated from available knowledge of the food and fiber source used.

Column 12: Transit Time — Hours and Transit Method

Transit time, the time it takes a substance to pass through the gut, can be measured using a number of techniques, in the majority of which an oral dose of inert marker is given with food and its appearance in feces is noted. Values for transit time obtained are very dependent on the method used. Colored dyes give short transit times since it is difficult to detect other than the "first appearance" of marker in feces. Methods which measure mean transit time are probably most accurate, while the radio-opaque pellet technique of Hinton et al.[88] gives values which are about 20% greater than the mean transit time methods. Values in this column must be interpreted, therefore, in the light of the method used and are not directly comparable with one another.

Transit Methods

I. Hinton, Lennard-Jones, and Young (1969)[88]
II. Cummings, Jenkins, and Wiggins (1975 and 1976)[89-90]
III. Colored dyes — "first apperance" method[91-93]
IV. ^{51}Cr sodium chromate[94]
V. Cr_2O_6 chromic oxide

Column 13: Fat (g/day)

Note that various methods are used to recover fat, including those which measure total lipid, triglycerides, and fatty acids and fatty acids alone (after hydrolysis); millimoles converted to milligrams by factor × 280.

Column 14: N (g/day)

This is usually measured by the Kjeldahl technique. Note variable conversion factors used by authors to convert fecal N to "protein" (from 5.75 to 6.25).

Column 15: Neutral Steroids (mg/day)

See original papers for methodology which affects results especially in early (pre-1970) papers. Millimoles converted to milligrams by factor × 386.

Column 16: Acid Steroids (mg/day)

See notes for Column 15. Millimoles converted to milligrams by factor × 400.

Column 17: Energy (kcal/day)

Total fecal energy excretion, usually measured by calorimetry.

Column 18: Comments, Notes, Other Data Available

This column includes special notes about the studies and lists other data available from related publications of the same study.

Other Data Available From Study

A	=	Digestibility (fecal excretion) of fiber
B	=	Volatile fatty acids
C	=	Calcium, magnesium, phosphorus (including phytate)
D	=	Iron, zinc, copper, and other trace elements
E	=	Blood lipids
F	=	Intestinal motility
G	=	Polyethylene glycol, Cr_2O_6, used as markers
H	=	Sodium, potassium, chloride, bicarbonate, ash, or other electrolytes
J	=	Microflora
K	=	Glucose tolerance
L	=	Bile composition and bile acid kinetics
M	=	Breath CH_4, and H_2.
N	=	Hematology

TABLES 4.4.12 TO 4.4.15 (1986–1992)

These additional tables detail papers on the effects of dietary fiber on bowel habit and fecal composition published between 1986 and 1992, and also include one or two additional reports omitted from the earlier survey. As before, the criteria for inclusion are that the studies have been undertaken in adults, contain quantitative data of an experimental, not observational, nature, and must include, as a minimum, fecal weights. There may be some publications that do not appear in these tables but which fit the criteria for inclusion. Such omissions are inadvertent and the author apologizes to anyone whose work has been so excluded.

While in 1985 it appeared that everything that could be said about dietary fiber and bowel habit had been said, papers still continue to appear on this topic at a steady rate. Some of them add little to what is already known, although there is clearly now an increased interest in forms of dietary fiber other than bran. This is seen in the papers on different plant gums and legumes, especially soya. The impetus for these studies is partly commercial, since few investigators use these studies to cast light on the unresolved question as to how dietary fiber works. Some progress has been made in this area, by study of the physical properties of fiber in relation to its effect on fecal composition, but a number of important questions remain unanswered.[220,247,248]

The revised version of Table 4.4.1 shows average increases in fecal weight (g per day per g fiber fed) for the major sources of dietary fiber, ranked according to their effectiveness. Thirty-seven additional papers have been added to the original compilation of about 80, detailing a total of approaching 150 individual dietary studies of assorted fiber sources. These additional data have not made a great deal of difference to the overall rankings, and the message remains the same. Dietary fiber is laxative, but the significant differences among the results confirm that not all fibers are the same, and one cannot really generalize about the whole group. Therefore, a single number on a food label for fiber is going to give the consumer very little useful information about its laxative effects, without some additional information. Wheat products, usually bran, remain unequivocally at the top of the league, although a small number of studies of methylcellulose suggest it is equally, if not more, effective as a laxative. With regard to wheat, there are now enough studies of both raw and cooked products to show a statistically significant difference in favor of raw bran (7.2 g/g raw vs. 4.9 cooked, t = 2.65, p = 0.012). The disadvantage of raw bran, of course, is its high content of phytate.

Fruits and vegetables remain second in the table, well ahead of the rest. While many people believe fruits and vegetables contain mainly soluble fiber with little potential to alter bowel habit, in fact this is clearly not the case. Many fruits and vegetables contain significant amounts of insoluble fiber.[253,254] These studies were mostly done with foods rather than purified forms of fiber, which means that the subjects are eating intact cell walls, which probably contributes to the effect.

Gums and mucilages have risen up the list to third place, although they are well behind wheat, fruits, and vegetables. There is clearly a lot of commercial interest in adding these preprations to food due to their potential cholesterol lowering properties. However, wide differences in the fecal bulking properties of gums are evident. For example, guar is a poor bulker in general, giving increases of around 1.0 g/g,[220,225] while tragacanth seems to be the best at 6.4 g/g,[228] although this is only one study.

Cellulose, corn, and oats are all effective laxative substances and give similar effects, with the exceptions of methylcellulose and carboxymethylcellulose, which are better. The legumes, despite being a good source of insoluble fiber,[253] are poor fecal bulkers. Since they also frequently contain resistant starch,[255] this is hard to understand. Finally, pectin remains the least effective along with guar.

How reliable are these rankings? Within each group there is great variability, although despite this the overall differences are statistically significant (by ANOVAR F 4.78 p < 0.001). The variability is due in part to the inherent difference in individual responses and to varying experimental designs, some of which are uncontrolled diets. However, a major problem is lack of consistency in methodology for measurement of dietary fiber. In the earlier part of this chapter, 12 methods were listed as being used to measure fiber in the various studies. A further seven have been added for the present update as follows:

XIII.	Anderson, Sieling, and Chen[197]
XIV.	Mergenthaler and Scherz[199]
XV.	Meuser et al.[200]
XVI.	Prosky et al.[202-204]
XVII.	Slavin et al.[215]
XVIII.	Theander and Westerlund [231]
XIX.	Asp et al.[232]

In addition, a further seven methods or modifications to methods have been developed over this period.[239-245] Because these methods give widely differing results for the amount of dietary fiber in a food,[256] this creates a problem in comparing data.

What of the future? The emergence of starch as a fecal bulking agent [248-252] is probably the single most important discovery to challenge the role of fiber in the diet. At the very least, the amount and type of starch in experimental diets must be controlled (as must its processing) to eliminate this as a variable. More than likely, we shall have to re-evaluate the whole dietary fiber story in the light of emerging evidence of the importance of resistant starch.

Table 4.4.2 Effect of Wheat Fiber in Various Forms on Fecal Composition (See Also Table 4.4.10)

Literature Source / Diet / Fiber Source	Total Number of Subjects in Study (sex and age)	Study period	Fiber Intake (g/day) and Fiber Method	Days on Diet	Fecal Collection Period (days)	Number of Subjects Collecting Feces	Fecal Weight (g/day)	Moisture (%)	Fecal Solids (g/day)	Apparent Increase in Fecal Weight per Gram Dietary Fiber Fed	Transit Time (h) and Transit Method	Fat (g/day)	N (g/day)	Neutral Sterols (mg/day)	Acid Sterols (mg/day)	Energy (kcal/day)	Comments / Notes / Other Data Available
Cowgill and Anderson (1932)[58] Controlled diet Normal foods	5 M	Low fiber basal	5.2 —	14	14	5	116 (11)	77	27								Both brans equally effective A
		+ Whole bran, 1–1½ oz	—	14	14	5	193* (8)	79	40								
Low fiber or very low fiber		Low fiber basal	5.2	14	14	5	112 (7)	76	27								
		+ Acid-washed bran, 1–1½ oz	—	14	14	5	171* (13)	77	39								
Bran — whole or with weak acid					14	4	93 (7)	70	28								
		Very low fiber basal	3.1	14													
		+ Whole bran, 1–1½ oz	—	14	14	4	189* (22)	74	49								
		Very low fiber basal + Acid-washed bran, 1–1½ oz	3.1	14	14	4	93 (5)	76	22								
			—	14	14	4	185* (17)	76	44								
Cowgill and Sullivan (1933)[59] Controlled diet Normal foods	6 M	Basal	30–38 [a]	7	7	6	78 (15)										Constipated subjects Also studied effect of fruits and vegetables (see Table 4.4.8) Whole bran slightly better than breakfast bran but less palatable
		+ Bran	50	7	7	6	121* (6)										
Bran and breakfast bran (a commercial breakfast cereal)		+ High bran	90	7	7	6	187* (18)										
		+ Breakfast bran	90	7	7	6	176* (12)										

Table 4.4.2 (Continued) Effect of Wheat Fiber in Various Forms on Fecal Composition (See Also Table 4.4.10)

Literature Source Diet Fiber Source	Total Number of Subjects in Study (sex and age)	Study period	Fiber Intake (g/day) and Fiber Method	Days on Diet	Fecal Collection Period (days)	Number of Subjects Collecting Feces	Fecal Weight (g/day)	Moisture (%)	Fecal Solids (g/day)	Apparent Increase in Fecal Weight per Gram Dietary Fiber Fed	Transit Time (h) and Transit Method	Fat (g/day)	N (g/day)	Neutral Steroids (mg/day)	Acid Steroids (mg/day)	Energy (kcal/day)	Comments Notes Other Data Available
Williams and Olmsted (1936)[19,29,57] Controlled diet Normal foods excluding fruit and vegetables Bran, prepared by washing for 24 h in warm water, extracting with hot ethanol, and drying	3 M	Bran	= +24	6	7	3	+79[b]			3.2							Noted greater fiber digestibility than in normal subjects A Part of a larger study in which 9 other fiber sources fed (see Tables 4.4.4–4.4.7) A, B
McCance and Widdowson (1942)[95] Controlled diet Bread as 40 to 50% of energy intake Bread either white, brown, brown with dephytenized bran, or brown with dephytenized bran and mineral supplement	3 M, 3 F, 21–42	White		10	7	6	116										Laxative properties of brown breads similar C
		Brown		10	7	6	224										
		Brown dephytenized		10	7	6	209										
		Brown dephy-tenized + minerals		10	7	6	226										

Reference	Subjects	Diet		Days													Comments
Eastwood et al. (1973)[96]	8 M, 25–43	Basal / Ad lib diet	—	7	7	8	107 (15)	76	26 (3)		I 62					216 (46)	Cellulose also studied (see Table 4.4.4) E
		+ Bran, 16 g / Bran	+7c	21	7	8	174* (18)	76	41* (3)	9.5	43					207 (34)	
Connell and Smith (1974)[97]	10, 25–45	Cornflakes 1 oz / Ad lib diet	IV	28	7	8	119 (9)				93 (16)						
		Bran buds, 1 oz / Bran buds or cornflakes	+8	28	7	8	218* (20)			12.3	44* (4)						Study included additional group with diverticular disease (see Table 4.4.11)
Findlay et al. (1974)[98]	6, 28–36	Basal / Ad lib diet	—	7	7	6	120 (18)	72	33 (4)		I, IV 66 (18)					296 (32)	See original paper for comments on liquid and solid phases of gut contents F, G
		+ Bran, 20 g / Bran	+9c	35	7	6	183* (22)	74	46* (3)	7.2	50 (11)					352 (45)	
Walters et al. (1975)[107]	2 M, 3 F, 52–69	Basal	15	12	7	5	93 (10)	75	23 (1)			2.8 (0.2)	1.1 (0.2)	646 (73)	199 (44)	108 (6)	Two separate studies: one of bagasse biscuits in nuns living in a convent (see Table 4.4.7); the sec- ond an in- patient controlled diet study of wheat bran biscuits A, C–E, J
Southgate et al. (1976)[108]		+ Bran crisp-bread	28	12	7	5	166* (15)	77	38* (8)	5.5		3.8 (0.6)	1.6* (0.2)	675 (81)	195 (17)	166* (6)	
McLean Baird et al. (1977)[109] Controlled diet Hospital low fiber Bran crisp-bread (Energen)			IV														
Cummings et al. (1976)[99]	6 M, 21–25	Basal	17	21	7	6	79 (7)	73	21 (1)		II 58 (3)	1.7 (0.2)	1.2 (0.0)	602 (79)	199 (19)		B, C, E, H
Jenkins et al. (1975)[100] Controlled diet Normal foods		+ Fiber	45	21	7	6	228* (30)	80	45* (2)	5.3	40* (4)	2.7* (0.2)	2.0* (0.1)	820 (121)	279* (19)		

Table 4.4.2 (Continued) Effect of Wheat Fiber in Various Forms on Fecal Composition (See Also Table 4.4.10)

Literature Source	Diet / Fiber Source	Total Number of Subjects in Study (sex and age)	Study period	Fiber Intake (g/day) and Fiber Method	Days on Diet	Fecal Collection Period (days)	Number of Subjects Collecting Feces	Fecal Weight (g/day)	Moisture (%)	Fecal Solids (g/day)	Apparent Increase in Fecal Weight per Gram Dietary Fiber Fed	Transit Time (h) and Transit Method	Fat (g/day)	N (g/day)	Neutral Steroids (mg/day)	Acid Steroids (mg/day)	Energy (kcal/day)	Comments / Notes / Other Data Available
Whole meal bread, All Bran, bran, and bran biscuits																		
Fuchs et al. (1976)[101]	Basal	4 M, 2 F, 22–47		IV	21	3	6	103 (20)	73	28								Eating habits showed reduced eggs, butter, and breakfast meats with increased milk and fruit during bran period Stool pH unchanged Fecal anaerobe: aerobe ratio increased by bran E, J
Kahaner et al. (1976)[102]	All Bran, 3 oz			+23	21	3	6	226* (45)	74	59	5.3							
Floch and Fuchs (1977/78)[103,104] Ad lib diet All Bran (Kellogg's)																		
Reinhold et al. (1976)[105] Controlled diet Normal foods, 58 to 62% of energy as bread	White Bread 500 g	2 M, 24, 35	V	22d	20	—	2	244 (92)	91	21 (5)			2.3 (0.1)					A, C, D
Bread: white or basari (80 to 90% extraction)	Basari, 500 g			30d	20		2	403 (121)	90	40 (8)			2.9 (0.1)					

Reference	Subjects	Diet	Design	Fiber (g)	Days	n	(n)	Fecal wt (g/day)	%	Dry wt (g/day)	Transit	I / II	Other	Comments
Wyman et al. (1976)[106]	10 M, 11–41. Ad lib low fiber avoiding cereals, bread, fruit, and vegetables. Raw bran or All Bran (Kellogg's)	Basal	IV			5	10	131 (17)	75	30 (3)	14.4	65 (8) *(I)*		Stool weight not significantly increased by any treatment. Cooked bran thought to be less effective than raw bran
		Raw bran, 12 g		+3.6	14	5	10	183 (21)	76	42* (5)	4.7	53 (17)		
		Raw bran, 20 g		+5.9	14	5	10	159 (13)	76	38* (3)	2.2	48* (7)		
		All Bran, 13.2 g		+3.6	14	5	10	139 (9)	73	36 (3)	5.6	58 (6)		
		All Bran, 22 g		+5.8	14	5	10	164 (20)	77	35 (3)		50 (9)		
Kay & Truswell (1977)[110]	3 F, 3 M, 22–27. Controlled low fiber. Normal foods. White bread or coarse bran (Prewetts) made into bread and whole meal bread	Basal		3.7	14	6	5	125*	71	32			288 / 312	Study design was basal-fiber-basal. Steroid output also higher in second basal period. C, E
		+ Fiber (23–35 g bran)		8.6	21	6	5	225*	74	53*	5.3*		256 / 233	
Cummings et al. (1978)[18]	19 M, 20–38	Basal	III	22	21	7	6	95 (8)	72	27 (1)		73 (10) *(II)*	1.5 (0.1)	Part of a larger study in which fiber from carrot, cabbage, apple (see Table 4.4.7), and guar gum (see Table 4.4.5) were fed. J
Stephen and Cummings (1980)[25]	Controlled. Normal food. Bran prepared by extracting with ethanol and acetone	+ Bran, 30 g	V, VI, VII, XII	40	21	7	6	197* (13)	76*	46* (1)	5.7	43* (3)	2.0* (0.1)	
Farrell et al. (1978)[111]	14 M, 22–46. Controlled or specified menus	Basal		33	9	4	14	—	—	29 (1)		—	2.9 (0.4) / 1.6 (0.1) / 151 (6)	A, C–E, H
		+ Fiber		53	9	4	14			50* (1)			3.7* (0.3) / 2.0* (0.1) / 241* (6)	

Table 4.4.2 (Continued) Effect of Wheat Fiber in Various Forms on Fecal Composition (See Also Table 4.4.10)

Literature Source / Diet / Fiber Source	Total Number of Subjects in Study (sex and age)	Study period	Fiber Intake (g/day) and Fiber Method	Days on Diet	Fecal Collection Period (days)	Number of Subjects Collecting Feces	Fecal Weight (g/day)	Moisture (%)	Fecal Solids (g/day)	Apparent Increase in Fecal Weight per Gram Dietary Fiber Fed	Transit Time (h) and Transit Method	Fat (g/day)	N (g/day)	Neutral Steroids (mg/day)	Acid Steroids (mg/day)	Energy (kcal/day)	Comments Notes Other Data Available
Normal foods All bran, whole meal bread,bran, and bran biscuits																	
Mathur et al. (1978)[112]	10 M	Basal				10	255 (17)				I — 37 (2)						Significant effect of bran on patients with amoebic dysentery also noted in separate study
Ad lib diet Reground bran		+ Bran, 30 g		30		10	295* (14)			3.0c	32 (2)						
Cummings et al. (1979)[113] Controlled diet Normal food	4 M, 20–24	High protein	22, V	21	7	4	80 (11)	72	22 (2)		II — 70 (6)				221 (19)		No effect of protein intake on stool weight noted in other part of study C
Fiber from bran crispbread, whole meal bread, All Bran, and fine bran		High protein + Fiber	53	21	7	4	210* (9)	73	56* (1)	4.2	50* (7)				444* (27)		
Munoz et al. (1979)[114]	10 M, 19–54	Basal	V	28–30	12	6	64 (10)									275 (40)	Part of a larger study of corn bran, soybean hulls, etc. on various aspects of metabolism (see Tables 4.4.5 to 4.4.7) C–E, K
Bell et al. (1981)[115] Sandstead et al. (1979)[117,118]		Soft white wheat bran, 26 g	+ 11	28–30	12	6	99* (7)			3.2						328 (86)	
		Basal		28–30	12	9	81 (6)									530 (21)	
Munoz et al. (1978)[119] (1979)[120]		Hard red spring wheat bran, 26 g	+ 13	28–30	12	9	151* (8)			5.4						477 (107)	

Study	Subjects	Diet						Fecal wt (SD)	%		Transit				f	f	f	Comments
Huijbrechts et al. (1980)[122]	7, x̄ 22.5	Basal	V	31		4	4	194 (32)	74	42 (2)				18.8 (1.1)		17.3 (3.5)	10.7 (2.5)	Seven subjects studied for 4 weeks, then 4 for a further 4 weeks. Average weight of 4 subjects: 67.8 kg. No change in bile composition or kinetics after bran. L
Ad lib but semi-controlled. Normal food. AACC bran		+ Bran 0.5 g/kg (34 g)	45		56	4	4	273 (49)	76	62* (11)	5.8					11.9 (2.2)		
Smith et al. (1980)[123]	18 M, 19 F, x̄ 81, 65–96	Basal	+ 8			5	10	27		8			3.6			160		Elderly hospitalized subjects — also studied with ispaghula (see also Table 4.4.5). Also transit studies with radioisotope capsule, colonic pressures unchanged. C, F, H
Ad lib hospital diet. AACC bran		+ Fiber, 20 g			28	5	10	62		17	4.4		4.8			216		
Stasse-Wolthuis et al. (1980)[124] Stasse-Wolthuis (1979)[125,126]	40 M, 22 F, 18–28	Basal	VIIIa IX	18	35	7	16	89 (12)		22		II 67 (7)	1.7 (0.3)		597	288		Part of a larger study including pectin and the effects of fruits and vegetables (see Table 4.4.3). Blood pressure unchanged. C,E,H
Controlled diet. Normal food. Bran		+ Bran, 38 g	37		35	7	16	166*		36*	4.0	48*	2.9		629	254*		
Yu & Miller (1981)[127]	10 M, 20–35	Basal	V	18		6	10	143 (11)	74 (1)	36 (1)	4.5 (0.4)	III 32 (2)	1.9 (0.1)				179 (5)	Nitrogen balances

Controlled diet. Normal food. Hard and soft bran fed as bread

Table 4.4.2 (Continued) Effect of Wheat Fiber in Various Forms on Fecal Composition (See Also Table 4.4.10)

Literature Source / Diet / Fiber Source	Total Number of Subjects in Study (sex and age)	Study period	Fiber Intake (g/day) and Fiber Method	Days on Diet	Fecal Collection Period (days)	Number of Subjects Collecting Feces	Fecal Weight (g/day)	Moisture (%)	Fecal Solids (g/day)	Apparent Increase in Fecal Weight per Gram Dietary Fiber Fed	Transit Time (h) and Transit Method	Fat (g/day)	N (g/day)	Neutral Steroids (mg/day)	Acid Steroids (mg/day)	Energy (kcal/day)	Comments / Notes / Other Data Available
Controlled diet; Normal food; AACC bran added to food and cooked		+ Bran, 15 g	+ 6 (V)	18	6	10	172* (12)	75 (1)	43* (1)	4.8	29 (2) —	5.4 (0.6)	2.1* (0.1)			211* (5)	A, H
Van Dokkum et al. (1982)[128] (1983)[129]	12 M, x̄ 23	Basal	9	20	4	12	77		21		88		1.1		374		Mainly a study of mineral balance and fiber digestibility
		+ Coarse bran	22	20	4	12	140*		34*	4.8	52*		1.6*		322		
Controlled diet; Normal food		Coarse bran, low dose	22	20	4	12	137		34		77		1.3		324		Also studied coarse and fine brans (see Table 4.4.10)
		Coarse bran, high dose	35	20	4	4	202*		46	5.0	45*		1.8		355		
Breads containing coarse and fine bran		Coarse bran	22	20	4	4	158		35		35		1.8		316		A–E
		Whole meal bread	22			4	143		34		45		1.5		258		
Graham et al. (1982)[130]	11 F, 20–40	Basal	(X)	14	7	5	31 (9)	67	10								Constipated subjects; also studied with corn bran (see Table 4.4.6) which was more effective per gram material fed
Ad lib low-fiber diet; AACC bran		+ Bran, 20 g	+ 8	14	7	5	58*	72*	16*	3.4							

Study	Subjects	Diet													H
Andersson et al. (1983)[131]	5 M, 1 F		X								II				Principally a study of the effect of fiber or mineral balance, and which showed no effect C, D
		White bread	16	24	6	6	137 (38)	79	29 (5)		46 (17)				
Controlled diet Normal food		Brown bread	24	24	6	6	175* (50)	79	37* (6)	5.0	41 (13)				
Bread either white, brown, or whole meal with added phytic acid		Whole meal bread	31	24	6	6	236* (51)	80	47* (6)	6.4	39 (12)				
Eastwood et al. (1983)[24]	9 M, 26–44		XI								I				A study comparing in vitro and in vivo properties of potato and bran fiber (see Table 4.4.7) E
		Basal	19	7	7	8	120 (6)	72	33 (1)		55			220 (17)	
Ad lib diet Coarse bran		Bran, 16 g	27	21	7	8	183* (8)	75	46* (1)	7.9	49			212 (35)	
Stephen et al. (1986)[132]	19 M, 11 F		X								II				A dose–response study showing a linear increase in stool output with increasing doses of bran-enriched bread A, C–E
		Basal	20	21	6	7	114 (20)	75	28 (3)		66 (17)	2.3 (0.3)	1.5 (0.2)	125 (12)	
Controlled Normal food		+ Bran bread, 30 g	22	21	6	7	128* (22)	76	30* (2)	6.4	53 (12)	2.4 (0.3)	1.6 (0.2)	136* (12)	
Bran-enriched breads		Basal	21	21	6	8	130 (28)	78	29 (3)		68 (14)	2.8 (0.3)	1.5 (0.2)	135 (14)	
		+ Bran bread, 60 g	25	21	6	8	163* (27)	78	36* (3)	7.7	54* (10)	2.9 (0.5)	1.7* (0.2)	162* (14)	
		Basal	21	21	6	7	110 (15)	74	28 (3)		73 (15)	3.5 (0.7)	1.5 (0.2)	133 (18)	
		+ Bran bread, 110 g	30	21	6	7	145* (13)	75	36* (2)	4.4	59 (7)	3.7 (0.8)	1.6 (0.2)	163* (14)	
		Basal	24	21	6	8	173 (15)	79	37 (2)		39 (4)	4.3 (0.3)	2.1 (0.1)	178 (9)	
		+ Bran bread, 170 g	36	21	6	8	240* (14)	77	54* (2)	5.4	34 (3)	4.7 (0.3)	2.4* (0.1)	263* (9)	

a Milligrams of crude fiber per kilogram body weight per day.
b Figures are increases over basal diet period—fiber remaining in stool.
c Assumes bran is about 44% dietary fiber.
d Acid detergent fiber.
e Per gram of dietary fiber.
f Micromole per kilogram per day.
g A variety of fiber methods used (see paper).

Table 4.4.3 Effect of Purified Pectin on Fecal Composition

Literature Source / Diet / Fiber Source	Total Number of Subjects in Study (sex and age)	Study Period	Fiber Intake (g/day) and Fiber Method	Days on Diet	Fecal Collection Period (days)	Number of Subjects Collecting Feces	Fecal Weight (g/day)	Moisture (%)	Fecal Solids (g/day)	Apparent Increase in Fecal Weight per Gram Dietary Fiber Fed	Transit Time (h) and Transit Method	Fat (g/day)	N (g/day)	Neutral Steroids (mg/day)	Acid Steroids (mg/day)	Energy (kcal/day)	Comments / Notes / Other Data Available
Drasar and Jenkins (1976)[133] Ad lib diets Pectin–Bulmers NF	10 M, 22–25	Basal	III —	14	7	4	119 (22)										Also studied were guar gum and bananas (see Tables 4.4.5 and 4.4.8)
		+ Pectin 35 g	+32	14	7	4	148 (13)			0.9							
Durrington et al. (1976)[134] Ad lib diet Pectin–Bulmers NF	12 M, 22–45	Basal	III —	7	5	12	150 (10)				I 59 (9)						Serum cholesterol fell but not triglycerides E
		+ Pectin, 12 g	+10	21	5	12	186* (15)			3.6	44 (6)						
Kay and Truswell (1977)[135] Controlled diet Normal food Pectin–Bulmers NF	4 M, 5 F, 21–28	Basal	III —	14	6	9	140	71	40		III 34	3.8		335	265		Study design was control-test-control; data from first control period reported here. Serum cholesterol fell but not triglycerides
		+ Pectin, 15 g	+12	21	6	9	168	68*	52*	2.3	37	8.6		390*	371*		

Reference	Subjects	Diet													Remarks
Miettinen and Tarpila (1977)[136] Controlled diet Normal food Pectin–Firmagel Bucness Ltd.	5 F, 4 M, 33–60	Basal	III	14	3	9	200 (89)		36 (3)			3.1 (0.4)	585 (62)	342 (8)	E 2 Normal subjects, 6 hyperlipidemics, 1 diabetic, 1 diverticular disease Serum cholesterol decreased but not triglycerides Bile composition unchanged E, L
		+ Pectin, 40–5 g	+37g	14	3	9	269 (49)		46* (6)	1.9		3.9 (0.4)	642 (87)	537* (93)	
Cummings et al. (1979)[137] Controlled diet Normal food Pectin–Bulmers NF	5 M, 21–24	Basal	III 15	21	7	5	107 (25)	73	27 (3)		II 77 (18)	1.5 (0.1) / 1.3 (0.2)	239 (42)		After 3 weeks on pectin, changes in bowel habit somewhat greater than at 6 weeks Serum glutamyl transpeptidase unchanged A, C
		+Pectin, 36 g	48	42	7	5	123* (25)	72	31* (3)	0.5	70 (16)	2.7 (0.2) / 1.6* (0.2)	322* (37)		
Stasse-Wolthuis et al. (1980)[124]	40 M, 25 F, 18–28	Basal	VIII* IX 18	35	7	15	89 (9)	75	22 (5)	—	II 59 (6)	1.6 (0.5)	617	263	Part of a larger study including wheat bran and the effect of fruit and vegetables (see Tables 4.4.2 and 4.4.8) Blood pressure unchanged Serum cholesterol reduced C, E, H
Stasse-Wolthuis (1979)[125,126] Controlled diet Normal food Pectin–Bulmers NF		+ Pectin, 10 g	27	35	7	15	99	74	26	1.0	63	2.8*	669	398	
Spiller et al. (1980)[138] Ad lib diet but excluding certain high fiber foods Pectin–Sunkist	42, 23–60	Basal	III	14	7	12	55 (5)				I 118 (13)				Subjects selected for low stool weight and slow transit Cellulose also given (see Table 4.4.4) B
		+ Pectin, 6 g	+6	21	7	12	54 (8)			0	120 (17)				

Table 4.4.3 (Continued) Effect of Purified Pectin on Fecal Composition

Literature Source / Diet / Fiber Source	Total Number of Subjects in Study (sex and age)	Study Period	Fiber Intake (g/day) and Fiber Method	Days on Diet	Fecal Collection Period (days)	Number of Subjects Collecting Feces	Fecal Weight (g/day)	Moisture (%)	Fecal Solids (g/day)	Apparent Increase in Fecal Weight per Gram Dietary Fiber Fed	Transit Time (h) and Transit Method	Fat (g/day)	N (g/day)	Neutral Steroids (mg/day)	Acid Steroids (mg/day)	Energy (kcal/day)	Comments Notes Other Data Available
Ross and Leklem (1981)[139] Controlled diet Normal food Low fiber Pectin "slow set grade 200"	8 M, 20–27	Basal	III	22	6	8	105	70	31		III 32	5.1		866	425		No significant changes in fecal excretions, but fecal β-glucuronidase activity increased 35% while 7-α-dehydroxylase activity was unchanged
		+Pectin, 15 g	+12	22	6	8	126	74	33	1.5	34	4.9		863	464		
Judd and Truswell (1982)[140] Ad lib diets Pectin–Bulmers NF Either 37% (low) methoxy or 71% (high) methoxy	5 M, 5 F, 23–38	Low methoxy, 15 g	IV 34	21	7	10	124 (8)	72	34 (2)		III 25 (3)	6.2 (0.5)		399 (71)	412 (31)		Both pectins reduced blood cholesterol to a similar extent; triglycerides unchanged High methoxy pectin produced greater fecal bulk E
		High methoxy, 15 g	34	21	7	10	161* (21)	74	39* (2)		23 (3)	6.8 (0.8)		452 (60)	436 (51)		
			V														

Study	Subjects	Diet	Group								Comments
Fleming et al. (1983)[141] Marthinsen and Fleming (1982)[142] Fleming and Rodriguez (1983)[143] Pectin–Sigma	5 M, 21–32	Basal	V	0	9	3	5	54	14		Part of a study including cellulose, corn bran, and xylose (see Tables 4.4.4 to 4.4.6) Fecal pH unchanged Fecal mutagenic activity negligible in all diets A, B, M
		+ Pectin, 0.5 g/kg		+32[b]	9	3	5	86	22	1.0	
Hillman et al. (1983)[144] Ad lib diet Pectin, 9.3 g/kg, methoxyl	10 M, 20 F, 21–43	Basal	III		28	2	10	135 (21)		51 (7)	Cellulose and lignin also studied (see Tables 4.4.4 and 4.4.7) Stool pH unchanged
		+ Pectin, 12 g		+11	28	2	10	119 (25)	0	57 (4)	

[a] A variety of fiber methods used.
[b] Assumes average weight of subjects 70.0 kg and pectin 91% dietary fiber.

Table 4.4.4 Effect of Cellulose and Cellulose Derivatives on Fecal Composition

Literature Source / Diet / Fiber Source	Total Number of Subjects in Study (sex and age)	Study Period	Fiber Intake (g/day) and Fiber Method	Days on Diet	Fecal Collection Period (days)	Number of Subjects Collecting Feces	Fecal Weight (g/day)	Moisture (%)	Fecal Solids (g/day)	Apparent Increase in Fecal Weight per Gram Dietary Fiber Fed	Transit Time (h) and Transit Method	Fat (g/day)	N (g/day)	Neutral Sterols (mg/day)	Acid Sterols (mg/day)	Energy (kcal/day)	Comments / Notes / Other Data Available
Williams and Olmsted (1936)[9,29,57] Controlled diet Normal food Cellulose—celluflour commercially available	3 M	Celluflour	= + 12a	6	7	3	+ 15			1.2							Part of a larger study in which 9 other fiber sources fed (see Tables 4.4.2, 4.4.5, 4.4.6, and 4.4.7) A, B
Tainter (1943)[60] "Constant" diet Normal food Methylcellulose	—	Basal + Methylcellulose, 10 g	+ 10	7–14 7–14	7–14 7–14	—	127 232	81 82	24 41	10.5							Part of a study in which a variety of combinations of methylcellulose, magnesium oxide, and bran were tested for their laxative effect (see Table 4.4.9)
Berberian et al. (1952)[61] Ad lib diet Methylcellulose tablets	8	Control + Methylcellulose 4.5 g	+ 45	—	7 7	8 8	163 190	80 80	32 38	6.0							Further studies were undertaken in the same subjects with a combination of psyllium and methylcellulose (see Table 4.4.9)
Marks (1949)[145] Ad lib diet Sodium carboxymethyl cellulose (CMC)	38	Basal + CMC, 10 g + CMC, 20 g	+10 +20	7 7 7	7 7 7	—	100 140 180			4.0 4.0							An early study briefly described

Reference	Subjects	Diet													Comments
Eastwood et al. (1973)[96] Ad lib diet Cellulose (Whatman CFI)	8 M, 25–43	Basal		7	7	4	152 (16)	81	29 (4)	—	55			396	Bran also studied (see Table 4.4.2) E
		+Cellulose, 16 g	+16	21	7	4	221* (29)	74	57* (6)	4.3	36			478 (122)	
Ismail-Beigi et al. (1977)[146] Controlled diet Normal food 60% of energy from bread Cellulose—Whatman No. 3 taken with either white bread or Basari (80 to 90% extraction brown bread)	3M	Basal white bread	V	9–20	—	3	141 (24)		20 (1.5)						Cellulose caused increased fecal excretion of calcium, magnesium, and zinc and negative balances of all three C, D
		+Cellulose[b] 12 g	+12	9–20	—	3	223		32	6.8					
		Basal Basari bread		14		2	280 (112)								
		+Cellulose, 12 g	+12	14		2	482 (225)			16.8					
Slavin and Marlett (1980)[147,148] Controlled diet Normal food Cellulose—Solka floc®	7 F, 20–39	Basal	>9	20–30	5	7	75 (9)	75	19 (1.6)	—	102 (22)	2.8 (0.2)	1.3 (0.1)	103 (9)	Fecal calcium and magnesium excretion increased
		+Cellulose, 16 g	24	20–30	5	7	130* (11)	70	39* (3)	3.5	63 (10)	3.4 (0.3)	1.4 (0.1)	189 (12)	Fat, nitrogen, and energy digestibilities unaffected A, C
Spiller et al. (1980)[138] Ad lib diet but excluding certain high fiber foods Cellulose—Solka floc®	42, 23–60	Basal	—	14	7	13	64 (7)			—	122 (12)				Subjects selected for low stool weight and slow transit
		+Cellulose, 14 g	+14	21	7	13	97 (11)			2.3	62 (8)				Pectin also given (see Table 4.4.3) B
Fleming et al. (1983)[141] Marthinsen and Fleming (1982)[142] Fleming and Rodriguez (1983)[143] Controlled semipurified diets Cellulose—Alphacell from ICN	5 M, 21–32	Basal	>0	9	3	5	54		14						Part of a study including pectin, corn bran, and xylan (see Tables 4.4.3, 4.4.5, and 4.4.6) Fecal pH Fecal mutagenic activity negligible on all diets A, B, M
		+Cellulose 0.5 g/kg	+35 g°	9	3	5	106		42	1.5					

Table 4.4.4　(Continued) Effect of Cellulose and Cellulose Derivatives on Fecal Composition

Literature Source Diet Fiber Source	Total Number of Subjects in study (sex and age)	Study Period	Fiber Intake (g/day) and Fiber Method	Days on Diet	Fecal Collection Period (days)	Number of Subjects Collecting Feces	Fecal Weight (g/day)	Moisture (%)	Fecal Solids (g/day)	Apparent Increase in Fecal Weight per Gram Dietary Fiber Fed	Transit Time (h) and Transit Method	Fat (g/day)	N (g/day)	Neutral Steroids (mg/day)	Acid Steroids (mg/day)	Energy (kcal/day)	Comments Notes Other Data Available
Hillman et al. (1983)[144] Ad lib diet Cellulose— α-cellulose from Sigma	10 M, 20 F, 21–43	Basal + Cellulose, 15 g	— + 15	28 28	2 2	10 10	133 (21) 208* (30)			5.0	55 (6) 40*(4) =						Pectin and lignin also fed (see Tables 4.4.3 and 4.4.7) Stool pH fell
Wrick et al. (1983)[149] Van Soest et al. (1978)[150] Ehle et al. (1982)[151] Heller et al. (1980)[152] Van Soest (1981),[153] (1984)[154] Van Soest et al. (1983)[155] Controlled diet Normal food Low fiber Cellulose— Solka floc[c] baked into bread	24	Basal + Cellulose, 13–18 g day	<	24 24	7 7	12 12	102 137		25 33		56[d] 47						Part of a larger study in which coarse and fine bran and cabbage fiber were fed (see Tables 4.4.7 and 4.4.10) A, B

[a] Figures are increases over basal diet period—fiber remaining in stool.
[b] Cellulose taken with 150 g apple compote (90 g apple + 60 g syrup).
[c] Assumes average weight of subjects of 70 kg.
[d] Various transit methods used (see Van Soest et al. [1983]).[156]

Table 4.4.5 Effect of Plant Gums, Mucilages, and Other Polysaccharides on Fecal Composition

Literature Source / Diet / Fiber Source	Total Number of Subjects in Study (sex and age)	Study Period	Fiber Intake (g/day) and Fiber Method	Days on Diet	Fecal Collection Period (days)	Number of Subjects Collecting Feces	Fecal Weight (g/day)	Percent Moisture	Fecal Solids (g/day)	Apparent Increase in Fecal Weight per Gram Dietary Fiber Fed	Transit Time (h) and Transit Method	Fat (g/day)	N (g/day)	Neutral Steroids (mg/day)	Acid Steroids (mg/day)	Energy (kcal/day)	Comments / Notes / Other Data Available
Williams and Olmsted (1936)[9,29,57] Controlled diet Normal food Agar-agar	3 M	Agar-agar	= +16	6	7	3	+111[a]			8.7							Part of a larger study in which 9 other fiber sources were fed (see Tables 4.4.2, 4.4.4, 4.4.6, and 4.4.7) A, B
Gray and Tainter (1941)[7] Ad lib diet Karaya gum—sterculia urens	5 M	Basal		7	3	5	68		18(2)								A major early study of the laxative effects of plant gums including animal data and extensive in vitro studies
		+ Karaya, 5 g	+5	7	3	5	83 (17)		20 (40)	3.0							
Bassora gum (Imbicoll)		Basal		7	3	5	84		21 (2)								
Psyllium seed (back psyllium NF)		+ Imbicoll, 5 g	+5	7	3	5	135 (24)		31 (5)	10.2							
Ispaghula - from Plantago ovata (Konsyl Siblin)		Basal		7	3	5	96		20 (2)								
Psyllium - from Plantago loeflingii (mucilose)		+ Psyllium seed, 5 g	+5	7	3	5	118 (24)		26 (6)	4.4							
		Basal		7	3	5	96		20 (2)								
		+ Konsyl, 5 g	+5	7	3	5	122 (30)		22 (6)	5.2							
		Basal		7	3	5	96		22 (2)								

Table 4.4.5 (Continued) Effect of Plant Gums, Mucilages, and Other Polysaccharides on Fecal Composition

Literature Source Diet Fiber Source	Total Number of Subjects in Study (sex and age)	Study Period	Fiber Intake (g/day) and Fiber Method	Days on Diet	Fecal Collection Period (days)	Number of Subjects Collecting Feces	Fecal Weight (g/day)	Percent Moisture	Fecal Solids (g/day)	Apparent Increase in Fecal Weight per Gram Dietary Fiber Fed	Transit Time (h) and Transit Method	Fat (g/day)	N (g/day)	Neutral Sterols (mg/day)	Acid Sterols (mg/day)	Energy (kcal/day)	Notes Comments Other Data Available
Block (1947)[157] *Ad lib* diet	22 M, 18 F	+ Mucilose, 5 g	+5	7	3	5	110 (25)		17 (4)	2.8							Mental hospital patients Includes one of the earliest observations of the moderating effect of fiber on blood glucose K
		Basal		7	3	5	90		19 (2)								
		+Siblin, 5 g	+5	7	3	5	99 (37)		16 (4)	1.8							
Psyllium (Metamucil)		Basal		7	1	14	52 (6)										
		+Psyllium, 12 g	+12	7	1	14	63 (23)			0.9							
Drasar and Jenkins (1976)[133] *Ad lib* diets	10 M, 22–25	Basal	III	14	7	3	100										Also studied were pectin and banana (see Tables 4.4.3 and 4.4.8) Guar lowered blood cholesterol but did not produce a detectable change in the fecal microflora E, J
Guar gum (clear gum, Hercules Powder Co.)		+ Guar gum, 35 g	+30	14	7	3	204 (21)			3.5							
Cummings et al. (1978)[18] Controlled Normal food	19 M, 20–38	Basal	III 22	21	7	3	120 (20)	74	30 (3)								Part of a larger study in which fiber from bran, carrot, cabbage, and apple were studied (see Tables 4.4.2 and 4.4.7)
Guar gum (clear gum, Hercules Powder Co.)		+ Guar, 20g	39	21	7	3	139 (17)	74	35 (1)	1.1							

Reference / diet	Subjects	Diet	III								I				Comments
Prynne and Southgate (1979)[158] Controlled diet Normal food Ispaghula husk (Isogel)	2M, 2F, 28–31	Basal	20	21	5	4	162 (22)	77	37 (5)	3.2					Data also given for apparent digestibilities of N, fat, energy, and ash, none of which changed significantly. Great detail of nonstarch polysaccharide intakes and outputs. A
		+ Ispaghula, 25 g	44	21	5	4	242* (188)	82	43* (14)						
Spiller et al. (1979)[159] Ad lib low fiber-restricted diet Psyllium seed hydrocolloid	50, 25–65	Basal	—	21	7	10	58		19		—	1.0 (0.1)			Subjects selected for low stool weight and slow transit, "double blind parallel repeated measures" design. A cellulose-pectin biscuit also studied (see Table 4.4.9). C, H, N
		+ Psyllium powder, 20 g	+10	21	7	10	107		29	4.9	101 / 92	1.1 (0.2)			
Smith et al. (1980)[123] Ad lib hospital diet Ispaghula (Fybogel)	18 M, 29 F, 65–96	Basal	—	28	5	15	37		10				4.2	104	Elderly hospitalized subjects. Also studied with bran (see Table 4.4.2). Colonic motility (pressures) unchanged. Ispaghula and bran equally effective per gram of fiber fed. C, F, H
		+ Ispaghula, 10 g	+8	28	5	15	75		20	4.7			7.9	216	

Table 4.4.5 (Continued) Effect of Plant Gums, Mucilages, and Other Polysaccharides on Fecal Composition

Literature Source Diet Fiber Source	Total Number of Subjects in Study (sex and age)	Study Period	Fiber Intake (g/day) and Fiber Method	Days on Diet	Fecal Collection Period (days)	Number of Subjects Collecting Feces	Fecal Weight (g/day)	Percent Moisture	Fecal Solids (g/day)	Apparent Increase in Fecal Weight per Gram Dietary Fiber Fed	Transit Time (h) and Transit Method	Fat (g/day)	N (g/day)	Neutral Sterols (mg/day)	Acid Sterols (mg/day)	Energy (kcal/day)	Comments Notes Other Data Available
Eastwood et al. (1983)[160] Ad lib diet Gum Karaya (Sterculia urens from Nargina)	5 M	Basal	—	7	5	5	135	73	36		63	4.2				699	372	The gum had no discernable effect on anything
		+ Karaya, 10.5 g	+8	21	5	5	139	73	38	0.5	68	3.9				540	272	
Fleming et al. (1983)[141] Marthinsen and Fleming (1982)[142] Fleming and Rodriguez (1982)[143] Controlled semipurified diets Xylan (ICN)	5 M, 21-32	Basal	V 0	9	3	5	54		14									Part of a study including cellulose, corn bran, and pectin (see Tables 4.4.3, 4.4.4, and 4.4.6); fecal pH unchanged A, B, M
		+ Xylan, 0.5 g/kg	+35[b]	9	3	5	65		16	0.3								
Ross et al. (1983)[161] Ad lib diet Gum Arabic	5 M, 30–55	Basal	—		5	5	147		37		51					699	472	Serum cholesterol reduced and some changes in breath, H2 excretion Extensive breakdown of gum in gut A, B, E, H, K, M, N
		+ Gum Arabic, 25 g	25	21	5	5	161		52	0.6	71					779	424	

[a] Figures are increases over basal diet period—fiber remaining in stool.
[b] Assumes average weight of 70 kg and also that xylan was 100% dietary fiber.

Table 4.4.6 Effect of Oats and Corn Products on Fecal Composition

Literature Source Diet Fiber Source	Total Number of Subjects in Study (sex and age)	Study Period	Fiber Intake (g/day) and Fiber Method	Days on Diet	Fecal Collection Period (days)	Number of Subjects Collecting Feces	Fecal Weight (g/day)	Moisture (%)	Fecal solids (g/day)	Apparent Increase in Fecal Weight per Gram Dietary Fiber Fed	Transit Time (h) and Transit Method	Fat (g/day)	N (g/day)	Neutral Steroids (mg/day)	Acid Sterols (mg/day)	Energy (kcal/day)	Comments Notes Other Data Available
Williams and Olmsted (1936)[19,29,57] Controlled diet Normal food but excluding fruits and vegetables Corn germ meal prepared by washing for 24 h in warm water, extracting with hot ethanol, and drying	3 M	Corn germ meal, 55 g	II +26	6	7	3	+96[a]			4.6							Part of a larger study in which 9 other fiber sources fed (see Tables 4.4.2, 4.4.4, 4.4.5, and 4.4.7) A, B
Calloway and Kretsch (1978)[162] Kretsch et al. (1979)[163] Controlled egg-based high protein formula diet Cooked oat bran, either plain or toasted	6 M, 28–42	Formula diet	V 4	15	6	6	68 (10)	79	14 (1)		III 28 (10)	1.2 (0.3)	1.0 (0.1)		238 (24)	98 (16)	Subjects average weight, 72.8 kg. No difference between toasted and plain bran for any parameter. Principally a study of N balance which was not affected by oat bran. Blood lipids unchanged. Guatemalan diet also fed (see Table 4.4.8) A, E
		Oat bran[b] (toasted)	12	15	6	6	112* (16)	75	28* (3)	5.5	31 (7)	2.0* (0.4)	1.5* (0.2)		504* (37)	184* (27)	
		Oat brain (plain)	12	15	6	6	128* (29)	77	29* (2)	5.0	27 (6)	1.9* (0.3)	1.6* (0.2)		501 (62)	189* (41)	

Table 4.4.6 (Continued) Effect of Oats and Corn Products on Fecal Composition

Literature Source Diet Fiber Source	Total Number of Subjects in Study (sex and age)	Study Period	Fiber Intake (g/day) and Fiber Method	Days on Diet	Fecal Collection Period (days)	Number of Subjects Collecting Feces	Fecal Weight (g/day)	Moisture (%)	Fecal solids (g/day)	Apparent Increase in Fecal Weight per Gram Dietary Fiber Fed	Transit Time (h) and Transit Method	Fat (g/day)	N (g/day)	Neutral Sterols (mg/day)	Acid Steroids (mg/day)	Energy (kcal/day)	Comments Notes Other Data Available
Munoz et al. (1979)[114,120] Controlled diet Normal food Dry milled corn bran baked into bread	10 M, 19–54	Basal + Corn bran, 26 g	V	28–30	12	7	72 (10)								337 (68)		Part of a larger study including wheat bran and soybean hulls (see Table 4.4.2 and 4.4.7)
			+24	28–30	12	7	144* (10)			3.0					483 (52)		
Judd and Truswell (1982)[164] Controlled diet Normal food Rolled oats – served as porridge and substituted for flour in bread, cakes, and biscuits	6 M, 4 F, 24–37	Basal + Oats, 110–160 g	23 25ᶜ	21 21	6 6	10 10	114 125	74 73	29 34*	5.5		III 36 30	3.4 5.1*		282 315	230 372*	Study design was control-oats-control; data from first control period presented here. Blood cholesterol fell significantly E
Kirby et al. (1981)[165] Controlled diet	8 m, 35–62	Basal V	20	10	3	8	147 (14)			35 (2)					862 (68)	230 (33)	Serum cholesterol lowered

Study	Subjects	Diet										Comments
Controlled diet Normal food Oat bran—served as muffins or hot cereal	11 F, 20–40	+ Oat bran, 100 g	43	10	3	8	169* (16)		43* (2)	1.0	819 (61) 354* (28)	Glucose tolerance unaffected E, K
Graham et al. (1982)[130] Ad lib low fiber diet		Basal	X	14	7	6	31 (2)	65	11			Constipated subjects also studied with wheat bran which was less effective per gram material fed (see Table 4.4.2) H
Corn bran (G-60 grade Staley Mfg. Co.) fine particle size		+Corn bran, 20 g	17	14	7	6	82* (18)	66	28*	3.0		
Fleming et al. (1983)[141]	5 m, 21–32	Basal	0	9	3	5	54	14				Part of a study including cellulose, pectin, and xylose (see Tables 4.4.3–4.4.5) Fecal pH unchanged A, B, M
Marthinsen and Fleming (1982)[142] Fleming and Rodriguez (1983)[143] Controlled semipurified diets Corn bran (Quaker Oats)		+ Corn bran, 0.6 g/kg	+ 29[d]	9	3	3	139*	46	2.9			

a Figures are increases over basal diet period—fiber remaining in stool.
b Oat bran fed at 0.6 g/kg/day.
c Oatmeal diet contained only 2 g more dietary fiber because of substitutions—according to the authors.
d Assumes average weight of subjects of 70 kg.

Table 4.4.7 Effect of Miscellaneous Purified Forms of Fiber on Fecal Composition

Literature Source Diet Fiber Source	Total Number of Subjects in Study (sex and age)	Study Period	Fiber Intake (g/day) and Fiber Method	Days on Diet	Fecal Collection Period (days)	Number of Subjects Collecting Feces	Fecal Weight (g/day)	Moisture (%)	Fecal Solids (g/day)	Apparent Increase in Fecal Weight per Gram Dietary Fiber Fed	Transit Time (h) and Transit Method	Fat (g/day)	N (g/day)	Neutral Steroids (mg/day)	Acid Steroids (mg/day)	Energy (kcal/day)	Comments Notes Other Data Available
Williams and Olmsted (1936)[9,29,57] Controlled diet Normal food, excluding vegetables and fruit Carrots, cabbage, and peas obtained on the open market, chopped and washed in warm water for 24 h, then extracted with hot ethanol and dried Alfalfa leaf meal, cotton seed hull meal, and sugar beet pulp from Ralston Purina Co, then processed as other materials	3 M	Alfalfa leaf meal, 21 g	+13 =	6	7	3	+40 a			3.0							Also studied: cellulose, wheat bran, agar-agar, and corn germ meal (see Tables 4.4.2, 4.4.4, 4.4.5, and 4.4.6)
		Carrot, 38 g	+18	6	7	3	+90			5.6							A
		Cotton seed hulls, 25 g	+18	6	7	3	+16			2.1							
		Sugar beet pulp, 27 g	+15	6	7	3	+67			4.9							
		Canned peas, 27 g	+12	6	7	3	+28			3.3							
		Cabbage, 35g	+17	6	7	3	104			6.9							

Reference	Subjects	No.	Diet	Fiber (g)	Period (days)	Days	n	Fecal wt (g/day)	% water		Transit (days)					Notes
Walters et al. (1975)[107]	20 F, 25–72	I	Basal	18	—	7	9	88 (6)	75	22 (2)		47 (6)	4.3 (0.5)	420 (51)	156 (20)	Blood lipids and fecal microflora unchanged A separate study of bran also reported (see Table 4.4.2) E, J
McLean Baird (1977)[109]			+Bagasse, 10.5 g	27	84	7	9	140* (10)	76	33* (1)	5.8	37 (3)	6.7* (0.5)	377 (13)	234* (16)	Ad lib diet in convent Bagasse (sugar cane residue from Tate and Lyle) made into biscuits
Cummings et al. (1978)[18]	19 M, 20–38	II	Basal	22	21	7	6	88 (9)	70	26 (1)		80 (11)				Bran and guar gum also studied (see Tables 4.4.2 and 4.4.5) J
Stephen and Cummings (1980)[25]		III	+Cabbage, 30 g	40	21	7	6	143* (16)	75*	35 (6)	3.0	64* (8)				
			Controlled diet Basal	22	21	7	6	117 (7)	74	30 (1)		60 (9)				
			+Carrot, 30 g	42	21	7	6	189* (16)	79*	39* (2)	3.6	50 (6)				
			Basal	22	21	7	6	141 (20)	77	30 (2)		50 (9)				
Cabbage, carrot, and apple obtained commercially, dried, extracted with hot ethanol and acetone, then dried and ground			+Apple, 25 g	44	21	7	6	203* (29)	80*	37* (3)	2.8	43* (6)				
Munoz et al. (1979)[114,120]	10 M, 19–54	V	Basal		28–30	12	5	68 (9)						388 (51)		Also studied on bran and corn bran (see Tables 4.4.2 and 4.4.6) Plasma cholesterol unchanged but triglycerides fell with SBH C, D, E, K
Controlled diet Soybean hulls (SBH) and textured vegetable protein (TVP) fed as bread			+SBH, 26 g	+23	28–30	12	5	128* (16)			2.6			330 (87)		
			Basal		28–30	12	3	92 (10)								
			+TVP, 26 g	+4	28–30	12	3	102 (21)								
Eastwood et al. (1983)[24]	9 M, 26–44	XI	Basal	20	7	7	7	161 (26)	75 (1)	39 (5)		50 (11)	4.9 (0.9)	368 (116)		Also studied on bran (see Table 4.4.2)

Table 4.4.7 (Continued) Effect of Miscellaneous Purified Forms of Fiber on Fecal Composition

Literature Source / Diet / Fiber Source	Total Number of Subjects in Study (sex and age)	Study Period	Fiber Intake (g/day) and Fiber Method	Days on Diet	Fecal Collection Period (days)	Number of Subjects Collecting Feces	Fecal Weight (g/day)	Moisture (%)	Fecal Solids (g/day)	Apparent Increase in Fecal Weight per Gram Dietary Fiber Fed	Transit Time (h) and Transit Method	Fat (g/day)	N (g/day)	Neutral Sterols (mg/day)	Acid Sterols (mg/day)	Energy (kcal/day)	Comments Notes Other Data Available
Ad lib diet Potato concentrate purified by commercial company and either air or roller-dried or boiled; fed with either milk or soup		+ Roller-dried potato, 20 g	33	21	7	7	215 (44)	76 (2)	47 (6)	4.1	33 (5)	6.9				340 (84)	No significant effect on fecal composition or blood lipids A, E
		Basal	18	7	7	7	170 (32)	74 (1)	42 (6)		48 (8)	4.2 (0.8)				392 (50)	
		+ Air-dried potato, 20 g	28	21	7	7	207 (42)	75 (2)	47 (6)	3.7	42 (6)	4.7 (0.8)				392 (47)	
		Basal	—	7	7	5	204 (50)	78 (3)	39 (7)		35 (7)	3.5 (0.7)				352 (52)	
		+ Boiled potato, 20 g	—	21	7	5	231 (51)	78 (2)	47 (7)	2.7[b]	32 (10)	4.5 (0.7)				340 (59)	
			III								=						
Hillman et al. (1983)[144] Lignin — pure Aspen auto-hydrolyzed from Stake Technology Ltd.	10 M, 2 F, 21–43	Basal		28	2	10	139 (17)				50 (5)						Cellulose and pectin also studied (see Tables 4.4.3 and 4.4.4) Stool pH unchanged
		+ Lignin, 12 g	+12	28	2	10	177 (25)			3.2	40 (5)						

Reference	Subjects	Diet	Method[d]				n												Comments
Schweizer et al. (1983)[156] — Ad lib diet — Soya: a never-dried pulp obtained as a by-product of milk production; purified soya fiber obtained from soya flour by extraction	2 M, 4 F, 20-30	Basal	V, XI	14	14	7	6	129 (16)	77	28		I	62 (4)				735 (49)	242 (19)	Never-dried soya increased fecal deoxycholate while purified soya increased low-density lipoprotein cholesterol and altered glucose tolerance A, C, D, E, K
		+ Never-dried soya pulp, 54 g		33	21	7	6	153* (14)	77	34* (4)	1.3		44 (9)				726 (28)	294 (23)	
		+ Purified soya pulp, 26.5 g		34	21	7	6	178* (28)	77	39* (4)	2.4		59 (11)				764 (66)	215 (17)	
Tsai et al. (1983)[167] — Controlled diet — Normal food but low fiber — Soy polysaccharide[c]	14 M, 20-30	Basal		—	17		14	140 (11)	76	34 (3)		III	26 (3)	7.2 (0.8)	1.6 (0.2)	246 (59)	109 (8)	263 (32)	Fasting blood glucose fell but lipids unchanged C, D, E, H, K
		+ Soy, 25 g		—	17		14	176* (16)	78	39 (4)			29 (3)	5.7* (1.0)	1.9 (0.2)	289 (49)	118 (16)	279 (23)	
Wrick et al. (1983)[149,156] — Controlled diet — Normal food — Cabbage — ethanol extracted and incorporated into bread	24	Basal		—	24	7	12	102		25		V	56[d]						12 g cell wall material daily at first but increased later up to 24 g/day Bran and cellulose also fed (see Tables 4.4.4 and 4.4.10) A, B
		+ Cabbage		—	24	7	12	110		24			58						

a Stool weights are increased over basal period—fiber remaining.

b Assumes fiber intake increased by about 10 g.

c Soy polysaccharides "a fiber-rich product purified from soy bean cotyledon."

d Various transit methods used (see Van Soest et al., 1983).[156]

Table 4.4.8   Effect of Foods Containing Fiber on Fecal Composition

Literature Source / Diet / Fiber Source	Total Number of Subjects in Study (sex and age)	Study Period	Fiber Intake (g/day) and Fiber Method	Days on Diet	Fecal Collection Period (days)	Number of Subjects Collecting Feces	Fecal Weight (g/day)	Moisture (%)	Fecal Solids (g/day)	Apparent Increase in Fecal Weight per Gram Dietary Fiber Fed	Transit Time (h) and Transit Method	Fat (g/day)	N (g/day)	Neutral Steroids (mg/day)	Acid Steroids (mg/day)	Energy (kcal/day)	Comments Notes Other Data Available
Cowgill and Sullivan (1933)[59] Controlled diet Normal food Fruit and vegetables	6 M	Basal	—	7	7	6	78 (15)										Constipated subjects
		+ Fruit and vegetables	30–38[a]	7	7	5	165[a] (27)										Also studied effect of various brans (see Table 4.4.2)
			90														Noted greater digestibility of fiber than in healthy subjects
		+Fruit and vegetables and bran	108–113	7	7	3	193[a] (10)										A
McCance and Widdowson (1942)[168] Controlled diet Normal food Fruit-plums, greengages, pears, and damsons	2 M, 2 F, 27–41	Basal	—	7	7	4	155										A chance observation in a study of mineral balance on various breads
		+ Fruit, 31–183 g	14–28	7	7	4	156										Fruit had no effect
																	C
Antonis and Bersohn (1962)[169,170] Controlled diets Normal prison foods	58 M: 29 white, 29 black	High fat, high fiber	15	22–29[b]	7	22 Wh	236 (13)					2.1 (0.1)			479 (10)	463 (29)	Prisoners in South Africa
		High fat, low fiber	4	22–29	7	22 Wh	85* (6)					1.2* (0.1)			324* (31)	450 (38)	A very large study of the effect of diet, especially fat and fiber, on fecal lipids, blood lipids, and bile acids
		High fat, high fiber	15	22–29	7	21 Bl	259 (16)					4.4 (0.3)			590 (62)	517 (31)	
		High fat, low fiber	4	22–29	7	21 Bl	99* (6)					2.1* (0.2)			310* (27)	521 (31)	
		Low fat, high fiber	15	15–17	7	18 Wh	209 (13)					2.2 (0.1)			537 (35)	459 (28)	E

Reference / Diet description	Subjects	Diet	Fiber	Days	No.	Group	Fecal wt (g/day)	Water %	Dry wt (g/day)						Comments
Southgate and Durnin (1970)[28]	23 M, 26 W, 18–78	Low fat, low fiber	4	15–17	7	18 Wh	100* (9)				1.5* (0.1)	1.8 (0.1)	297* (25)	320* (25)	A large and detailed study of the energy value of the diet as influenced by fiber. A
		Low fat, high fiber	15	15–17	7	13 BI	240 (10)				2.6		543	393 (18)	
		Low fat, low fiber	4	15–17	7	13 BI	97* (7)				1.6* (0.1)		277* (24)	316* (20)	
Controlled diet normal food		Diet 1	III 9.7	10–14	7	c 12 YM	82 (6)	75	21 (1)		4.1 (0.3)			117 (6)	
		Diet 2	21.5	10–14	7	12 YM	163* (8)	76	38* (1)	8.3	6.4* (0.3)	2.2* (0.1)		206* (6)	
Diet 1: no fruit or vegetables except potato		Diet 1	6.2	10–14	7	14 YW	47 (3)	68	15 (0.8)		3.0 (0.2)	1.0 (0.1)		83 (4)	
Diet 2: contains fruit and vegetables and whole meal bread		Diet 2	16.2	10–14	7	14 YW	91* (5)	73	24* (1.0)	4.4	3.7* (0.2)	1.3* (0.1)		127* (5)	
Diet 3: contains larger amounts of fruit and vegetables		Diet 3	31.9	10–14	7	14 YW	181* (8)	78	40* (1.1)	5.2	6.2* (0.3)	2.2* (0.1)		210* (7)	
		Diet 1	9.6	10–14	7	11 EM	79 (11)	77	18 (1.0)		5.1 (0.3)	1.4 (0.1)		103 (5)	
		Diet 2	28.3	10–14	7	11 EM	140* (12)	77	32* (1.7)	3.3	5.4 (0.4)	2.0* (0.2)		164* (8)	
		Diet 1	7.4	10–14	7	12 EW	60 (5)	75	15 (0.8)		4.5 (0.3)	0.9 (0.1)		90 (5)	
		Diet 2	20.9	10–14	7	12 EW	130* (7)	79	28* (1.0)	5.1	4.8 (0.0)	1.4* (0.1)		150* (6)	
Drasar and Jenkins (1976)[133]	10 M, 22–25	Basal	IV	14	7	5	121 (15)								Also studied pectin and guar (see Tables 4.4.3 and 4.4.5). Blood lipids and fecal microflora unaffected. E, J
Ad lib diet		+ Banana, 1000 g	+34	14	7	5	170 (23)			1.4					
Bananas and Plantain banana		+ Plantain, 1000 g	+58	14	7	4	208 (46)			1.5					

Table 4.4.8 (Continued) Effect of Foods Containing Fiber on Fecal Composition

Literature Source / Diet / Fiber Source	Total Number of Subjects in Study (sex and age)	Study Period	Fiber Intake (g/day) and Fiber Method	Days on Diet	Fecal Collection Period (days)	Number of Subjects Collecting Feces	Fecal Weight (g/day)	Moisture (%)	Fecal Solids (g/day)	Apparent Increase in Fecal Weight per Gram Dietary Fiber Fed	Transit Time (h) and Transit Method	Fat (g/day)	N (g/day)	Neutral Steroids (mg/day)	Acid Steroids (mg/day)	Energy (kcal/day)	Comments / Notes / Other Data Available
Flynn, Beirn, and Burkitt (1977)[171]	48 M, 20–56	Basal[d]	5.6 (II)	—	—	5	149 (20)				46 (20) (I)						No change in blood lipids E, F
Ad lib diet Cooked potato		+ Potato, 860 g	7.3 (+8.6)[e]			5	249* (39)			11.6	33 (21)						
		Basal[d] (low fiber)	3.5			18	125 (15)				62 (18)						
		+Potato, 860 g	6.6 (+8.6)[e]			18	294* (24)			19.6	35* (24)						
Beyer and Flynn (1978)[172] Controlled diet Normal food Mixed sources	6 M, 21–29	Low fiber	1.1 (I)	5	5	6	51		15		48 (III)	2.5	1.1			63	
		Increased fiber	8.7	5	5	6	157		37	3.5[f]	12	6.1*	2.2*			140*	
Calloway and Kretsch (1978)[182] Controlled diet	6 M, 28–42	Formula diet	0 (V)	15	3	6	68 (26)	79	14 (3.2)			1.2 (0.7)	1.0 (0.3)		238 (58)	98 (40)	Also studied with oat bran (see Table 4.4.6)
Kretsch et al. (1978)[182] Controlled egg-based high protein formula diet		Guatemalan diet	89	15	3	6	327* (89)	81	62* (10)	2.9		1.9* (0.1)	3.4* (0.3)		502* (160)	348* (64)	A, E

Guatemalan diet contained mainly black beans and corn tortilla together with rice, bread, cheese, pumpkin, squash, and banana

Robertson et al. (1979)[173]	5	Basal	V 21 (14–33)	21	7	5	142 (37)	75	35 (6)		— 72 (12)	2.7 (0.4)	602 (73)	271 (29)	Serum cholesterol fell
Ad lib diet Raw carrot		+ Carrot	+6	21	7	5	177* (33)	76	42 (6)	5.8	55 (14)	3.5 (0.7)	645 (96)	389 (33)	Breath hydrogen excretion increased C, E, H, M
Stasse-Wolthuis et al. (1979)[174]	23 M, 23 F, 20–27	Low fiber	III[g], VIII, IX 12	21	3–5	43	69 (8)	74	18 (2)		= 55 (3)	1.2 (0.1)			Diets were fed at either high or low cholesterol (about 200 and 600 mg/day)
Controlled diet Normal food Mixed fiber sources		High fiber	33	21	3–5	43	184* (11)	76	44* (7)	3.5	37* (2)	2.5* (0.1)			Serum cholesterol fell in both groups with fiber but results confounded by changes in fat intake C, E, H

Table 4.4.8 (Continued) Effect of foods Containing Fiber on Fecal Composition

Literature Source Diet Fiber Source	Total Number of Subjects in Study (sex and age)	Study Period	Fiber Intake (g/day) and Fiber Method	Days on Diet	Fecal Collection Period (days)	Number of Subjects Collecting Feces	Fecal Weight (g/day)	Moisture (%)	Fecal Solids (g/day)	Apparent Increase in Fecal Weight per Gram Dietary Fiber Fed	Transit Time (h) and Transit Method	Fat (g/day)	N (g/day)	Neutral Steroids (mg/day)	Acid Steroids (mg/day)	Energy (kcal/day)	Comments Notes Other Data Available
Stasse-Wolthuis et al. (1979)[124-126] Controlled diet Normal food Fruit and vegetables	40 M, 22 F, 18–28	Low fiber	18[g]	35	7	15	89 (10)		23		I 66 (10)	2.2 (0.5)			682	364	Also studied with pectin and wheat bran (see Tables 4.4.2 and 4.4.3) Serum cholesterol changes not significant No change in blood pressure C, E, H
		+ Fruit and vegetables, 1065 g	43	35	7	15	138*		32*	2.0	53*	2.9			888	290	
Kelsay et al. (1978)[175-178] Controlled diet Low fiber with fruit and vegetable juices then with whole fruit and vegetables (no cereals)	12 M, 37–58	Low fiber	> 4	26	7	12	89 (9)	73	23 (2)		III 52 (4)	4.9 (0.5)	1.3 (0.1)			117	Blood pressure unchanged except in those in whom diastolic was 80 mm + Mineral balances became "lower" A, C, D
		High fiber	24	26	7	12	209* (9)	75	52* (2)	6.0	38* (4)	6.4* (0.4)	2.6* (0.2)			255*	
Kelsay et al. (1981)[179]	12 M, 35–49	Low fiber	> 2	21	7	12	87 (5)	74	23 (1)		III 30 (3)	4.8 (0.4)	1.4 (0.1)			113 (6)	Latin square design

Controlled diet Low fiber with fruit and vegetable juice then increasing amounts of fruit and vegetables		+ Fruit and vegetables	10	21	7	12	127* (8)	75	32* (2)	4.9	27 (2)	5.4 (0.4)	1.8 (0.1)	162* (10)	Blood pressure unchanged
		+ Fruit and vegetables	19	21	7	12	171* (12)	75	42* (2)	2.5	27 (2)	6.0 (0.4)	2.3 (0.1)	209* (11)	Calcium, magnesium, and copper balance unchanged
		+ Fruit and vegetables	26	21	7	12	274* (26)	78	50* (3)	5.8	31 (4)	6.2 (0.1)	2.6 (0.2)	255* (16)	Zinc balance "decreased" A, C, D
Leeds et al. (1982)[180]	8 F, 21–36	Basal	IV 22	14	14	6–8	115 (15)		31		III 53 (8)				All subjects noted marked increase in flatulence Noticeable effect of menstruation on transit time
		+ Haricot beans, 450 g	49	14	14	6–8	150* (14)		38	1.3	45 (6)				

a Milligrams of crude fiber per kilogram body weight per day.
b Weeks on diet (data are from Table 4.4.5).
c YM, young men; YW, young women; EM, elderly men; EW, elderly women.
d Subjects divided into those consuming more than 5 g crude fiber per day (average 5.6 g/day) and those consuming less (average 3.5 g/day).
e Dietary fiber equivalent.
f Dietary fiber values calculated from food tables (IV).
g A variety of fiber metods used (see paper).

Table 4.4.9　Effects of Mixed Sources of Fiber on Fecal Composition

Literature Source / Diet / Fiber Source	Total Number of Subjects in Study (sex and age)	Study Period	Fiber Intake (g/day) and Fiber Method	Days on Diet	Fecal Collection Period (days)	Number of Subjects Collecting Feces	Fecal Weight (g/day)	Moisture (%)	Fecal Solids (g/day)	Apparent Increase in Fecal Weight per Gram Dietary Fiber Fed	Transit Time (h) and Transit Method	Fat (g/day)	N (g/day)	Neutral Sterols (mg/day)	Acid Sterols (mg/day)	Energy (kcal/day)	Comments / Notes / Other Data Available
Berberian et al. (1952)[61] *Ad lib* diet — Tablets containing 0.4 g methylcellulose and 0.1 g psyllium	8	Basal		—	7	8	163	80	32								Also studied with pure methylcellulose (see Table 4.4.4)
		+6 Tablets	+3		7	8	184	81	35	7							
		+9 Tablets	+4½		7	8	213	82	38	11.1							
Tainter (1943)[60]	—	Basal		7–14	7–14	—	127	81	24								Also studied with pure methylcellulose (see Table 4.4.4)
"Constant" diets, normal foods — Various combinations of methylcellulose (MC), bran (B), and magnesium oxide (MO)		35% MC 65% B	3.2*	7–14	7–14		145	78	31	5.6							
		5 g	6.4	7–14	7–14		160	81	31	5.2							Magnesium oxide providing significant additional laxation
		10 g / 3.5% MO 35% MC 61.5% B	6.2	7–14	7–14		179	81	35	8.4							
		10 g / 10% MO 45% MC 45% B	6.5	7–14	7–14		177	83	30	7.7							
		10 g / 10% MO 90% MC / 10 g	9	7–14	7–14		231	84	36	11.6							
Raymond et al. (1977)[81] Controlled formula diets	3 F, 5 M, 19–67	Low cholesterol basal	V 0	28	7	6	177 (46)	82	32 (2)		—			505 (41)	194 (23)		Hospitalized subjects, 5 with lipid disorders, 3 normals
		+ Fiber	60	28	7	6	239* (35)	77	54* (9)	1.0	60 (9) / 35* (8)			656 (75)	266 (47)		

Reference / Age	Diet		Days		n	Fecal wt (g/day)							Comment
	High cholesterol basal + Fiber	0	28	7	6	192 (41)	89	22 (2)		66 (11)		1189 (84) 423 (122)	No decrease in plasma cholesterol E
		60	28	7	6	286* (21)	77	66* (4)	1.6	46* (9)		1152 (57) 401 (89)	
Spiller et al. (1979)[159] 50, 25–65	Basal		21	7	16	62		17		95	0.9 (0.1)		Subjects selected for low stool weight and slow transit. "Double-blind parallel repeated measures" design. Also studied with psyllium (see Table 4.4.5) C, H, N
Ad lib but low fiber-restricted diets	+ Cellulose-pectin	+20	21	7	16	106		31	2.2	69	1.1 (0.1)		
Cellulose-pectin biscuit											(0.1)		
Spiller et al. (1982)[121] 22, 24–57	V Basal		28	5	11	100 (16)				—			Considerable individual variation in responses noted
Ad lib low fiber normal food diet	Low fiber	+2	28	5	11	114 (18)				77 (12) 70 (12)			
Low fiber bar containing mainly oats and rice.	High fiber	+10	28	5	11	146* (25)				70 (14)			
High fiber bar containing soy and corn bran, peanut butter, oats, carrots, prunes, pectin, rice, etc.													

* Assumes bran about 44% fiber.

Table 4.4.10 Effects of Particle Size on Fecal Composition

Literature Source Diet Fiber Source	Total Number of Subjects in Study (sex and age)	Study Period	Fiber Intake (g/day) and Fiber Method	Days on Diet	Fecal Collection Period (days)	Number of Subjects Collecting Feces	Fecal Weight (g/day)	Moisture (%)	Fecal Solids (g/day)	Apparent Increase in Fecal Weight per Gram Dietary Fiber Fed	Transit Time (h) and Transit Method	Fat (g/day)	N (g/day)	Neutral Steroids (mg/day)	Acid Steroids (mg/day)	Energy (kcal/day)	Comments Notes Other Data Available
Macrae et al. (1942)[182] Semicontrolled diet; mainly bread (74% of energy intake) White bread and whole meal bread made from either medium or fine-ground flour	6	White bread (530–630 g)	0.9 I	10	7	6	62		18			2.7	1.4			99	A study of the digestibility of the nutrients in bread
		Medium whole meal	11.7	10	7	6	283*		69*			4.9*	2.3*			325*	Fineness of grinding made no significant difference to energy or nitrogen utilization but medium flour produced significantly greater stool bulk than fine flour
		Fine whole meal	12.0	10	7	6	232*		69*			4.5*	2.3*			317*	
Brodribb and Groves (1978)[183] Ad lib diet with either coarse bran or same bran finely milled	9 M, 12 F	Basal	III	7	7	21	140										Coarse bran increased stool weight significantly more than fine bran
		+ Coarse bran, 20 g	+10	14	7	21	219			8.0							
		+ Fine bran, 20 g	+9	14	7	21	199			6.6							

Reference / diet	No. subjects	Diet									Transit	I		Comments
Heller et al. (1980)[152] Controlled diet; Normal food; AACC white wheat bran fed whole and after fine grinding, in bread	24	Basal	V		14	4	8								Also studied with cabbage and cellulose (see Tables 4.4.4 and 4.4.7). Coarse bran produced greater fecal bulk, high moisture content, and faster transit than fine bran; fiber digestibility less in coarse bran; dietary changes during the study made comparisons with basal diet difficult
		Coarse bran, 32 g		+12	14	4	8	123	74	31				37	
		Fine bran		+12	14	4	8	108	72	29				56	
Smith et al. (1981)[184] Ad lib diet; Canadian red spring wheat bran (CRSW) or French soft wheat bran (FSW) in either coarse or fine form	24[b]	Basal	III	—	7	7	6	80 (6)					56 (11)		Coarse brans both produced significantly greater effects on bowel habit. Effects on motility not great. F
		+ Fine CRSW, 20 g		+58	28	7	6	92 (11)			2.1	51 (12)		
		Basal		—	7	7	6	96 (6)					61 (6)		
		+ Coarse CRSW		+7.5	28	7	6	123* (11)			3.6	21* (9)		
		Basal		—	7	7	6	81 (11)					54 (8)		
		+ Fine FSW, 20 g		+59	28	7	6	102 (6)			3.6	41 (5)		
		Basal		—	7	7	6	68 (9)					48 (8)		
		+ Coarse FSW, 20 g		+6.9	28	7	6	106* (6)			5.5	20* (7)		
Van Dokkum et al. (1982)[128] (1983)[129] Controlled diet; Normal food; Breads containing coarse and fine brans	12 M, 23	Coarse bran	V	22	20	4	12	126		33	1.7	44		327	(See also Table 4.4.2). Fecal weight significantly lower with fine bran than coarse bran. A, B, C, D, E, N
		Fine bran		22	20	4	4	102*		29	1.6	62		315	

a Various transit methods used (see papers).

b Patients with diverticular disease.

Table 4.4.11 Effects of Fiber on Fecal Composition in Patients With Diverticular Disease (See Also Table 4.4.10)

Literature Source Diet Fiber Source	Total Number of Subjects in Study (sex and age)	Study Period	Fiber Intake (g/day) and Fiber Method	Days on Diet	Fecal Collection Period (days)	Number of Subjects Collecting Feces	Fecal Weight (g/day)	Moisture (%)	Fecal Solids (g/day)	Apparent Increase in Fecal Weight per Gram Dietary Fiber Fed	Transit Time (h) and Transit Method	Fat (g/day)	N (g/day)	Neutral Steroids (mg/day)	Acid Steroids (mg/day)	Energy (kcal/day)	Comments Notes Other Data Available
Findlay et al. (1974)[98] Ad lib diet Coarse bran	7 30–84	Basal + Bran, 20 g	— 9ᵃ	7 35	7 7	7 7	84 101 (19)	70 74	23 24 (3)	1.9	I, IV 93 58* (8)				273 241 (85)		Study included a control group of healthy subjects (see Table 4.4.2) Effect of bran on fecal weight only one-third that seen in controls Intraluminal pressure in response to food reduced by bran. F, G
Parks (1974)[185, 186] Out-patient semicontrolled diet Lower residue than with addition of 40 g bran, fruit, vegetables, and whole meal bread	11 M, 10 F	Low fiber High fiber	III — +12	4 4	6 6	21 21	96 176*	77 78	20 34	6.7	I, IV 44 37*	2.0 2.0					Similar value for transit by both methods Increased abdominal discomfort noted in early weeks

Reference / Diet	Subjects	Treatment	Change	Days	n		Fecal wt	Transit				Remarks
Brodribb and Humphreys (1976)[187] Ad lib diet Coarse bran	10 M, 30 F, 25–85	Basal			4	40	66		—			Colonic motility in response to eating reduced. Patients had lower basal fiber intakes than health controls. F, K
		+ Bran, 24 g	+10	8[b]	4	40	89*	2.3	I			
Taylor and Duthie (1976)[188] Ad lib diet High fiber diet Normacol (an ispaghula derivative) Bran tablets	20	Basal			5	20	79 (7)		97 (7)			Bran was the most effective of the three treatments
		High fiber diet		28	5	5	102 (16)		76* (7)			
		Normacol		28	5	5	105* (13)		72* (11)			
		Bran tablets (9)	−8	28	5	10	121* (7)		56* (4)			
Eastwood et al. (1978)[189] Ad lib diet Coarse bran Ispaghula (Fybogel) Lactulose	31, 32–84	Basal			7	7	82	2.4	I, IV 88		268	Bran reduced postprandial motility while ispaghula increased basal pressures. C, F, H
		+ Bran, 20 g	+9	28	7	7	103		50*	2.8	164	
		Basal			7	14	75	4.7	62	2.8	145	
		+ Ispaghula, 7 g	+7	28	7	14	108		72		226	
		Basal			7	10	95	3.2	48	3.4	206	
		Lactulose, 20–40 ml	+20	28	7	10	160*		40	3.2	218	

Table 4.4.11 (Continued) Effects of Fiber on Fecal Composition in Patients With Diverticular Disease (See Also Table 4.4.10)

Literature Source	Diet Fiber Source	Total Number of Subjects in Study (sex and age)	Study Period	Fiber Intake (g/day) and Fiber Method	Days on Diet	Fecal Collection Period (days)	Number of Subjects Collecting Feces	Fecal Weight (g/day)	Moisture (%)	Fecal Solids (g/day)	Apparent Increase in Fecal Weight per Gram Dietary Fiber Fed	Transit Time (h) and Transit Method	Fat (g/day)	N (g/day)	Neutral Steroids (mg/day)	Acid Steroids (mg/day)	Energy (kcal/day)	Comments Notes Other Data Available
Tarpila et al. (1978)[190]	Bran rusks 6 per day	11 M, 11 F; 35–64	Time zero control	— (III)	c	3	11	167 (20)		33 (4)			5.3 (1.1)		733 (106)	330 (48)		No effect on biliary cholesterol saturation; Biliary deoxycholate decreased by bran. No consistent cholesterol-lowering effect; E, L
			High fiber			3	11	215 (28)		38 (4)			4.2 (0.7)		816 (133)	475 (82)		
			6 Months control			3	11	155 (19)		29 (2)			4.2 (0.5)		697 (93)	320 (49)		
			High fiber			3	11	272* (24)		55* (5)			6.9* (1.4)		883 (147)	384 (61)		
			12 Months control			3	11	179 (35)		37 (6)			5.5 (1.4)		709 (91)	346 (89)		
			High fiber			3	11	265 (44)		47 (7)			5.0 (0.9)		541 (46)	240 (39)		
Ornstein et al. (1981)[191]	Ad lib diet Bran crisp bread Ispaghula (Fybogel) Placebo	22 M	Placebo	17.5 (III)	d	7	57	119 (6)				50 (4) (II)						Fiber supplement conferred no benefit on symptoms but did relieve constipation
			Bran	22.2	4	7	57	137* (7)			3.9	45 (4)						
			Ispaghula	24.2	4	7	57	161 (8)			6.3	47 (4)						

a   Assumes bran about 44% fiber.

b   After 8-month treatment, patients showed satisfactory clinical response.

c   Some 22 patients allocated to control or high fiber diet and followed for 12 months.

d   Four months on each diet; 58 patients divided into 3 groups, each of which took all 3 treatments in random order.

Table 4.4.12 Effects of Cereal Products on Fecal Composition

Literature Source / Diet / Fiber Source	Total Number of Subjects in Study (sex and age)	Study Period	Fiber Intake (g/day) and Fiber Method	Days on Diet	Fecal Collection Period (days)	Number of Subjects Collecting Feces	Fecal Weight (g/day)	Moisture (%)	Apparent Increase in Fecal Weight per Gram Dietary Fiber Fed	Fecal Solids (g/day)	Transit Time (h) and Transit Method	Fat (g/day)	N (g/day)	Neutral Steroids (mg/day)	Acid Steroids (mg/day)	Energy (kcal/day)	Comments / Notes / Other Data Available
Fedail et al. (1984)[192] Wheat bran Sorghum barn	10 M 23 (22–24)	Basal	X 20	21	3	10	138 (14)				II 31 (2)						Sudan medical students Symptom diary Stool consistency
		Sorghum	+ 2.5	21	3	10	173 (15)		14.0		30 (1)						
		Wheat	+ 7.9	21	2	10	221a (31)		10.5		26a (1)						
Eastwood et al. (1986)[193] Ad lib diet White or Whole meal bread	14 M 14 F 69 (50–82)	Ad lib	IV 13–14		7	28	74 (5)	72		21 (1.4)	I 80 (5.8)	2.5 (0.2)		640 (60)	266 (31)		Long-term study in the community
		+ White bread	12–14	182	7	28	80 (4.8)	75		20 (1)	76 (6.4)	3.1 (0.3)		640 (48)	243 (23)		
		+ Whole meal bread	22–23	182	7	28	101a (5.9)	73	3.4	27a (1.3)	74 (5.9)	3.6 (0.3)		720 (84)	232 (19)		
Marlett et al. (1986)[194] Ad lib diet AACC wheat bran	5 F 2 M 59–76	Ad lib	V 8.5	11	9	7	122 (44)	76		29 (5)							Dietary compliance study
		+ Bran	20.9	22	9	7	170a (52)	74	3.9	44a (6)							
Mallet et al. (1987)[195] Ad lib diet Wheat bran	3 M 3 F 22–26	Ad lib	IV 16–21	21	5	6	44 (12)										Study of fecal flora and enzymes. J, Ammonia. Also pectin (see Table 4.4.14) g fecal weight/g fiber based on average of 3 control periods
		Bran	+ 13	21	5	6	137 (30)		4.4								
		Ad lib		21	5	6	92 (27)										

Table 4.4.12 (Continued) Effects of Cereal Products on Fecal Composition

Literature Source / Diet / Fiber Source	Total No. Subjects in Study (sex and age)	Study Period	Fiber Intake (g/day) and Fiber Method	Days on Diet	Fecal Collection Period (days)	No. Subjects Collecting Feces	Fecal Weight (g/day)	Moisture (%)	Fecal Solids (g/day)	Apparent Increase in Fecal Weight per Gram Dietary Fiber Fed	Transit Time (h) and Transit Method	Fat (g/day)	N (g/day)	Neutral Sterols (mg/day)	Acid Sterols (mg/day)	Energy (kcal/day)	Comments / Notes / Other Data Available
Reddy et al. (1987)[196] Ad lib Mixed grain bread	8 M 7 F	Ad lib	IV, XIII		2	15	151 (18)	75	38 (4)								Fecal mutagenesis pH
		+ Bread	+ 11g	28	2	15	228 (21)	77	52 (5)	7.0							
Wisker et al. (1988)[198] Controlled diet Wheat/Rye	6 F 23–27	Low	XIV, XV, and X 19.7	21	5	6	144 (17)					2.4 (0.2)	1.7 (0.2)			144 (17)	Study of energy metabolism Body weight A
		High	48.3	21	5	6	329ᵃ (39)			6.5		4.2 (0.2)	2.9 (0.3)			307 (41)	
Spiller et al. (1986)[201] Semi-controlled Wheat bread	36 F 19.8 18–32	Basal	V, XVI 15 (3)	13	5	36	73 (6)	73	20 (1.5)	—	77 (8)			641 (86)	58 (7.9)		Dose response study H, L
		B	+ 5.7	13	5	12	95ᵃ (10)	74	25ᵃ (2.2)	3.8	58 (5)			568 (72)	80 (13)		
		C	+ 17.1	13	5	12	139ᵃ (12)	76	34ᵃ (2.6)	3.8	58 (10)			550 (93)	96 (14)		
		D	+ 28.5	13	5	12	212 (17)	77	49ᵃ (3.2)	4.9	50 (5)			492 (65)	92 (9)		
Stevens et al. (1988)[205] Semi-controlled AACC Bran	12 F 29 22–38	Basal	V, XVI 21	7	7	12	79 (8)	75	20 (1)		I–V 70 (6.3)						Also psyllium (Table 4.4.14) Stool consistency
		Bran	40	14	7	12	135ᵃ (9)	75	34ᵃ (2)	2.9	47ᵃ (3.2)						
Villaume et al. (1988)[206] Controlled diet Wheat bran	5	Basal		21		5	77	62	29								Letter 2 diet periods at 1 year interval A, K
		+ Bran	+ 8.8	49		5	95	65	33	2.0							
Melcher et al. (1991)[207]	14 M 10 F	Ad lib	XVI	7	7	24	155 (18)	74	40 (4.1)		II						Consistency M

Reference / Diet	Subjects	Diet	Fibre (g/day)				Fecal wt (g/day) (SE)	% water	Dry wt (g/day) (SE)	Transit (days)						Comments
Ad lib Fiber-One (Wheat and corn bran)	20–36	+ Fiber-One	+ 240	13	13	24	287a (21)	74	74 (4.3)	5.5						Dose-response study. Fecal weight on control periods varied (see original paper)
Jenkins et al. (1987)[208]	34 M 39 F	Ad lib	XVI													
Ad lib diet Bran Flakes and All Bran	29 18–61	Bran Flakes, 30 g	5.6	14	3		124 (12)									
		60	9.5	14	3		136 (13)									
							137 (5)									
		All Bran 30	11.2	14	3		138 (11)									
		60	19.0	14	3		168 (7)			2.7						
		90	28.4	14	3		212 (14)									
Anderson et al. (1984)[209] Controlled diet Oats (and Beans)	20 M 34–66	Control	XIII / 19		3		134 (27)	80	27 (4)	2.0				719 (140)	109 (37)	Also beans (see Table 4.4.13) Hypercholesterolemic volunteers E, K
		Oats	47		3		191a (20)	78	42a (4)					829 (9)	180 (43)	
Miyoshi et al. (1987)[210] Controlled diet Rice	5 M 21.4	Polished rice	V / 6.2	14		5	125 (19)	80	25 (1.3)		III / 26 (5.2)	2.3 (0.3)	1.5 (0.1)	106 (13)		C, E, H, N Blood urea
		Brown rice	15.0	8		5	192a (23)	73	51a (9)	7.6	24a (1.9)	10.6a (2.1)	2.4a (0.4)	249a (34)		
Miyoshi et al. (1986)[211] Controlled diet	5 M 20.2	Brown rice	V / 30.1	14		5	238a (20)	77	54a (4)	5.5	III / 27 (0.2)	12a (1.1)	2.5 (0.2)	278 (30)		A, E, N Blood Urea Proteins
		Polished rice	14.8	14		5	154 (22)	81	29 (3)		28 (0.3)	2.5 (0.2)	2.0 (0.2)	140 (12)		

Table 4.4.12 (Continued) Effects of Cereal Products on Fecal Composition

Literature Source / Diet / Fiber Source	Total Number of Subjects in Study (sex and age)	Study Period	Fiber Intake (g/day) and Fiber Method	Days on Diet	Fecal Collection Period (days)	Number of Subjects Collecting Feces	Fecal Weight (g/day)	Moisture (%)	Fecal Solids (g/day)	Apparent Increase in Fecal Weight per Gram Dietary Fiber Fed	Transit Time (h) and Transit Method	Fat (g/day)	N (g/day)	Neutral Sterols (mg/day)	Acid Sterols (mg/day)	Energy (kcal/day)	Comments / Notes / Other Data Available
Kaneko et al. (1986)[212] Controlled diet Rice (Agar)	5 F 18–20	A B C D	V 18.2 11.8 16.2	5 5 5 5	5 5 5 5	5 5 5 5	276 (27) 120 (9.4) 126 (14) 242 (15)		44 (4.4) 19 (1.5) 25 (2.9) 41 (2.5)	8.6 7.5		21 (3.5) 6.3 (0.7) 7.8 (0.6) 24 (1.2)	1.7 (0.3) 0.7 (0.1) 1.0 (0.1) 1.8 (0.3)				Diets A: High fiber, low protein brown rice B: Semi-purified low protein agar C: Low fiber, normal protein white rice D: High fiber, normal protein brown rice pH, fecal cholesterol C, A
Sugawara et al. (1991)[213] Controlled diet Corn residue	6 26–32	Basal Corn Basal	V, XVI + 4.2	10 10 10	6 6 6	6 6 6	115 (4.5) 128 (7.3) 117 (4.0)	79 (1.3) 79 (1.8) 78 (1.4)	24 26 26	2.8							pH Fecal ammonia and enzymes J

a Significantly different from control.

Table 4.4.13 Effect of Legumes on Fecal Composition

Literature Source / Diet / Fiber Source	Total Number of Subjects in Study (sex and age)	Study Period	Fiber Intake (g/day) and Fiber Method	Days on Diet	Fecal Collection Period (days)	Number of Subjects Collecting Feces	Fecal Weight (g/day)	Moisture (%)	Fecal Solids (g/day)	Apparent Increase in Fecal Weight per Gram Dietary Fiber Fed	Transit Time (h) and Transit Method	Fat (g/day)	N (g/day)	Neutral Steroids (mg/day)	Acid Steroids (mg/day)	Energy (kcal/day)	Comments / Notes / Other Data Available
Slavin et al. (1985)[214] Controlled diets Soya	16 M 20–34		V, XVII								>						Liquid diets with added soya fiber. Fecal consistency See also Reference 216
		Ensure		10	5		67 (5)		19		72						
		Enrich 30 g soya	+25	10	5		115 (13)		29	1.9	48						
		Ensure 30 g soya	+25	10	5		100 (10)		25	1.3	57						
		Ensure 60 g soya	+50	10	5		150 (20)		30	1.7	51						
		Ad lib					145 (13)				55						
Kurpad et al. (1988)[217] Ad lib diet	6 M		IV								=						A, H
		Ad lib			3	6	196 (23)	87	25 (5.8)		27 (5.9)		3.5 (0.7)				
		Beans (haricot)	+18	7	3	6	216 (31)	86	29 (3.1)	1.1	33 (6.6)		3.3 (0.4)				
Anderson et al. (1984)[209] Controlled diet	20 M 34–66		XIII														See also Table 4.4.12 (Oats) E, K
		Control	19		3		132 (23)	80	31 (7)					878 (206)	154 (37)		
		Beans (Oats)	47		3		140 (14)	77	32 (3)	0.3				894 (184)	108[a] (20)		
Fleming et al. (1985)[218] Ad lib diet	12 M 21–35		III														B, M pH
		Ad lib		23	3		172 (12)	78	38 (21)		42 (3)						
		Red kidney beans	+8.4	23	3		198[a] (12)	78	44 (12)	3.1	41 (3)						

[a] Significantly different from control.

Table 4.4.14 Effect of Gums and Mucilages and Other Purified Sources on Fecal Composition

Literature Source / Diet / Fiber Source	Total Number of Subjects in Study (sex and age)	Study Period	Fiber Intake (g/day) and Fiber Method	Days on Diet	Fecal Collection Period (days)	Number of Subjects Collecting Feces	Fecal Weight (g/day)	Moisture (%)	Fecal Solids (g/day)	Apparent Increase in Fecal Weight per Gram Dietary Fiber Fed	Transit Time (h) and Transit Method	Fat (g/day)	N (g/day)	Neutral Sterols (mg/day)	Acid Sterols (mg/day)	Energy (kcal/day)	Comments / Notes / Other Data Available
Abraham and Mehta (1988)[219]	7 M 31.8 26–38		V														Fiber from psyllium measured by Englyst method[82] E, K Retinyl esters Glucagon
Controlled diet		Basal		21	5	7	104 (24)	75	26 (3)					556 (44)	289 (93)		
Psyllium		Psyllium	+ 18	21	5	7	223 (39)	84	36 (5)	6.6				732 (100)	320 (89)		
Tomlin and Read (1988)[220]	6 M 1F		X														In vitro fermentation Data read from graphs Fiber data by Englyst[82]
		Control		7	7	7	160				51						
		Ispaghula	+ 12.8	7	7	7	214a			4.2	46						
Semi-controlled Guar		Control		7	7	7	160				51						
Ispaghula		Guar	+ 13.5	7	7	7	173			1.0	40						
Xanthan gum		Control		7	7	7	159				51						
		Xanthan	+ 14.0	7	7	7	186			1.9	53						
Rasmussen et al. (1987)[221]	6 M 3 F 30.3	Ad lib	X		3		178 (20)										In vitro fermentation B Fiber by Englyst[82]
Ad lib		Ispaghula	+ 25	14	3		276a (15)			3.9							
Ispaghula Lactulose		Lactulose	+ 30	14	3		200 (26)			0.7							
Miettenen et al. (1989)[222]	9																Patients with lipid disorders Also guar study with diverticular disease patients E
Controlled diet		Basal			3		159 (26)	78	35 (4)			3 (1)		787 (103)	346 (64)		
Plantago ovata		Plantago	+ 25	11	3		251a (39)	84	39 (4)	3.7		4a (1)		759 (96)	468a (72)		
Hamilton et al. (1988)[223]	44 F 6 M	Placebo	X		7	9	101										Data read from graphs

Reference	Treatment	Dose (g)	n	Age	Days	No.	Fecal wt (SD)	% water	col b	Transit	col d	col e (pH)	col f	col g	Comments
Ad lib Methylcellulose	M-C 2 g	+2	27	18–70	7	20	115			7.0					Also constipated subjects studied with psyllium and methyl cellulose. See also Reference 224.
	M-C 4 g	+4			7	21	154[a]			12.2					
Perragini et al. (1986)[225] Controlled diet Guar	Basal	22	6 M	21–28	14	6	68 (6)			0.8	= 46 (3.5)				E, M, A
	Guar	+10			14	6	76 (14)				54 (7.2)				
Anderson et al. (1986)[226] *Ad lib* diet Carboxymethyl-cellulose	*Ad lib*		5 M	38 (24–58)	7	5	140 (33)	73	38 (7)	6.8	− 53 (10)	5.3 (0.8)	672 (120)	364 (77)	B, E, K, M, N. Blood biochemistry
	CMC	+15			23	5	242 (20)	75	60 (5)		46 (10)	7.8 (0.8)	728 (160)	664 (116)	
Eastwood et al. (1987)[227] *Ad lib* Xanthan gum	*Ad lib*		5 M	35 (26–50)	7	5	187 (27)	76	44 (3)	4.8	= 56 (12)	7.8 (2.2)	560 (80)	347 (39)	B, E, K, M, N. Blood biochemistry. Immunoglobulins
	Xanthan	10.4 to 12.9			23	5	242 (39)	79	51 (6)		45 (10)	8.1 (1.4)	600 (40)	656 (116)	
Eastwood et al. (1984)[228] *Ad lib* Tragacanth	Control		5 M	36 (21–57)	7	5	125 (18)	74	32 (5)	6.4	46	3.9 (1)	386 (66)	368 (36)	B, E, K, M, N. Blood biochemistry
	Gum	9.9			21	5	188[a] (26)	75	46[a] (6)		36	7.0 (1.4)	521 (111)	752 (112)	
Tomlin and Read (1988)[229] *Ad lib* Ispaghula (I) Polydextrose (P)	Basal		12 M	20–30	10		171			1.5	= 54				Stool consistency. Medians, not means
	I 7g	+6			10		180[a]				59				
	P 30g	+30			10		174[a]				59				
	I 2g and P 30 g	+32			10		183[a]				59				
	Basal				10		220			5.7	33				
	I 7g	+6			10		254[a]				35				
	I 2g and P 10 g	+12			10		236[a]				36				
Stevens et al. (1988)[205] Semi-controlled Psyllium	Basal	21	12 F	29 (22–38)	7	12	79 (8)	75	20 (1)	4.4	I–V 70 (6.3)				Also bran (see Table 4.4.12)
	Psyllium	40			14	12	163[a] (11)	80	33[a] (1)		59[a] (3)				
Mallet et al. (1987)[195] *Ad lib* Pectin	*Ad Lib*	16–21	3 M 3 F	22–26	21	6	103 (18)			6.8					Also bran (see Table 4.4.12). Mainly study of fecal flora. See notes to Table 4.4.12
	Pectin	+16			21	6	93[a] (36)								

[a] Significantly different from control.

Table 4.4.15 Effect of Foods and Mixed Diets on Fecal Composition

Literature Source / Diet / Fiber Source	Total Number of Subjects in Study (sex and age)	Study Period	Fiber Intake (g/day) and Fiber Method	Days on Diet	Fecal Collection Period (days)	Number of Subjects Collecting Feces	Fecal Weight (g/day)	Moisture (%)	Fecal Solids (g/day)	Apparent Increase in Fecal Weight per Gram Dietary Fiber Fed	Transit Time (h) and Transit Method	Fat (g/day)	N (g/day)	Neutral Steroids (mg/day)	Acid Steroids (mg/day)	Energy (kcal/day)	Comments / Notes / Other Data Available
Allinger et al. (1989)[230,246] Ad lib Vegetarian	6 M 20 F 44 27–61	Ad lib	XVIII XIX 20	91	2		118	72	33								Fecal pH L Urinary N, K, Na
		Vegetarian	30	91	2		176ª	78	38ª	5.8							
Kesaniemi et al. (1990)[233] Semi-controlled Mixed foods	34 M 50 47–55	Basal	IV 12	56	3		144 (18)	71	33 (1)					2268 (115)	1351 (83)		E Biliary lipids Cholesterol kinetics
		High fiber	26	56	3		197ª (10)	78	43ª (2)	3.6				2088 (102)	1391ª (91)		
Tinker et al. (1991)[234] Ad lib (grape juice) Prunes	41 M	Grape	XVI 18	28	3		171 (5)	77	40 (1)						501 (54)		E
		Prunes	24	28	3		209ª (7)	78	47ª (1)	6.3					518 (67)		
Forsum et al. (1990)[235]	21	A	XVII 57.6	20	5	5	288 (62)	80	58 (8.9)	4.7							A Fecal biomass

Study / Diet	Subjects	Diet												Comments
Controlled diet Mixed sources		B$_1$	71.4	20	5	5	179 (19)	80	36 (1.7)	1.8				A
		B$_2$	55.0	20	5	5	108 (21)	77	25 (1.5)	0.8				B$_1$, B$_2$ = digestible fibers
		C	12.0	20	5	6	74 (9)	72	21 (2.4)					C = low fiber
Ghoos et al. (1988)[236] Semi-controlled Mixed sources	11 F 14 M 45.8 47.8	Low	13.2		3	25	136 (15)	85	20 (1.7)				115 (18)	E, L Monastery
		High	23.2		3	26	288[a] (25)	86	39 (3.5)				393 (44)	
Miles et al. (1988)[237] Controlled Fruit and vegetables	12 M 41	High	37	42	7						4.3 (0.4)	2.6 (0.2)	249 (18)	A Digestible energy Metabolizable energy Week 5 values used
		Low	26	42	7						3.5 (0.3)	1.6 (0.1)	134 (9)	
Reddy et al. (1988)[238] Low fat/high fiber	11 F 46–67	Ad lib	XIII 17		2		86 (26)							Also follow up at one year
		Low fat/high fiber	37	26	2		145[a] (18)			3.0				Fecal steroids pH E

[a] Significantly different from control.

REFERENCES

1. Burne, J., *A Treatise on the Causes and Consequence of Habitual Constipation*, Longman, Orme, Brown, Green & Longmans, London, 1840.
2. Hertz, A. F., *Constipation and Allied Intestinal Disorders*, Oxford Medical Publ., 1909.
3. Dimock, E. M., The Treatment of Habitual Constipation by the Bran Method, M.D. thesis, University of Cambridge, Cambridge, U.K., 1936.
4. Porges, M., Treatment of constipation with Normacol, *Med. J. Rec.*, 128, 87, 1928.
5. Morgan, H., The laxative effect of a regenerated cellulose in the diet, *JAMA*, 102, 995, 1934.
6. Ivy, A. C. and Isaacs, B. L., Karaya gum as a mechanical laxative: an experimental study on animals and man, *Am. J. Dig. Dis.*, 5, 315, 1938.
7. Gray, H. and Tainter, M. L., Colloid laxatives available for clinical use, *Am. J. Dig. Dis.*, 8, 130, 1941.
8. Tainter, M. L. and Buchanan, O. H., Quantitative comparisons of colloidal laxatives, *Ann. N.Y. Acad. Sci.*, 58, 438, 1954.
9. Williams, R. D. and Olmsted, W. H., The effect of cellulose, hemicellulose and lignin on the weight of the stool: a contribution to the study of laxation in man, *J. Nutr.*, 11, 433, 1936.
10. Burkitt, D. P., Related disease—related causes, *Lancet*, ii, 1229, 1969.
11. Burkitt, D. P., The aetiology of appendicitis, *Br. J. Surg.*, 58, 595, 1971.
12. Burkitt, D. P., Epidemiology of cancer of the colon and rectum, *Cancer*, 28, 3, 1971.
13. Burkitt, D. P., Varicose veins, deep vein thrombosis and haemorrhoids: epidemiology and suggested aetiology, *Br. Med. J.*, 2, 556, 1972.
14. Burkitt, D. P., Walker, A. R. P., and Painter, N. S., Effect of dietary fibre on stools and transit times, and its role in the causation of disease, *Lancet*, ii, 1408, 1972.
15. Painter, N. S., Diverticular disease of the colon, *Br. Med. J.*, ii, 475, 1968.
16. Painter, N. S., Diverticular disease of the colon: a disease of this century, *Lancet*, 2, 586, 1969.
17. Painter, N. S., Almeida, A. L., and Colebourne, K. W., Unprocessed bran in the treatment of diverticular disease of the colon, *Br. Med. J.*, 2, 137, 1972.
18. Cummings, J. H., Southgate, D. A. T., Branch, W., Houston, H., Jenkins, D. J. A., and James, W. P. T., Colonic response to dietary fibre from carrot, cabbage, apple, bran and guar gum, *Lancet*, i, 5, 1978.
19. Stephen, A. M. and Cummings, J. H., Water holding by dietary fibre in vitro and its relationship to faecal output in man, *Gut*, 20, 722, 1979.
20. Eastwood, M. A., Brydon, W. G., and Tadesse, K., Effect of fiber on colonic function, in *Medical Aspects of Dietary Fiber*, Spiller, G. A. and Kay, R. M., Eds., Plenum Press, New York, 1980, 1.
21. Robertson, J. A. and Eastwood, M. A., An examination of factors which may affect the water holding capacity of dietary fibre, *Br. J. Nutr.*, 45, 83, 1981.
22. Robertson, J. A. and Eastwood, M. A., A method to measure the water-holding properties of dietary fibre using suction pressure, *Br. J. Nutr.*, 46, 247, 1981.
23. Robertson, J. A. and Eastwood, M. A., An investigation of the experimental conditions which could affect water-holding capacity of dietary fibre, *J. Sci. Food Agric.*, 32, 819, 1981.
24. Eastwood, M. A., Robertson, J. A., Brydon, W. G., and MacDonald, D., Measurement of water-holding properties of fibre and their faecal bulking ability in man, *Br. J. Nutr.*, 50, 539, 1983.
25. Stephen, A. M. and Cummings, J. H., Mechanisms of action of dietary fibre in the human colon, *Nature (London)*, 284, 283, 1980.
26. Cummings, J. H., Dietary fibre, *Br. Med. Bull.*, 37, 65, 1981.
27. Cummings, J. H., Polysaccharide fermentation in the human colon, in *Colon and Nutrition*, Kasper, H. and Goebell, Eds., MTP Press, Lancaster, 1982, 91.
28. Southgate, D. A. T. and Durnin, J. V. G. A., Calorie conversion factors. An experimental measurement of the factors used in the calculation of the energy value of human diets, *Br. J. Nutr.*, 24, 517, 1970.
29. Williams, R. D. and Olmsted, W. H., The manner in which food controls the bulk of the feces, *Ann. Intern. Med.*, 10, 717, 1936.
30. Cummings, J. H., Short chain fatty acids in the human colon, *Gut*, 22, 763, 1981.
31. Stephen, A. M. and Cummings, J. H., The microbial contribution to human faecal mass, *J. Med. Microbiol.*, 13, 45, 1980.
32. Stephen, A. M., Dietary Fibre and Human Colonic Function, Ph.D. thesis, University of Cambridge, Cambridge, U.K., 1980.

33. Mason, V. C., Some observations on the distribution and origin of nitrogen in sheep faeces, *J. Agric. Sci. Camb.*, 73, 99, 1969.
34. Mason, V. C. and Palmer, R., The influence of bacterial activity in the alimentary canal of rats on faecal nitrogen excretion, *Acta Agric. Scand.*, 23, 141, 1973.
35. Bastedo, W. A., Food and bulk producing drugs in constipation, *Rev. Gastroenterol. N.Y.*, 2, 279, 1935.
36. Stein, D. and Gelehrter, J., Effects of hydrogels on the configuration and function of the colon, *Rev. Gastroenterol. N.Y.*, 7, 39, 1940.
37. Fantus, B., Kopstein, G., and Schmidt, H. R., Roentgen study of intestinal motility as influenced by bran, *JAMA*, 114, 404, 1940.
38. Fantus, B., Wozasek, O., and Steigmann, F., Studies on colonic irritation. Examination of feces, *Am. J. Dig. Dis.*, 8, 296, 1941.
39. Fantus, B., Wozasek, O., and Steigmann, F., Studies on colonic irritation. Effect of bran, *Am. J. Dig. Dis.*, 8, 298, 1941.
40. Fantus, B. and Frankl, W., The mode of action of bran. I. Effect of bran upon composition of stools, *J. Lab. Clin. Med.*, 26, 1774, 1941.
41. Fantus, B. and Frank, W., The mode of action of bran. II. Influence of size and shape of bran particles and of crude fiber isolated from bran. A preliminary report, *Rev. Gastroenterol.*, 8, 277, 1941.
42. Werch, S. C. and Ivy, A. C., On the fate of ingested pectin, *Am. J. Dig. Dis.*, 8, 101, 1941.
43. Wozasek, O. and Steigmann, F., Studies on colon irritation. III. Bulk of feces, *Am. J. Dig. Dis.*, 9, 423, 1942.
44. Streicher, M. H. and Quirk, L., Constipation: clinical and roentgenologic evaluation of the use of bran, *Am. J. Dig. Dis.*, 10, 179, 1943.
45. Machle, W., Heyroth, F. F., and Witherup, S., The fate of methyl-cellulose in the human digestive tract, *J. Biol. Chem.*, 153, 551, 1944.
46. Streicher, M. H. and Quirk, L., Constipation: further clinical evidence of the use of bran as a dietary laxative agent, *Am. J. Dig. Dis.*, 11, 259, 1944.
47. Hoppert, C. A. and Clark, A. J., Digestibility and effect on laxatives of crude fibre and cellulose in certain common foods, *J. Am. Dietet. Assoc.*, 21, 157, 1945.
48. Blake, A. D., Clinical evaluation of a new laxative, *Am. J. Dig. Dis.*, 15, 336, 1948.
49. Schweis, K., The use of methylcellulose as a bulk laxative, *N.Y. State J. Med.*, 48, 1822, 1948.
50. Schultz, J., Carboxymethylcellulose as a colloid laxative, *Am. J. Dig. Dis.*, 16, 319, 1949.
51. Bargen, J. A., A method of improving function of the bowel: the use of methylcellulose, *Gastroenterology*, 13, 275, 1949.
52. Cass, L. J. and Wolf, L. P., A clinical evaluation of certain bulk and irritant laxatives, *Gastroenterology*, 20, 149, 1952.
53. Olmsted, W. H., Duden, C. W., Whitaker, W. M., and Parker, R. F., A method for the rapid distillation of the lower volatile fatty acids from stools, *J. Biol. Chem.*, 85, 115, 1929–1930.
54. Olmsted, W. H., Curtis, G., and Timm, O. K., Cause of laxative effect of feeding bran pentosan and cellulose to man, *Proc. Soc. Exp. Biol. Med.*, 32, 141, 1934.
55. Olmsted, W. H., Curtis, G., and Timm, O. K., Stool VFA. IV. The influence of feeding bran, pentosan, and fiber to man, *J. Biol. Chem.*, 108, 645, 1935.
56. Williams, R. D. and Olmsted, W. H., A biochemical method for determining indigestible residue (crude fiber) in faeces. Lignin, cellulose and non-water soluble hemicellulose, *J. Biol. Chem.*, 108, 653, 1935.
57. Olmsted, W. H., Williams, R. D., and Bauerlein, T., Constipation: the laxative value of bulky foods, *Med. Clin. N. Am.*, 20, 449, 1936.
58. Cowgill, G. R. and Anderson, W. E., Laxative effects of wheat bran and washed bran in healthy men. A comparative study, *JAMA.* 98, 1866, 1932.
59. Cowgill, G. R. and Sullivan, A. J., Further studies on the use of wheat bran as a laxative, *JAMA*, 100, 795, 1933.
60. Tainter, M. L., Methyl cellulose as a colloid laxative, *Proc. Soc. Exp. Biol. Med.*, 54, 77, 1943.
61. Berberian, D. A., Pauly, R. J., and Tainter, M. L., Comparison of a plain methyl cellulose with a compound bulk laxative tablet, *Gastroenterology*, 20, 143, 1952.
62. Cummings, J. H., Cellulose and the human gut, *Gut*, 25, 805, 1984.
63. Analytical Methods Committee, Determination of the crude fibre in national flour, *Analyst*, 68, 276, 1943.

64. AOAC, Official Methods of Analysis of the Association of Official Analytical Chemists, 11th ed., Horwitz, W., Ed., AOAC, Washington, D.C., 1970, 129.

65. Southgate, D. A. T., Determination of carbohydrates in foods. II, Unavailable carbohydrates, *J. Sci. Food Agric.*, 20, 331, 1969.

66. Southgate, D. A. T., The analysis of dietary fibre, in Fiber in *Human Nutrition*, Spiller, G. A. and Amen, R. J., Eds., Plenum Press, New York, 1976, 73.

67. Southgate, D. A. T., Determination of Food Carbohydrates, Applied Science, London, 1976.

68. Southgate, D. A. T., Bailey, B., Collinson, E., and Walker, A. F., A guide to calculating intakes of dietary fibre, *J. Hum. Nutr.*, 30, 303, 1976.

69. Southgate, D. A. T., Bailey, B., Collinson, E., and Walker, A. F., Dietary fiber analysis tables, *Am. J. Clin. Nutr.*, 31, S281, 1978.

70. Southgate, D. A. T., Use of the Southgate method for unavailable carbohydrates in the measurement of dietary fiber, in *The Analysis of Dietary Fiber in Food*, James, W. P. T. and Theander, O., Eds., Marcel Dekker, New York, 1981, 1.

71. Paul, A. A. and Southgate, D. A. T., *McCance and Widdowson's The Composition of Foods*, Her Majesty's Stationery Office, London, 1978.

72. Van Soest, P. J., Use of detergents in the analysis of fibrous feeds. II. A rapid method for the determination of fiber and lignin, *J. Assoc. Off. Agric. Chem.*, 46, 829, 1963.

73. Van Soest, P. J., Non-nutritive residues. A system for the replacement of crude fibre, *J. Assoc. Off. Agric. Chem.*, 49, 546, 1966.

74. Van Soest, P. J., Development of comprehensive system of feed analyses and its application to forages, *J. Anim. Sci.*, 26, 119, 1967.

75. Van Soest, P. J. and Wine, R. H., Use of detergents in the analysis of fibrous feeds. IV. Determination of plant cell wall constituents, *J. Assoc. Off. Agric. Chem.*, 50, 50, 1967.

76. Goering, H. K. and Van Soest, P. J., Forage Fiber Analysis: Apparatus, Reagents, Procedures and some Applications, Agriculture Handbook No. 379, Agriculture Research Service, U.S. Department of Agriculture, Washington, D.C., 1970, 1.

77. Crampton, E. W. and Maynard, L. A., The relation of cellulose and lignin content to the nutritive value of animal feeds, *J. Nutr.*, 15, 383, 1938.

78. O'Shea, J., Ribiero, M. A. do V., and Moran, M. A., Relationships between digestibility (in vitro), crude fibre and cellulose content of some animal feeds, *Ir. J. Agric. Res.*, 7, 173, 1968.

79. McCance, R. A., Widdowson, E. M., and Shackleton, L. R. B., *The Nutritive Value of Fruits, Vegetables and Nuts*, His Majesty's Stationery office, London, 1936.

80. Katan, M. B. and von de Bovenkamp, P., Determination of total dietary fiber by difference and of pectin by calorimetry or copper titration, in *Analysis of Dietary Fiber in Human Foods*, James, W. P. T. and Theander, O., Eds., Marcel Dekker, New York, 1981.

81. Englyst, H., Wiggins, H. S., and Cummings, J. H., Determination of the non-starch polysaccharides in plant foods by gas-liquid chromatography of constituent sugars as alditol acetates, *Analyst*, 107, 307, 1982.

82. Englyst, H. N. and Cummings, J. H., Simplified method for measurement of total non-starch polysaccharides by gas-liquid chromatography of constituent sugars as alditol acetates, *Analyst*, 109, 937, 1984.

83. Schweitzer, T. F. and Wursch, P., Analysis of dietary fiber, in *Analysis of Dietary Fiber in Foods*, James, W. P. T. and Theander, O., Eds., Marcel Dekker, New York, 1981, 203.

84. Schweitzer, T. F. and Wursch, P., Analysis of dietary fibre, *J. Sci. Food Agric.*, 30, 613, 1979.

85. Angus, R., Sutherland, T. M., and Farrell, D. J., A simplified method for determining fibre in foods, *Proc. Nutr. Soc. Aust.*, 2, 90, 1977.

86. Trowell, H., Crude fibre, dietary fibre and atherosclerosis, *Atherosclerosis*, 16, 138, 1972.

87. Trowell, H., Southgate, D. A. T., Wolever, T. M. S., Leeds, A. R., Gassull, M. A., and Jenkins, D. J. A., Dietary fibre redefined, *Lancet*, i, 967, 1976.

88. Hinton, J. M., Lennard-Jones, J, E., and Young, A. C., A new method of studying gut transit times using radio-opaque markers, *Gut*, 10, 842, 1969.

89. Cummings, J. H. and Wiggins, H. S., Transit through the gut measured by analysis of a single stool, *Gut*, 17, 219, 1975.

90. Cummings, J. H., Jenkins, D. J. A., and Wiggins, H. S., Measurement of the mean transit time of dietary residue through the human gut, *Gut*, 17, 210, 1976.

91. Mulinos, M. G., The value of elective drugs in the treatment of constipation, *Rev. Gastroenterol.*, 2, 292, 1935.

92. Davignon, J., Simmonds, W. S., and Ahrens, E. H., Usefulness of chromic oxide as an internal standard for balance studies in formula-fed patients and for assessment of colonic function, *J. Clin. Invest.*, 47, 127, 1968.

93. Sharpe, S. J. and Robinson, M. F., Intermittent and continuous faecal markers in short-term metabolic balance studies in young women, *Br. J. Nutr.*, 24, 489, 1970.

94. Hansky, J. and Connell, A. M., Measurement of gastrointestinal transit using radioactive chromium, *Gut*, 3, 187, 1962.

95. McCance, R. A. and Widdowson, E. M., Mineral metabolism on dephytenized bread, *J. Physiol.*, 101, 304, 1942.

96. Eastwood, M. A., Kirkpatrick, J. R., Mitchell, W. D., Bone, A., and Hamilton, T., Effects of dietary supplements of wheat bran and cellulose on faeces and bowel function, *Br. Med. J.*, iv, 392, 1973.

97. Connell, A. M. and Smith, C. L., The effect of dietary fibre on transit time, in *Proc. 4th Int. Symp. GI Motility*, Mitchell Press, Vancouver, Canada, 1974, 365.

98. Findlay, J. M., Mitchell, W. D., Smith, A. N., Anderson, A. J. B., and Eastwood , M. A., Effects of unprocessed bran on colon function in normal subjects and in diverticular disease, *Lancet*, i, 146, 1974.

99. Cummings, J. H., Hill, M. J., Jenkins, D. J. A., Pearson, J. R., and Wiggins, H. S., Changes in fecal composition and colonic function due to cereal fiber, *Am. J. Clin. Nutr.*, 29, 1468, 1976.

100. Jenkins, D. J. A., Hill, M. J., and Cummings, J. H., Effect of wheat fiber on blood lipids, fecal steroid excretion and serum iron, *Am. J. Clin. Nutr.*, 28, 1408, 1975.

101. Fuchs, H.–M., Dorfman, S., and Floch, M. H., The effect of dietary fiber supplementation in man. II. Alteration in fecal physiology and bacterial flora, *Am. J. Clin. Nutr.*, 29, 1443, 1976.

102. Kahaner, N., Fuchs, H., and Floch, M. H., The effect of dietary fiber supplementation in man. I. Modification of eating habits, *Am. J. Clin. Nutr.*, 29, 1437, 1976.

103. Floch, M. H. and Fuchs, H.-M., Effect of dietary fiber supplementation in man, *Am. J. Clin. Nutr.*, 30, 833, 1977.

104. Floch, M. H. and Fuchs, H.-M., Modifications of stool content by increased bran intake, *Am. J. Clin. Nutr.*, 31, S185, 1978.

105. Reinhold, J. G., Faradji, B., Abadi, P., and Ismail-Beigi, F., Decreased absorption of calcium, magnesium, zinc and phosphorus by humans due to increased fiber and phosphorus consumption as wheat bread, *J. Nutr.*, 106, 493, 1976.

106. Wyman, J. B., Heaton, K. W., Manning, A. P., and Wicks, A. C. B., The effect of intestinal transit and the feces of raw and cooked bran in different doses, *Am. J. Clin. Nutr.*, 29, 1474, 1976.

107. Walters, R. L., Baird, I. M., Davies, P. S., Hill, M. J., Drasar, B. S., Southgate, D. A. T., Green, J., and Morgan, B., Effects of two types of dietary fibre on faecal steroid and lipid excretion, *Br. Med. J.*, 2, 536, 1975.

108. Southgate, D. A. T., Branch, W. J., Hill, M. J., Drasar, B. S., Walters, R. L., Davies, P. S., and Baird, I. M., Metabolic responses to dietary supplements of bran, *Metabolism*, 25, 1129, 1976.

109. Baird, I. M., Walters, R. L., Davies, P. S., Hill, M. J., Drasar, B. S., and Southgate, D. A. T., The effects of two dietary fiber supplements on gastrointestinal transit, stool weight and frequency, and bacterial flora, and fecal bile acids in normal subjects, *Metabolism*, 26, 117, 1977.

110. Kay, R. M. and Truswell, A. S., The effect of wheat fibre on plasma lipids and faecal steroid excretion in man, *Br. J. Nutr.*, 37, 227, 1977.

111. Farrell, D. J., Girle, L., and Arthur, J., Effects of dietary fibre on the apparent digestibility of major food components and on blood lipids in men, *Aust. J. Exp. Biol. Med. Sci.*, 56, 469, 1978.

112. Mathur, M. S., Ram, H., and Chadda, V. S., Effect of bran on intestinal transit time in normal Indians and in intestinal amoebiasis, *Am. J. Proct. Gastroent. Colon Rect. Surg.*, 29, 30, 1978.

113. Cummings, J. H., Hill, M. J., Jivraj, T., Houston, H., Branch, W. J., and Jenkins, D. J. A., The effect of meat protein and dietary fiber on colonic function and metabolism. I. Changes in bowel habit, bile acid excretion and calcium absorption, *Am. J. Clin. Nutr.*, 32, 2086, 1979.

114. Munoz, J. M., Sandstead, H. H., Jacob, R. A., Logan, G. M., Reck, S. J., Klevay, L. M., Dintzis, F. R., Inglett, G. E., and Shuey, W. C., Effects of some cereal brans and textured vegetable protein on plasma lipids, *Am. J. Clin. Nutr.*, 32, 580, 1979.

115. Bell, E. W., Emken, E. A., Klevay, L. M., and Sandstead, H. H., Effects of dietary fiber from wheat, corn and soy hull bran on excretion of fecal bile acids in humans, *Am. J. Clin. Nutr.*, 34, 1071, 1981.

116. Sandstead, H. H., Munoz, J. M., Jacob, R. A., Klevay, L. M., Reek, S. J., Logan, G. M., Dintzis, F. R., Inglett, G. E. , and Shuey, W. C., Influence of dietary fiber on trace element balance, *Am. J. Clin. Nutr.*, 31, S180, 1978.

117. Sandstead, H. H., Klevay, L. M., Jacob, R. A., Munoz, J. M., Logan, G. M., Reck, S. J., Dintzis, F. R., Inglett, G. E., and Shuey, W. C., Effects of dietary fiber and protein level on mineral element metabolism, in *Dietary Fibers: Chemistry and Nutrition*, Inglett, G. E. and Falkehag, S. I., Eds., Academic Press, New York, 1979, 147.

118. Sandstead, H., Klevay, L., Jacob, R., Munoz, J., Johnson, L., Dintzis, F., and Inglett, G., Mineral requirements: influence of fiber and protein, *Am. J. Clin. Nutr.*, 32, 933, 1979.

119. Munoz, J. M., Sandstead, H. H., Jacob, R. A., Logan, G. M., Jr., and Kelvay, L. M., Effects of dietary fiber on plasma lipids of normal men, *Am. J. Clin. Nutr.*, 31, 696, 1978.

120. Munoz, J. M., Sandstead, H. H., and Jacob, R. A., Effect of dietary fiber on glucose tolerance of normal men, *Diabetes*, 28, 496, 1979.

121. Spiller, G. A., Wong, L. G., Whittam, J. H., and Scala, J., Correlation of gastrointestinal transit time to fecal weight in adult humans and the levels of fiber intake, *Nutr. Rep. Int.*, 25, 23, 1982.

122. Huijbregts, A. W. M., van Berge-Henegouwen, G. P., Hectors, M. P. C., von Schaik, A., and van der Werf, S. D. J., Effects of a standard wheat bran preparation on biliary lipid composition and bile acid metabolism in young healthy males, *Eur. J. Clin. Invest.*, 10, 451, 1980.

123. Smith, R. G., Rowe, M. J., Smith, A. N., Eastwood, M. A., Drummond, E., and Brydon, W. G., A study of bulking agents in elderly patients, *Age Aging*, 9, 267, 1980.

124. Stasse-Wolthuis, M., Albers, H. F. F., van Jeveren, J. C. C., Wil de Jong, J., Hautvast, J. G. A. J., Hermus, R. J. J., Katan, M. B., Brydon, W. G., and Eastwood, M. A., Influence of dietary fiber from vegetables and fruits, bran or citrus pectin on serum lipids, fecal lipids, and colonic function, *Am. J. Clin. Nutr.*, 33, 1745, 1980.

125. Stasse-Wolthuis, M., Katan, M. B., Hermus, R. J. J., and Hautvast, J. G. A. J., Increase of serum cholesterol in man fed a bran diet, *Atherosclerosis*, 34, 87, 1979.

126. Stasse-Wolthuis, M., Effect of a natural high fibre diet on blood lipids and intestinal transit in man, *Qual. Plant.*, 29, 31, 1979.

127. Yu, M. H. M. and Miller, L. T., Influence of cooked wheat bran on bowel function and fecal excretion of nutrients, *J. Food Sci.*, 216, 720, 1981.

128. Van Dokkum, W., Wesstra, A., and Schippers, F. A., Physiological effects of fibre-rich types of bread. I. The effect of dietary fibre from bread on the mineral balance of young men, *Br. J. Nutr.*, 47, 451, 1982.

129. Van Dokkum, W., Pikaar, N. A., and Thissen, J. T. N. M., Physiological effects of fibre-rich types of bread. II. Dietary fibre from bread: digestibility by the intestinal microflora and water-holding capacity in the colon of human subjects, *Br. J. Nutr.*, 50, 61, 1983.

130. Graham, D., Moser, S. E., and Estes, M. K., The effect of bran on bowel function in constipation, *Am. J. Gastroenterol.*, 77, 599, 1982.

131. Andersson, H., Navert, B., Bingham, S. A., Englyst, H. N., and Cummings, J. H., The effects of breads containing similar amounts of phytate but different amounts of wheat bran on calcium, zinc and iron balance in man, *Br. J. Nutr.*, 50, 503, 1983.

132. Cummings, J. H., Stephen, A. M., Wayman, B., Englyst, H. N., and Wiggins, H. S., The effect of age, sex and level of intake on the colonic response in man to wholemeal bread with added wheat bran, *Br. J. Nutr.*, 56, 349, 1986.

133. Drasar, B. S. and Jenkins, D. J. A., Bacteria, diet and large bowel cancer, *Am. J. Clin. Nutr.*, 29, 1410, 1976.

134. Durrington, P. N., Manning, A. P., Bolton, C. H., and Hartog, M., Effect of pectin on serum lipids and lipoproteins, whole-gut transit-time, and stool weight, *Lancet*, 2, 394, 1976.

135. Kay, R. M. and Truswell, A. S., Effect of citrus pectin on blood lipids and fecal steroid excretion in man, *Am. J. Clin. Nutr.*, 30, 171, 1977.

136. Miettinen, T. A. and Tarpila, S., Effect of pectin on serum cholesterol, fecal bile acids and biliary lipids in normolipidemic and hyperlipidemic individuals, *Clin. Chim. Acta*, 79, 471, 1977.

137. Cummings, J. H., Southgate, D. A. T., Branch, W. J., Wiggins, H. S., Houston, H., Jenkins, D. J. A., Jivraj, T., and Hill, M. J., The digestion of pectin in the human gut and its effect on calcium absorption and large bowel function, *Br. J. Nutr.*, 41, 477, 1979.

138. Spiller, G. A., Chernoff, M. C., Hill, R. A., Gates, J. E., Nassar, J. J., and Shipley, E. A., Effect of purified cellulose, pectin, and a low-residue diet on fecal volatile fatty acids, transit time, and fecal weight in humans, *Am. J. Clin. Nutr.*, 33, 754, 1980.

139. Ross, J. K. and Leklem, J. E., The effect of dietary citrus pectin on the excretion of human fecal neutral and acid steroids and the activity of 7 α–dehydroxylase and β–glucuronidase, *Am. J. Clin. Nutr.*, 34, 2068, 1981.

140. Judd, P. A. and Truswell, A. S., Comparison of the effects of high- and low-methoxyl pectins on blood and faecal lipids in man, *Br. J. Nutr.*, 48, 451, 1982.

141. Fleming, S. E., Marthinsen, D., and Kuhnlein, H., Colonic function and fermentation in men consuming high fiber diets, *J. Nutr.*, 113, 2535, 1983.

142. Marthinsen, D. and Fleming, S. E., Excretion of breath and flatus gases by humans consuming high fiber diets, *J. Nutr.*, 112, 1133, 1982.

143. Fleming, S. E. and Rodriguez, M. A., Influence of dietary fiber on fecal excretion of volatile fatty acids by human adults, *J. Nutr.*, 113, 1613, 1983.

144. Hillman, L., Peters, S., Fisher, A., and Pomare, E. W., Differing effects of pectin, cellulose and lignin on stool pH, transit time and weight, *Br, J. Nutr.*, 50, 189, 1983.

145. Marks, M. M., Cellulose esters in the treatment of constipation, *Am. J. Dig. Dis.*, 16, 215, 1949.

146. Ismail-Beigi, F., Reinhold, J. G., Faraji, B., and Abadi, P., Effects of cellulose added to diets of low and high fiber content upon the metabolism of calcium, magnesium, zinc and phosphorus by man, *J. Nutr.*, 107, 510, 1977.

147. Slavin, J. L. and Marlett, J. A., Influence of refined cellulose on human bowel function and calcium and magnesium balances, *Am. J. Clin. Nutr.*, 33, 1932, 1980.

148. Slavin, J. C. and Marlett, J. A., Effect of refined cellulose on apparent energy, fat and nitrogen digestibilities, *J. Nutr.*, 110, 2020, 1980.

149. Wrick, K. L., Robertson, J. B., Van Soest, P. J., Lewis, B. A., Rivers, J. M., Roe, D. A., and Hackler, L. R., The influence of dietary fiber source on human intestinal transit and stool output, *J. Nutr.*, 113, 1464, 1983.

150. Van Soest, P. J., Robertson, J. B., Roe, D. A., Rivers, J., Lewis, B. A., and Hackler, L. R., The role of dietary fiber in human nutrition, in *Proc. Cornell Nutrition Conference for Feed Manufacturers*, Canada, 1978, 5.

151. Ehle, F. R., Robertson, J. B., and Van Soest, P. J., Influence of dietary fibers on fermentation in the human large intestine, *J. Nutr.*, 112, 158, 1982.

152. Heller, S. N., Hackler, L. R., Rivers, J. M., Van Soest, P. J., Roe, D. A., Lewis, B. A., and Robertson, J., Dietary fiber: the effect of particle size of wheat bran on colonic function in young adult men, *Am. J. Clin. Nutr.*, 33, 1734, 1980.

153. Van Soest, P. J., Some factors influencing the ecology of gut fermentation in man, in *Banbury Report No. 7: Gastrointestinal Cancer: Endogenous Factors*, Bruce, W. R., Correa, P., Lipkin, M., Tannenbaum, S. R., and Wilkins, T. D., Eds., Cold Spring Harbor Laboratory, Cold Spring Harbor, N.Y., 1981, 61.

154. Van Soest, P. J., Some physical characteristics of dietary fibre and their influence on the microbial ecology of the human colon, *Proc. Nutr. Soc.*, 43, 25, 1984.

155. Van Soest, P. J., Horrath, P. J., McBurney, M. I., and Allen, M. S., *Unconventional Sources of Dietary Fiber, Symposium Series 214*, Furda, I., Ed., American Chemical Society, Washington, D.C., 1983, 135.

156. Van Soest, P. J., Uden, P., and Wrick, K. L., Critique and evaluation of markers for use in humans and farm and laboratory animals, *Nutr. Rep. Int.*, 27, 17, 1983.

157. Block, L. H., Management of constipation with a refined psyllium combined with dextrose, *Am. J. Dig. Dis.*, 14, 64, 1947.

158. Prynne, C. J. and Southgate, D. A. T., The effects of a supplement of dietary fibre on faecal excretion by human subjects, *Br. J. Nutr.*, 41, 495, 1979.

159. Spiller, G. A., Shipley, E. A., Chernoff, M. C., and Cooper, W. C., Bulk laxative efficacy of a psyllium seed hydrocolloid and of a mixture of cellulose and pectin, *J. Clin. Pharmacol.*, 19, 313, 1979.

160. Eastwood, M. A., Brydon, W. G., and Anderson, D. M. W., The effects of dietary gum karaya (sterculia) in man, *Toxicol. Lett.*, 17, 159, 1983.

161. Ross, A. H., McLean, Eastwood, M. A., Brydon, W. G., Anderson, J. R., and Anderson, D. M. W., A study of the effects of dietary gum arabic in humans, *Am. J. Clin. Nutr.*, 37, 268, 1983.

162. Calloway, D. H. and Kretsch, M. J., Protein and energy utilization in men given a rural Guatemalan diet and egg formulas with and without added oat bran, *Am. J. Clin. Nutr.*, 31, 1118, 1978.

163. Kretsch, M. J., Crawford, L., and Calloway, D. H., Some aspects of bile acid and urobilinogen excretion and fecal elimination in men given a rural Guatemalan diet and egg formulas with and without added oat bran, *Am. J. Clin. Nutr.*, 32, 1492, 1979.

164. Judd, P. A. and Truswell, A. S., The effect of rolled oats on blood lipids and fecal steroid excretion in man, *Am. J. Clin. Nutr.*, 34, 2061, 1982.

165. Kirby, R. W., Anderson, J. W., Sieling, B., Rees, E. D., Lin Chen, W.-J., Miller, R. E., and Kay, R. M., Oat-bran intake selectively lowers serum low-density lipoprotein cholesterol concentrations of hyper-cholesterolemic men, *Am. J. Clin. Nutr.*, 34, 824, 1981.

166. Schweizer, T. F., Bekhechi, A. R., Koellreutter, B., Reimann, S., Pometta, D., and Bron, B. A., Metabolic effects of dietary fiber from dehulled soybeans in humans, *Am. J. Clin. Nutr.*, 38, 1, 1983.

167. Tsai, A. C., Mott, E. L., Owen, G. M., Bennick, M. R., Lo, G. S., and Steinke, F. H., Effects of soy polysaccharide on gastrointestinal functions, nutrient balance, steroid excretions, glucose tolerance, serum lipids, and other parameters in humans, *Am. J. Clin. Nutr.*, 38, 504, 1983.

168. McCance, R. A. and Widdowson, E. M., Mineral metabolism of healthy adults on white and brown bread dietaries, *J. Physiol.*, 101, 44, 1942.

169. Antonis, A. and Bersohn, I., The influence of diet on serum lipids in South African white and Bantu prisoners, *Am. J. Clin. Nutr.*, 10, 485, 1962.

170. Antonis, A. and Bersohn, I., The influence of diet on fecal lipids in South African white and Bantu prisoners, *Am. J. Clin. Nutr.*, 11, 143, 1962.

171. Flynn, J. F., Beirn, S. F. O., and Burkitt, D. P., The potato as a source of fiber in the diet, *Ir. J. Med. Sci.*, 146, 285, 1977.

172. Beyer, P. L. and Flynn, M. A., Effects of high- and low-fiber diets on human feces, *J. Am. Dietet. Assoc.*, 72, 271, 1978.

173. Robertson, J., Brydon, W. G., Tadesse, K., Wenham, P., Walls, A., and Eastwood, M. A., The effect of raw carrot on serum lipids and colon function, *Am. J. Clin. Nutr.*, 32, 1889, 1979.

174. Stasse-Wolthuis, M., Hautvast, J. G. A. J., Hermus, R. J. J., Katan, M. B., Bausch, E., Rietberg-Brussard, J. H., Velema, J. P., Zondervan, J. H., Eastwood, M. A., and Brydon, W. G., The effect of a natural high-fiber diet on serum lipids, fecal lipids, and colonic function, *Am. J. Clin. Nutr.*, 32, 1881, 1979.

175. Kelsay, J. L., Behall, K. M., and Prather, E. S., Effect of fiber from fruits and vegetables on metabolic responses of human subjects. I. Bowel transit time, number of defecations, fecal weight, urinary excretions of energy and nitrogen and apparent digestibilities of energy, nitrogen and fat, *Am. J. Clin. Nutr.*, 31, 1149, 1978.

176. Kelsay, J. L., Behall, K. M., and Prather, E. S., Effect of fiber from fruits and vegetables on metabolic responses of human subjects. II. Calcium, magnesium, iron and silicon balances, *Am. J. Clin. Nutr.*, 32, 1876, 1979.

177. Kelsay, J. L., Jacob, R. A., and Prather, E. S., Effect of fiber from fruits and vegetables on metabolic responses of human subjects. III. Zinc, copper and phosphorus balances, *Am. J. Clin. Nutr.*, 32, 2307, 1979.

178. Kelsay, J. L., Goering, H. K., Behall, K. M., and Prather, E. S., Effect of fiber from fruit and vegetables on metabolic responses of human subjects: fiber intakes, fecal excretions and apparent digestibilities, *Am. J. Clin. Nutr.*, 34, 1849, 1981.

179. Kelsay, J. L., Clark, W. M., Herbst, B. J., and Prather, E. S., Nutrient utilization by human subjects consuming fruits and vegetables as sources of fiber, *J. Agric. Food Chem.*, 29, 461, 1981.

180. Leeds, A. R., Khumalo, T. D., Ndaba, G., and Lincoln, D., Haricot beans, transit time and stool weight, *J. Plant Foods*, 4, 33, 1982.

181. Raymond, T. L., Connor, W. E., Lin, D. S., Warner, S., Fry, M. M., and Connor, S. L., The interaction of dietary fibers and cholesterol upon the plasma lipids and lipoproteins, sterol balance, and bowel function in human subjects, *J. Clin. Invest.*, 60, 1429, 1977.

182. Macrae, T. F., Hutchinson, J. C. D., Irwin, J. O., Bacon, J. S. D., and McDougall, E. I., Comparative digestibility of wholemeal and white breads and the effect of the degree of fineness and grinding on the former, *J. Hyg. Camb.*, 42, 423, 1942.

183. Brodribb, A. J. M. and Groves, C., Effect of bran particle size on stool weight, *Gut*, 19, 60, 1978.

184. Smith, A. N., Drummond, E., and Eastwood, M. A., The effect of coarse and fine Canadian Red Spring Wheat and French Soft Wheat bran on colonic motility in patients with diverticular disease, *Am. J. Clin. Nutr.*, 34, 2460, 1981.

185. Parks, T. G., The effect of low and high residue diet on the rate of transit and composition of the feces, in *Proc. 4th Int. Symp. GI Motility*, Mitchell Press, Vancouver, Canada, 1974.

186. Parks, T. G., Diet and diverticular disease, *Proc. R, Soc. Med.*, 67, 1037, 1974.

187. Brodribb, A. J. M. and Humphreys, D. M., Diverticular disease: three studies. I. Relation to other disorders and fibre intake. II. Treatment with bran. III. Metabolic effects of bran in patients with diverticular disease, *Br. Med. J.*, 1, 424, 1976.

188. Taylor, I. and Duthie, H. L., Bran tablets and diverticular disease, *Br. Med. J.*, 1, 988, 1976.

189. Eastwood, M. A., Smith, A. N., Brydon, W. G., and Pritchard, J., Comparison of bran, ispaghula and lactulose on colon function in diverticular disease, *Gut*, 19, 1144, 1978.

190. Tarpila, S., Miettinen, T. A., and Metsaranta, L., Effects of bran on serum cholesterol, faecal mass, fat, bile acids and neutral sterols, and biliary lipids in patients with diverticular disease, *Gut*, 19, 137, 1978.

191. Ornstein, M. H., Littlewood, E. R., Baird, I., McLean, Fowler, J., North, W. R. S., and Cox, A. G., Are fibre supplements really necessary in diverticular disease of the colon? A controlled clinical trial, *Br. Med. J.*, 282, 1353, 1981.

192. Fedail, S. S., Badi, S. E. M., and Musa, A. R. M., The effects of sorghum and wheat bran on the colonic functions of healthy Sudanese subjects, *Am. J. Clin. Nutr.*, 40, 776, 1984.

193. Eastwood, M. A., Elton, R. A., and Smith, J. H., Long term effect of whole meal bread on stool weight, transit time, fecal bile acids, fats, and neutral sterols, *Am. J. Clin. Nutr.*, 43, 343, 1986.

194. Marlett, J. A., Balasubramanian, R., Johnson, E. J., and Draper, N. R., Determining compliance with a dietary fiber supplement, *J. Natl. Cancer Inst.*, 76, 1065, 1986.

195. Mallett, A. K., Rowland, I. R., and Farthing, M. J., Dietary modification of intestinal bacterial enzyme activities—potential formation of toxic agents in the gut, *Scand. J. Gastroenterol.*, 129 (Suppl. 22), 251, 1987.

196. Reddy, B. S., Sharma, C., Simi, B., Engle, A., Laakso, K., Puska, P., and Korpela, R., Metabolic epidemiology of colon cancer: effect of dietary fiber on fecal mutagens and bile acids in healthy subjects, *Cancer Res.*, 47, 644, 1987.

197. Anderson, J. W., Sieling, B., and Chen, W.-J. L., Plant Fiber and Food, University of Kentucky, Lexington, 1980.

198. Wisker, E., Maltz, A., and Feldheim, W., Metabolizable energy of diets low or high in dietary fiber from cereals when eaten by humans, *J. Nutr.*, 118, 945, 1988.

199. Mergenthaler, E. and Scherz, H., Beitrage zur Analytik von als Lebensmittelzusatzstoffen verwendeten Polysacchariden, *Z. Lebens. Unter. Forsch.*, 162, 25, 1976.

200. Meuser, F., Suckow, P., and Kulikowski, W., Verfahren zur Bestimmung von unloslichen und loslichen Ballaststoffen in Lebensmittein, *Z. Lebens. Unters. Forsch.*, 181, 101, 1985.

201. Spiller, G. A., Story, J. A., Wong, L. G., Nunes, J. D., Alton, M., Petro, M. S., Furumoto, E. J., Whittam, J. H., and Scala, J., Effect of increasing levels of hard wheat fiber on fecal weight, minerals and steroids and gastrointestinal transit time in healthy young women, *J. Nutr.*, 116, 778, 1986.

202. Prosky, L., Asp, N.-G., Furda, I., Devries, J. W., Schweizer, T. F., and Harland, B. F., Vitamins and other nutrients. Determination of total dietary fiber in foods, food products, and total diets: interlaboratory study, *J. Assoc. Off. Anal. Chem.*, 67, 1044, 1984.

203. Prosky, L., Asp, N.-G., Furda, I., Devries, J. W., Schweizer, T. F., and Harland, B. F., Vitamins and other nutrients. Determination of total dietary fiber in foods and food products: collaborative study, *J. Assoc. Off. Anal. Chem.*, 68, 677, 1985.

204. Prosky, L., Asp, N.-G., Schweizer, T. F., Devries, J. W., and Furda, I., Determination of insoluble, soluble and total dietary fiber in foods and food products: interlaboratory study, *J. Assoc. Off. Anal. Chem.*, 71, 1017, 1988.

205. Stevens, J., Van Soest, P. J., Robertson, J. B., and Levitsky, D. A., Comparison of the effects of psyllium and wheat bran on gastrointestinal transit time and stool characteristics, *J. Am. Diet. Assoc.*, 88, 323, 1988.

206. Villaume, C., Bam, H. W., and Mejean, L., Physico-chemical properties of wheat bran and long term physiological effects in healthy man, *Diabete Metab.*, 14, 664, 1988.

207. Melcher, E. A., Levitt, M. D., and Slavin, J. L., Methane production and bowel function parameters in healthy subjects on low and high fiber diets, *Nutr. Cancer*, 16, 85, 1991.

208. Jenkins, D. J. A., Peterson, R. D., Thorne, M. J., et al., Wheat fiber and laxation: dose response and equilibration time, *Am. J. Gastroenterol.*, 82, 1259, 1987.

209. Anderson, J. W., Story, L., Sieling, B., Chen, W.-J. L., Petro, M. S., and Story, J., Hypocholesterolemic effects of oat-bran or bean intake for hypercholesterolemic men, *Am. J. Clin. Nutr.*, 40, 1146, 1984.

210. Miyoshi, H., Okuda, T., Okuda, K., and Koishi, H., Effects of brown rice on apparent digestibility and balance of nutrients in young men on low protein diets, *J. Nutr. Sci. Vitaminol.* (Tokyo), 33, 207, 1987.

211. Miyoshi, H., Okuda, T., Oi, Y., and Koishi, H., Effects of rice fiber on fecal weight, apparent digestibility of energy, nitrogen and fat, and degradation of neutral detergent fiber in young men, *J. Nutr. Sci. Vitaminol.* (Tokyo), 32, 581, 1986.

212. Kaneko, K., Nishida, K., Yatsuda, J., Osa, S., and Koike, G., Effect of fiber on protein, fat and calcium digestibilities and fecal cholesterol excretion, *J. Nutr. Vitaminol.* (Tokyo), 32, 317, 1986.

213. Sugawara, M., Sato, Y., Yokoyama, S., and Mitsuoka, T., Effect of corn fiber residue supplementation on fecal properties, flora, ammonia and bacterial enzyme activities in healthy humans, *J. Nutr. Sci. Vilaminol.* (Tokyo), 37, 109, 1991.

214. Slavin, J. L., Nelson, N. L., McNamara, E. A., et al., Bowel function of healthy men consuming liquid diets with and without dietary fiber, *J. Parent. Entr. Nutr.*, 9, 317, 1985.

215. Slavin, J. L., Marlett, J. A., and Neilson, M. J., Determination and apparent digestibility of neutral detergent fiber monosaccharides in women, *J. Nutr.*, 113, 2353, 1983.

216. Fischer, M., Adkins, W., Hall, L., et al., The effects of dietary fibre in a liquid diet on bowel function of mentally retarded individuals, *J. Ment. Defic. Res.*, 29, 373, 1985.

217. Kurpad, A. V., Holmes, J., and Shetty, P. S., Effect of fibre supplementation and activated charcoal on faecal parameters and transits in the tropics, *Indian J. Gastroenterol.*, 7, 199, 1988.

218. Fleming, S. E., O'Donnell, A. U., and Perman, J. A., Influence of frequent and long-term bean consumption on colonic function and fermentation, *Am. J. Clin. Nutr.*, 41, 909, 1985.

219. Abraham, Z. D. and Mehta, T., Three-week psyllium husk supplementation: effect of plasma cholesterol concentrations, fecal steroid excretion, and carbohydrate absorption in men, *Am. J. Clin. Nutr.*, 47, 67, 1988.

220. Tomlin, J. and Read, N. W., The relation between bacterial degradation of viscous polysaccharides and stool output in human beings, *Br. J. Nutr.*, 60, 467, 1988.

221. Rasmussen, H. S., Holtug, K., Andersen, J. R., Krag, E., and Mortensen, P. B., The influence of ispaghula husk and lactulose on the in vivo and the in vitro production capacity of short-chain fatty acids in humans, *Scand. J. Gastroenterol.*, 22, 406, 1987.

222. Miettinen, T. A. and Tarpila, S., Serum lipids and cholesterol metabolism during guar gum, plantago ovata and high fibre treatments, *Clin. Chem. Acta*, 183, 253, 1989.

223. Hamilton, J. W., Wagner, J., Burdick, M. A., and Bass, P., Clinical evaluation of methylcellulose as a bulk laxative, *Dig. Dis. Sci.*, 33, 993, 1988.

224. Marlett, J. A., Li, B. U. K., Patrow, C. J., and Bass, P., Comparative laxation of psyllium with and without senna in an ambulatory constipated population, *Am. J. Gastroent.*, 82, 333, 1987.

225. Penagini, R., Velio, P., Vigorelli, R., Bozzani, A., Castagnone, D., Ranzi, T., and Bianchi, P. A., The effect of dietary guar on serum cholesterol, intestinal transit, and fecal output in man, *Am. J. Gastroent.*, 81, 123, 1986.

226. Anderson, D. M. W., Eastwood, M. A., and Brydon, W. G., The dietary effects of sodium carboxy-methylcellulose in man, *Food Hydrocolloids*, 1, 37, 1986.

227. Eastwood, M. A., Brydon, W. G., and Anderson, D. M. W., The dietary effects of xanthan gum in man, *Food Add. Contam.*, 4, 17, 1987.

228. Eastwood, M. A., Brydon, W. G., and Anderson, D. M. W., The effects of dietary gum tragacanth in man, *Toxicol. Lett.*, 21, 73, 1984.

229. Tomlin, J. and Read, N. W., A comparative study of the effects on colon function caused by feeding ispaghula husk and polydextrose, *Aliment. Pharmacol. Therap.*, 2, 513, 1988.

230. Allinger, U. G., Johansson, G. K., Gustafsson, J. A., and Rafter, J. J., Shift from a mixed to a lactovegetarian diet: influence on acidic lipids in fecal water—a potential risk factor for colon cancer, *Am. J. Clin. Nutr.*, 50, 992, 1989.

231. Theander, O. and Westerlund, E., Studies on dietary fiber. 3. Improved procedures for analysis of dietary fiber, *J. Agric. Food Chem.*, 34, 330, 1986.

232. Asp, N.-G., Johansson, C.-G., Hallmer, H., and Siljestrom, M., Rapid enzymatic assay of insoluble and soluble dietary fiber, *J. Agric. Food Chem.*, 31, 476, 1983.

233. Kesaniemi, Y. A., Tarpila, S., and Miettinen, T. A., Low vs high dietary fiber and serum, biliary, and fecal lipids in middle aged men, *Am. J. Clin. Nutr.*, 51, 1007, 1990.

234. Tinker, L. F., Schneeman, B. O., Davis, P. A., Gallaher, D. D., and Waggoner, C. R., Consumption of prunes as a source of dietary fiber in men with mild hypercholesterolemia, *Am. J. Clin. Nutr.*, 53, 1259, 1991.

235. Forsum, E., Eriksson, C., Goranzon, H., and Sohostrom, A., Composition of faeces from human subjects consuming diets based on conventional foods containing different kinds and amounts of dietary fibre, *Br. J. Nutr.*, 64, 171, 1990.

236. Ghoos, Y., Rutgeerts, P., Vantrappen, G., Hiele, M., and Schurmans, P., The effect of long-term fibre and starch intake by man on faecal bile acid excretion, *Eur. J. Clin. Invest.*, 18, 128, 1988.

237. Miles, C. W., Kelsay, J. L., and Wong, N. P., Effect of dietary fiber on the metabolizable energy of human diets, *J. Nutr.*, 118, 1075, 1988.

238. Reddy, B. S., Engle, A., Simi, B., O'Brien, L. T., Barnard, R. J., Pritikin, N., and Wynder, E. L., Effect of low fat, high carbohydrate, high fiber diet on fecal bile acids and neutral sterols, *Prev. Med.*, 17, 432, 1998.

239. Mongeau, R. and Brassard, R., A rapid method for the determination of soluble and insoluble dietary fiber: comparison with AOAC total dietary fiber procedure and Englyst's method, *J. Food Sci.*, 51, 1333, 1986.

240. Neilson, M. J. and Marleft, J. A., A comparison between detergent and nondetergent analyses of dietary fiber in human foodstuffs, using high-performance liquid chromatography to measure neutral sugar composition, *J. Agric. Food Chem.*, 31, 1342, 1983.

241. Englyst, H. N. and Hudson, G. J., Colorimetric method for routine measurement of dietary fibre as nonstarch polysaccharides. A comparison with gas-liquid chromatography, *Food Chem.*, 24, 63, 1987.

242. Marlett, J. A., Analysis of dietary fiber, *Animal Feed Sci. Tech.*, 23, 1, 1989.

243. Li, B. W. and Cardozo, M. S., Simplified method for the determination of total dietary fiber and its soluble and insoluble fractions in foods, in *New Developments in Dietary Fiber*, Furda, I. and Brine, C. J., Eds., Plenum Press, New York, 1990, 283.

244. Jeraci, J. L. and Van Soest, P. J., Improved methods for analysis and biological characterization of fiber, in *New Developments in Dietary Fiber*, Furda, I. and Brine, C. J., Eds., Plenum Press, New York, 1990, 245.

245. Lee, S. C. and Hicks, V. A., Modifications of the AOAC total dietary fiber method, in *New Developments in Dietary Fiber*, Furda, I. and Brine, C. J., Eds., Plenum Press, New York, 1990, 237.

246. Johansson, G. K., Ottova, L., and Gustafsson, J. A., Shift from a mixed diet to a lactovegetarian diet: influence on some cancer-associated intestinal bacterial enzyme activities, *Nutr. Cancer*, 14, 239, 1990.

247. Adiotomre, J., Eastwood, M. A., Edwards, C. A., and Brydon, W. G., Dietary fiber: in vitro methods that anticipate nutrition and metabolic activity in humans, *Am. J. Clin. Nutr.*, 52, 128, 1990.

248. Kurpad, A. V. and Shetty, P. S., Effects of antimicrobial therapy on faecal bulking, Gut, 27, 55, 1986.

249. Shetty, P. S. and Kurpad, A. V., Increasing starch intake in the human diet increases fecal bulking, *Am. J. Clin. Nutr.*, 43, 210, 1986.

250. Tomlin, J. and Read, N. W., The effect of resistant starch on colon function in humans, *Br. J. Nutr.*, 64, 589, 1990.

251. Cummings, J. H., Beatty, E. R., Kingman, S., Bingham, S. A., and Englyst, H. N., Laxative properties of resistant starches, *Gastroenterology*, 102, A548, 1992.

252. Flourie, B., Florent, C., Jouany, J. P., Thivend, P., Etanchaud, F., and Rambaud, J. C., Colonic metabolism of wheat starch in healthy humans. Effects on fecal outputs and clinical symptoms, *Gastroenterology*, 90, 111, 1986.

253. Englyst, H. N., Bingham, S. A., Runswick, S. A., Collinson, E., and Cummings, J. H., Dietary fibre (non-starch polysaccharides) in fruit, vegetables and nuts, *J. Hum. Nutr. Dietet.*, 1, 247, 1988.

254. Englyst, H. N., Bingham, S. A., Runswick, S. A., Collinson, E., and Cummings, J. H., Dietary fibre (non-starch polysaccharides) in cereal products, *J. Hum. Nutr. Dietet.*, 2, 253, 1989.

255. Englyst, H. N., Kingman, S. M., and Cummings, J. H., Classification and measurement of nutritionally important starch fractions, *European J. Clin, Nutr.*, 1992 (in press).

256. Wood, R., Englyst, H. N., Southgate, D. A. T., and Cummings, J. H., Determination of dietary fibre—collaborative trials Part IV. A comparison of the Englyst and Prosky procedures for measurement of soluble, insoluble and total dietary fibre, *J. Assoc. Publ. Analysts*, 1992 (in press).

Correlations of Transit Time to a Critical Fecal Weight (CFW) and to Substances Associated with Dietary Fiber

Gene A. Spiller and Monica Spiller

THE CONCEPT OF CRITICAL FECAL WEIGHT (CFW)

The correlation of transit time (TT) to fecal wet weight (FWW) is important, as it gives a simple method to help individuals determine whether their diet supplies enough fiber and enough of the right kind of fiber. In a more general way, it is useful in arriving at desirable recommendations for fiber intake on various diet patterns and for different populations.

Several studies[1-5] have shown that (1) TT decreases rapidly as FWW increases to about 200 g/d and (2) beyond FWWs of about 200 g/d there is little change in TT as FWW increases. The line correlating TT to FWW becomes practically asymptotic to the abscissa for this FWW. Figures 4.5.1 and 4.5.2 summarize these concepts. When data correlating TT to FWW are presented for individual subjects (Figure 4.5.2), one finds a wide scatter of points correlating TT to FWW below FWW values of about 180 g/d; many values for TT are as high as 4 or 5 days. This indicates that as FWW values increase, there is a critical fecal wet weight (CFW) of about 200 g/d, beyond which practically no TT is greater than 2 days. While we do not know the ideal transit time for humans, it may be reasonable to assume that extremely long transit times are not desirable, and that a more predictable colon function is preferable.

EPIDEMIOLOGICAL CORRELATIONS

A well-executed epidemiological study[6] on two Scandinavian populations showed lower colon cancer incidence in the population with an average FWW of 200 g/d compared to the group with an average of 150 g/d. This supports the concept that there is a CFW, that its value is in the range of 200 g/d for adults, and that the CFW is a basic physiological concept.

0-8493-2387-8/01/$0.00+$1.50

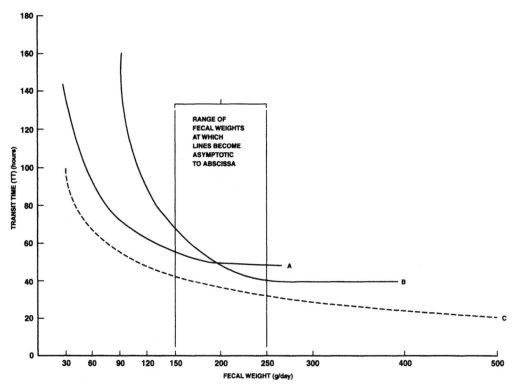

Figure 4.5.1 Correlation of transit time to fecal weight in three different studies. Curve A is from Spiller et al.,[2] curve B is from Connell,[8] and curve C is from Burkitt et al.[1]

CORRELATION OF CFW TO LEVELS OF DIETARY FIBER AND ASSOCIATED COMPOUNDS

The amount of fiber needed to achieve the CFW appears to be in the range of 35 to 45 g/d, as long as enough cereal fiber is included (probably 60 to 70%), especially wheat-type fiber. Wheat-type fibers are high in water-insoluble fractions. The question of how much of the water-soluble fibers we need in relation to their effect on lipid and carbohydrate metabolism has not yet been answered, but it is certainly logical to assume that a fraction of the fiber should be of the water-soluble type, perhaps 30 to 40%. Pharmacological uses of dietary fiber and their effective levels are not part of these considerations. It also appears that other substances present in plant foods, such as tartaric acid in grapes and raisins, may decrease the amount of fiber needed to achieve a desirable TT.

TARTARIC ACID: EXAMPLE OF FACTORS THAT WORK WITH DIETARY FIBER TO AFFECT COLON FUNCTION

Many plant foods contain substances other than dietary fiber that affect colon function. A typical example of such compounds in common foods is tartaric acid, which is present in grapes and their products such as sun-dried raisins and in tamarinds. The effect of various amounts of raisin on TT is greater than expected by their fiber content,[7] and tartaric acid appears to play an important role. When 120 g of raisins were fed, subjects' TT decreased from 42 hours at baseline to 28 hours after a week of adaptation to the raisin diet. When the same subject consumed the amount of tartaric

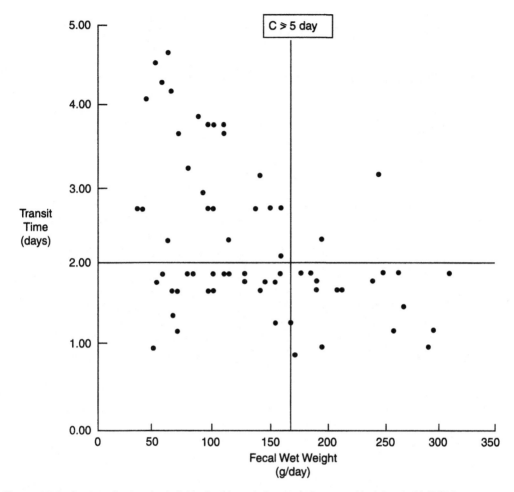

Figure 4.5.2 Scatter of points for individual subjects below and above a critical threshold (CFW).

acid equivalent to that present in the raisins, the TT decreased from 42 to 31 hours. In addition, on both the raisins and the tartaric acid, feces were softer and easier to eliminate. While tartaric acid affected TT, it did not significantly affect FWW, which was increased by the raisins. This example was used to emphasize the importance of considering dietary fiber when present in whole foods as part of a complex matrix of bioactive compounds.

More studies are needed to determine other non-fiber substances in plant foods that may work together with fiber to normalize colon function.

OVERALL DIETARY PATTERN AND TRANSIT TIME

Part of any recommendation on the intake of dietary fiber to obtain ideal transit times should include the importance of eating a variety of dietary fibers. In this way, both water-insoluble and water-soluble components will be represented.

The data on dietary fiber content of various foods, as presented in the Appendixes of this Handbook, indicate that it is difficult to obtain sufficient dietary fiber from a single food (except for concentrated sources) and that the easiest way to obtain a reasonable amount of dietary fiber in the daily diet is to consume a diversity of unrefined plant foods, such as whole grain products, in the form of breads and prepared cereals, whole grains such as brown rice, whole corn and oats, beans, nuts, vegetables, and fruits. Some Asian populations obtain additional dietary fiber from sea vegetation. Whole grain wheat deserves a special mention as a high source of insoluble dietary fiber, while beans and oats deserve a special mention as a source of good mixtures of water-soluble and water-insoluble fiber. The use of concentrated sources such as wheat bran (for the wheat-type fiber portion) or oat bran offers additional assurance of a sufficient daily intake of particular fiber types. In bread selection great care should be taken, as there is a tremendous diversity of breads on the market; the amount and type of dietary fiber may vary greatly according to the level of extraction and type of flours used.

REFERENCES

1. Burkitt, D. P., Walker, A. R. P., and Painter, N. S., Dietary fiber and disease, *JAMA*, 229, 1068, 1974.
2. Spiller, G. A., Chernoff, M. C., Shipley, E. A., Beigler, M. A., and Briggs, G. M., Can fecal weight be used to establish a recommended intake of dietary fiber (plantix)?, *Am. J. Clin. Nutr.*, 39, 659, 1977.
3. Spiller, G. A., Shiplet, E. A., and Blake, J. A., Recent progress in dietary fiber (plantix) in human nutrition, *CRC Crit. Rev. Food Sci. Nutr.*, 10, 31, 1978.
4. Spiller, G. A., Wong, L. G., Whittam, J. H., and Scala, J., Correlation of gastrointestinal transit time to fecal weight in adult humans at two levels of fiber intake, *Nutr. Rep. Int.*, 25, 23, 1982.
5. Spiller, G. A., Story, J. A., Wong, L. G., Nunes, J. D., Alton, M., Petro, M. S., Furarnoto, E. J., Whittam, J. H., and Scala, J., Effect of increasing levels of hard wheat fiber on fecal weight, minerals and steroids and gastrointestinal transit time in healthy young women, *J. Nutr.*, 116, 778, 1986.
6. International Agency for Cancer Research, Dietary fiber, transit time, fecal bacteria and colon cancer in two Scandinavian populations, *Lancet*, i, 207, 1977.
7. Spiller, G. A., Bruce, B. and Spiller, M., Effect of tartrate and dietary fiber in sun-dried raisins on colon function in healthy adults, *J. Am. Coll. Nutr.*, 14, 536, 1995.
8. Connell, A. H., Fiber, bulk and colonic activity, in *Fiber Deficiency and Colonic Disorders*, Reily, R. W. and Kirsner, J. B., Eds., Plenun Press, New York, 1975, 81.

Influences of Fiber on the Ecology
of the Intestinal Flora

Margo N. Woods and Sherwood L. Gorbach

INTRODUCTION

A variety of environmental and physiological conditions are known to influence microbial composition and metabolic activities of the intestinal microflora.[1–3] Among the recognized factors within the bowel lumen are

1. Diet, substrata, and nutrient availability
2. Redox potential
3. Gas composition
4. Acidity or pH
5. Osmotic and ionic effects
6. Surface tension and liquid flow
7. Endogenous and exogenous substances that may inhibit bacterial growth (bile salts, volatile and nonvolatile fatty acids, bacteriocides, intestinal antibodies, and drugs)
8. Bacterial interactions and competition
9. Intestinal motility

Individual microbial species vary in their sensitivity to changes in these parameters. The composition of the flora itself can affect many of these factors. Fiber has the potential to influence most of the factors listed above. This complex interactive system is only now being explored, and only partial data are available in humans.

INTESTINAL BACTERIA

Bacteria are distributed throughout the intestine, but the major concentration reside in the large bowel. The upper bowel, including the stomach, duodenum, and jejunum, has a sparse microflora derived largely from the oral cavity. The bacteria are washed down in a wave-like fashion, along with saliva. The organisms are found in the upper bowel in relatively low concentrations, up to 10^5 colony-forming units (CFU) per milliliter. The ileum is a transitional zone, with a flora containing elements from the upper intestine, along with some coliforms and anaerobes from the colon. Across the ileocecal valve there is a marked increase in numbers and types of bacteria, which remain fairly consistent throughout the large bowel. Total concentrations are 10^{11} to 10^{12} CFU per gram, approaching the theoretical limit of forms that can be accommodated in that mass.

Although over 400 species of anaerobic bacteria are present in the large intestine of a human being, five genera account for the majority of the viable forms: *Bacteroides, Eubacterium, Bifidobacterium, Lactobacillus,* and *Gram-positive cocci.*[4] The first four are saccharolytic, indicating that they can break down various complex carbohydrates present in the intestine and colon. The majority of microorganisms present in the large intestine have a strictly anaerobic metabolism, and the number of facultative anaerobes are several orders of magnitude lower than those of the obligate anaerobes.[5–7] Bacteria account for 35 to 50% of volume of the contents of the human colon or 41 to 57% of the dry weight.[8,9]

Another way of describing the intestinal flora is by morphological characteristics. Six major categories are listed in Table 4.6.1, including an example of typical species found in the human intestine.

Table 4.6.1 Morphologic Characteristics of Human Intestinal Microflora

- Gram-negative anaerobic nonsporing rods
  Bacteroides
  Fusobacterium
- Gram-negative facultative rods
  Enterobacteriaceae
- Gram-positive cocci
  Streptococcus – facultative bacteria
  Peptostreptococcus – anaerobic bacteria
- Gram-negative anaerobic cocci – minor contribution to flora in man
- Gram-positive nonsporing rods
  Bifidobacterium – anaerobic bacteria
  Lactobacillus – facultative or anaerobic bacteria
  Eubacterium – anaerobic bacteria
- Gram-positive spore-forming anaerobic rods
  Clostridium

When evaluating the composition of the intestinal flora, it is useful to keep in mind some general considerations regarding classifications of the most typical intestinal flora as harmful/pathogens, neutral/potentially harmful, and healthful/beneficial flora.[4] Some of the general harmful effects that can be caused by bacteria include (1) production of toxins, (2) diarrhea/constipation, (3) infection, (4) liver damage, (5) encephalopathy, and (6) increased cancer risk.[4] A number of health-promoting actions have also been associated with some intestinal flora, and they include (1) inhibition of growth of harmful bacteria, (2) decreasing gas formation, (3) stimulation of immune functions, (4) improved absorption of nutrients (calcium, zinc, and iron), and (5) synthesis of B-vitamins that are available to the host. *Bifidobacteria* and *Lactobacillus* are the two common microflora most often described as desirable.

Table 4.6.2 Division of Common Bacteria into Harmful, Neutral, or Beneficial

Harmful/Pathogens (Some Species)	Neutral/Potentially Harmful	Healthful/Beneficial
Ps-Aeruginosa	Peptostreptococci	Bifidobacteria[a]
Proteus	E. coli	Lactobacilli
Staphlococci	Streptococci	Eubacteria[a]
Clostridia	Bacteroides[a]	
Veillonellae	Fusobacteria[a]	
	Enterococci	

Source: From Gibson, G. R. and Roberfroid, M. B., *J. Nutr.*, 125, 1401, 1995. With permission.

[a] Genera that account for the majority of viable bacterial forms found in the large intestine.[4,20]

Table 4.6.2 lists some common bacteria in each of the three categories of desirability of the microflora. A number of studies have looked at the advantageous physiological characteristics of *Bifidobacteria* and *Lactobacillus*.[10,11] *Bifidobacteria* may constitute up to 25% of the total population in the gut of adults.[12] *Bifidobacteria* produce strong acids and metabolic products (acetate, lactate) that lower gut pH and exert an antibacterial effect directly.[13] It has also been reported that *Bifido-bacteria* excrete a metabolic end product inhibitory to a number of pathogenic bacteria.[14,15] An increase in *Bifidobacteria* also results in lower levels of the bacterial enzymes glucosidase and β-glucuronidase in the bacterial milieu, which results in lower levels of secondary bile acids in the intestinal lumen.[16,17] These secondary bile acids have been reported to be co-carcinogens.[18,19]

Understanding the factors that encourage the presence of these "beneficial" vs. "potentially harmful" intestinal flora provides many useful research questions. Enhancing beneficial bacteria has become a new food technology and market opportunity termed *probiotics*. Probiotics are defined as live microbial food supplements which beneficially affect the host animal by improving its intestinal microbial balance.[11,21,22] Probiotics are reported to have many positive effects on numerous medical conditions, as reviewed by Goldin and Gorbach.[19] Alternatively, investigations into intestinal conditions, intestinal bacterial substrates, and food intake patterns that affect type and prevalence of intestinal organisms offer a second approach to enhancing beneficial bacteria. A non-digestible food ingredient that beneficially affects the host by selectively stimulating the growth and/or activity of one or a limited number of bacteria in the colon and thus improve host health is termed a *prebiotic*.[4] Certain dietary fibers have been labeled prebiotics, notably the fructooligosaccharides.[4]

An example of the changes observed in the predominant bacterial groups in eight volunteers fed a strictly controlled diet for 45 days is shown in Table 4.6.3. During days 0–15, the diet was supplemented with 15 g of sucrose, and during days 16–30, the supplementation was 15 g of oligofructose.[20]

Table 4.6.3 Percentage of Microflora from Humans on Two Different Diets

Bacterial Group	Sucrose	Oligofructose
Bacteroides	72%	16%
Bifidobacteria	17%	82%
Fusobacteria	9%	1%
Clostridia	2%	1%

Note: The four groups represented were taken as 100% of the fecal flora.

Source: From Roberfroid, M. B. et. al., *J. Nutr.*, 128, 11, 1998. With permission.

DIETARY FIBER

Definitions of fiber are broad but, as stated earlier in this text, it is generally agreed to include the components of plant cells which are "resistant to hydrolysis by the digestive enzymes of humans."[23] Food components that are included in this definition are presented below:

- Resistant starch
- Non-starch polysaccharides (NSP)
  - Cellulose
  - Hemicellulose
  - Pectin
  - Gums
- Non-carbohydrate aromatic polymers
  - Lignin
- Non-digestible oligosaccharides
  - Fructooligosaccharides
  - Galactooligosaccharides
  - Glucooligosaccharides

Most of these food components or undigested residues are good substrates for intestinal flora. Estimates of daily intake of dietary fiber in the U.S. as NSP + lignin are 8–18 g/day,[24] while non-digested carbohydrates account for 10–60 g/day.[3] Resistant starch provides 8–40 g/day of substrate to the large intestine,[25] and oligosaccharides provide 1–10 g of substrate per day.[25]

Foods in our usual diet that are high in dietary fiber include fruits, vegetables, whole grains, and legumes. These provide pectins, hemicellulose, cellulose, and lignin. Pectins and hemicellulose are generally considered soluble fiber, have higher water-holding capacity, form gels in the intestines, and are in higher quantities in fruits, vegetables, and legumes. Oat bran is a good example of a soluble fiber. Insoluble fibers, cellulose and lignin, are not water-soluble, have a lower water-holding capacity, and are derived from the tougher structural components of plants. These are more prevalent in grains. Wheat bran is an example of an insoluble fiber. There is great variation in fiber amount and type within each food group, however. The fructooligosaccharides are the most widely studied of the oligosaccharides. They are naturally found in such foods as garlic, onion, leek, artichoke, asparagus, banana, and wheat.[25] They are defined by the degree of polymerization (DP). If the DP is <9, then they are termed *oligofructose*, and with an average DP of 12 (but up to 60), they are termed *inulin*. Inulin is obtained by hot water extraction of chicory root and, as such, is an ingredient in a number of food products due to its fat-like properties and its sweet taste (1/3 the sweetness of sugar). Inulin is on the "Generally Recognized As Safe" (GRAS) list.

As can be seen, dietary fiber includes a heterogeneous mixture of materials. Its physiological effects depend on specific properties, some of which can influence the intestinal flora. Among these properties are the following:

1. *Particle size:* Particle size determines the surface area of the fiber and alters its susceptibility to digestion, binding properties, water-holding properties, and transit time in the bowel.
2. *Cation-exchange characteristics:* The ability to bind endogenous and exogenous materials in the intestine is related to the ionic binding properties of the fiber, which appear to be influenced by the amount of lignin present. The binding capacity of fiber may determine its availability for metabolism by the flora.
3. *Water-holding capacity:* The swelling and permeability properties can influence the ability of bacteria to infiltrate and digest the fiber by changing the surface area available for digestion and the speed of transport through the intestine.
4. *Digestibility or degradability:* This depends on the composition of the fiber.
   A. Lignin — not digested by the flora
   B. Cellulose — 30 to 50% digested by the flora
   C. Hemicellulose — 50 to 80% digested by the flora
   D. Pectin and gums — 90 to 100% digested by the flora
   E. Non-digestible oligosaccharides — 95 to 100% digested by the flora

Most of the research investigating the effect of dietary fiber on intestinal and fecal flora has been carried out with wheat bran, pectin, and inulin (fructooligosaccharides). This is in contrast to information on hemicellulose, cellulose, or lignin, which are difficult to obtain in their pure form with their physiological properties intact. Pectin is used widely in the food industry to obtain certain properties of texture and binding. Standardized forms of wheat bran have also been developed to facilitate studies investigating their potential benefits. Studies on fructooligosaccharides, which are readily available, have been used for some time in food manufacturing. They are available under the product names of RAFTILOSE® (oligofructose) and RAFTILINE® (inulin). It is of interest to note that the direction of this research appears to be determined by the availability of pure or standardized forms of the dietary components and their usefulness to the food industry. If benefits are observed, the addition of these fiber components to standard food products would allow labeling of their health benefits and advertising as "functional foods." An alternative approach is the investigation of specific, commonly consumed foods that contain high levels of these specific types of fiber and their role in supporting and/or maintaining health or markers of health.

In order to evaluate the potential benefit or harm of specific dietary fibers on the intestinal flora, one needs to identify criteria that are generally accepted as "beneficial" vs. "undesirable." The factors given below, which represent our current understanding of the biochemistry and physiology of intestinal flora, will be the focus for the evaluation and rating of the cited literature.

1. **Increase in the bacteria generally recognized as desirable.** An increase in *Bifidobacteria* or *Lactobacillus* and/or the decrease of bacteria generally recognized as "neutral or potentially harmful" (*Bacteroides* and *Fusobacteria*) is considered desirable. Justification of this position was previously stated and is related to the ability of *Bifidobacteria* to decrease pathogenic organisms and promote physiological properties such as increased immune response. A rating of 1^+ indicates a higher level or increase of one or both of the "desirable" microflora and/or a lower level or decrease in the "undesirable." A rating of 1^- would indicate the reverse, and 1^0 would indicate no difference.

2. **Change in intestinal pH.** A decrease in the pH of the intestinal contents is deemed to support an increase in bifidobacteria and to generally decrease pathogens. Therefore, such a change caused by the presence of specific fibers or fiber in general would be considered a beneficial change. A rating of 2^+ would indicate a lower intestinal or fecal pH. A rating of 2^- would indicate a higher pH, and 2^0 would indicate no difference.

3. **Production of short-chain fatty acids (SCFAs).** The increase in SCFAs is generally agreed to be beneficial, since they decrease the pH, act as antibacteriacidals, and serve as substrates for colonic cells. The most typical acids formed are acetic, lactic, butyric, and proprionic. A rating of 3^+ would indicate a higher level or increase in SCFA. A rating of 3^- would indicate a lower level or decrease, and 3^0 would indicate no difference.

4. **Production of immunostimulants.** It has been reported and previously stated that *Bifidobacteria* excretes a metabolic product that results in the decrease in pathogenic flora.[14,15] A decrease in known pathogens could be an indicator of this capability. A rating of 4^+ would indicate that the results of the study supported the excretion or presence of a metabolite that decreased known microbial pathogens. (No study reported in Tables 4.6.4 or 4.6.5 supplied data on this topic.)

5. **Changes in bacterial enzymes.** A decrease in bacterial glucuronidase and/or glycosidase would be considered a positive change, due to their association with decreased absorption of intestinal cholesterol and other steroids. A decrease in 7-α-hydroxylase would also be considered a positive observation, since it would indicate a decrease in formation of secondary bile acids (lithocholic and deoxycholic acids), which are considered co-carcinogens.[2,19] A rating of 5^+ would indicate a lower level or decrease in one or both of these enzymes. A rating of 5^- would indicate a higher level or increase in the enzyme, and 5^0 would indicate no change.

A reasonable number of human experiments have been performed with fiber sources such as wheat bran ($N = 8$ studies). Thus, there is more information on the effect of wheat bran on the intestinal flora. Fructooligosaccharides have also been studied in a reasonable number of controlled experiments ($N = 8$ studies).

Two approaches have been taken in studies of fiber and its effect on the intestinal microflora. In the first approach, the intestinal flora has been measured in people eating customary diets with different levels of fiber intakes (Table 4.6.4). For example, vegetarians and non-vegetarians, or Western and Japanese people eating their customary diet, have been studied. The second approach involves a defined diet or a controlled diet in a study population to which the fiber of interest is added as a supplement (Table 4.6.5).

Evaluation of data from Table 4.6.4 indicates that the Western-type or high-risk diets (high fat, low fiber) generally showed higher levels of *Bacteroides* and sometimes lower levels of *Bifidobacteria*. Four studies reported on bacterial enzymes. The Western diet, omnivore diet, or high-risk diet (high fat, low fiber) reported higher levels of β-glucuronidase or dehydrogenation or steroids and increased secondary bile acids.

Table 4.6.4 Fecal Microflora in Different Human Populations

Western Diet (N)	Non-Western Diet (N)	Fecal Microflora Characteristics	Score[a]	Ref.
Western	Vegetarian	No change in predominant fecal flora	1°	26
English	Ugandans (48)	English had 30-fold more Bacteroids and 4-fold more *Bifidobacterium*; Ugandans had significantly greater numbers of *Streptococci, Enterococci, Lactobacilli*, and yeasts	1+	27
British (91), American (34)	Ugandans, South Indians, Japanese	British and Americans had greater numbers of Bacteroides and a higher ratio of anaerobes	1+	28
British	Strict vegetarians	Vegetarians had fewer isolates of Bacteroides that could dehydrogenate bile acids	5+	29
Western (17)	Japanese, Seventh-Day Adventists (11), American vegetarians (12), Chinese (11)	Westerners had greater conversion of bile acids to secondary bile acids and 2.5 times more β-glucuronidase activity	5+	30
American diet in Japanese (1)	Japanese diet in Japanese (1)	Western diet resulted in disappearance of *Fusobacterium* (10-month study)	—	31
High risk	Low risk	High-risk populations had higher levels of *Clostridium paraputrificum* which was able to dehydrogenate steroids	5+	32
Western Japanese (18)	Traditional Japanese (15)	Traditional diets have more aerobes and facultative bacteria, higher *Streptococcus faecalis*, and fewer *Bifidobacterium*; Western diet eliminated *Eubacterium contortum*	1+	33
North American	Japanese, Hawaiian (20)	No consistent pattern between types or numbers in fecal samples; great differences between individuals	1°	34
High-risk colon cancer	Low-risk colon cancer	High-risk group had more anaerobes (Bacteroides and *Fusobacterium*); low-risk had more *Eubacterium*	1°	35
Non-Seventh-Day Adventists	Seventh-Day Adventists	Seventh-Day Adventists had higher Lactobacillus and lower *Clostridium perfringens* than the U.S. population. *Clostridium septum, C. tertim*, and *Fusobacterium* were lower in the Adventist group	1+	36
Nonvegetarian-Seventh-Day Adventists	Adhering and nonadhering Seventh-Day Adventists showed little differences	1°		
High-risk colon cancer, urban Danes, Copenhagen	Low risk colon cancer, rural Finns	High-risk group had higher ratio of anaerobes due to decrease in aerobes (*Enterococcus, Streptococcus*, and *Lactobacillus*)	—	37
England (36), Scotland (11), Wales (65), U.S. (8)	Japan, Hong Kong, Uganda	Western population had greater numbers of *Clostridium paraputrificum* than non-Western groups	1+	38
High risk, U.S.	Low risk, Africa	Western population had higher levels of Bacteroides and *Bifidobacterium*	1°	39
U.S. (15)	Lacto-ovo vegetarians (13), Vegetarians (17)	Fecal bacterial enzymes, β-glucuronidase, nitroreductase, and azo-reductase were higher in the omnivores compared to the vegetarian groups; 7-α-dehydroxylase was higher in omnivores compared to lacto-ovo vegetarians	5+	40

[a] A positive sign indicates more "desirable" microflora characteristics in the Non-Western Diet group compared to the Western diet group.

Table 4.6.5 Effect of Various Fiber on Fecal Microflora

Diet and Fiber	Amount	Duration	No. of subjects	Fecal Microflora Characteristics	Score[a]	Ref.
				Low-Residue Diets		
Low-residue diet	—	21–56 days	6 astronauts	No significant change in fecal flora; decrease in *Enterococci* in low-residue diet	1°	41
Low-residue diet (glucose-base)	—	15 days	11	Diverse microbial population reduced to bacteroids, coliforms, and *Enterococci*	1-	42
Vivonex low-residue diet	—	9 days	3	Disappearance of *Bifidobacterium* and increase in *E. coli*; decrease in very oxygen-sensitive anaerobes	1-	43
Chemically defined diet	—	10 days	3	*Enterobacteria* increased, *Enterococci* and other lactic acid bacteria decreased in number	—	44
Elemental-low residue	—	12 days	14	Decrease in *Enterococci*; no change in total anaerobes, aerobes, or coliforms	—	45
Low-residue diet	—	7 days	10	No change in fecal flora	1°	46
				Usual Diet with Fiber Supplement		
American diet plus Laminarin Xylan Guar gum Psyllium hydrocolloid	— — — —		*In vitro* incubation of colon flora	Plant sources cited resulted in induction of enzymes in *Bacteroides* species that were capable of degrading the polysaccharides	5°	47
American diet plus All Bran	1 oz	3 weeks	6	No significant difference in qualitative or quantitative count of bacteria; ratio of anaerobes to aerobes appeared to increase.	1°	48
British diet plus Carrots	200 g, raw	3 weeks	5	Total breath hydrogen increased twofold by the third week; no change was seen until 10 days after the start of eating carrots; this suggests an increase in bacteria capable of digesting carrots or an induction of enzymes present in the flora	—	49
British diet plus Wheat bran Cabbage	18 g DF 18 g DF	3 weeks	6	Cabbage stimulated growth of intestinal flora	—	50
Western diet plus Bran Wheat germ	30 g 30 g	1–2 months	4 5	Addition of fiber led to a reduction of fecal 7-α-dehydroxylase activity	5+	40

Table 4.6.5 (Continued) Effect of Various Fiber on Fecal Microflora

Diet and Fiber	Amount	Duration	# of subjects	Fecal Microflora Characteristics	Score[a]	Ref.
British diet plus Coarse bran	12–26 g	14–70 days	24	Fecal samples from persons on fiber-supplemented diets showed no difference in the *in vitro* digestibility of the individual fiber; this might suggest that endogenous sources of nutrients and not diet are the energy source of flora; however, increased volatile fatty acids were observed in fecal samples of persons on the fiber diets for more than two weeks.	3+	51
Western diet plus Wheat bran	1 oz	14-Mar	7	No change in flora; no change in ability to digest bran	1°	52
British diet plus Pectin Guar Plantains Bananas	35 g/day 35 g/day 1000 g/day 1000 g/day	2 weeks	4 3 5 4	No significant difference in composition of flora	1°	53
American diet plus All Bran	3 oz/day (27 g dietary fiber)	3 weeks	6	Increase in anaerobes in high-fat diet; no change in aerobes; slight increase in *Streptococcus* during fiber supplement; slight decrease in *Lactobacillus* during fiber supplementation	1−	54
British diet plus Wheat bran	11.7 g of crude fiber	3 weeks	4	No change in relative number of the following: *Enterobacteria, Enterococcus, Lactobacillus, Clostridium, Bacteroides, Bifidobacterium, Eubacterium,* or *Streptococcus*	1°	55
Western diet plus Bran Bagasse	39 g 10.5 g	12 weeks	20 20	No change in composition of the bacteria; increase in total bacteria excreted associated with increase in stool weight	1°	56
British diet plus Gum arabic (GA)	25 g	7-day control; 21-day test diet	5	Flora not tested — effect on metabolism tested; GA caused a significant increase in breath hydrogen after chronic but not acute treatment with GA; this suggests increases in number of flora capable of metabolizing GA or induction of bacterial enzymes	—	57
American diet plus Pectin	15 g	21 days	6	Pectin caused a decrease in anaerobic/aerobic ratio from 3.6 to 2.6 ($p < .01$); 7-α-dehydroxylase increased and cholesterol dehydrogenase decreased, but neither reached significance	5−	58

Diet	Amount	Duration	Subjects	Effect		Ref.
Basal diet (12% protein, 33% fat, 260 mg cholesterol, 5 g NDF) plus Pectin	15 g	18-day cycles	8 (M)	35% increase of β-glucuronidase on pectin diet	5-	59
				No effect of pectin on 7-α-dehydroxylase (question of adequacy of fiber supplementation and wash-out times)	5°	
Basal diet (.8 g kg wgt of egg albumin, 30% fat and 0 gm DF) plus	(30–40 g 1 day)	9-day cycles	5 (M)	Only pectin decreased fecal pH	2+	60
Cellulose	0.5 g/kg wgt			Indirect effect on flora via changes of pH which can affect species and enzymatic activity	2+	
Pectin	0.5 g/kg wgt			Pectin decreased fecal pH	2+	
Xylan	0.5 g/kg wgt					
Corn Bran	0.6 g/kg wgt					
Controlled diet (3×3 design)			12 females	SCFA production		61
Low-fiber diet	20 g	3 weeks		Baseline		
High-fiber/high-protein	34 g	3 weeks		NC	3°	
High-figer/low-protein	36 g	3 weeks		NC	3°	
Barley fiber	23 g	3 weeks		Decrease in total SCFA	3-	
Oligosaccharides (Fructooligosaccharides)						
Japanese diet plus Oligofructose (OF) (neosugar)	8 g/day	2 weeks	—	Tenfold increase in Bifidobacteria; decrease in C. perfringens	1+	62
Japanese diet plus Oligofructose	8 g/day	5 weeks	Hyperlipidemics	Fivefold increase in Bifidobacteria after oligofructose and decrease in Bacteroides and Eubacteria	1+	63
Sucrose (placebo)	8 g/day	5 weeks				
Typical Western diet plus Oligofructose	4 g/day	15 days		Significant increase in Bifidobacteria with oligofructose	1+	64
Controlled diet plus Oligofructose	15 g/day	15 days	8	Increase of Bifidobacteria; decrease in Bacteroides	1+	65
Inulin	15 g/day	15 days	8	Increase of Bifidobacteria; decrease in Bacteroides	1+	
			4	Increase in Bifidobacteria with BFM	1+	
Typical diet (France) +BFM[b] Inulin	18 g/day	38 days	12	No increase in Bifidobacteria with BFM and inulin, only BFM alone; no change in pH, nitrate reductase, nitro-reductase or azoreductase	1°, 2°, 5°	66
placebo		12 days				

Table 4.6.5 (Continued) Effect of Various Fiber on Fecal Microflora

Diet and Fiber	Amount	Duration	# of subjects	Fecal Microflora Characteristics	Score	Ref.
Typical diet (American) plus						
Inulin	20 g	1–8 days	10	Increased *Bifidobacteria* and decreased *Enterobacteria*	1[+]	67
	40 g	9–19 days	10			
Lactore	20 g	1–8 days	15	Decreased *Lactobacilli* and increased *Enterococci*	1[-]	
	40 g	9–19 days	15	No change in pH or β-glucosidase or β-glucuronidase	2[*], 5[°]	
Controlled diet — baseline		2 weeks	8 (M+F)			
plus Fn type oligosaccharide (RAFTILOSE®)	8 g/day	2 weeks		Increased *Bifidobacteria*; decreased pH	1[+], 2[+]	68
Usual diet plus oligofructose	8 g/day	3 weeks		Increased *Bifidobacteria*; decreased pH	1[+], 2[+]	
Controlled diet (CD)		1–6 days	12	Increased *Bifidobacteria* on CD	1[+]	69
plus oligofructose (OF) (neosugar)	4 g/day	7–32 days		Increased *Bifidobacteria* by one log	1[+]	
				OF decreased β-glucuronidase	5[+]	
				OF decreased glycocholic acid hydroxylase	5[+]	
				OF resulted in no change in nitroreductase	5[°]	

[a] A positive sign indicates that the tested fiber supplement restulted in more "desirable" microflora characteristics.
[b] Bifidoborterium of fermented milk.

In Table 4.6.5, the use of low-residue diets caused a decrease in *Bifidobacteria* and a general indication of a rise of less desirable microflora. Studies of fiber supplementation with wheat bran indicated no change or a decrease in beneficial bacteria (*Lactobacillus*). One study with bran[40] reported a reduction of fecal 7-α-dehydroxylase. Studies using oligosaccharides ($N = 8$) resulted in seven of the eight studies reporting an increase in the desirable over the undesirable microflora. The one study that did not report an increase in *Bifidobacteria* with inulin was designed to deliver inulin in a probiotic of *Bifidobacteria*. The addition of inulin with the probiotic did not increase *Bifidobacteria* over the level achieved with the probiotic alone. Four studies reported on changes in pH: two saw a decrease, and two failed to see a decrease. Two studies of fructooligosaccharides reported on fecal enzymes, and only one study[69] reported a decrease in β-glucuronidase.

Additional studies are needed to clarify the effect of fiber, including oligosaccharides, on bacterial enzymes, to determine the amount necessary to elicit desirable effects and the equivalent intake of usual foods (whole wheat, wheat bran, fruit, vegetable, etc.) that produce similar results.

REFERENCES

1. Simon, G. L. and Gorbach, S. L., Intestinal flora in health and disease, *Gastroenterology*, 86, 174, 1984.
2. Goldin, B. R., Lichtenstein, A. H., and Gorbach, S. L., The role of intestinal flora, in *Modern Nutrition in Health and Disease*, 8th ed., Shils, M. and Young, V., Eds., Lea & Febiger, Philadelphia, 1994, chapter 38, 569–582.
3. Cummings, J. H. and Macfarlane, G. T., A review: the conditions and consequences of bacterial fermentation in the human colon, *J. Appl. Bacteriol.*, 70, 443, 1991.
4. Gibson, G. R. and Roberfroid, M. B., Dietary modulation of the human colonic microbiota: introducing the concept of prebiotics, *J. Nutr.*, 125, 1401, 1995.
5. Finegold, S. M., Flora, D. J., Attebury, H. R., and Sutter, L. V., Fecal bacteriology of colonic polyp patients and control patients, *Cancer Res.*, 35, 3407, 1975.
6. Moore, W. E. C. and Holdeman, L. V., Identification of anaerobic bacteria, *Am. J. Clin. Nutr.*, 25, 1306, 1972.
7. Reddy, B. S., Weisburger, J. H., and Wynder, E. L., Effects of high risk and low risk diets for colon carcinogenesis on fecal microflora and steroids in man, *J. Nutr.*, 105, 878, 1975.
8. Salyer, A. A., Energy sources of major intestinal fermentative anaerobes, *Am. J. Clin. Nutr.*, 32, 258, 1979.
9. Stephen, A. N. and Cummings, J. H., The microbial contribution to human fecal mass, *J. Med. Microbiol.*, 13, 45, 1980.
10. Tamura, Z., Nutriology of bifidobacteria, *Bifidobacteria Microflora*, 2, 3, 1983.
11. Fuller, R., Ed., *Probiotics, The Scientific Basis*, Chapman and Hall, London, 1992.
12. Finegold, S. M., Sutter, V. L., and Mattisen, G. E., Normal indigenous intestinal flora, in *Human Intestinal Microflora in Health and Diseases*, Hentges, D. J., Ed., Academic Press, New York, 1983, 3–31.
13. Rasic, J. L., The role of dairy foods containing bifido and acidophilic bacteria in nutrition and health, *N. Europ. Dairy J.*, 4, 80, 1983.
14. Gibson, G. R. and Wang, X., Inhibitory effects of *bifidobacteria* on other colonic bacteria, *J. Appl. Bacteriol.*, 77, 412, 1994.
15. Gibson, G. R. and Wang, X., Bifidogenic properties of different types of fructooligosaccharides, *Food Microbiol.*, 11, 491, 1994.
16. Marteau, P., Pochart, P., Flourie, B., Pellier, P., Santos, L., Desjeux, G. F., and Rombaud, J. C., Effects of chronic indigestion of a fermented dairy product containing *Lactobacillus* acidophilus and *Bifidobacterium* bifidum on metabolic activities of the colonic flora in humans, *Am. J. Clin. Nutr.*, 52, 685, 1990.
17. Kulkami, N. and Reddy, B. S., Inhibitory effect of *Bifidobacterium longum* cultures on the azoxymethane-induced aberrant crypt foci formation and fecal bacterial β-glucuronidase, *Proc. Soc. Exp. Biol. Med.*, 207, 278, 1994.

18. Mallett, A. K. and Rowland, I. R., Factors affecting the gut microflora, in *Role of the Gut Flora in Toxicity and Cancer*, Rowland, I. R., Ed., Academic, London, 1988, 347–382.
19. Goldin, B. R. and Gorbach, S. L., Probiotics for humans, in *Probiotics. The Scientific Basis*, Fuller, R., Ed., Chapman and Hall, London, 1992, 3555–376.
20. Roberfroid, M. B., Van Loo, J. A. E., and Gibson, G. R., The bifidogenic nature of chicory inulin and its hydrolysis products, *J. Nutr.*, 128, 11, 1998.
21. Fuller, R., Probiotics in man and animals, *J. Appl. Bacteriol.*, 66, 365, 1989.
22. Fuller, R., Probiotics in human medicine, *Gut*, 32, 439, 1991.
23. Trowell, H., Definition of fiber, *Lancet*, 1, 503, 1974.
24. Federation of American Societies for Experimental Biology, Life Sciences Research Office, For the U.S. population, daily dietary fiber intake in grams, on 1 day, by sex, age, and race/ethnicity, in *Third Report on Nutrition Monitoring in the United States: Volume 2*, U.S. Government Printing Office, Washington, D.C., 1988–1991, 154.
25. Van Loo, J., Coussement, P., Leenhees, L. D., Huebrege, H., and Smits, G., On the presence of inulin and oligofructose as natural ingredients on the Western diet, *Crit. Rev. Food Service Nutr.*, 35, 525, 1995.
26. Moore, W. E. C., Cato, E. P., and Holdeman, L. V., Anaerobic bacteria of the gastrointestinal flora and their occurrence in clinical infections, *J. Infect. Dis.*, 119, 641, 1969.
27. Aries, V., Crowther, J. S., Drasar, B. S., Hill, M. J., and Williams, R. E. O., Bacteria and aetiology of cancer of the large bowel, *Gut*, 10, 334, 1969.
28. Hill, M. J., Drasar, B. S., Aries, V., Crowther, J. S., Hawksinth, G., and Williams, R. E. O., Bacteria and aetiology of cancer of the large bowel, *Lancet*, 1, 95, 1971.
29. Aries, V. C., Crowther, J. S., Drasar, B. S., Hill, M. J., and Ellis, F. R., The effect of a strict vegetarian diet on the faecal flora and faecal steroid concentration, *J. Pathol. Bacteriol.*, 103, 54, 1971.
30. Reddy, B. S. and Wynder, E. L., Large bowel carcinogenesis: fecal constituents of populations with diverse incidence rates of colon cancer, *J. Natl. Cancer Inst.*, 40, 1437, 1973.
31. Ueno, K. et al., Comparison of characteristics of gram-negative anaerobic bacilli isolated from feces of individuals in Japan and the United States, in *Anaerobic Bacteria: Role in Disease*, Balowz, A., DeHaan, R. M., Dowell, V. R., Jr., and Gage, L. B., Eds., Charles C. Thomas, Springfield, IL, 1974, 135.
32. Hill, M. J., Steroid nuclear dehydrogenation and colon cancer, *Am. J. Clin. Nutr.*, 27, 1475, 1974.
33. Finegold, S. M., Attebury, H. R., and Sutter, V. L., Effect of diet on human fecal flora: comparison of Japanese and American diets, *Am. J. Clin. Nutr.*, 27, 1456, 1974.
34. Moore, W. E. C. and Holdeman, L. V., Human fecal flora: the normal flora of 20 Japanese-Hawaiians, *Appl. Microbiol.*, 27, 961, 1974.
35. Peach, S., Fernandez, F., Johnson, K., and Drasar, B. S., The non-sporing anaerobic bacteria in human faeces, *J. Med. Microbiol.*, 7, 213, 1974.
36. Finegold, S. M., Sutter, V. L., Sugihara, P. T., Elder, H. A., Lehmann, S. M., and Phillips, R. L., Fecal microbial flora in Seventh-Day Adventist population and control subjects, *Am. J. Clin. Nutr.*, 30, 1781, 1977.
37. International Agency for Research of Cancer, Intestinal Microbiology Group, Dietary fibre, transit-time, faecal bacteria, steroids, and colon cancer in two Scandinavian populations, *Lancet*, 2, 207, 1977.
38. Drasar, B. S., Goddard, P., Heaton, S., Peach, S., and West, B., Clostridia isolated from faeces, *J. Med. Microbiol.*, 9, 63, 1976.
39. Moore, W. E. C., Cato, E. P., and Holdeman, L. V., Some current concepts in intestinal bacteriology, *Am. J. Clin. Nutr.*, 31, 533, 1978.
40. Goldin, B. R., Swenson, L., Dwyer, J., Sexton, M., and Gorbach, S. L., Effect of diet and *Lactobacillus acidophilus* supplements on human fecal bacterial enzymes, *J. Natl. Cancer Inst.*, 64, 255, 1980.
41. Cordaro, J. T., Sellers, W. M., Bull, R. J., and Schmidt, J. P., Study of man during a 56-day exposure to an oxygen-helium atmosphere at 258 mmHg total pressure, *Aerospace Med.*, 37, 594, 1966.
42. Winitz, M., Adams, R. F., Seedman, D. A., Davis, P. N., Jayko, L. G., and Hamilton, J. A., Studies in metabolic nutrition employing chemically defined diets. II. Effects on gut microflora populations, *Am. J. Clin. Nutr.*, 23, 546, 1970.
43. Attebery, W. R., Sutter, V. L., and Finegold, S. M., Effect of a partially chemically defined diet on normal human fecal flora, *Am. J. Clin. Nutr.*, 25, 1391, 1972.
44. Crowther, J. S., Drasar, B. S., Goddars, P., Hill, M. J., and Johnson, K., The effect of a chemically defined diet of the faecal flora and faecal steroid concentrations, *Gut*, 14, 790, 1973.

45. Burnside, G. and Deurode, G. J., Effects of an elemental diet of human fecal flora, *Gastroenterology*, 66, 210, 1974.
46. Bounous, G. N. and Cohn, I., Stability of normal human fecal flora during a chemically defined, low residue liquid diet, *Ann. Surg.*, 181, 58, 1975.
47. Salyer, A. A., Palmer, J. K., and Wilkins, T. D., Degradation of polysaccharides by intestinal bacterial enzymes, *Am. J. Clin. Nutr.*, 31, S128, 1978.
48. Floch, M. J. and Fuchs, H. M., Modification of stool content by increased bran intake, *Am. J. Clin. Nutr.*, 31, S185, 1978.
49. Robertson, J., Brydon, W. G., Tadesse, K., Wenham, P., Wallks, A., and Eastwood, M. A., The effect of raw carrot on serum lipids and colon function, *Am. J. Clin. Nutr.*, 32, 1889, 1979.
50. Stephen, A. M. and Cummings, J. H., Mechanism of action of dietary fiber in the human colon, *Nature* (*London*), 284, 283, 1980.
51. Ehle, F. R., Robertson, J. B., and Van Soest, P. J., Influence of dietary fiber on fermentation in the human large intestine, *J. Nutr.*, 112, 158, 1982.
52. Hirschberg, N. and Fantus, B., Mode of action of bran: III. Bacterial action on bran, *Rev. Gastroenterology*, 9, 370, 1942.
53. Drasar, B. S. and Jenkins, D. J. A., Bacteria, diet and large bowel cancer, *Am. J. Clin. Nutr.*, 29, 1410, 1976.
54. Fuchs, H. M., Dorfman, S., and Floch, M. H., The effect of dietary fiber supplementation in man. II. Alteration in fecal physiology and bacterial flora, *Am. J. Clin. Nutr.*, 29, 1443, 1976.
55. Drasar, B. S., Jenkins, D. J. A., and Cummings, J. H., The influence of a diet rich in wheat fibre on the human faecal flora, *J. Med. Microbiol.*, 9, 423, 1976.
56. McLean-Baird, I., Walters, R. L., Davies, P. S., Hill, M. J., Drasar, B. S., and Southgate, D. A. T., The effect of two dietary fiber supplements on gastrointestinal transit, stool weight, and frequency, and bacterial flora, and fecal bile acids in normal subjects, *Metabolism*, 26, 117, 1977.
57. McLean Ross, A. W., Eastwood, M. A., Anderson, J. R., and Anderson, D. M. W., A study of the effects of dietary gum arabic in humans, *Am. J. Clin. Nutr.*, 37, 368, 1983.
58. Doyle, R. B., Wolfman, M., Vargo, D., and Floch, M. H., Alteration in bacterial flora induced by dietary pectin, *Am. J. Clin. Nutr.*, 34, 635, 1981.
59. Ross, J. K. and Leklem, J. E., The effect of dietary citrus pectin on the excretion of human fecal neutral and acid steroids and the activity of 7-α-dehydroxylase and β-glucuronidase, *Am. J. Clin. Nutr.*, 34, 2068, 1981.
60. Fleming, S. E., Marthinsen, D., and Kuhnlein, H., Colonic function and fermentation in men consuming high fiber diets, *J. Nutr.*, 113, 2535, 1983.
61. Daniel, M., Wisker, E., Rave, G., and Feldheim, W., Fermentation in human subjects of non-starch polysaccharides in mixed diets, but not in a barley fiber concentrate, could be predicted by *in vitro* fermentation using human fecal inocula, *J. Nutr.*, 127, 1981, 1997.
62. Hidaka, H., Eida, T., Takizawa, T., Tokunaga, T., and Tashiro, Y., Effects of fructooligosaccharides on intestinal flora and human health, *Bifid Microflora*, 5, 37, 1986.
63. Hidaka, H., Tashiro, Y., and Toshiaki, E., Proliferation of bifidobacteria by oligosaccharides and their useful effect on human health, *Bifid Microflora*, 10, 65, 1991.
64. Williams, C., Witherly, S., and Buddington, R., Influence of dietary neosugar on selected bacterial groups of the human faecal microbiota, *Microb. Eco. Health Dis.*, 7, 91, 1993.
65. Gibson, G. R., Beatty, E. R., Wang, S., and Cummings, J. H., Selective stimulation of *Bifidobacteria* in the human colon by oligofructose and inulin, *Gastroenterology*, 108, 975, 1995.
66. Bouhnik, Y., Flourie, B., Andriew, C., Bisetti, N., Briet, N., and Rambaud, J.-C., Effects of *Bifidobacterium* sp. fermented milk ingested with or without inulin on colonic *bifidobacteria* and enzymatic activities in healthy humans, *Eur. J. Clin. Nutr.*, 50, 269, 1996.
67. Kleesen, B., Sykura, B., Sunft, H.-J., and Blaut, M., Effects of inulin and lactose on fecal microflora, microbial activity, and bowel habit in elderly constipated persons, *Am. J. Clin. Nutr.*, 65, 1397, 1997.
68. Menne, E., Guggenbuhl, N., and Roberfroid, M., Fn-type chicory inulin hydrolysate has a prebiotic effect in humans, *J. Nutr.*, 130, 1197, 2000.
69. Buddington, R. K., Williams, C. H., Chen, S.-C., and Witherly, S. A., Dietary supplement of neosugar alters the fecal flora and decreases activities of some reductive enzymes in human subjects, *Am. J. Clin. Nutr.*, 63, 709, 1996.

Interaction between Human Gut Bacteria and Dietary Fiber Substrates

Betty A. Lewis, Mary Beth Hall, and Peter J. Van Soest

Dietary fiber plays an important physiological and nutritional role in human diets. It encompasses a wide range in its chemical composition and physical characteristics.[1-3] Each source of dietary fiber has an intrinsic property that is based on its chemical composition and physical properties and which determines the biological and fermentive properties, i.e., the maximum limit for the rate and extent of fermentation for a specific substrate under optimal environmental conditions.[4,5] The effects of different dietary fibers on human intestinal bacteria are further complicated since these dietary fibers also affect environmental conditions throughout the GI tract.[5-8] Attempts to understand interactions between dietary fiber and intestinal bacteria also have to consider how responses of the GI tract will affect the fermentation.[8] The presence of dietary fiber in the human diet could affect intestinal bacteria directly through catabolite regulation and indirectly through physical changes in the GI tract environment. The amount of fiber fermented, the amount of microbial organic matter produced, and the amount of water held by each fraction must be considered in order to predict the effect of dietary fiber on colonic contents.[9] References 10–12 give more detailed information about the bacteria and the intestinal environment.

Intrinsic properties of cereal brans have received considerable attention, but other sources of dietary fiber, which include vegetables, fruits, plant gums, bacterial and wood-derived polysaccharides, and chemically and physically modified polysaccharides, offer a wide variety of properties.[13-15] Mucopolysaccharides from sloughed epithelial cells and secreted mucin glycoproteins are carbohydrates supplied by the host that are available to intestinal bacteria.[16,17] However, *in vitro* studies with *Bacteroides* species suggest that these host substances are not an important energy source for the bacteria.[18,19] The *Bacteroides*, numerically a major bacterial genus in the colon, may utilize low levels of a variety of polysaccharides *in vivo* rather than a single source. Some of the predominant anaerobic species found in the human intestine which have been studied in pure culture with carbohydrate substrates are summarized in Table 4.7.1. It is apparent that the colonic bacterial species vary in their specificity for different polysaccharides.[20] Thus, some *Bacteriodes* species can utilize different types of polysaccharides, while other species are more limited. In a study based on DNA homologies of fecal bacteria, the colon of each person evaluated had a bacterial population specific for that individual.[21]

The mechanism by which colonic bacteria digest a particular polysaccharide depends on the structure of the polysaccharide and the bacterial species.[20] Several polysaccharide-degrading enzymes have been isolated from colonic *Bacteroides* species, revealing aspects of their mode of

0-8493-2387-8/01/$0.00+$1.50

Table 4.7.1   Some of the Predominant Anaerobic Bacterial Species Found in the Human Intestine and Studied in Pure Cultures with Selected Carbohydrates

Substrate	Degradability	Bacterial Species[a]
Cellulose	Partially fermentable	1
Methyl and carboxymethyl cellulose	Partially fermentable or unfermentable	N.K.
Hemicellulose	Partially fermentable	3,4,5,8,11,13
Pectin	Highly fermentable	4,5,6,8,10,15
Cereal gums	Highly fermentable	2,6,7,9
Guar gum, locust bean gum	Highly fermentable	5,7,11,16
Arabinogalactans	Partially fermentable	5,6,7,8,9,10,14
Maillard polymer	Unfermentable	N.K.
Algal gum	Unfermentable	N.K.
Mucopolysaccharide	Highly fermentable	4,5,6,10
Mucin glycoprotein	Partially fermentable	Few *Bacteroides* strains: 12, 17

[a] Adapted from Reference 20: 1, *Bacteroides* sp.; 2, *B. distansnis*; 3, *B. eggerthii*; 4, *B. fragilis* subspecies; 5, *B. ovatus*; 6, *B. thetaiotaomicron*; 7, *B. uniformis*; 8, *B. vulgatus*; 9, *B.* "*T4-1*"; 10, *B.* "*3452A*"; 11, *Bifidobacterium adolescentis*; 12, *B. bifidum*; 13, *B. infantis*; 14, *B. longum*; 15, *Eubacterium eligens*; 16, *Ruminococcus albus*; and 17, *R. torques*. N.K., not known.

action. Thus, *B. thetaiotaomicron* degrade starch,[22] laminaran,[23] polygalacturonic acid,[24] and chondroitin sulfate[25] by induced enzymes that are cell-associated rather than extracellular. These glycanases, either soluble or membrane bound, appear to be located in the periplasmic space of the cell. They degrade the polysaccharides directly to mono- and oligosaccharides. Proteins bound to the outer cell surface of the bacteria may act as receptors to bind and facilitate transport of the polysaccharide into the cellular periplasmic space where the glycanases are located.[26] Although the neutral polysaccharides are hydrolyzed to mono- and oligosaccharides, the acidic polysaccharides are broken down by lyase enzymes which cleave glycosidic bonds by a β-elimination reaction, giving rise to C4-C5-unsaturated uronic acid oligosaccharides. In both cases the oligosaccharides are further digested to the sugars by intracellular glycosidases. Not all polysaccharides are digested to mono- and oligosaccharides by the glycanases, however. The viscous guar galactomannan was digested only to high molecular weight fragments,[27] which may be related to the distribution of branches or to the high viscosity. Aspects of the mechanisms by which colonic bacteria utilize polysaccharides have been reviewed.[28]

Person-to-person variation in the microbial fermentation of dietary fiber as shown in Table 4.7.2 was the most consistent result reported when mixed cultures of human fecal bacteria were incubated with various dietary fibers.[29,30] Variation in the microbial fermentation of different sources of dietary fiber among people reflects responses by the bacteria and responses by the intestinal tract in a particular individual. This variation was dramatic with Solka floc® as the source of dietary fiber,[29-31] with fermentation ranging from 0 to 40%. Solka floc is a processed wood cellulose, which has been used as a source of dietary fiber for human and animal experimental diets and is commercially available for food-processing applications. The chemical and biological properties of Solka floc are different from native vegetable and forage celluloses.[32] Mixed rumen bacteria incubated with Solka floc usually demonstrate an 18- to 24-h lag before significant fermentation is observed.[4,5]

Rumen bacteria and human fecal bacteria that ferment dietary fiber have many similarities in respect to nutritional requirements, volatile fatty acid production, and fermentation balances.[33-36] However, human fecal, bovine ruminal, and equine cecal bacteria differed in their ability to ferment fiber from various sources (Table 4.7.3).[4] Some humans also produce methane gas.[36]

The source of fiber supplement can have both short- and long-term effects on digestibility of other fiber sources. Ehle et al.[30] reported that the source of dietary fiber (coarse white wheat bran, AACC-certified food grade R07-3691; cabbage; and Solka floc) in the diet was a significant factor

Table 4.7.2   Concentration (g/g) of Various Neutral Detergent Fibers Remaining after Incubation with Inoculum from Three Human Donors at Various Times in Batch Culture

Substrate[a]	Hours	Human Donor					
		1	SD	2	SD	3	SD
Cabbage	6	0.58[b]	0.03	0.56	0.02	0.39	0.05
Wheat bran	6	0.69	0.02	0.86	0.01	0.72	0.02
Alfalfa	6	0.85	0.01	0.83	0.02	0.89	0.02
Cabbage	24	0.10	0.01	0.20	0.03	0.17	0.02
Wheat bran	24	0.56	0.04	0.53	0.03	0.53	0.04
Alfalfa	24	0.61	0.03	0.65	0.02	0.59	0.05
Cabbage	48	0.05	0.02	0.07	0.01	0.14	0.05
Wheat bran	48	0.56	0.02	0.53	0.03	0.53	0.01
Alfalfa	48	0.59	0.04	0.60	0.04	0.54	0.03
Solka floc®	48	1.00	0.01	0.99	0.03	0.77	0.02

[a] Ethanol-extracted cabbage, coarse white wheat bran (AACC-certified RO7 3691), Solka floc® (food grade cellulose), and alfalfa hay.
[b] $n = 3$, replicates.

Table 4.7.3   Effect of Inoculum Source on the Fermentation of Neutral Detergent Fibers of Various Substrates

Inoculum:	Fermentation (%)				
		Bovine		Equine	
Source:	Human Feces	Concentrate-Fed Rumen	Hay-Fed Rumen	Hay-Fed Cecum	Hay- and Grain-Fed Cecum
Substrate					
Alfalfa	38	53	57	49	50
Timothy	1	40	50	32	27
Wheat bran[a]	53	56	71	—	—
Cabbage[b]	91	91	91	—	—
Wheat straw	0	31	42	—	—

[a] Coarse white wheat bran (AACC-certified food grade RO7-3691).
[b] Ethanol-extracted cabbage, see Ehle et al.[30]

Source: Jeraci, J. L., Interactions between Rumen or Human Fecal Inocula and Fiber Substrates, Master's thesis, Cornell University, Ithaca, NY, 1981. With permission.

influencing the *in vitro* fermentation of coarse white wheat bran, ethanol-extracted cabbage, Solka floc, and alfalfa hay when incubated with the respective human fecal bacteria. No long-term microbial adaptation to these fiber-supplemented diets was observed, since fermentation values obtained from 12 individuals who received a single fiber supplement for an extended period of time (approximately 70 days) did not differ from fermentation values obtained in another 12 individuals who received a different fiber supplement every 2 weeks. In the same study, the apparent *in vivo* fermentation of neutral detergent fiber (NDF) was significantly affected by the source of dietary fiber in the fiber-supplemented diets. Estimates of the apparent *in vivo* fermentation were confounded by the quantity of microbial organic matter and the presence or lack (for cabbage) of unfermented residue from the diet in the feces. However, the true calculated *in vivo* fermentation of NDF was affected by the source of dietary fiber. Regardless of the dietary fiber source, ingestion of Solka floc in any 2-week period resulted in the carryover effect of depressed fermentation of NDF in all future periods.

The observation that previous exposure to Solka floc depressed the fermentation of other dietary fiber substrates was confirmed with *in vitro* techniques.[8,37] Fermentations with human fecal bacteria showed a 36-h depression of pectin fermentation in batch culture only when the bacterial inoculum came from a continuous culture that received Solka floc as the substrate. A selective depression of

Solka floc fermentation in the batch culture flasks was not observed when bacteria received Solka floc or pectin as the continuous culture substrate. This would suggest that certain modified or highly crystalline sources of cellulose may generate unexpected artifacts in fiber digestion studies. Although colonic fermentation of the hydrated and less lignified cellulose of plant foods has been well established for humans,[32,38] fermentation of the more crystalline isolated celluloses (Solka floc, filter paper) by fecal bacteria has been demonstrated for only 20 to 30% of the subjects studied.[30–32,39]

Resistance of polysaccharides to fermentation has also been related to binding to other components in the plant cell wall and to branching patterns of polysaccharides, in addition to intra- and intermolecular H-bonding with consequent lack of hydration and solubility.

Significant amounts of starch (20%) may survive digestion and absorption in the small intestine.[40] The proportion of dietary starch passing the ileum is related to the plant source, food-processing effects, diet portion, and individual variation. This resistant or nondigested starch, like other nondigestible polysaccharides, is fermented to short-chain fatty acids (SCFA) and the gases hydrogen, methane, and carbon dioxide. Recent studies have shown differences among human subjects in the rate at which the fecal bacteria ferment the starch and in the relative proportions of the individual SCFA formed.[41,42] Weaver et al.[43] observed significantly higher proportions of acetate and lower proportions of butyrate to total SCFA in subjects with polyps or colon cancer. Butyrate, the predominant energy source for colonocytes, may play a regulatory role in the pathogenesis of colon cancer.

In vitro systems have been evaluated as models for fermentation of fiber in the large intestine.[8,44] Human feces afford an adequate and representative inoculum for *in vitro* systems and have been used in many studies of colonic fermentation.[9,45,46] In an *in vitro* system, SCFA production from fermentation of ileal effluents was significantly correlated with SCFA production from dietary fiber isolates but not with the SCFA production from whole foods.[47]

REFERENCES

1. Eastwood, M. A., The physiological effect of dietary fiber: an update, *Ann. Rev. Nutr.*, 12, 19, 1992.
2. Selvendran, R. R. and MacDougall, A. J., Cell-wall chemistry and architecture in relation to sources of dietary fibre, *Eur. J. Clin. Nutr.*, 49, S3, S27, 1995.
3. Van Soest, P. J. and Robertson, J. B., Chemical and physical properties of dietary fibre, in *Dietary Fibre, Proc. Miles Symp. 1976*, Halfax, Nova Scotia, Nutr. Soc. Canada, Hawkins, W. W., Ed., Miles Laboratories, Ltd., Rexdale, Ontario, 13.
4. Jeraci, J. L., *Interactions between Rumen or Human Fecal Inocula and Fiber Substrates*, Master's thesis, Cornell University, Ithaca, NY, 1981.
5. Van Soest, P. J., *Nutritional Ecology of the Ruminant*, 2nd ed., Cornell University Press, Ithaca, NY, 1994.
6. Stevens, C. E., Physiological implications of microbial digestion in the large intestine of mammals: relation to dietary factors, *Am. J. Clin. Nutr.*, 31 (suppl.), S161, 1978.
7. Spiller, G. A., Chernoff, M. C., Hill, R. A., Gates, J. E., Nassar, J. J., and Shipley, E. A., Effect of purified cellulose, pectin, and a low-residue diet on fecal volatile fatty acids, transit-time, and fecal weight in humans, *Am. J. Clin. Nutr.*, 33, 754, 1980.
8. Jeraci, J. L., Use of the High Fiber Chemostat System to Study Interactions among Gut Microflora, Ph.D. thesis, Cornell University, Ithaca, NY, 1984.
9. McBurney, M. I., Horvath, P. J., Jeraci, J. L., and Van Soest, P. J., Effect of in vitro fermentation using human faecal inoculum on the water-holding capacity of dietary fibre, *Br. J. Nutr.*, 53, 17, 1985.
10. Roth, H. P. and Mehlman, M. A., Eds., Symposium on role of dietary fiber in health, *Am. J. Clin. Nutr.*, 31 (suppl.), 1978.
11. Hentges, D. J., Ed., *Human Intestinal Microflora in Health and Disease*, Academic Press, New York, 1983.
12. Cummings, J. H. and Macfarlane, G. T., The control and consequences of bacterial fermentation in the human colon, *J. Appl. Bacteriol.*, 70, 443, 1991.

13. Cummings, J. H., Hill, M. J., Jenkins, P. J. A., Pearson, J. R., and Wiggins, H. S., Changes in fecal composition and colonic function due to cereal fiber, *Am. J. Clin. Nutr.*, 29, 1468, 1976.

14. Van Soest, P. J., Horvath, P. J., McBurney, M. I., Jeraci, J. L., and Allen, M., Some in vitro and in vivo properties of dietary fibers from noncereal sources, in *Unconventional Sources of Dietary Fiber*, Series 214, Furda, I., Ed., American Chemical Society, Washington, D.C., 1983.

15. Horvath, P. J., The Measurement of Dietary Fiber and the Effects of Fermentation, Ph.D. thesis, Cornell University, Ithaca, NY, 1984.

16. Savage, D. C., Factors involved in colonization of the gut epithelial surface, in Symp. on Role of Dietary Fiber in Health, Roth, H. P. and Mehlman, M. A., Eds., *Am. J. Clin. Nutr.*, 31 (suppl.), S131, 1978.

17. Salyers, A. A., O'Brien, M., and Schmetter, B., Catabolism of mucopolysaccharides, plant gums, and Maillard products by human colonic *Bacteroides*, in *Unconventional Sources of Dietary Fiber*, Series 214, Furda, I., Ed., American Chemical Society, Washington, D.C., 1983.

18. Salyers, A. A. and McCarthy, R. E., Assessing the importance of host-derived polysaccharides as carbon sources for bacteria growing in the human colon, *Anim. Feed Sci. Tech.*, 23, 109, 1989.

19. Salyers, A. A., Activities of polysaccharide-degrading bacteria in the human colon, in *Dietary Fiber: Chemistry, Physiology, and Health Effects*, Kritchevsky, D., Bonfield, C., and Anderson, J. W., Eds., Plenum Press, New York, 1990, 187.

20. Salyers, A. A., Energy sources of major intestinal fermentative anaerobes, in 5th Int. Symp. on Intestinal Microecology, Luckey, T. D., Ed., *Am. J. Clin. Nutr.*, 32, 158, 1979.

21. Johnson, J. L., Specific strains of *Bacteroides* species in human fecal flora as measured by deoxyribonucleic acid homology, *Appl. Environ. Microbiol.*, 39, 407, 1980.

22. Smith, K. and Salyers, A. A., Purification and characterization of enzymes involved in starch utilization by *Bacteroides thetaiotaomicron*, *J. Bacteriol.*, 173, 2962, 1991.

23. Salyers, A. A., Palmer, J. K., and Wilkins, T. D., Laminarinase (β-glucanase) activity in *Bacteroides* from the human colon, *Appl. Environ. Microbiol.*, 33, 1118, 1977.

24. McCarthy, R. E., Kotarski, S. F., and Salyers, A. A., Location and characteristics of enzymes involved in the breakdown of polygalacturonic acid by *Bacteroides thetaiotaomicron*, *J. Bacteriol.*, 161, 493, 1985.

25. Salyers, A. A. and O'Brien, M., Cellular location of enzymes involved in chondroitin sulfate breakdown by *Bacteroides thetaiotaomicron*, *J. Bacteriol.*, 143, 772, 1980.

26. Cheng, Q., Yu, M. C., Reeves, A. R., and Salyers, A. A., Identification and characterization of a *Bacteriodes* gene, *csuF*, which encodes an outer membrane protein that is essential for growth on chondroitin sulfate, *J. Bacteriol.*, 177, 3721, 1995.

27. Gherardini, F. C. and Salyers, A. A., Characterization of an outer membrane mannanase from *Bacteriodes ovatus*, *J. Bacteriol.*, 169, 2031, 1987.

28. Salyers, A. A., Polysaccharide utilization by human colonic bacteria, in *New Developments in Dietary Fiber*, Furda, I. and Brine, C. J., Eds., Plenum Press, New York, 1990, 151.

29. Jeraci, J. L., Robertson, J. B., and Van Soest, P. J., A human fecal inoculum in the in vitro fermentation procedure, *J. Anim. Sci. Suppl.*, 51, 206, 1980.

30. Ehle, F. R., Robertson, J. B., and Van Soest, P. J., Influence of dietary fibers on fermentation in the human large intestine, *J. Nutr.*, 112, 158, 1982.

31. Betian, H. G., Linehan, B. A., Bryant, M. P., and Holdeman, L. V., Isolation of a cellulolytic *Bacteroides* sp. from human feces, *Appl. Environ. Microbiol.*, 33, 1009, 1977.

32. Van Soest, P. J., Jeraci, J. L., Foose, T., Wrick, K., and Ehle, F. R., Comparative fermentation of fibre in man and other animals, in *Proc. Dietary Fibre in Human and Animal Nutrition Symp.*, Wallace, G. and Bell, L., Eds., The Royal Society of New Zealand, Palmerston North, N.Z., 1982.

33. Bryant, M. P., Nutritional features and ecology of predominant anaerobic bacteria of the intestinal tract, *Am. J. Clin. Nutr.*, 27, 1313, 1974.

34. Miller, T. L. and Wolin, M. J., Fermentations by saccharolytic intestinal bacteria, in 5th Int. Symp. on Intestinal Microecology, Luckey, T. D., Ed., *Am. J. Clin. Nutr.*, 32, 164, 1979.

35. Smith, C. J. and Bryant, M. P., Introduction to metabolic activities of intestinal bacteria, in 5th Int. Symp. on Intestinal Microecology, Luckey, T. D., Ed., *Am. J. Clin. Nutr.*, 32, 149, 1979.

36. Wolin, M. J. and Miller, T. L., Carbohydrate fermentation, in *Human Intestinal Microflora in Health and Disease*, Hentges, D. J., Ed., Academic Press, New York, 1983, 147.

37. Jeraci, J. L. and Horvath, P. J., In vitro fermentation of dietary fiber by human fecal organisms, *Anim. Feed Sci. Tech.*, 23, 121, 1989.
38. Cummings, J. H., Microbial digestion of complex carbohydrates in man, *Proc. Nutr. Soc.*, 43, 35, 1984.
39. Wedekind, K. J., Mansfield, H. R., and Montgomery, L., Enumeration and isolation of cellulolytic and hemicellulolytic bacteria from human feces, *Appl. Environ. Microbiol.*, 54, 1530, 1988.
40. Stephen, A. M., Haddad, A. C., and Phillips, S. F., Passage of carbohydrates into the colon, *Gastroenterology*, 85, 589, 1983.
41. Weaver, G. A., Krause, J. A., Miller, T. L., and Wolin, M. J., Constancy of glucose and starch fermentations by two different human faecal microbial communities, *Gut,* 30, 19, 1989.
42. Scheppach, W., Fabian, C., Sachs, M., and Kasper, H., The effect of starch malabsorption on fecal short-chain fatty acid excretion in man, *Scand. J. Gastroenterol.*, 23, 755, 1988.
43. Weaver, G. A., Krause, J. A., Miller, T. L., and Wolin, M. J., Short chain fatty acid distributions of enema samples from a sigmoidoscopy population: an association of high acetate and low butyrate ratios with adenomatous polyps and colon cancer, *Gut,* 29, 1539, 1988.
44. Macfarlane, S., Quigley, M. E., Hopkins, M. J., Newton, D. F., and Macfarlane, G. T., Polysaccharide degradation by human intestinal bacteria during growth under multi-substrate limiting conditions in a three-stage continuous culture system, *FEMS Microbiol. Ecology*, 26, 231, 1998.
45. McBurney, M. I. and Thompson, L. U., Effect of human faecal inoculum on in vitro fermentation variables, *Br. J. Nutr.*, 58, 233, 1987.
46. McBurney, M. I. and Thompson, L. U., Dietary fiber and energy balance: integration of the human ileostomy and in vitro fermentation models, *Anim. Feed Sci. Tech.*, 23, 261, 1989.
47. McBurney, M. I., Thompson, L. U., Cuff, D. J., and Jenkins, D. J. A., Comparison of ileal effluents, dietary fibers, and whole foods in predicting the physiological importance of colonic fermentation, *Am. J. Gastroenterol.*, 83, 536, 1988.

Effects of Dietary Fiber on Digestive Enzymes

Barbara O. Schneeman and Daniel Gallaher

Dietary fibers affect the functioning of the GI tract as indicated by a lower digestibility and availability of nutrients from high-fiber diets. Assimilation of nutrients from diets requires the movement of the bolus of food through the gut, the enzymatic hydrolysis of complex nutrients to simpler compounds, and absorption of these compounds into and through the small intestinal cells. The presence of dietary fibers can alter these processes, resulting in a slower rate of nutrient absorption and a shift in the site of absorption to the more distal areas of the small intestine. In this chapter, the effects of dietary fibers on digestive enzyme activity and on the intestinal contents are reviewed.

Table 4.8.1 presents the effects of various fiber sources on amylase, lipase, trypsin, chymotrypsin, or pepsin activity *in vitro*. The enzymes were derived from human samples or from commercial enzyme preparations. In general, commercial lipase or amylase is of porcine origin, and -trypsin and chymotrypsin are of bovine origin. Discrepancies are most likely due to the enzyme source or to the method of incubating the fiber and enzyme and reporting values. As shown in Table 4.8.2, lipase inhibitory activity is associated with several cereals.

Addition of fiber sources to an *in vitro* protein digestibility test can lead to reductions in the percentage of digestible casein (Table 4.8.3), indicating that fibers can interfere with proteolytic enzyme activity. Other *in vitro* data indicate that certain foods which contain fiber may slow starch or carbohydrate hydrolysis (Table 4.8.4). For both carbohydrates and protein, the change in *in vitro* digestibility was dependent on the source of fiber (Tables 4.8.3 and 4.8.4). The data in Table 4.8.4 indicate that the physical state of the plant cell wall rather than simply the presence of dietary fiber may be important in slowing the rate of carbohydrate hydrolysis. Grinding brown rice or lentil samples significantly increased the percentage of starch hydrolyzed in a 30-minute period.[11] These results indicate that the physical state of the food or of the cell wall layers can slow the penetration of digestive enzymes.[11,13] Tinker and Schneeman[14] demonstrated *in vivo* that the consumption of the viscous polysaccharide, guar gum, slows the disappearance of starch from the small intestine of rats. An interference with starch hydrolysis by amylase may contribute to this effect. These studies suggest that slowing enzymatic hydrolysis in the intestine could contribute to the apparent slower rate of nutrient assimilation associated with certain fiber-rich foods or diets.

The activity of digestive enzymes *in vivo* has been estimated (Table 4.8.5). Both rat studies, collecting total intestinal contents, and human studies based on a sample of duodenal aspirate indicate that within the intestinal contents pancreatic enzyme activities are either similar or significantly higher when a fiber supplement is added to a basal diet. In pancreatic duct cannulated rats, instillation of a pectin test diet reduced amylase and chymotrypsin secretion; however, infusion of

Table 4.8.1   Percent of Control Enzyme Activity In Vitro

Fiber Source	Amylase	Lipase	Trypsin	Chymotrypsin	Pepsin	Ref.
Alfalfa		48.6	63.0*	93.9		1c
Alfalfa	87.3	72.8	29.0*	51.6*		2d
Oat bran	72.6	83.83	94.9	71.3		2
Wheat bran	8.0					1
Wheat bran		82.1	96.1	90.8		1
Wheat bran	66.9*	85.9	93.8	76.2		2
Rice bran		70.0	92.1	90.1		1
Safflower meal		44.6*	56.3*	90.1		1
Xylan	32.7*	31.0*	11.2*	20.0*		2
Xylan		20.8*	91.8	98.5		1
Cellulose	20.4*	4.6*	55.3*	52.9*		2
Cellulose		9.9*	87.5	78.3*		1
Pectin		113.0	105.0	105.0		1
Pectin	148.0*	123.0	100.0	129.0*		2
Pectin-HMa	50.0	20.0	40.0	20.0		4+e
Pectin-LMb	0.0	5.0	12.0	25.0		4+
Pectin					98.0	5+c
Guar gum	54.0					3+e
Guar gum	60.0	45.0	90.0	95.0		4+
Guar gum			74.0			6+c
Carob bean Gum			121.0			6+
Na-alginate			89.0			6+
Agar-agar			101.0			6+
Carrageenan					74.0	5+
Carrageenan			Inhibits			7+c
Carrageenan					Inhibits	8+c
Carrageenan			59.0			6+
Psyllium	59.0					3+
Lignin	100.0					3+

Note: An asterisk means that there was a significant change from control. A plus sign in the reference column indicates that a statistical analysis was not reported in these studies.

a High methoxy.
b Low methoxy.
c Commercial enzyme source was used.
d Human pancreatic juice was used.
e Human duodenal juice was used.

Table 4.8.2   Pancreatic Lipase Inhibition by Cereals, In Vitro

Cereal Source	Lipase Inhibitory Activitya (IU/g)
French soft wheat	25.6 ± 1.1
French durum wheat	33.6 ± 1.0
Scandinavian soft wheat	43.3 ± 4.1
North American hard wheat	37.9 ± 1.1
Barley (8 varieties)	23.5 ± 2.0
White sorghum (5 varieties)	22.4 ± 4.8
Red sorghum (4 varieties)	3.3 ± 1.5
Millet (6 varieties)	37.3 ± 3.3

a Defined by Borel et al. (1989) as the mg of material that decrease lipase activity by 50% under their experimental conditions.

Source: Adapted from Cara et al.[9]

Table 4.8.3   Decrease in *In Vitro* Casein Digestibility^a Due to Fiber Addition

Fiber Source	Decrease Digestibility of Casein	Fiber: Protein (wt:wt)
Holocellulose	1.66	0.4
Lignin	1.36	0.4
Citrus pectin	4.03	0.4
Xylan	5.34	0.4
Karaya gum	4.42	0.4
Wheat bran	0.15	0.5
Brown rice	7.64	0.5
Cooked broccoli	8.93	0.5
Cooked blackeyed peas	9.35	0.5
Canned corn	14.86	0.5

[a] Enzyme mixture was trypsin, chymotrypsin, and peptidase followed by a bacterial protease.

Source: Adapted from Gagne, C. M. and Acton, J. C., *J. Food Sci.*, 48, 734, 1983. With permission.

Table 4.8.4   *In Vitro* Carbohydrate Hydrolysis of Foods

Product	% Starch Hydrolyzed in 30 min	% Carbohydrate Released in 3 h	Ref.
Wheat			
Rolled	5.1		11[a]
Cooked, rolled	45.8		11[a]
White bread	77.6		11[a]
Whole meal bread	80.1		11[a]
Whole meal bread		27	12[b]
Rice			
Cooked, brown	17.6		11[a]
Cooked, ground brown	68.2		11[a]
Cooked, white	30.8		11[a]
Cooked, ground white	71.8		11[a]
Rye, rolled	11.9		11[a]
Barley, rolled	13.5		11[a]
Oats, rolled cooked	68		11[a]
Maize, cooked rneal	71.5		11[a]
Brown lentils			
Whole	12.1		13[a]
Ground	60.9		13[a]
Lentils, ground cooked		15	12[b]
Soybeans, ground cooked		6	12[b]

[a] Enzyme source is commercial α-amylase and amyloglucosidase.
[b] Enzyme source is human saliva and jejunal juice.

a pectin alone (i.e., not in a test diet) did not change basal pancreatic protein secretion from basal values.[17] In contrast, two viscous polysaccharides, konjac mannan and Na-alginate, have been reported to increase pancreatic output,[18] although this response could be due to long-term adaptation to continual feeding and not a change in the acute response. The data in Table 4.8.5 illustrate an interesting point: although various fibers may interfere with digestive enzyme activity based on *in vitro* evidence, they do not reduce the total amount of measurable digestive enzyme activity in the gut contents. The only reported significant decrease in enzyme activity occurred in pancreatectomy

Table 4.8.5 *In Vivo* Pancreatic Enzyme Activity: Values Expressed as Percentage of Fiber-Free Treated Controls

Fiber Source	Amylase	Lipase	Trypsin	Chymotrypsin	Protease	Species	Ref.
Total Units in Intestinal Contents (% Control)							
Apple pectin	119	193*			142*	Rat	18
Carrageenan	121	203*			140*		
Na-alginate	111	208*			136*		
Locust gum	104	167*			134*		
Xanthan gum	109	303*			142*		
Guar gum	115	321*			161*		
Cellulose	142	89.5	114	69.6		Rat	15
Wheat bran	71	172*	101	80.4			
Pectin	152*	216*	240*	138*			
Guar gum	141*	218*			159*		
Total Units in Ileostomy Fluid (% Control)							
Pectin	883	359*	151			Rat	19
Wheat bran	488	187	180*				
Units per ml of Intestinal Fluid (% Control)							
Pectin	175*	144	154	130		Human	16
Carob flour	179*	218*	228	163*			
Pectin[a]	53*	37*	37*			Human	20
Wheat bran[b]	48*	45	65				
Rate of Pancreatic Secretion (% Control)							
Pectin	47.8*	61.5			44.9*	Rat	16
Carob flour	91.4	108			63.6		
Carrageenan	56.8	51.4			51.3		
Guar gum	67.2	114			102		
Pectin	122	125			185	Rat	18
Carrageenan	115	132			217*		
Na-alginate	155*	109			170		
Locust gum	153*	160			208*		
Xanthan gum	173*	155			205*		
Guar gum	232*	186*			250*		
Cellulose Pectin	No change in pancreatic protein secretion from baseline					Rat	17

Note: * The value was reported as different from the fiber-free treated control.

[a] Pancreatectomized patients who received a pancreatic enzyme supplement.
[b] Chronic pancreatitis patients who did not receive an enzyme supplement.

or pancreatitis patients, who cannot respond effectively by increasing secretion.[20] Enzyme activity from intestinal contents is typically measured under *in vitro* conditions that optimize activity and thus may not reflect the physiologically available activity within the gut contents. To answer the question of whether fiber sources cm slow the rate of substrate hydrolysis, *in vivo* studies have been conducted that estimate the rate or extent of lipid and carbohydrate disappearance from the gastrointestinal tract.

Table 4.8.6 summarizes several studies conducted in humans and rats to determine if fiber supplements will delay the absorption of lipid. The physiological importance of *in vitro* lipase inhibition by wheat bran and wheat germ has been studied extensively.[9,25] Borel et al.[25] reported that feeding wheat bran or wheat germ decreases gastrointestinal lipolysis of fats, resulting in lower intestinal absorption of cholesterol and fatty acids. Experimental evidence suggests that *in vitro* inhibition of lipase by cereal fractions may be due to a protein fraction.[9] However, *in vivo* reductions

Table 4.8.6 Effect of Fiber Sources on Lipid Digestion and Absorption

Fiber Source	Dose	Results	Ref.
		Human Studies	
Pectin	5 g	Triolein breath test indicated a 30% reduction in lipid digestibility in pancreatectomized patients receiving enzyme replacement	20
Pectin	15 g/day	Fat excretion in ileostomy fluid increased by 36%	21
Wheat bran	20 g	Triolein breath test indicated up to a 30% reduction in lipid digestibility in pancreatitis patients	20
Wheat bran	16 g/day	No change in fat excretion in ileostomy fluid	22
		Animal Studies	
Cellulose	20%	Intestinal disappearance of triolein reduced by 20–30% for 5-h period after meal compared to fiber-free group	23
Cellulose	10%	Lymphatic appearance of triolein was not lower than fiber-free adapted rats; appearance of cholesterol was lower at 4 h but not at 24 h after lipid infusion	33
Wheat bran	10%	Delayed the disappearance of triglyceride from the gastrointestinal tract	25
Wheat bran	20%	1.6-fold nonsignificant increase in the excretion of fat in ileostomy fluid	19
Wheat germ	10%	Delayed the disappearance of triglyceride from the gastrointestinal tract	25
Guar gum	5%	Lymphatic appearance of triolein and cholesterol was lower than fiber-free adapted rats at 4 h after lipid infusion; only cholesterol appearance was lower at 24 h	33
Guar gum	5%	Intestinal disappearance of cholesterol and triolein was 20–25% lower than cellulose at 2 h after meal	24
Pectin	5%	Lymphatic appearance of triolein and cholesterol was lower than fiber-free adapted rats at 4 h after lipid infusion; only cholesterol appearance was lower at 24 h	33
Pectin	5%	Threefold significant increase in the excretion of fat in ileostomy fluid	19
Konjac mannan	5%	Intestinal disappearance of cholesterol and triolein was 40% lower than cellulose at 2 h after meal	24
Chitosan	5%	Intestinal disappearance of cholesterol and triolein did not differ from cellulose at 2 h after meal	24
Psyllium husk	5%	Lymphatic appearance of triolein and cholesterol was lower than fiber-free treatment at 4 and 24 h after lipid infusion	33

of lipid digestion may be due to interference with micelle formation as well as direct inhibition of lipolytic activity. The results summarized in Table 4.8.6 indicate that sources of viscous polysaccharides reduce the overall rate of lipid digestion.

The change in the activity of small intestinal brush order enzymes with fiber treatments in animals is shown in Table 4.8.7. Two of the studies tend to report increases in enzyme activity due to the fiber supplement where a change in activity was observed, and two studies reported decreases with pectin treatment. One study reported that thymidine kinase activity was higher than the fiber-free control in rats fed alfalfa, guar gum, or psyllium, but not in those fed cellulose or pectin. This apparent discrepancy is most likely due to factors such as feeding very high levels of fiber, use of weanling animals that may be unable to adapt to high fiber intakes, not fasting the animals prior to killing them for collection of intestinal mucosa, or differences in the site of tissue sampling. In Table 4.8.8, we have summarized a variety of reasons that will lead to different observations when examining digestive enzyme adaptation and activity.

In altering digestion and absorption in the small intestine, another effect of dietary fiber could be to alter the composition of the intestinal contents. Table 4.8.9 gives the effect of several fibers on viscosity of human duodenal juice, and Figure 4.8.1 presents the viscosity of gastric and intestinal

Table 4.8.7   Small Intestinal Enzyme Activity: Change in Enzyme Activity

Fiber Source	Peptidase	Sucrase	Lactase	Maltase	Thymidine Kinase	Ref.
Pectin	↑	NC	–	–	–	26
Pectin	–	↓	↓	NC	–	27
Pectin	–	↑	↑	↑	–	28
Pectin	↓[a]	–	–	–	–	29
Pectin	–	NC	–	–	NC	30
Cellulose	↑	NC	–	–	–	26
Cellulose	–	NC	NC	NC	–	27
Cellulose	–	NC	NC	NC	–	28
Cellulose	–	NC	–	–	NC	30
Oat bran	NC	NC	–	–	–	26
Wheat bran	NC	NC	–	NC	–	31
Alfalfa	–	–	–	–	↑[b]	30
Guar gum	–	↑[a]	–	–	↑[a,b]	30
Psyllium	–	↑[a]	–	–	↑[a,b]	30

Note: ↑,↓ = direction of change from control; NC = no change; – = not determined.

[a] Proximal intestine.
[b] Distal intestine.

Table 4.8.8   Reasons for Differences in Enzyme Values

Use of weanling vs. adult animals
Level and type of fiber added
Protein content of the diet
Fasting or fed state at time of killing
Methodology differences relative to sample preparation and analysis
Method of expressing units relative to volume of sample, milligrams of tissue, protein, or DNA

Table 4.8.9   Effect of Dietary Fiber on Viscosity of Duodenal Juice (mPa)

Duodenal juice	30
LM-pectin (2.5 g%)	40
HM-pectin (1.5 g%)	200
Guar gum (0. 15 g%)	500
Wheat bran (1.5 g%)	90

Source: Adapted from Isaksson, G., et al., *Gastroenterology*, 82, 918, 1982.

contents of rats fed different fiber sources. In addition, it has been reported that addition of fiber to a basal diet will increase the volume and weight of intestinal content in rats.[15,31,32] Sandberg et al.[21,22] reported that the wet weight of ileostomy fluid was increased by 94 g/d due to wheat bran and by 314 g/d due to pectin. The greater volume or viscosity of intestinal contents will have an impact on the interaction of substrates and enzymes as well as on the movement of nutrients to sites for absorption.

Hydrolysis of triglycerides in the stomach and small intestine is related to the surface area available. The lipase enzymatic systems act at this interface to release free fatty acids, diglycerides, and monoglycerides. The amount of surface area available is determined by the size of lipid droplets and/or micelles.[34] Pasquier et al.[35,36] have demonstrated *in vitro* that viscous polysaccharides increase the size of lipid droplets under conditions that mimic the stomach or small intestine. Under conditions that mimic gastric contents, a threefold increase in droplet size was associated

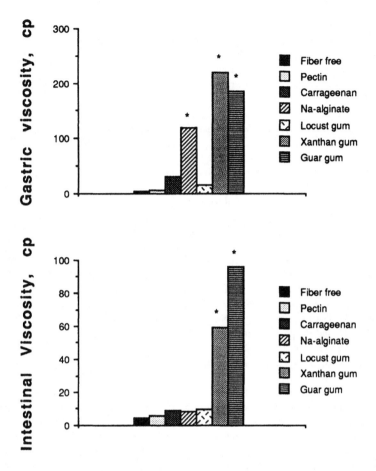

Figure 4.8.1 Gastric and intestinal viscosity in rats fed different fiber sources. *Value differs significantly from the fiber-free control group ($p < 0.05$). (Data adapted from Ikegami et al., 1990.[18])

with reduced surface area and about a 30% reduction in the extent of triglyceride hydrolysis. Likewise, with conditions that mimic the duodenum *in vitro*, triglyceride hydrolysis was inversely correlated with viscosity and an increase in viscosity resulted in larger lipid droplets. The effects of viscous polysaccharides on *in vitro* lipid emulsification and hydrolysis have been confirmed *in vivo* in rat studies.[34]

REFERENCES

1. Schneeman, B. O., Effect of plant fiber on lipase, trypsin, and chymotrypsin activity, *J. Food Sci.*, 43, 634, 1978.

2. Dunaif, G. and Schneeman, B. O., The effect of dietary fiber on human pancreatic enzyme activity in vitro, *Am. J. Clin. Nutr.*, 34, 10349, 1981.

3. Hansen, W. E. and Schulz, G., The effect of dietary fiber on pancreatic amylase activity in vitro, *Hepato-Gastroenterology*, 29, 157, 1982.

4. Isaksson, G., Lundquist, I., and Ihse, I., Effect of dietary fiber on pancreatic enzyme activity in vitro, *Gastroenterology*, 82, 918, 1982.

5. Houck, J. C., Bhayana, J., and Lee, T., The inhibition of pepsin and peptic ulcers, *Gastroenterology*, 39, 196, 1960.

6. Harmuth-Hoene, A. E. and Schwerdtfeger, E., Effect of indigestible polysaccharides on protein digestibility and nitrogen retention in growing rats, *Nutr. Metab.*, 23, 399, 1979.
7. Gatfield, I. L. and Stute, R., Enzymatic reactions in the presence of polymers. The competitive inhibition of trypsin by A-carrageenan, *FEBS Lett.*, 28, 29, 1972.
8. Anderson, W., Baille, A. J., and Harthill, J. E., Peptic inhibition by macroanions, *J. Pharm. Pharmacol.*, 20, 715, 1968.
9. Cara, R., Borel, P., Armaud, M., Lafont, H., Lesgards, G., and Lairon, D., Milling and processing of wheat and other cereals affect their capacity to inhibit lipase in vitro, *J. Food Sci.*, in press.
10. Gagne, C. M. and Acton, J. C., Fiber constituents and fibrous food residues effects on the in vitro enzymatic digestion of protein, *J. Food Sci.*, 48, 734, 1983.
11. Snow, P. and O'Dea, K., Factors affecting the rate of hydrolysis of starch in food, *Am. J. Clin. Nutr.*, 34, 2721, 1981.
12. Jenkins, D. J. A., Rate of digestion of foods and postprandial glycaemia in normal and diabetic subjects, *Br. Med. J.*, 281, 14, 1980.
13. Wong, S. and O'Dea, K., Importance of physical form rather than viscosity in determining the rate of starch hydrolysis in legumes, *Am. J. Clin. Nutr.*, 37, 66, 1983.
14. Tinker, L. F. and Schneeman, B. O., The effect of guar gum or wheat bran on the disappearance of ^{14}C-labelled starch from the rat gastrointestinal tract, *J. Nutr.*, 119, 403, 1989.
15. Schneeman, B. O., Forman, L. P., and Gallaher, D., Pancreatic and intestinal enzyme activity in rats fed various fiber sources, in *Fiber in Human and Animal Nutrition*, Wallace, G. and Bell, L., Eds., Bulletin 20, The Royal Society of New Zealand, 1983, 139.
16. Sommer, H. and Kasper, H., The effect of dietary fiber on the pancreatic excretory function, *Hepato-Gastroenterology*, 27, 477, 1980.
17. Schneeman, B. O., Acute pancreatic and biliary response to protein, cellulose and pectin, *Nutr. Rep. Int.*, 20, 45, 1979.
18. Ikegami, S., Tsuchihashi, N., Harada, H., and Innami, S., Effects of viscous indigestible polysaccharides on pancreatic biliary secretion and digestive organs in rats, *J. Nutr.*, 120, 353, 1990.
19. Isaksson, G., Asp, N.-G., and Ihse, I., Effects of dietary fiber on pancreatic enzyme activities of ileostomy evacuates and on excretion of fat and nitrogen in the rat, *Scand. J. Gastroenterol.*, 18, 417, 1983.
20. Isaksson, G., Lundquist, I., Akesson, B., and Ihse, I., Effects of pectin and wheat bran on intraluminal pancreatic enzyme activities and on fat absorption as examined with the triolein breath test in patients with pancreatic insufficiency, *Scand. J. Gastroenterol.*, 19, 467, 1984.
21. Sandberg, A.-S., Ahderinne, R., Andersson, H., Hallgren, B., Hasselblad, K., Isaksson, B., and Hultén, L., The effects of citrus pectin on the absorption of nutrients in the small intestine, *Human Nutrition: Clinical Nutrition*, 37C, 171, 1983.
22. Sandberg, A.-S., Andersson, H., Hallgren, B., Hasselblad, K., Isaksson, B., and Hulten, L., Experimental model for in vivo determination of dietary fibre and its effects on the absorption of nutrients in the small intestine, *Br. J. Nutr.*, 45, 283, 1981.
23. Gallaher, D. and Schneeman, B. O., Effect of dietary cellulose on site of lipid absorption, *Am. J. Physiol.*, 249, G184, 1985.
24. Ebihara, K. and Schneeman, B. O., Interaction of bile acids, phospholipids, cholesterol, and triglycerides with dietary fibers in the small intestine of rats, *J. Nutr.*, 119, 1100, 1989.
25. Borel, P., Lairon, D., Senft, M., Chantan, M., and Lafont, H., Wheat bran and wheat germ: effect on digestion and intestinal absorption of dietary lipids in the rat, *Am. J. Clin. Nutr.*, 49, 1192, 1989.
26. Farness, P. L. and Schneeman, B. O., Effects of dietary cellulose, pectin and oat bran on the small intestine in the rat, *J. Nutr.*, 112, 1315, 1982.
27. Thomsen, L. L. and Tasmen-Jones, C., Disaccharide levels of the rat jejunum are altered by dietary fibre, *Digestion*, 23, 252, 1982.
28. Schwartz, S. E., Starr, C., Backman, S., and Holtzapple, P. G., Dietary fiber decreases cholesterol and phospholipid synthesis in rat intestine, *J. Lipid. Res.*, 24, 746, 1983.
29. Brown, R. C., Kelleher, J., and Losowsky, M. S., The effect of pectin on the structure and function of the rat small intestine, *Br. J. Nutr.*, 42, 357, 1979.

30. Calvert, R., Schneeman, B. O., Satchithanandam, S., Cassidy, M., and Vahouny, G. V., Dietary fiber and intestinal adaptation: effects on intestinal and pancreatic digestive enzyme activities, *Am. J. Clin. Nutr.*, 41, 1249, 1985.

31. Stock-Damgé, C., Aprahamian, M., Raul, F., Humbert, W., and Bouchet, P., Effects of wheat bran on the exocrine pancreas and the small intestinal mucosa in the dog, *J. Nutr.*, 114, 1076, 1984.

32. Poksay, K. S. and Schneeman, B. O., Pancreatic and intestinal response to dietary guar gum in rats, *J. Nutr.*, 113, 1544, 1983.

33. Vahouny, G. V., Satchithanandam, S., Chen, I., Tepper, S. A., Kritchevsky, D., Lightfoot, F. G., and Cassidy, M. M., Dietary fiber and intestinal adaptation: effects on lipid absorption and lymphalic transport in the rat, *Am. J. Clin. Nutr.*, 47, 201, 1988.

34. Lairon, D., Soluble fiber and dietary lipids, *Adv. Exp. Med. Biol.*, 427, 99–108, 1997.

35. Pasquier, B., Armand, M., Castelain, C., Guillon, F., Borel, B., Lafont, H., and Lairon, D., Emulsification and lipolysis of triacylglycerols are altered by viscous soluble dietary fibres in acidic gastric medium *in vitro*, *Biochem. J.*, 314, 269–275.

36. Pasquier, B., Armand, M., Guillon, F., Castelain, C., Borel, B., Barry, J. L., Pieroni, G., and Lairon, D., Viscous soluble dietary fibres alter emulsification and lipolysis of triacylglycerides in duodenal medium *in vitro*, *J. Nutr. Biochem.*, 7, 293–302, 1996.

The Source of Dietary Fiber Influences — Short-Chain Fatty Acid Production and Concentrations in the Large Bowel

H. Kobayashi and Sharon E. Fleming

Short-chain fatty acids (SCFA), also referred to as volatile fatty acids, primarily include acetate, propionate, and butyrate, which compose more than 80% of all SCFAs. They are produced from carbohydrates or dietary fiber which cannot be degraded by human digestive enzymes, but which are hydrolyzed and fermented by intestinal microflora in the large bowel.[47] Carbohydrate and dietary fiber affect colonic metabolism and the luminal environment, since they stimulate SCFA production, absorption, and excretion which, in turn, affect characteristics such as luminal and fecal pH.

This chapter summarizes data which show the effects due to dietary fiber on SCFA production and excretion, and on fecal pH. Since SCFA production cannot easily be measured directly in humans due to difficulties obtaining human colonic contents, animal models are widely used. Data from various strains of rats, pigs, and humans are included. Data from ruminant animals, dog, cats, and rabbits are excluded due to important differences from humans in their intestinal physiology and functions. In the previous edition,[48] the summarized data illustrated the importance of intestinal microflora on SCFA production and of having internal consistency within each experiment regarding gender of animal due to differences between gender in SCFA production, absorption, and excretion. These earlier data showed also that the age of animal used in experiments might affect SCFA production, absorption, and excretion. In this edition, we extended the data from studies conducted from 1990 to the present.

DURATION OF FEEDING DIETARY FIBER

The studies reported in the previous edition of this review[48] generally showed that increasing the duration of dietary fiber consumption increased SCFA concentration in the intestinal lumen, increased SCFA digesta pool size, and increased SCFA absorption. Of the three more recent studies (Table 4.9.1), two studies showed increases in SCFA concentration in cecal digesta production with increasing duration of dietary fiber consumption,[1,2] while one study showed a possible decrease in SCFA excretion in feces with increased exposure to fiber.[3] Decreased fecal excretion may be due to increased SCFA absorption, as shown in an earlier rat study.[48]

0-8493-2387-8/01/$0.00+$1.50

Table 4.9.1 Influence of the Duration of Feeding on SCFA Concentrations in Luminal Contents and Feces

Animal Model	Specimen and Diet	Duration of Feeding				Comments	Ref.
Rats, male Wistar, 115 g	Cecal contents (Mean, $n = 6$, μmol/g wet contents)	2 wk	8 wk	27 wk			1
	Acetate Control	44.0	55.9	47.6			
	Fructooligosaccharide	55.2a	53.3	69.5a		↑ duration → ↑ [Ac] for FOSb at 27 wks	
	Propionate Control	12.0	16.5	19.2			
	Fructooligosaccharide	14.7	14.5	17.4		↑ duration → ↑ [Pr] at 27 wks	
	Butyrate Control	4.9	5.3	4.7			
	Fructooligosaccharide	13.5a	25.3a	15.3a		↑ duration → may ↑ [Bu] for FOS at 8 wks, then ↓ [Bu] at 27 wks	
	Total SCFA Control	62.0	79.4	73.2			
	Fructooligosaccharide	83.8a	94.2a	103.5a		↑ duration → ↑ [total SCFA]	
Rats, male Wistar, 115 g	Cecal contents (Mean, $n = 6$, μmol/g wet)	0.5 mo	2 mo	6 mo			2
	Acetate Control	44.0	55.9	47.6			
	Resistant potato starch	64.9a	66.8	94a		↑ duration → ↑ [Ac]	
	Propionate Control	12.0	16.5	19.2			
	Resistant potato starch	12.9	16.4	21.3		↑ duration → ↑ [Pr]	
	Butyrate Control	4.9	5.3	4.7			
	Resistant potato starch	11.2a	31.4a	45.4a		↑ duration → ↑ [Bu]	
	Total SCFA Control	62.0	79.4	73.2			
	Resistant potato starch	90.3a	115.9a	162.3a		↑ duration → ↑ [total SCFA]	
Rats, male Sprague-Dawley 40–60 g	Feces (Mean ± SEM, $n = 10$, μmol/g wet)	4 wk	8 wk	12 wk	16 wk		3
	Acetate Wheat bran	24.3 ± 10.9	17.7 ± 3.7	14.4 ± 1.7	15.7 ± 1.7		
	Oat bran	28.3 ± 2.6	32.1 ± 2.8	20.5 ± 2.8	26.3 ± 2.5		
	Propionate Wheat bran	4.2 ± 1.4	2.4 ± 0.6	2.1 ± 0.4	2.4 ± 0.3		
	Oat bran	8.7 ± 1.1	7.1 ± 1.3	5.4 ± 0.8	5.3 ± 1.1		
	Butyrate Wheat bran	7.5 ± 2.5	4.3 ± 1.3	4.9 ± 1.0	4.6 ± 1.1		
	Oat bran	16.2 ± 2.9	18.5 ± 2.2	11.9 ± 2.3	12.6 ± 2.0		
	Total SCFA Wheat bran	37.4 ± 13.7	25.4 ± 5.4	23.1 ± 3.0	23.8 ± 3.0	↑ duration → may ↓ SCFA excretion	
	Oat bran	55.5 ± 4.8	60.2 ± 4.9	40.5 ± 5.5	46.7 ± 4.7	Differences between diets were statistically significant	

a Significantly different from control group $p < 0.05$.
b FOS = fructooligosaccharides.

CONCENTRATION OF FIBER IN DIET

The influence of the amount of fiber ingested was evaluated by increasing the concentration of fiber in the diet (Table 4.9.2). In one of the two recent studies, SCFA concentrations in rat cecal contents were increased in a dose-dependent manner with increasing dietary concentrations of both inulin and resistant starch.[4] With both of these fiber sources, the molar ratios of propionate and butyrate increased, whereas the molar ratio of acetate decreased with increasing dietary fiber concentrations. In the one human study, fecal SCFA concentrations were increased by increasing the vegetable fiber, but not the wheat bran, concentration in the diet.[5] Both studies were conducted for only 1 week; thus, caution should be used in extrapolating these findings to physiological situations. The reader is referred to the earlier review, since the effects of concentration of fiber on SCFA production and excretion was more thoroughly studied in the previous years.

THE EFFECTS OF FIBER ON SCFA CONCENTRATIONS ARE OBSERVED ALONG THE LENGTH OF THE LARGE BOWEL

The SCFA concentrations in intestinal segments including the cecum, proximal colon, and distal colon, and in excreted feces, are reported for several fiber sources (Table 4.9.3). Although not the purpose of this review, SCFA concentrations were highest in the contents of the cecum and lowest in feces,[2,3,6-8,10,12] with only one exception.[9] Differences among segments in the molar ratios of the three major SCFAs are worth noting. In the one study where these were reported, acetate constituted a greater proportion of the three SCFAs in contents of the distal colon than in the cecum or proximal colon; this increase was offset by a decrease in the proportion of propionate, whereas butyrate percentages were unchanged.[12] Calculations performed on original data indicated, however, that differences between segments in molar percentages of the three SCFAs were not consistent. By comparing data within the study, it appears that the source of dietary fiber may play a role in determining the longitudinal gradient in molar percentages among the three major SCFAs. Specifically, the proportion of acetate was higher in the cecum than the distal colon for treatments including cellulose,[8] pectin,[8] and psyllium;[10] was similar for treatments including potato starch,[2] wheat bran,[3,9] oat bran,[8] and pectin;[9] and was lower in the cecum than the distal colon for treatments including rolled oats[12] and wheat bran.[12] Some inconsistencies among studies are evident.

In most,[2,3,6-9,11] but not all,[10,11] studies, the effects of a dietary fiber on SCFA concentrations were consistent along the length of the large bowel. As one example, when compared to a low-fiber diet, a high-fiber diet caused total SCFA concentrations to be higher in lumenal contents of both the cecum and colon of rats.[7] Similarly, potato starch increased the concentrations of acetate and butyrate in the intestinal contents of both the proximal and distal colon of rats,[2] and differences for pectin and oat bran vs., cellulose were consistent among the cecum, proximal colon, and distal colon contents of rats.[8] As a result, it is possible to use data from one segment to predict the relative differences among dietary fibers in another segment. Unfortunately, insufficient data are available to conclude that differences in fecal SCFA concentrations can equally well predict dietary differences in the luminal contents of the cecum or colon.

THE SOURCE OF FIBER INFLUENCES SCFA PRODUCTION

Comparisons among fiber sources have been made most commonly by feeding diets that contain equivalent concentrations of fiber but which differ in the source from which the fiber is derived (Tables 4.9.3 and 4.9.4). Based on earlier studies, it was noted that feeding cellulose resulted in lower SCFA production than pectin, oat bran, wheat bran, and psyllium.[48] In several recent studies, data suggest that cellulose consumption may depress cecal SCFA concentrations below those

Table 4.9.2 Influence of the Dietary Fiber Concentration on SCFA Concentration in Cecal Contents and Fecal Fluid

Animal Model	Fiber	Specimen/Data	Source (and Level) of Fiber in Diet				Comments	Ref.
Rats, male Wistar, 200 g, fed 7 days	Inulin	Cecal contents Mean ± SEM, n = 10						4
		SCFA conc, mM	Fiber free 101 ± 7	Inulin (3.75%) 104 ± 6	Inulin (7.5%) 117 ± 6	Inulin (15%) 129 ± 8[a]	↑ [fiber] → ↑ [SCFA]	
		Molar Ratio (Ac:Pr:Bu)	69:24:07	60:29:11	50:33:17	43:37:20	↑ [fiber] → ↓ %Ac, ↑ %Bu	
	Resistant starch	SCFA conc, mM	Fiber free 101 ± 7	Resistant starch (5%) 114 ± 6	Resistant starch (10%) 149 ± 9[a]	Resistant starch (20%) 173 ± 10[a]	↑ [fiber] → ↑ [SCFA]	
		Molar Ratio (Ac:Pr:Bu)	69:24:07	61:26:13	56:27:17	53:30:17	↑ [fiber] → ↓ %Ac, ↑ %Bu	
Human, fed 8 days	Wheat bran	Fecal dyalysate fluid Mean ± SEM, n = 9						5
		SCFA conc, mM	Fiber free 58.2 ± 3.6	Wheat bran (10g) 99.3 ± 3.6	Wheat bran (30g) 75.5 ± 3.4		No change in [SCFA]	
		Molar Percentage (Ac/Pr/Bu)	55/23/9	55/22/14	52/22/16		No change in molar percentage	
	Veg fiber	SCFA conc, mM		Vegetable fiber (10g) 74.5 ± 4.1	Vegetable fiber (30g) 90.0 ± 4.1		↑ [fiber] → ↑ [SCFA]	
		Molar Percentage (Ac/Pr/Bu)		58/22/10	60/22/12		No change in molar percentage	

Note: Ac = acetate; Pr = propionate; Bu = butyrate.

[a] Significant differences from fiber-free group.

Table 4.9.3 Influence of the Source of Dietary Fiber on SCFA Concentrations and Proportions in Various Intestinal Segments

Animal Model	Specimen/Intestinal Segment	Source (and Level) of Fiber in Diet			Comments	Ref.
		Basal	Wheat Bran (10%)	Ispagula (5%)		
Rats, male Wistar, 150 g, fed 28 days	Luminal contents Mean ± SEM, n = 9–20, μmol/g dry Total SCFA					6
	Cecal	441 ± 17.9	380 ± 23.4	517 ± 26.7*	[Total SCFA] higher for ispagula in cecum	
	Proximal colon	201 ± 16.5	218 ± 24.9	326 ± 20.2*	[Total SCFA] higher for ispagula in prox. colon	
	Distal colon	158.5 ± 15.7	120.4 ± 12.1	180 ± 16.4	No differences among fibers in distal colon	
Rats, male Wistar, fed 18 mo	Luminal contents Mean ± SEM, n = 10, μmol/g dry Total SCFA	Low fiber (17 g NSP/kg)	High fiber (133 g NSP/kg)			7
	Cecum	60.2 ± 10.3	296.6 ± 18.4*		[Total SCFA] higher for high-fiber diet in cecum	
	Colon	24.7 ± 3.5	135.9 ± 12.1*		[Total SCFA] higher for high-fiber diet in colon	
Rats, male Wistar, 115 g	Luminal contents Mean, n = 6, μmol/g wet	Basal	Potato starch			2
	Acetate					
	Proximal colon	29.6	66.3*			
	Distal colon	15.5	52.7*			
	Propionate					
	Proximal colon	11.9	16.6			
	Distal colon	6.8	10.9			
	Butyrate					
	Proximal colon	2.8	30.5*			
	Distal colon	1.7	25.2*			
	Total SCFA					
	Proximal colon	45.3	114.5*		Potato starch increases the conc. of each SCFA in both the proximal and distal colon	
	Distal colon	24.5	89.5*			

Table 4.9.3 (Continued)   Influence of the Source of Dietary Fiber on SCFA Concentrations and Proportions in Various Intestinal Segments

Animal Model	Specimen/Intestinal Segment	Source (and Level) of Fiber in Diet			Comments	Ref.
Rats, male Sprague-Dawley 40–60 g	Colonic contents, Mean ± SEM, $n = 11$, μmol/g	Wheat bran	Oat bran		[SCFA] are similar for wheat and oat bran at both the proximal and distal colon	3
	Acetate					
	Proximal colon	29.2 ± 2.6	27.1 ± 2.5			
	Distal colon	24.2 ± 2.6	23.8 ± 2.9			
	Propionate					
	Proximal colon	4.9 ± 0.6	6.7 ± 0.6			
	Distal colon	4.6 ± 0.6	7.0 ± 0.7			
	Butyrate					
	Proximal colon	9.6 ± 1.8	17.2 ± 1.7			
	Distal colon	8.2 ± 1.8	19.0 ± 2.0			
	Total SCFA					
	Proximal colon	45.4 ± 4.1	53.5 ± 4.0			
	Distal colon	38.7 ± 4.1	53.5 ± 4.6			
†Rats, male Sprague-Dawley, 270–320 g, fed 4 wk	Luminal contents, Mean ± SEM, $n = 19$–20, μmol/g	Cellulose (6%DF)	Pectin (6%DF)	Oat bran (6%DF)		8
	Acetate				[Ac] for pectin and oat bran > cellulose at all three sites	
	Cecum	28.8 ± 1.3[c]	52.3 ± 2.0[a]	36.6 ± 2.6[b]		
	Proximal colon	13.3 ± 0.8[b]	31.7 ± 1.7[a]	28.8 ± 1.7[a]		
	Distal colon	5.8[c]	13.6 ± 0.6[b]	21.4 ± 1.0[a]		
	Propionate				[Pr] for pectin and oat bran > cellulose at all three sites	
	Cecum	5.9[b]	7.9[a]	7.2[a]		
	Proximal colon	4.2[b]	6.7[a]	6.7[a]		
	Distal colon	1.9[c]	3.9 ± 0.3[b]	4.9 ± 0.3[a]		
	Butyrate				[Bu] for oat bran > cellulose and oat bran at all three sites	
	Cecum	1.7[b]	1.3[b]	11.8[a]		
	Proximal colon	0.8[b]	1.25[b]	5.4[a]		
	Distal colon	0.6[c]	1.9[b]	5.2 ± 0.3[a]		
	Total SCFA				[total SCFA] for pectin and oat bran > cellulose at all three sites	
	Cecum	37.9 ± 1.3[b]	62.8 ± 2.6[a]	57.6 ± 2.6[a]		
	Proximal colon	20 ± 1.25[b]	40.8 ± 1.7[a]	42.5 ± 1.7[a]		
	Distal colon	9.7 ± 0.3[c]	21.4 ± 1.0[b]	33.1 ± 1.3[a]		

9

†Rats, male Sprague-Dawley, 200–230 g body wt, fed 3 wk

Luminal contents
Mean ± SEM, $n = 10$, mmol/l

	Fiber-free (8% DF)	Pectin (8% DF)	Wheat bran	
Acetate				
Cecum	39.1 ± 11.2	53.0 ± 19.5	64.2 ± 14.0	In prox. colon only, [Ac] for pectin > fiber-free
Proximal colon	55.8 ± 11.2[b]	92.1 ± 11.2[a]	72.6 ± 14.0[a,b]	
Distal colon	44.7 ± 11.2	36.3 ± 5.6	37.7 ± 8.4	
Propionate				In prox. and distal colon, [Pr] for pectin > fiber-free
Cecum	9.5 ± 3.6	9.2 ± 4.9	9.0 ± 2.1	
Proximal colon	1.5 ± 0.8[b]	13.3 ± 7.4[a]	10.8 ± 3.1[a,b]	
Distal colon	0.3 ± 0.1[b]	5.1 ± 1.5[a]	3.1 ± 1.5[a,b]	
Butyrate				At all 3 sites, [Bu] for wheat bran > fiber-free and pectin
Cecum	4.7 ± 1.0[b]	2.5 ± 0.8[b]	1.6 ± 3.3[a]	
Proximal colon	1.6 ± 0.8[b]	3.1 ± 2.0[b]	12.4 ± 2.4[a]	
Distal colon	0.4 ± 0.4[b]	3.1 ± 1.4[b]	11.6 ± 2.7[a]	
Total SCFA				In prox. colon only, [total SCFA] for pectin and wheat bran > fiber-free
Cecum	45 ± 13[a]	65 ± 23[a,b]	92 ± 18[b]	
Proximal colon	60 ± 10[b]	110 ± 40[a]	97 ± 20[a]	
Distal colon	45 ± 10	43 ± 7	53 ± 13	

10

†Rats, male Sprague-Dawley, 208–234 g body wt, fed 2 wk

Luminal contents and feces
Mean, μmol/g wet

	Low Amylose Starch		High Amylose Starch		
	Alone	with Psyllium	Alone	with Psyllium	
Acetate					
Cecum	35.3[b]	29.3[a]	34[b]	29.3[a]	Psyllium → ↓ [Ac] in cecum ↑ [Ac] in feces
Proximal colon	26	30	31.3	26	
Distal colon	13.3	23.3	16.6	23.3	
Fecal	12.6[a]	23.6[b]	18[a,b]	22.6[b]	
Propionate					
Cecum	14.2[b]	10.3[a]	14.2[b]	12.4[b]	With low amylose, psyllium → ↓ [Pr] in cecum ↑ [Pr] in feces
Proximal colon	10.7	5	10.7	4.6	
Distal colon	4.6	7.5	8.9	6	
Fecal	1.1[a]	5.3[b]	5.3[b]	8.5[b]	
Butyrate					
Cecum	4[a]	4[a]	9.3[b]	8.7[b]	Psyllium had little or no effect on [Bu] at all sites
Proximal colon	3.1	3.6	7.1	4.9	
Distal colon	2.2	1.8	5.3	6.4	
Fecal	0.4[a]	0.9[a]	2.7[b]	5.3[c]	

Table 4.9.3 (Continued) Influence of the Source of Dietary Fiber on SCFA Concentrations and Proportions in Various Intestinal Segments

Animal Model	Specimen/Intestinal Segment	Source (and Level) of Fiber in Diet				Comments	Ref.
	Total SCFA						11
	Cecum	53.3[b,c]	43.3[a]	57.8[c]	50[b]	Psyllium → ↓ [total SCFA] in cecum	
	Proximal colon	40	37.8	48.9	35.6	↑ [total SCFA] in feces	
	Distal colon	21.1	32.2	31.1	35.6		
	Fecal	14.4[a]	24.4[b]	26.7[b]	36.7[c]		
Rats, male Sprague-Dawley, 40–60 g, fed 38 wk	Luminal contents Mean + SD, n = 5, μmol/g wet	**Cellulose (6 g/100 g diet)**		**Pectin (6 g/100 g diet)**			
	Acetate						
	Proximal colon	21.8 ± 2.32		50.7 ± 5.1		[Ac] for pectin > cellulose at both sites	
	Distal colon	15.3 ± 1.3		29.1 ± 3.6			
	Propionate						
	Proximal colon	4.79 ± 0.39		4.22 ± 0.21		[Pr] for pectin and cellulose similar at both sites	
	Distal colon	2.68 ± 0.34		3.01 ± 0.15			
	Butyrate						
	Proximal colon	4.22 ± 0.19		4.68 ± 0.30		[Bu] for pectin and cellulose similar at both sites	
	Distal colon	3.86 ± 0.28		4.36 ± 0.26			
†Pigs, fed 34 days	Luminal contents Mean, n = 4 Molar percentage (Ac/Pr/Bu)	**Wheat Flour**					12
		Alone	w/Aleurone	w/Pericarp	w/Bran		
	Cecum	51/40/6	44/40/6	51/40/7	56/36/7	Adding wheat bran to wheat flour did not, substantially change the percentages of the three SCFAs	
	Proximal colon	55/31/6	55/31/8	51/36/7	56/34/8		

THE SOURCE OF DIETARY FIBER INFLUENCES

12

†Pigs, fed 42 days	Wheat Flour		Rolled Oats		
	Alone	& Oat Bran	Alone	& Oat Bran	
Distal colon	70/18/6	59/26/6	63/23/7	69/19/7	In comparison to the cecum and prox. colon, the distal colon appeared to have higher % Ac and lower % Pr
Luminal contents Mean, n = 4					
Total SCFA (mmol/l)					
Cecum	100.5	117.8	133	144.9	Adding oat bran to wheat flour or rolled oats tended to increase [SCFA] in cecum, but decrease [SCFA] in distal colon contents
Proximal colon	91.9	108.1	143.8	121.1	
Distal colon	54.1	51.9	75.7	60.5	
Molar percentage (Ac/Pr/Bu)					
Cecum	55/34/6	50/38/8	52/38/7	53/31/11	Adding oat bran did not consistently influence percentages of the three SCFAs
Proximal colon	60/23/8	57/26/8	52/34/9	55/28/12	In comparison to the cecum, the distal colon tended to have higher % Ac and lower % Pr
Distal colon	69/14/6	66/15/9	58/22/9	61/19/10	

* Significantly different from basal group p < 0.05.
† Data was extrapolated from the original graphs.
a,b,c Values in a row with different superscripts are significantly different at $p < 0.05$.

observed for animals fed a fiber-free diet.[15,16] More recent studies confirmed previous observations[48] that, in comparison to cellulose, pectin ingestion increased luminal SCFA concentrations and pool size.[8,15] This study extended our knowledge by showing that cecal SCFA concentration and pool size was higher also for pea fiber than cellulose.[14]

In comparison to a cellulose diet, the cereal fibers oat bran and corn bran resulted in higher luminal propionate concentration in pigs[21] and higher concentrations of each of the three major SCFAs when this comparison was made using rats.[8] When compared to methylcellulose consumption, cecal SCFA concentrations in rats were higher for diets containing both rice bran and wheat bran.[17]

The results of these most recent studies show that water-dispersible fibers such as inulin, pectin, indigestible dextrins, and ispagula provide higher luminal SCFA concentrations than do cereal fibers or brans from wheat, oats, and corn.[6,14,18,19] Furthermore, it appears that fiber from chicory, carrots, and cocoa might respond similarly to inulin.[14,18] Among the cereal fibers, wheat bran, corn bran, and oat bran may support similar luminal SCFA concentrations, while rice bran might support higher concentrations.[3,14,17,21]

Dietary Fiber Source Influences Fecal SCFA Excretion

The generalizations that were made earlier regarding the influence of various sources of dietary fibers on luminal concentrations of SCFA appear to apply, but to a more limited extent to fecal excretion of SCFA (Table 4.9.5). In particular, there is evidence that fecal excretion of SCFA is increased when water-dispersible compounds such as ispagula,[6,27] inulin,[24] galactooligosaccharides,[24] senna,[25] and resistant starch[26] are consumed. By contrast, wheat bran had little or no effect on fecal SCFA excretion.[6,22,23,25]

Many Dietary Fiber Sources Reduce Luminal pH

The effect of the dietary fiber on luminal pH has been studied most commonly in rats, although fecal pH data are also available for humans (Table 4.9.6). In general, wheat bran did not have a consistent significant effect on either luminal or fecal pH using rats,[9,28] pigs,[12] or humans.[25] Also, cellulose consumption did not appear to lower luminal pH.[29] Luminal and fecal pH, however, appeared to be reduced following consumption by rats of dietary fibers including fructooligosaccharides,[1] galacto-oligosaccharides,[29] inulin,[4,14] pectin,[8,9] psyllium,[21] oat bran,[8,12] and following consumption of diets high in resistant starch.[4,13,26] Results using inulin and resistant starch suggest that there is a dose–response relationship such that increasing fiber consumption shows further decreases in luminal pH.[4] Results of another study suggest that there may be a threshold, however, after which further increases in fiber intake do not further influence fecal pH.[30] Overall, the pH values of control treatments, even when compared within a specific site, varied considerably among the experiments. If one focuses simply on the absolute pH values, rather than on the significance of differences between a specific fiber treatment and a control, then it appears that luminal pH values of 6 or less can be attained by feeding water-dispersible but fermentable constituents including inulin, galactooligosaccharides, resistant starch and, in some cases, fructooligosaccharides.

In Vitro SCFA Production Varies with the Source of the Dietary Fiber

Since it is difficult to examine the fermentation dynamics within the intestine of humans or animals, *in vitro* fermentation systems have been developed and utilized to study the influence of dietary fiber (substrate) on SCFA production (Table 4.9.7). Many research groups presented data for SCFA as a function of fermentation time.[6,21,22,34,35,37,40–46] In general, time-dependent increases in SCFA production were observed. Since SCFA production tended to level off after a 24-hour incubation period, data are presented only for this later time point in an attempt to simplify this presentation.

Table 4.9.4 Influence of the Source of Dietary Fiber on SCFA Concentration, or Quantity, in Cecal Contents

Animal Model	Specimen/Data	Source of DF (Level)				Comments	Ref.
		Control	Pea starch	Potato starch	Resistant starch		
Rats, male Wistar, 75 ± 5 g, fed 12 days	Cecal contents; Mean ± SEM, $n = 7$						13
	SCFA conc. mmol/l	58 ± 4[a]	76 ± 5[a,b]	85 ± 4[b]	61 ± 4[a]	[SCFA] for potato starch > resistant starch	
	SCFA pool, μmol	48 ± 6[a]	78 ± 10[a]	150 ± 19[b]	153 ± 15[b]	SCFA pools for potato and resistant > pea starch	
	Molar percentage (Ac/Pr/Bu)	72/21/4	69/19/5	71/15/10	72/16/8	Molar ratios not different	
Rats, male Fischer, 10 wk, 280 g, fed 8 wk	Cecal contents; Mean ± SEM, $n = 6$, μmol/g wet	Inulin	Carrot	Cocoa			14
	Acetate	31.42 ± 1.91[a]	32.66 ± 3.04[a]	32.16 ± 0.65[a]		[Ac] for Inulin, carrot, and cocoa > others	
	Propionate	8.65 ± 0.26	8.80 ± 0.55	8.71 ± 0.21			
	Butyrate	14.83 ± 0.88[a]	3.66 ± 0.27[b]	4.16 ± 0.30[b]		[Bu] higher for inulin than others	
	Total SCFA	55.83 ± 2.69[a]	46.02 ± 3.66[a,b]	45.99 ± 0.97[a,b]			
		Wheat bran	Pea	Oat			
	Acetate	28.40 ± 1.53[a,b]	23.91 ± 1.22[b]	23.27 ± 1.29[b]			
	Propionate	9.42 ± 0.41	9.44 ± 0.26	9.15 ± 0.35			
	Butyrate	4.14 ± 0.33[b]	3.12 ± 0.60[b]	3.20 ± 0.29[b]			
	Total SCFA	43.20 ± 2.11[b]	37.62 ± 1.84[b]	36.81 ± 1.65[b]			
Rats, male Sprague-Dawley, 150–200 g, fed 4 wk	Cecal contents; Mean ± SEM, $n = 5$	Control	Cellulose (30% DF)	Pectin (30% DF)	Pea fiber (30% DF)		15
	Total SCFA, mmol/l	37.1 ± 2.3[a]	15.7 ± 2.7[b]	45.9 ± 3.2[a]	46.3 ± 3.6[a]	Cellulose had lowest conc. of all SCFAs	
	Acetate, μmol/animal	48.9 ± 3.4[c]	21.9 ± 2.8[d]	386.4 ± 58.2[a]	167.4 ± 8.7[b]		
	Propionate, μmol/animal	18.4 ± 1.4[c]	9.5 ± 1.6[d]	121.4 ± 20.6[a]	51.3 ± 5.7[b]	Pectin had greatest [Ac] and [Pr]	
	Butyrate, μmol/animal	3.3 ± 0.3[b,c]	1.7 ± 0.3[c]	7.1 ± 2.5[b]	25.4 ± 1.6[a]	Pea fiber had greatest [Bu]	
	Total SCFA, μmol/animal	70.6 ± 4.9[c]	33.1 ± 4.6[d]	515 ± 78[a]	244 ± 12.8[b]		

Table 4.9.4 (Continued)   Influence of the Source of Dietary Fiber on SCFA Concentration, or Quantity, in Cecal Contents

Animal Model	Specimen/Data	Source of DF (Level)				Comments	Ref.
†Rats, male Sprague–Dawley, 125–150 g, fed 22 days	Cecal contents Mean ± SE, n = 6 Conc, μmol/g	Fiber-free	Maize husk (100 g/kg)	Acid-treated Maize husk (100 g/kg)		Higher amount of SCFA for maize husk groups. Acid treating husks increased SCFA concs. and pools	16
	Acetate	33.9 ± 5.3	32.7 ± 1.8	40.5 ± 2.4			
	Propionate	17.3 ± 1.8[b]	16.1 ± 0.6[b]	23.2 ± 2.4[a]			
	Butyrate	7.1 ± 1.2[c]	10.7 ± 0.6[b]	14.3 ± 0.6[a]			
	Pool, μmol/ cecum						
	Acetate	41.1 ± 6.9[c]	85.7 ± 6.9[b]	116.6 ± 6.9[a]			
	Propionate	24.0 ± 2.7[c]	39.4 ± 2.7[b]	68.6 ± 6.9[a]			
	Butyrate	10.3 ± 1.7[c]	27.4 ± 1.7[b]	37.7 ± 3.4[a]			
Rats, male Sprague–Dawley, 208–234 g, fed 2 wk	Cecal contents Mean, n = 8 Molar percentage (Ac:Pr:Bu)	Low Amylose Starch 66:26:8	Low Amylose/ Psyllium (1.5%) 68:24:9	High Amylose Starch 59:25:16	High Amylose/ Psyllium (1.5%) 58:25:17	High amylose starch had lower % Ac and higher % Bu	10
Rats, male Sprague–Dawley, 150–200 g, fed 4 wk	Cecal contents Mean ± SEM, n = 8, mmol/l	Fiber-free	Methyl-cellulose	Parboiled rice bran	Coarse WB	Low levels of all SCFAs were seen for methylcellulose. [Pr] was significantly higher for no-fiber group. [Bu] rice and wheat bran > others	17
	Acetate	70.0 ± 3.9[c]	13.1 ± 0.7[a]	67.0 ± 3.0[c]	32.9 ± 2.0[b]		
	Propionate	23.5 ± 1.5[c]	4.9 ± 0.3[a]	16.0 ± 1.0[b]	13.6 ± 0.9[b]		
	Butyrate	5.3 ± 0.6[a]	1.6 ± 0.3[a]	18.0 ± 1.0[b]	15.2 ± 0.9[b]		
Rats, male Sprague–Dawley, 152 g, fed 4 wk	Cecal contents Mean, n = 8, mmol/g wet	Fiber-free	Chicory (1%)	Chicory (5%)	Inulin (5%)	[Pr] for chicory and inulin > fiber-free group	18
	Acetate	55.2	41.6	51.5	40.9		
	Propionate	24.8[c]	28.0[b,c]	33.6[a]	31.5[a,b]		
	Butyrate	9.1	7.8	9.0	8.0		

	Control	Indigestible dextrin (5%)	Pectin (5%)	Corn fiber (5%)	Ref
Rats, male Sprague-Dawley, 6 wks old, fed 8 wk					19
Cecal contents Mean ± SEM, $n = 7-9$, μmol/cecum					
Acetate	48.8 ± 7.8[a]	93.4 ± 7.1[b]	96.8 ± 13.5[b]	64.1 ± 7.8[a]	
Propionate	18.5 ± 1.5[a]	40.5 ± 2.2[b]	45.2 ± 8.1[b]	22.6 ± 2.7[a]	
Butyrate	8.4 ± 1.1[a]	19.7 ± 1.6[b]	21.2 ± 3.5[b]	12.7 ± 2.3[a]	Output of each SCFA for dextrin and pectin > others

	Casein/Starch	Casein/Wheat	Chickpea/Wheat		Ref
Rats, male Sprague-Dawley, 5 wks old, fed 28 wk					20
Cecal contents Mean ± SD, $n = 18$, μmol/g					
Acetate	148.3 ± 31.0[f]	169.4 ± 43.9[f]	231.8 ± 48.0[e]		
Propionate	31.3 ± 10.9[g]	51.0 ± 18.9[f]	78.2 ± 17.8[e]		
Butyrate	29.1 ± 10.5[g]	59.0 ± 16.4[f]	81.5 ± 19.0[e]		
Total SCFA	208 ± 43	279 ± 72	390 ± 66		Chickpea had highest [Ac], [Pr], and [Bu]

	Cellulose (7%)	Oat bran (7%)	Corn bran (7%)	Corn bran (13%)	Ref
Pigs, male, Hanford Miniature, ~5 mo old, 40 kg body wt					21
Cecal digesta Mean ± SEM, $n = 5$ SCFA conc., mmol/l					
Acetate	37.9 ± 1.7	42.6 ± 3.6	55.4 ± 4.3	47.1 ± 3.7	
Propionate	14.9 ± 1.0[a]	25.7 ± 3.0[b]	23.7 ± 3.1[b]	20.1 ± 2.8[a,b]	[Pr] for oat and corn bran > cellulose
Butyrate	3.9 ± 0.5	9.2 ± 2.3	6.4 ± 0.7	5.9 ± 1.0	
Total SCFA	58.5 ± 3.5[a]	81.4 ± 8.6[a,b]	88.5 ± 7.2[b]	72.6 ± 8.0[a,b]	[total SCFA] for 7% corn bran > cellulose
Molar ratio (Ac:Pr:Bu)	67:26:07	55:33:12	65:28:07	64:27:08	Oat bran had lower % Ac and higher % Bu than others
SCFA pool, mmol/animal					
Acetate	25.2 ± 2.3	27.9 ± 2.1	21.8 ± 5.2	22.1 ± 3.5	
Propionate	10.0 ± 1.2[a,b]	17.0 ± 2.3[b]	9.1 ± 2.0[a,b]	9.0 ± 1.2[a]	
Butyrate	2.6 ± 0.5[a]	5.5 ± 0.7[b]	2.5 ± 0.7[a]	2.7 ± 0.5[a]	Bu and total SCFA pools for oat bran > corn bran
Total SCFA	39.0 ± 4.0[a,b]	52.9 ± 3.8[b]	34.6 ± 7.3[a]	33.3 ± 4.6[a]	

a,b,c,d Values in a row with different superscripts are significantly different at $p < 0.05$.
e,f,g Values in a row with different superscripts are significantly different at $p < 0.001$.
† Data was extrapolated from the original graphs.

Table 4.9.5　Influence of the Source of Dietary Fiber on Fecal Excretion of SCFA

Animal Model	Specimen/Data	Source (and Level) of Fiber in Diet	Comments	Ref.
Rats, male Wistar, 150 g, fed 28 days	Feces Mean ± SEM, n = 9–20 Total SCFA, μmol/day	Basal — 127.4 ± 11.4 Wheat bran (10%) — 287 ± 51.3 Ispagula (5%) — 572.6 ± 54.7	SCFA excretion for ispagula > wheat bran > basal	6
Rats, male Sprague-Dawley, 220 g, fed 2 wk	Feces n = 8 Molar percentage (Ac/Pr/Bu)	Low-amylose starch — 90/6/3 Low-amylose and psyllium — 76/21/3 High-amylose starch — 70/21/11 High amylose and psyllium — 66/24/14	Psyllium reduced % Ac and increased % Pr or Bu	10
Pigs, barrow Cross-bred, 50–85 kg, fed > 7 days	Feces Mean ± SD, n = 5 Total SCFA (mmol/kg dry) Molar percentage (Ac/Pr/Bu)	Low-fiber (56g NSP/kg) — 248 ± 61.6 — 60/21/6 Oat bran (93g NSP/kg) — 270 ± 62.7 — 57/21/9 Wheat bran (102g NSP/kg) — 252 ± 66.2 — 63/21/6	Oat bran gave significantly higher % Bu	22
Humans, 12 male, 12 pre-menopausal female, 33 ± 2 yr old	Feces Mean ± SEM, n = 24 Concentration (mmol/l) 　Acetate 　Propionate 　Butyrate Output (mmol/d) 　Acetate 　Propionate 　Butyrate	**Elemental** / **Wheat bran (30 g DF/d)** Concentration: Acetate: 60.7 ± 4.6 / 64.2 ± 3.9 Propionate: 14.2 ± 1.2 / 14.3 ± 1.2 Butyrate: 19.2 ± 2.4 / 21.3 ± 1.9* Output: Acetate: 10.21 ± 1.62 / 16.82 ± 2.13* Propionate: 2.34 ± 0.38 / 3.86 ± 0.60* Butyrate: 3.07 ± 0.51 / 5.35 ± 0.66*	Wheat bran → ↑ [Bu] Wheat bran → ↑ fecal output of Ac, Pr, and Bu	23
Humans, 12 male, 23 ± 3 yr, fed 3 wk	Feces Mean ± SD, n = 12 mmol/100 g dry 　Acetate 　Propionate 　Butyrate	**Control** / **Inulin (15 g/d)** / **Fructooligo-saccharides (15 g/d)** / **Galactooligo-saccharides (15 g/d)** Acetate: 854 ± 541 / 1181 ± 355* / 1058 ± 444 / 1246 ± 698* Propionate: 671 ± 297 / 795 ± 300 / 707 ± 297 / 679 ± 293 Butyrate: 313 ± 177 / 401 ± 179 / 318 ± 105 / 369 ± 199	Acetate excretion for inulin and GOS > control and FOS	24

Subjects	Sample	Treatment	Acetate	Propionate	Butyrate	Total SCFA	Effect	Ref
Humans, 3 male, 10 female, fed 9 days	Feces, Mean, $n = 13$, μmol/g wet	Control	72.9	24.0	69.0	95.0		25
		Wheat bran (28.3 ± 8.7 g/d)	81.0	21.9	79.4	113.0		
		Control	63.9	18.4	16.6	111.0	Senna → ↑ fecal [Ac], [Pr], and [Bu]	
		Senna	138.2*	40.3*	59.1*	202.0*		
		Control	79.8	27.2	24.8	152.0	Loperamide → ↓ fecal [Pr] and [Bu]	
		Loperamide	51.6	16.6*	6.0*	82.0*		
Humans, 10 male, fed 4 days	Feces, Mean, $n = 10$, mmol/kg dry	Low-resistant starch (fresh maize porridge)	65.8	24.8	17.6	116.1	Highly resistant starch treatment had higher excretion of Ac and Bu	26
		Highly resistant starch (stale maize porridge)	93.9*	43.1	35.1*	182.6*		
Humans, 5 male, 2 female, 21–25 yr old, fed 15 days	Fecal water, Mean ± SEM, $n = 7$, mmol/l	Placebo	25.7 ± 2.3	7.5 ± 1.3	7.3 ± 1.0	44.7 ± 4.4	Ispagula increased fecal [Ac] and [Pr]	27
		Ispagula (18g/d)	60.1 ± 6.3	24.9 ± 5.4	11.1 ± 2.0	100.9 ± 12.6		

Note: NSP = non-starch polysaccharide; GOS = galactooligosaccharides; FOS = fructodigosaccharides.

* Significant difference from control at $p < 0.05$.

Table 4.9.6 Influence of the Source of Dietary Fiber on Luminal and Fecal pH

Animal Model	Specimen/Data	Source (and Level) of Fiber in Diet	Comments	Ref.
Rats, male Wistar, 115 g, fed 27 wk	Cecal contents; Mean pH, $n = 6$	Basal / FOS (9 g/100 g): 7.5 / 6.6	FOS → may ↓ fecal pH at all timepoints	1
Rats, male, fed 17 days	Cecal contents; Mean pH, $n = 4$; 4 h post-feeding; 16 h post-feeding	Basal / Wheat Bran (200 g/kg diet): 6.1 / 5.9; 5.9 / 6		28
Rats, male, Wistar, 115 g, fed 0.5 or 6 mo	Cecal contents; Mean pH, $n = 6$; 0.5 mo; 6 mo	Basal / Resistant starch from potato: 7.5 / 6.4; 7.5 / 6.4	Resistant potato starch → ↓ pH in cecum	2
Rats, male Wistar, 75 ± 5 g, fed 12 days	Cecal contents; Mean pH ± SEM, $n = 7$	Control 7.8 ± 0.1^c; Pea starch 7.2 ± 0.0^b; Potato starch 6.5 ± 0.1^a; Resistant starch from wheat 7.0 ± 0.1^b	Each starch → ↓ pH in cecum	13
Rats, male Wistar, 200 g, fed 7 days	Cecal contents; Mean pH ± SEM, $n = 10$	Fiber-free 7.02 ± 0.08; Inulin (3.75%) 6.40 ± 0.11*; Inulin (7.5%) 5.93 ± 0.13*; Inulin (15%) 5.34 ± 0.08*; Res starch (5%) 6.58 ± 0.06*; Res starch (10%) 5.99 ± 0.09*; Res starch (20%) 5.61 ± 0.08*	↑ Inulin → ↓ pH in cecum; ↑ Resistant starch → ↓ pH in cecum	4
Rats, male, 8 wk old, fed 9 mo	Cecal contents; Mean pH, $n = 39$	Low-Fat: Low-Cellulose 6.5 / High-Cellulose 6.5 / Low-GOS 6.3 / High-GOS 5.8**; Medium-Fat: Low-Cellulose 6.6 / High-Cellulose 6.4 / Low-GOS 6.2 / High-GOS 5.8**	Cellulose did not influence cecal pH at any fat level; GOS → ↓ pH in cecum at all fat levels	29

Animal / Study	Measurement / Site	High-Fat		High-Fat		Comments	Ref
		Low-Cellulose 6.5	High-Cellulose 6.4	Low-GOS 6.2	High-GOS 5.8**		
Rats, male Fischer, 280 g, fed 8 wk	Cecal contents, Mean pH ± SEM, n = 6	Inulin 5.9 ± 0.1[a]	Carrot 6.3 ± 0.1[b]	Cocoa 6.5 ± 0.1[b]		Cecal pH was lowest for the inulin-fed group	14
		Wheat bran 6.3 ± 0.1[b]	Pea 6.3 ± 0.1[b]	Oat 6.5 ± 0.1[b]			
†Rats, male Sprague-Dawley, 270–300 g, fed 4 wk	Luminal content, Mean pH ± SEM, n = 19–20	Cellulose (6%DF)	Pectin (6%DF)	Oat bran (6%DF)		Cecal pH for pectin and oat bran < cellulose; Prox. colon pH for pectin and oat bran < cellulose; Distal colon pH for oat bran < pectin and cellulose	8
	Cecum	7.11 ± 0.08[a]	6.67 ± 0.06[b]	6.57 ± 0.06[b]			
	Proximal colon	6.72 ± 0.03[a]	6.36 ± 0.06[b]	6.30 ± 0.04[b]			
	Distal colon	7.22 ± 0.03[a]	7.05 ± 0.03[a]	6.97 ± 0.11[b]			
Rats, male Sprague-Dawley, 208–234 g, fed 2 wk	Feces and colonic digesta, Mean pH ± SEM	Low-amylose	Low-amylose and psyllium	High-amylose	High-amylose and psyllium	Psyllium → ↓ in fecal pH	21
	Cecum	7.5[b]	7.3[b]	6.9[a]	7.0[a]		
	Proximal colon	7.7	7.4 ± 0.1	6.9	6.8 ± 0.2		
	Distal colon	7.7	7.0 ± 0.1	6.6	6.3 ± 0.1		
	Feces	7.5[c]	7.3[b]	7.3[b]	6.7[a]		
†Rats, male Sprague-Dawley, 200–220 g, fed 8 wk	Luminal contents, Mean pH ± SEM, n = 10	Fiber-free	Pectin (8% DF)	Wheat bran (8% DF)		Pectin → ↓ pH in cecum and prox. colon; Wheat bran → ↓ pH in cecum only	9
	Cecum	7.35 ± 0.05[a]	6.34 ± 0.05[c]	6.74 ± 0.08[b]			
	Proximal colon	6.98 ± 0.08[a]	6.16 ± 0.03[b]	6.55 ± 0.18[a,b]			
	Distal colon	7.27 ± 0.05	7.03 ± 0.03	7.27 ± 0.05			
Rats, male Sprague-Dawley, 40–60 g, fed 38 wk	Luminal contents, Mean pH ± SE, n = 5	Cellulose	Pectin				11
	Proximal colon	6.66	6.67				
	Distal colon	6.85	6.81				

Table 4.9.6 (Continued) Influence of the Source of Dietary Fiber on Luminal and Fecal pH

Animal Model	Specimen/Data	Source (and Level) of Fiber in Diet				Comments	Ref.
Pigs, male Hanford miniature, ~5 months old, 40 kg	Cecal digesta Mean pH ± SEM, $n = 5$	Cellulose	Oat bran	Corn bran		Cecal pH was lower for oat than corn bran at 0~4 hr	21
	0~4 h postprandial	6.47 ± 0.30[a,b]	6.14 ± 0.27[a]	6.92 ± 0.23[b]			
	8~12 h postprandial	6.51 ± 0.09	6.04 ± 0.37	6.31 ± 0.45			
†Pigs, fed 34 days	Luminal content Mean pH, $n = 4$	Wheat flour	Wheat flour + wheat bran				12
	Cecum	5.97	5.78				
	Proximal colon	6.71	5.91				
	Distal colon	6.77	6.52				
†Pigs, fed 42 days	Luminal content Mean, $n = 4$	Wheat flour	Wheat flour and oat bran	Rolled oats	Rolled oats and oat bran	Oat bran, when added to wheat flour, may lower pH at all three sites	12
	Cecum	6.65	5.91	5.91	5.66		
	Proximal colon	7.26	6.52	5.91	5.91		
	Distal colon	6.77	6.09	6.28	6.28		
Humans, 3 male, 10 female, fed 9 days	Feces and colon Mean pH ± SD, $n = 13$	Control	Wheat Bran			Wheat bran may lower pH in mid- and distal colon	25
	Mid-colon	6.83 ± 0.39	6.59 ± 0.48				
	Distal colon	7.08 ± 0.47	6.88 ± 0.43				
	Feces	6.82 ± 0.73	6.80 ± 0.52				
		Control	Senna			Senna may lower pH at all sites	
	Mid-colon	6.85 ± 0.48	6.39 ± 0.48				
	Distal colon	7.14 ± 0.52	6.66 ± 0.48				
	Feces	6.99 ± 0.67	6.70 ± 0.35				

Subjects	Sample	Statistic					Comments	Ref
Humans, male, 22 ± 1 yr old, fed 4 wk	Mid-colon	Mean pH ± SEM, n = 9	Control 6.89 ± 0.46	Loperamide 6.96 ± 0.39			Fiber appears to have a threshold effect on pH	30
	Distal colon		7.11 ± 0.25	7.15 ± 0.37				
	Feces		6.89 ± 0.42	7.22 ± 0.53				
	Feces		Low-fiber (16 g/d) 6.9 ± 0.1[a]	Medium-fiber (30 g/d) 6.5 ± 0.1[b]	High-fiber (42 g/d) 6.6 ± 0.1[b]			
Humans, male, 23 ± 3 yr old, fed 3 wk	Feces	Mean pH ± SD, n = 12	Control 6.83 ± 0.19	Inulin (15 g/d) 6.70 ± 0.46	FOS (15 g/d) 6.88 ± 0.23	GOS (15 g/d) 6.72 ± 0.48		24
Humans, male, fed 3 days	Feces	Mean pH, n = 14	Maize porridge — Fresh 6.7	Maize porridge — Stale 5.91*			↑ Starch resistance → ↓ fecal pH	26
Humans, female	Feces	Mean fiber intake ± SEM, n = 18-22	White omnivore 16.6 ± 0.97 g/d[a]	Indian vegetarians 16.2 ± 1.17 g/d[a]	White vegetarian 29.3 ± 2.57 g/d[b]		Fecal pH was lowest for Indian vegetarians	31
		Mean pH, (95% CI)	6.65 (6.40–6.91)[a]	6.18 (5.91–6.45)[b]	6.55 (6.27–6.82)[a]			

Note: GOS = galactooligosaccharides; FOS = fructooligosaccharides.

[a,b,c] Different superscripts within row indicate significant differences between diets at $p < 0.05$.
* Significantly different from fiber-free group at $p < 0.05$.
** Significantly different at $p < 0.01$.
† Data was extrapolated from the original graphs.

Table 4.9.7 Influence of the Source of Dietary Fiber on SCFA Production In Vitro

Animal model	Inoculum		Source (and Level) of Fiber in Diet				Comments	Ref.
Rats, male Wistar, 190 g, 24 h incubation	Cecal content Mean ± SD, n = 6 μmol/mg substrate		Agiolax	Cenat	Metamucil	Fibra Kneipp		32
		Acetate	3.4 ± 0.5	2.9 ± 0.2	7.1 ± 0.3	4.8 ± 0.2		
		Propionate	2.5 ± 0.2	2.1 ± 0.1	5.6 ± 0.1	2.4 ± 0.1		
		Butyrate	0.6 ± 0.04	0.5 ± 0.02	0.8 ± 0.04	0.8 ± 0.08		
		Total SCFA	6.5 ± 0.7	5.5 ± 0.2	13.5 ± 0.4	8.0 ± 0.3		
			Humamil	Fibra Leo	Fybogel	Fibraplan	Metamucil, Humamil, Fybogel, and Fibraplan, which are mainly soluble fiber components, produced more SCFA than others.	
		Acetate	9.2 ± 1.3	6.0 ± 0.2	7.3 ± 0.3	6.4 ± 0.3		
		Propionate	5.0 ± 0.6	2.9 ± 0.1	5.4 ± 0.2	4.9 ± 0.2		
		Butyrate	1.0 ± 0.1	1.0 ± 0.02	0.5 ± 0.04	0.4 ± 0.02		
		Total SCFA	15.2 ± 1.9	9.9 ± 0.3	13.2 ± 0.5	11.6 ± 0.5		
Rats, male Sprague-Dawley, 6 wk old, 24 h incubation	Cecal contents Mean ± SEM, n = 8		Control	Citrus pectin (5%)	Indigestible dextrin (5%)	Corn fiber (5%)	SCFA for control and pectin > corn and dextrin	18
		Total SCFA, mM	10.59 ± 0.37[a]	10.88 ± 0.46[a]	7.20 ± 0.62[b]	1.83 ± 0.19[c]		
		Molar ratio (Ac:Pr:Bu)	15:27:58	49:05:56	38:19:43	64:11:25	% of the 3 SCFAs differed greatly among treatments	
†Rats, female Sprague-Dawley, 24 h incubation	Cecal contents Mean, n = 5		Ileal digesta from pigs consuming				SCFA for oat bran > wheat bran	33
		Total SCFA, μmol	Oat bran 3319[a]	Wheat bran 1617				
Pigs, barrows, 50 kg body wt, 24 h incubation	Feces Mean, n = 6 mol/g substrate organic matter		Cellulose	Beet pulp	Citrus pulp	Citrus pectin	Cellulose had the lowest SCFA production	34
		Acetate	0.03[a]	2.97[b]	3.97[c]	4.13[c]		
		Propionate	0.03[a]	1.41[b]	1.48[b]	1.97[c]		
		Butyrate	0.00[a]	0.54[b]	0.78[c]	0.92[c]		
		Total SCFA	0.06[a]	4.93[b]	6.23[c]	7.02[c]		

35 — Humans, 24 h incubation

Feces	Apple fiber	Pea fiber
Mean ± SEM, $n = 4$ Total SCFA, mmol/g	75.2 ± 5.7	54.6 ± 2.7
Molar percentage (Ac/Pr/Bu)	68/16/13	66/18/11

SCFA production from apple fiber > pea fiber

36 — Humans, 24 h incubation

Feces Mean ± SEM, $n = 12$ mmol/g organic matter	β-Glucan	Mixed fiber	Psyllium
Acetate	5.22 ± 0.32[b]	2.86 ± 0.05[c]	3.12 ± 0.05[a]
Propionate	1.77 ± 0.21[b]	0.89 ± 0.03[c]	1.49 ± 0.03[a]
Butyrate	1.23 ± 0.04[b]	0.60 ± 0.02[a]	0.45 ± 0.03[c]
Total SCFA	8.24 ± 0.27[b]	4.50 ± 0.05[c]	5.57 ± 0.10[a]

Mixed fiber contains pea fiber, oat fiber, sugar beet fiber, and xanthan gum. Total SCFA production for β-glucan > psyllium > mixed fiber

37 — †Humans, 24 h incubation

Feces Mean, $n = 2$, mmol/l	Wheat bran	Sugar beet	Maize	Pea
Acetate	44	88	24	48
Propionate	17.6	33.6	11.2	12.8
Butyrate	18	20	7.3	12.2

[Ac] and [Pr] were highest for sugar beet

[Bu] wheat bran and sugar beet > maize and pea

38 — Humans, 28-42 yr old, 24 h incubation

Feces Mean, $n = 3$ mmol/g original org. matter	Williamson oat fiber	Canadian Harvest oat fiber	Corn bran
Acetate	0.28[a]	0.48[a]	0.45[a]
Propionate	0.09[a]	0.16[a,b]	0.16[a,b]
Butyrate	0.12[a]	0.13[a]	0.11[a]
Total SCFA	0.48[a]	0.77[a]	0.71[a]
Molar ratio (Ac:Pr:Bu)	56[a,b]:19[c,d]:25[e]	62[a,b]:21[c,d]:17[c,d]	62[a,b]:22[c,d]:16[c,d]

	Wheat bran fiber	Xanthan gum	Gum karaya
Acetate	1.23[a,b]	3.05[b]	5.28[d,e]
Propionate	0.24[a,b,c]	0.59[b,c,d]	0.90[d,e]
Butyrate	0.52[b,c]	0.27[a,b]	0.68[c,d]
Total SCFA	1.99[a,b]	3.91[b,c]	6.86[d]
Molar ratio (Ac:Pr:Bu)	61[a,b]:13[b]:26[e]	78[c]:16[b,c]:7[a]	79[c]:12[b]:9[a,b]

Production of SCFA and ratios among the 3 major SCFAs were significantly influenced by the fiber source

Table 4.9.7 (Continued) Influence of the Source of Dietary Fiber on SCFA Production In Vitro

Animal model	Inoculum	Source (and Level) of Fiber in Diet				Comments	Ref.
Humans, 3 male, 25–41 yr old, 24 h incubation	Feces	Oat bran fiber	Soy fiber	Guar gum			39
	Mean, n = 6 mmol/g dry substrate matter						
	Acetate	2.4[b,c]	3.82[c,d]	3.59[c,d]			
	Propionate	0.78[c,d,e]	1.24[e]	2.32[f]			
	Butyrate	0.89[d,e]	1.09[e,f]	0.95[d,e,f]			
	Total SCFA	4.08[b,c]	6.14[c,d]	6.85[d]			
	Molar ratio (Ac:Pr:Bu)	59[a,b]:19[c,d]:22[d,e]	62[a,b]:20[c,d]:18[c,d]	53[a,e]:33[e]:14[b,c]			
		Gum arabic	Citrus pectin				
	Acetate	6.38[e]	5.7[d,e]				
	Propionate	2.02[f]	0.45[a–d]				
	Butyrate	1.24[f]	1.22[f]				
	Total SCFA	9.64[e]	7.37[d]				
	Molar ratio (Ac:Pr:Bu)	66[b]:21[c,d]:13[a,b,c]	77[c]:6[a]:17[c,d]				
Humans, 3 male, 25–41 yr old, 24 h incubation	Feces	Williamson oat fiber	Canadian Harvest oat fiber	Gum arabic	Carboxymethyl-cellulose	Gum arabic and soy fiber produced the highest amounts of SCFA	39
	Mean, n = 6 mmol/g dry substrate matter						
	Acetate	0.26	0.52	5.38	0.27		
	Propionate	0.07	0.16	1.87	0.08		
	Butyrate	0.09	0.19	0.93	0.05		
	Total SCFA	0.42	0.87	8.19	0.41		
		Soy fiber	Psyllium				
	Acetate	3.71	2.10				
	Propionate	1.12	0.72				
	Butyrate	0.92	0.18				
	Total SCFA	5.75	3.00				
Humans, 4 male, 35–61 yr old, 24 h incubation	Feces	Fig	Oat	Soy fibrium	Pea		40
	Mean ± SEM, n = 6 mmol/g of dietary fiber						
	Acetate	2.55 ± 0.06	1.32 ± 0.05	1.19 ± 0.08	1.46 ± 0.11		
	Propionate	0.33 ± 0.01	0.96 ± 0.01	1.14 ± 0.05	0.42 ± 0.01		
	Butyrate	0.04 ± 0.002	0.38 ± 0.01	0.22 ± 0.01	0.11 ± 0.01		
	Total SCFA	2.92[h]	2.66[i]	2.55[i]	1.99[i]		

Humans, 4 male, 35–61 yr old, 24 h incubation — Feces; Mean ± SEM, $n = 6$, mmol/g polysaccharide

	Apple	Corn	Wheat	Pear	
Acetate	1.06 ± 0.03	0.76 ± 0.02	0.62 ± 0.01	0.66 ± 0.02	There were significant differences among substrates for total SCFA production, and it appeared that differences were present also for each of the the 3 major SCFAs
Propionate	0.41 ± 0.01	0.21 ± 0.01	0.36 ± 0.01	0.24 ± 0.01	
Butyrate	0.09 ± 0.002	0.16 ± 0.01	0.11 ± 0.003	0.05 ± 0.002	
Total SCFA	1.56[k]	1.13[l]	1.09[l]	0.95[m]	

[40]

Humans, 3 donors, av. 43 yr old, 24 h incubation — Feces; Mean, $n = 9$, mmol/g organic matter

	Starch (whole)	Resistant Starch	Pectin	β-glucan	
Acetate	2.39 ± 0.07	1.30 ± 0.04	5.18 ± 0.20	2.41 ± 0.04	In comparison to uncooked (whole) starch, total SCFA production was lower for resistant starch and higher for pectin and β-glucan
Propionate	0.96 ± 0.01	0.89 ± 0.02	0.76 ± 0.05	1.69 ± 0.06	
Butyrate	1.00 ± 0.02	1.23 ± 0.05	0.57 ± 0.02	1.44 ± 0.01	
Total SCFA	4.35	3.42*	6.51*	5.54*	

	Methycellulose 15	Methycellulose 1500	Methycellulose 4000	
Acetate	0.00[a]	−0.06[b]	−0.03[a]	Viscosity for methyl-cellulose 15 > 1500 > 4000
Propionate	0.01[a]	−0.01[a]	0.00[a]	
Butyrate	0.02[a,b]	−0.01[a]	0.03[a,b]	Negative values indicate that SCFA production was lower than in controls, but differences not significant
Total SCFA	0.04[a]	−0.08[a]	0.00[a]	

	Pectin	Psyllium	Solka Floc®	
Acetate	5.48[c]	0.83[b]	0.01[a]	There were significant differences among substrates for production of individual and total SCFA; production was highest for pectin
Propionate	0.79[b]	0.65[b]	0.02[a]	
Butyrate	1.53[d]	0.24[c]	0.01[a]	
Total SCFA	7.81[c]	1.72[b]	0.04[a]	

[41]

Humans, 3 donors, 24 h incubation — Feces; Mean, $n = 3$, μmol/g substrate

	Soy fiber	Sugarbeet fiber	Pea fiber	Citrus pectin	
Acetate	1385[b]	1074[b]	564[a]	5765[c]	Ac, Pr, and Bu production for citrus pectin > pea and sugarbeet
Propionate	400[b]	77[a]	127[a]	453[b]	
Butyrate	158[b,c]	9[a]	70[a,b]	182[c]	

[42]

Table 4.9.7 (Continued) Influence of the Source of Dietary Fiber on SCFA Production In Vitro

Animal model: Humans, 3 donors, 24 h incubation
Inoculum: Feces, Mean, $n = 3$, μmol/g substrate
Ref.: 42

	Gum arabic	Oat fiber	Apple pectin	Corn fiber
Acetate	4593[b]	68[a]	5620[b]	401[a]
Propionate	1758[c]	55[a]	793[b]	188[a]
Butyrate	585[b]	10[a]	472[b]	47[a]

Animal model: Human, 3 donors, 24 h incubation
Inoculum: Feces, Mean ± SE, $n = 2$, mg/ml
Ref.: 43

	Glucose	Soy Oligosaccharide	Fructo-oligosaccharide	Hydrolyzed Guar Gum
Acetate	30.5 ± 1.6	17.7 ± 1.3*	22.7 ± 1.2*	19.2 ± 0.4*
Propionate	8.9 ± 0.1	11.7 ± 0.2*	9.8 ± 0.7	19.8 ± 0.3*
Butyrate	4.6 ± 0.1	12.2 ± 2.5*	6.0 ± 0.4	15.5 ± 0.03*
Total SCFA	44.0 ± 1.6	41.8 ± 1.4	38.6 ± 2.3	54.6 ± 0.7*

	Cellulose	Powdered Cellulose	Methyl Cellulose	Psyllium Husk
Acetate	13.4 ± 0.6*	11.0 ± 0.3*	22.1 ± 0.8*	12.5 ± 0.2*
Propionate	21.0 ± 0.5*	14.8 ± 0.2*	10.4 ± 0.1*	14.3 ± 0.3*
Butyrate	3.4 ± 0.02	7.5 ± 0.1	10.6 ± 0.5	16.8 ± 0.5*
Total SCFA	38.3 ± 1.1	33.5 ± 0.01*	43.1 ± 0.2	43.6 ± 0.9

	Inulin	Hydrolyzed Inulin
Acetate	19.4 ± 0.4*	21.7 ± 0.9*
Propionate	13.9 ± 0.1*	11.4 ± 0.2*
Butyrate	11.3 ± 0.2*	8.3 ± 0.7
Total SCFA	44.7 ± 0.21	41.4 ± 0.01

Comments (Ref. 43): All treatments → ↓ Ac prod. All treatments (except FOS) → ↑ Pr prod. Bu prod. increased by soy, guar, psyllium, and inulin

Animal model: Human, 3 male, 28–40 yr old, 48 hr incubation
Inoculum: Feces, Mean, $n = 6$, mmol/g substrate
Ref.: 44

Corn Fiber Fractions

	Original material	Total dietary fiber residue	Cell wall polysaccharides
Acetate	2.24[d,e]	1.75[e]	5.60[a]
Propionate	0.56[g]	0.50[g]	2.58[a]
Butyrate	0.74	0.38	0.7

Comments (Ref. 44): Ac and Pr from cell wall polysacc. > TDF fraction

Humans, 3 male, 32 ± 5 yr old, 24 h incubation

Oat bran fractions	Original material	Total dietary fiber residue	Cell wall polysaccharides		Ref
Acetate	4.43[b]	3.17[b,c]	4.93[a,b]	Pr from Cell wall polysacc. > TDF fraction	34
Propionate	1.60[b,c]	1.15[d,e]	1.65[b]		
Butyrate	1.43	0.85	0.91		

Wheat bran fractions	Original material	Total dietary fiber residue	Cell wall polysaccharides	
Acetate	2.85[c,d]	2.28[d,e]	4.27[b]	Ac and Pr from cell wall polysacc. > TDF fraction
Propionate	0.91[e,f]	0.58[f,g]	1.27[c,d]	
Butyrate	0.96	0.72	0.84	

Feces, Mean, n = 6 mmol/g substrate org matter

	Cellulose	Beet pulp	Citrus pulp	Citrus pectin	
Acetate	−0.03[a]	2.04[b]	2.68[b]	2.80[b,c]	SCFA prod. for cellulose < other treatments
Propionate	0.02[a]	0.97[b]	1.04[b]	1.05[b]	
Butyrate	0.00[a]	0.42[b]	0.61[c]	0.96[d]	
Total SCFA	0.00[a]	3.43[b]	4.32[b]	4.81[b,c]	

Humans, 2 donors, 24 h incubation

Feces, Mean ± SE, n = 2–7

	No fiber	Himanthalia elongata	Laminaria digitata	Undaria pinnatifida		Ref
Total SCFA, mmol/l	10.6 ± 1.7[d]	39.5 ± 0.6[c]	54.6 ± 1.0[b]	46.2 ± 2.7[b,c]	In comparison to the no-fiber treatment, all fibers except for fucans produced more total SCFA	45
Molar % (Ac/Pr/Bu)	—	73/15/10	69/19/9	75/14/9		

	Alginates	Fucans	Laminarans	Sugar beet
Total SCFA, mmol/l	54.3 ± 3.6[b]	11.4 ± 1.5[d]	87.6 ± 3.6[a]	73.1[a]
Molar % (Ac/Pr/Bu)	80/14/5	—	60/23/16	66/19/12

Table 4.9.7 (Continued) Influence of the Source of Dietary Fiber on SCFA Production In Vitro

Animal model	Inoculum	Source (and Level) of Fiber in Diet				Comments	Ref.
		Corn	Oat	Rice	Wheat		
Humans, 3 donors, 24 h incubation	Feces Mean ± SEM, $n = 6$ mmol/g organic matter						46
	Acetate	1.63 ± 0.21[a]	3.89 ± 0.49[b]	1.75 ± 0.21[a]	3.42 ± 0.11[b]	Ac production for oat and wheat > corn and rice	
	Propionate	0.60 ± 0.09[a]	1.20 ± 0.08[b]	0.90 ± 0.10[a,b]	1.02 ± 0.04[b]	Pr production for oat and wheat > corn	
	Butyrate	0.55 ± 0.03[b]	1.37 ± 0.28[c,d]	0.78 ± 0.15[a,b]	1.58 ± 0.07[c]	Bu production for oat and wheat > corn and rice	
	Total SCFA	2.78 ± 0.28[a]	6.45 ± 0.33[b]	3.42 ± 0.45[a]	6.01 ± 0.07[b]	Total SCFA prod. for oat and wheat > corn and rice	
		Broccoli	Cabbage	Carrot	Lettuce		
	Acetate	4.38 ± 0.87[b]	4.53 ± 0.53[b]	4.10 ± 0.82[b]	4.23 ± 0.84[b]	SCFA production vegetables > corn and rice	
	Propionate	1.31 ± 0.22[b]	1.24 ± 0.12[b]	1.21 ± 0.09[b]	1.03 ± 0.21[b]		
	Butyrate	1.14 ± 0.23[a,c,d]	1.45 ± 0.09[c,d]	1.15 ± 0.06[a,c,d]	1.01 ± 0.17[a,d]		
	Total SCFA	6.82 ± 1.29[b]	7.22 ± 0.59[b]	6.46 ± 0.92[b]	6.27 ± 1.20[b]		

Note: Solka Floc®, registered trademark of Fiber Sales and Development Corp., St. Louis, MO.

[a,b,c,d,e,f,g] Different superscripts within row (or within individual or for Total SCFA) indicate significant difference between diets at $p < 0.05$.

[h,i,j,k,l,m] Different superscripts within row indicate significant differences, between diets at $p < 0.01$.

[†] Data were extrapolated from the original graphs.

[*] Significant difference from control treatment.

In vitro, SCFA production appears to be higher for water-dispersible sources of dietary fiber than for fibers composed of a heterogeneous mix of water-dispersible and -indispersible compounds. More specifically, fibers derived from citrus or sugar beets produced more SCFA *in vitro* than did cellulose or corn bran.[18,34,38,41,42] Also, a range of plant gums appeared to produce more SCFA *in vitro* than did cereal fibers derived from oats, corn, or wheat.[38,39,42] Results with three different types of cereal suggest that SCFA production arises primarily from the cell wall polysaccharides of the brans rather than from the total dietary fiber residue.[44] In a separate study, vegetables were shown to support higher SCFA production *in vitro* than cereals. Taken together, it appears that foods rich in water-dispersible cell wall polysaccharides support greater SCFA production than do foods rich in cellulose, lignin, or other water-indispersible but structurally important components.

SUMMARY

It is now evident that the quantity and source of fiber affect SCFA production and absorption, and luminal pH. Since SCFA transport from the lumen to the mesenteric and portal blood supply is strongly dependent on luminal SCFA concentration, SCFA absorption will increase along with increased SCFA production. Given these kinetics, luminal SCFA concentrations will be attenuated by absorption. Thus, changes in luminal concentration will almost certainly underestimate the effect of the dietary component on SCFA production *in vivo*. While a standard *in vitro* system is useful to determine SCFA production under defined and rigorously controlled conditions, this approach is unable to consider fully aspects of the physiological situation, including differences in residence time, interaction effects with other luminal constituents, etc.

Much interest has been focused on the physiological roles of SCFA for the intestine and also for other tissues and cells. The importance of fiber in the diet evolved from viewing this as a nonnutritional and noncaloric substance to valuing dietary fiber as an important substance able to effect the health of the intestine as well as lipid metabolism, carbohydrate metabolism, and prevention of cancer development. As more information becomes available, identifying the precise mechanism by which dietary fiber and SCFA exert their physiological effects, differences among fibers will be able to be more effectively exploited to optimize health and prevent disease.

REFERENCES

1. Balay, G. L. et al., Prolonged intake of fructo-oligosaccharides induces a short-term elevation of lactic acid-producing bacteria and a persistent increase in cecal butyrate in rats, *J. Nutr.*, 129, 2231, 1999.
2. LeBlay, G. et al., Enhancement of butyrate production in the rat caecocolonic tract by long-term ingestion of resistant potato starch, *Br. J. Nutr.*, 82, 419, 1999.
3. Zoran, D. L. et al., Wheat bran diet reduces tumor incidence in a rat model of colon cancer independent of effects on distal luminal butyrate concentrations, *J. Nutr.*, 127, 2217, 1997.
4. Younes, H. et al., Fermentable carbohydrate exerts a urea-lowering effect in normal and nephrectomized rats, *Am. J. Physiol.*, 272, G515, 1997.
5. Fredstrom, S. B. et al., Apparent fiber digestibility and fecal short-chain fatty acid concentrations with ingestion of two types of dietary fiber, *JPEN*, 18, 14, 1994.
6. Edwards, C. A. and Eastwood, M. A., Comparison of the effects of ispaghula and wheat bran on rat caecal and colonic fermentation, *Gut*, 33, 1229, 1992.
7. Edward, C. A., Wilson, R. G., Hanlon, L., and Eastwood, M. A., Effect of the dietary fibre content of lifelong diet on colonic cellular proliferation in the rat, *Gut*, 33, 1076, 1992.
8. Zhang, J. and Lupton, J. R., Dietary fibers stimulate colonic cell proliferation by different mechanisms at different sites, *Nutr. Cancer*, 22, 267, 1994.
9. Lupton, J. R. and Kurtz, P. P., Relationship of colonic luminal short-chain fatty acids and pH to in vivo cell proliferation in rats, *J. Nutr.*, 123, 1522, 1993.

10. Morita, T. et al., Psyllium shifts the fermentation site of high-amylose cornstarch toward the distal colon and increases fecal butyrate concentration in rats, *J. Nutr.*, 129, 2081, 1999.

11. Zoran, D. L. et al., Diet and carcinogen alter luminal butyrate concentration and intracellular pH in isolated rat colonocytes, *Nutr. Cancer*, 27, 222, 1997.

12. Bachknudsen, K. E. et al., Gastrointestinal implications in pigs of wheat and oat fractions, *Br. J. Nutr.*, 65, 233, 1991.

13. Berggren, A., Bjorck, I. M. E., and Nyman, E. M. G. L., Short-chain fatty acid content and pH in caecum of rats fed various sources of starch, *J. Sci. Food Agric.*, 68, 241, 1995.

14. Roland, N. et al., Comparative study of the fermentative characteristics of inulin and different types of fibre in rats inoculated with a human whole faecal flora, *Br. J. Nutr.*, 74, 239, 1995.

15. Stark, A. H. and Madar, Z., In vitro production of short-chain fatty acids by bacterial fermentation of dietary fiber compared with effects of those fibers on hepatic sterol synthesis in rats, *J. Nutr.*, 123, 2166, 1993.

16. Hara, H. et al., Evaluation of fermentability of acid-treated maize husk by rat caecal bacteria in vivo and in vitro, *Br. J. Nutr.*, 71, 719, 1994.

17. Folino, M. M. A. and Young G. P., Dietary fibers differ in their effects on large bowel epithelial proliferation and fecal fermentation-dependent events in rats, *J. Nutr.*, 125, 1521, 1995.

18. Kim, M. and Shin, H. K., The water-soluble extract of chicory influences serum and liver lipid concentrations, cecal short-chain fatty acid concentrations and fecal lipid excretion in rats, *J. Nutr.*, 128, 1731, 1998.

19. Kishimoto, Y., Wakabayashi, S., and Takeda, H., Hypocholesterolemic effect of dietary fiber: relation to intestinal fermentation and bile acid excretion, *J. Nutr. Sci. Vitaminol.*, 41, 151, 1995.

20. McIntosh, G. H., Wang Y. H. A., and Royle, P. J., A diet containing chickpeas and wheat offers less protection against colon tumors than a casein and wheat diet in dimethylhydrazine-treated rats, *J. Nutr.*, 128, 804, 1998.

21. Fleming, S. E., Fitch, M. D., and DeVries, S., The influence of dietary fiber on proliferation of intestinal mucosal cells in miniture swine may not be mediated primarily by fermentation, *J. Nutr.*, 122, 906, 1992.

22. Christensen, D. N. et al., Integration of ileum cannulated pigs and in vitro fermentation to quantify the effect of diet composition on the amount of short-chain fatty acids available from fermentation in the large intestine, *J. Sci. Food Agric.*, 79, 755, 1999.

23. Jenkins, D. J. A. et al., Physiological effects of resistant starches on fecal bulk, short chain fatty acids, blood lipids and glycemic index, *J. Am. Coll. Nutr.*, 17, 609, 1998.

24. Dokkum, V. et al., Effect of nondigestible oligosaccharides on large-bowel functions, blood lipid concentrations and glucose absorption in young healthy male subjects, *Eur. J. Clin. Nutr.*, 53, 1, 1999.

25. Lewis, S. J. and Heaton, K. W., Increasing butyrate concentration in the distal colon by accelerating intestinal transit, *Gut*, 41, 245, 1997.

26. Ahmed, R. et al., Fermentation of dietary starch in humans, *Am. J. Gastroenterology*, 95, 1017, 2000.

27. Marteau, P. et al., Digestibility and bulking effect of ispaghula husks in healthy humans, *Gut*, 35, 1747, 1994.

28. Mathers, J. C. and Tagny, J. M. F., Diurnal changes in large-bowel metabolism: short-chain fatty acids and transit time in rats fed on wheat bran, *Br. J. Nutr.*, 71, 209, 1994.

29. Wijnands, M. V. W. et al., A comparison of the effects of dietary cellulose and fermentable galacto-oligosaccharide, in a rat model of colorectal carcinogenesis: fermentable fibre confers greater protection than non-fermentable fibre in both high and low fat backgrounds, *Carcinogenesis*, 20, 651, 1999.

30. Haack, V. S. et al., Increasing amounts of dietary fiber provided by foods normalizes physiological response of the large bowel without altering calcium balance or fecal steroid excretion, *Am. J. Clin. Nutr.*, 68, 615, 1998.

31. Reddy, S., Faecal pH, bile acid and sterol concentrations in premenopausal Indian and white vegetarians compared with white omnivores, *Br. J. Nutr.*, 79, 495, 1998.

32. Goni, I. et al., In vitro fermentation and hydration properties of commercial dietary fiber-rich supplements, *Nutr. Res.*, 18, 1077, 1998.

33. Monsma, D. J. et al., In vitro fermentation of swine ileal digesta containing oat bran dietary fiber by rat cecal inocula adapted to the test fiber increases propionate production but fermentation of wheat bran ileal digesta does not produce more butyrate, *J. Nutr.*, 130, 585, 2000.

34. Sunvold, G. D. et al., In vitro fermentation of cellulose, beet pulp, citrus pulp, and citrus pectin using fecal inoculum from cats, dogs, horses, humans, and pigs and ruminal fluid from cattle, *J. Anim. Sci.*, 73, 3639, 1995.

35. Guillon, F. et al., Characterisation of residual fibres from fermentation of pea and apple fibres by human faecal bacteria, *J. Sci. Food Agric.*, 68, 521, 1995.

36. McBurney, M. I., Potential water-holding capacity and short-chain fatty acid production from purified fiber sources in a fecal incubation system, *Nutr.*, 7, 421, 1991.

37. Salvador, V. et al., Sugar composition of dietary fibre and short-chain fatty acid production during in vitro fermentation by human bacteria, *Br. J. Nutr.*, 70, 189, 1993.

38. Bourquin, L. D. et al., Fermentation of various dietary fiber sources by human fecal bacteria, *Nutr. Res.*, 16, 1119, 1996.

39. Bourquin, L. D. et al., Fermentation of dietary fibre by human colonic bacteria: disappearance of, short-chain fatty acid production from, and potential water-holding capacity of various substrates, *Scand. J. Gastroenterology*, 28, 249, 1993.

40. Casterline, J. L., Jr., Oles, C. J., and Ku, Y., In vitro fermentation of various food fiber fraction, *J. Agric. Food Chem.*, 45, 2463, 1997.

41. Campbell, J. M. et al., Psyllium and methylcellulose fermentation properties in relation to insoluble and soluble fiber standards, *Nutr. Res.*, 17, 619, 1997.

42. Titgemeyer, E. C. et al., Fermentability of various fiber sources by human fecal bacteria in vitro, *Am. J. Clin. Nutr.*, 53, 1418, 1991.

43. Velazquez, M. et al., Effect of oligosaccharides and fibre substitutes on short-chain fatty acid production by human faecal microflora, *Anaerobe*, 6, 87, 2000.

44. Bourquin, L. D. et al., Short-chain fatty acid production and fiber degradation by human colonic bacteria: effects of substrate and cell wall fractionation procedures, *J. Nutr.*, 122, 1508, 1992.

45. Michel, C. et al., In vitro fermentation by human faecal bacteria of total and purified dietary fibres from brown seaweeds, *Br. J. Nutr.*, 75, 263, 1996.

46. McBurney, M. I. and Thompson, L. U., Fermentative characteristics of cereal brans and vegetable fibers, *Nutr. Cancer*, 13, 271, 1990.

47. Vanderhoof, J. A., Immunonutrition: the role of carbohydrates, *Nutr.*, 14, 595, 1998.

48. Fleming, S. E., Influence of dietary fiber on the production, absorption, or excretion of short chain fatty acids in humans, in *CRC Handbook of Dietary Fiber in Human Nutrition*, 2nd ed., Spiller, G. A., Ed., CRC Press, Boca Raton, FL, 1993, 387.

Effects of Dietary Fiber on Fecal and Intestinal Luminal Mutagens

Hugh J. Freeman

Human feces contain mutagens and have been assessed by a variety of short-term *in vitro* methods.[1-6] Fecal mutagenic activity has been postulated to influence colon cancer risk, and this activity may be modulated by the diet. Generally, methods employed to measure mutagenic activity have involved bacterial mutation assays; these are based on a qualitative relationship between carcinogenicity and DNA damage. They are sensitive and rapidly performed.[7] Initially, the presence of mutagenic activity was shown in feces from healthy human male volunteers consuming a "Western diet."[1] It was subsequently claimed that stool samples contain both volatile and nonvolatile *N*-nitroso compounds[8] as well as nitrite and nitrates;[9] however, the precise nature of the compound or compounds in feces causing bacterial mutations was not known. Using a different approach, genotoxic effects of human feces were demonstrated using induction of chromosome damage in cultured Chinese hamster ovary cells as the indicator of mutagenic activity.[10] Later, fecal extracts from both carnivorous and herbivorous animals were demonstrated[11] with high chromosome damaging potency observed in three carnivorous species examined. It was noted that the chromosome aberrations seen were comparable to those in mammalian cells exposed to 250 to 400 rads of X-rays as well as to several known carcinogens.[11]

Subsequent studies focused on changes induced in mutagen levels of feces by altered diets or lifestyles. For example, ingestion of antioxidants such as ascorbic acid or tocopherol caused a reduction in fecal mutagenic activity followed by a gradual return to control values over a 1-month period.[12] Later, fecal mutagens were defined in a single stool sample from each individual in groups of South Africans (i.e., urban whites, urban blacks, and rural blacks) with differing colon cancer risks.[13] Urban whites, a high colon cancer risk population, had a significantly higher percentage of mutagen-positive stools compared to two low-risk black populations. Later, it was suggested that bacterial flora are involved in the formation of this mutagenic activity.[14] Others[15] examined fecal mutagens in three groups: Seventh-Day Adventists living in New York consuming an ovo-lacto vegetarian diet (milk and milk products but no fish, poultry, or meat) with a low colon cancer risk, inhabitants of Kuopio, Finland with a low risk, and omnivorous New Yorkers, a high-risk group. The Finns consumed more milk, dairy products, and fiber but less animal fat than New Yorkers. No Adventist sample was mutagenic; however, positive activity was observed in 13% of Finnish samples compared to 22% of New Yorkers. In Vancouver, Canada, fecal mutagens were determined in strict vegetarians, ovo-lacto vegetarians, and nonvegetarians[16] using the fluctuation test for weak mutagens.[17] Because this bacterial assay method is extremely sensitive compared to the method used in earlier studies,[1,12–15] virtually all samples showed mutagenic activity. Ovo-lacto vegetarians and strict vegetarians had significantly lower levels of fecal mutagens than nonvegetarians, and the presence of at least two fecal mutagens was suggested. Later, it was shown that formula-fed individuals with consistent nutrient levels had fecal mutagenic activities that did not vary significantly within an individual; however, there were significant differences between subjects on identical diets, suggesting that long-term dietary and possibly genetic factors influence mutagen levels.[18] The effects of short-term dietary modification on fecal mutagens were also assessed:[9] two dietary regimes were used, a low colon cancer risk non-meat diet was consumed for 2 weeks, followed by 2 weeks on a high-risk beef diet. Within a 2-week period, mutagen levels increased on the high-meat diet. More recent studies have shown that fecal mutagen levels are lower in a rural low-risk colon cancer population (i.e., Kuopio, Finland) compared to an urban high-risk colon cancer population (i.e., Helsinki, Finland).[20] Multiple types of mutagens may be present, as shown in a New York population consuming a high-fat, low-fiber "mixed" Western diet. Fecal mutagenic activities were determined after a period of supplementation with high fat and high fiber. Although no significant change was seen in the high-fat group, high-fiber feeding reduced fecal mutagenic activities.[22] Human studies have demonstrated that only specific sources of ingested dietary fibers, such as wheat bran or cellulose, reduce the production and/or excretion of fecal mutagens.[23] In addition, a shift from a well-balanced mixed diet to a lacto-vegetarian diet reduced direct-acting mutagen activities in human urine and feces, measured with the fluctuation assay for weak mutagens, possibly related to higher water content in feces from dilution of fecal mutagens.[24] Finally, *in vitro* studies have shown a dietary fiber–induced reduction in fecapentaene excretion, a potent mutagen present in human feces related to fecapentaene fiber adsorption.[25]

Studies specifically focused on the effect of dietary fibers *per se* are limited.[26] Extracts were obtained from fecal pellets and the luminal contents along the length of the GI tract in rats fed either a chemically defined fiber-free diet or nutritionally and calorically equivalent diets with differing amounts of purified cellulose or pectin (4.5 or 9%) or a mixture of cellulose and pectin (4.5% each). Mutagenicity was measured using the fluctuation test for weak mutagens[17] with *Salmonella typhimurium* TA 98 and TA 1535 as tester strains. Over a 6-week period only the high-cellulose diet influenced fecal mutagen levels; significant reduction was observed with the TA 1535 strain. Analysis of the contents of the stomach, distal small bowel, cecum, and colon after 8 weeks on the fiber-free diet revealed that the distal small bowel had a several-fold-higher mutagen concentration than any other site. These activities were significantly reduced by ingestion of either the cellulose or pectin single-fiber diet. Previous studies using chemically induced animal models demonstrate protective effects for some dietary fibers in rats exposed to exogenously administered chemical carcinogens (see Chapter 5.9). This study further extended these observations to endogenous mutagenic activities and provided strong evidence that these mutagens are formed within the small bowel. Subsequently, they are presented to the cecum and colon in high concentrations. Some studies have explored possible mechanisms for these dietary effects on mutagens. These have revealed that different fiber sources including corn bran, wheat bran, and alfalfa directly bind carcinogens in a pH-dependent manner, optimally in the pH range of 4 to 6 found in the human GI tract and apparently through a mechanism of cation exchange.[27–30] Alternatively, specific types of dietary fibers, such as pure cellulose, have been shown to alter colonic bacterial enzyme activities important in mutagen metabolism, in experimental colon cancer[31] as well as in humans on high-fiber diets.[32] This differed from effects of the purified fiber, lignin, that did not lead to reduced levels of colon cancer in chemically treated rats.[33] Finally, some recent studies have explored the effects of luminal mutagenic activities on the colonic mucosa *per se*. Surrogate endpoint biomarkers for colon cancer risk in both rats and humans have been evaluated.[34] In these studies, both wheat bran fiber supplementation and phytic acid (inositol hexaphosphate) resulted in decreased formation of aberrant crypt foci.[34,35]

REFERENCES

1. Bruce, W. R., Varghese, A. J., Furrer, R., and Land, P. C., A mutagen in feces of normal humans, in *Origins of Human Cancer*, Book C, Cold Spring Harbor Conferences on Cell Proliferation, vol. 4, Hiatt, H. H., Watson, J. D., and Winsten, J. A., Eds., Cold Spring Harbor Laboratory, Cold Spring Harbor, NY, 1977, 1641.
2. Stich, H. F. and Kuhnlein, U., Chromosome breaking activity of human feces and its enhancement by transition metals, *Int. J. Cancer*, 24, 284, 1979.
3. de Vet, H. C. W., Sharma, C., and Reddy, B. S., Effect of dietary fried meat on fecal mutagenic and co-mutagenic activity in humans, *Nutr. Rep. Int.*, 23, 653, 1981.
4. Nader, C. J., Potter, C. D., and Weller, R. A., Diet and DNA-modifying activity in human fecal extracts, *Nutr. Rep. Int.*, 23, 113, 1981.
5. Venitt, S., Faecal mutagens in the aetiology of colonic cancer, in *Colonic Carcinogenesis, Falk Symposium 31*, Malt, R. A. and Williamson, R. C. N., Eds., MTP Press, Lancaster, England, 59, 1982.
6. Wilkins, T. D., Lederman, R. L., van Tassell, R. L., Kingston, D. G. I., and Henion, J., Characterization of a mutagenic bacterial product in human feces, *Am. J. Clin. Nutr.*, 33, 2513, 1980.
7. Ames, B. N., McCann, J., and Yamasaki, E., Methods for detecting carcinogens and mutagens with the Salmonella/mammalian microsome mutagenicity test, *Mutat. Res.*, 31, 347, 1975.
8. Wang, T., Kakizoe, T., Dion, P., Furrer, R., Varghese, A. J., and Bruce, W. R., Volatile nitrosamines in normal human feces, *Nature (London)*, 276, 280, 1978.
9. Tannenbaum, S. R., Fett, D., Young, V. R., Land, P. C., and Bruce, W. R., Nitrite and nitrate are formed by endogenous synthesis in human intestine, *Science*, 200, 1487, 1978.
10. Stich, H. F., Wei, L., and Lam, P., The need for a mammalian test system for mutagens: action of some reducing agents, *Cancer Lett.*, 5, 199, 1978.
11. Stich, H. F., Stich, W., and Acton, A. B., Mutagenicity of fecal extracts from carnivorous and herbivorous animals, *Mutat. Res.*, 78, 105, 1980.
12. Bruce, W. R., Varghese, A. J., Wang, S., and Dion, P., The endogenous production of nitroso compounds in the colon and cancer at that site, in *Naturally Occurring Carcinogens — Mutagens and Modulators of Carcinogenesis*, Miller, E. C., Ed., University Park Press, Baltimore, 221, 1979.
13. Erhrich, M., Aswell, J. E., van Tassell, R. L., Walker, A. R. P., Richardson, N. J., and Wilkins, T. D., Mutagens in feces of 3 South African populations at different levels of risk for colon cancer, *Mutat. Res.*, 64, 231, 1979.
14. Lederman, M., van Tassell, R., West, S. E. H., Erhrich, M. F., and Wilkins, T. D., In vitro production of human fecal mutagen, *Mutat. Res.*, 79, 115, 1980.
15. Reddy, B. S., Sharma, C., Darby, L., Laakso, K., and Wynder, E. L., Metabolic epidemiology of large bowel cancer. Fecal mutagens in high- and low-risk populations for colon cancer, *Mutat. Res.*, 72, 511, 1980.
16. Kuhnlein, U., Bergstrom, D., and Kuhnlein, H., Mutagens in feces from vegetarians and nonvegetarians, *Mutat. Res.*, 85, 1, 1981.
17. Green, M. H. L. and Muriel, W. J., Mutagen testing using TRP+ reversion in *Escherichia coli*, *Mutat. Res.*, 38, 3, 1976.
18. Kuhnlein, H. V. and Kuhnlein, U., Mutagens in feces from subjects on controlled formula diets, *Nutr. Cancer*, 2, 119, 1981.
19. Kuhnlein, H. V., Kuhnlein, U., and Bell, P. A., The effect of short-term dietary modifications on human fecal mutagenic activity, *Mutat. Res.*, 113, 1, 1983.
20. Reddy, B. S., Sharma, C., Mathews, L., Engle, A., Laakso, K., Choi, K., Puska, P., and Korpella, R., Metabolic epidemiology of colon cancer: fecal mutagens in healthy subjects from rural Kuopio and urban Helsinki, Finland, *Mutat. Res.*, 152, 97, 1985.
21. Reddy, B. S., Sharma, C., Mathews, L., and Engle, A., Fecal mutagens from subjects consuming a mixed-Western diet, *Mutat. Res.*, 135, 11, 1984.
22. Venitt, S., Bosworth, D., and Aldrick, A. J., Pilot study of the effect of diet on the mutagenicity of human faeces, *Mutagenesis*, 1, 353, 1986.
23. Reddy, B. S., Engle, A., Katsifis, S., Simi, B., Bartram, H. P., Perrino, P., and Mahan, C., Biochemical epidemiology of colon cancer: effect of types of dietary fiber on fecal mutagens, acid, and neutral sterols in healthy subjects, *Cancer Res.*, 49, 4629, 1989.

24. Johansson, G., Holmen, A., Persson, L., Hogstedt, R., Wassen, C., Ottova, L., and Gustafsson, J. A., The effect of a shift from a mixed diet to a lacto-vegetarian diet on human urinary and fecal mutagenic activity, *Carcinogenesis*, 13, 153, 1992.

25. de Kok, T. M., van Iersel, M. L., ten Hoor, F., and Kleinjans, J. C., In vitro study on the effects of fecal composition on fecapentaene kinetics in the large bowel, *Mutat. Res.*, 302, 103, 1993.

26. Kuhnlein, U., Gallagher, R., and Freeman, H. J., Effects of purified cellulose and pectin fiber diets on mutagenicity of feces and luminal contents of stomach, small and large bowel in rats, *Clin. Invest. Med.*, 6, 253, 1983.

27. Barnes, W. S., Maiello, J., and Weisburger, J. H., In vitro binding of the food mutagen 2-amino-3-methylimidazo(4,5-f)quinoline to dietary fibers, *J. Natl. Cancer Inst.*, 70, 757, 1983.

28. Morotomi, M. and Mutai, M., In vitro binding of potent mutagenic pyrolysates to intestinal bacteria, *J. Natl. Cancer Inst.*, 77, 195, 1986.

29. Takeuchi, M., Hara, M., Inoue, T., and Kada, T., Adsorption of mutagens by refined wheat bran, *Mutat. Res.*, 204, 263, 1988.

30. Roberton, A. M., Harris, P. J., Hollands, H. J., and Ferguson, L. R., A model system for studying the adsorption of a hydrophobic mutagen to dietary fibre, *Mutat. Res.*, 244, 173, 1990.

31. Freeman, H. J., Effects of differing purified cellulose, pectin, and hemicellulose fiber diets on fecal enzymes in 1,2-dimethylhydrazine-induced rat colon carcinogenesis, *Cancer Res.*, 46, 5529, 1986.

32. Reddy, B. S., Engle, A., Simi, B., and Goldman, M., Effect of dietary fiber on colonic bacterial enzymes and bile acids in relation to colon cancer, *Gastroenterology*, 102, 1475, 1992.

33. Cameron, I. L., Hardman, W. E., and Heitman, D. W., The nonfermentable dietary fiber lignin alters putative colon cancer risk factors but does not protect against DMH-induced colon cancer in rats, *Nutr. Cancer*, 28, 170, 1997.

34. Earnest, D. L., Einspahr, J. G., and Alberts, D. S., Protective role of wheat bran fiber: data from marker trials, *Am. J. Med.*, 106, 32S, 1999.

35. Reddy, B. S., Prevention of colon carcinogenesis by components of dietary fiber, *Anticancer Res.*, 19, 3681, 1999.

CHAPTER **4.11**

Effect of Dietary Fiber and Foods on Carbohydrate Metabolism

Thomas M. S. Wolever and David J. A. Jenkins

INTRODUCTION

This chapter will review the relationship between gastrointestinal events and carbohydrate metabolism in the short and long terms, beginning with the effects of dietary fiber and including the extension of this to more recent work on the glycemic index of foods where fiber, food form, and the so-called "antinutrients" all combine to produce the glycemic response typical of the whole food.

ADDITION OF FIBER TO SINGLE TEST MEALS

There is evidence that the viscosity of purified dietary fiber is directly related to its effect on glucose tolerance.[1,16] Guar, pectin, psyllium, and other viscous fibers have been shown to flatten postprandial blood glucose and insulin responses more consistently than wheat bran and other nonviscous fibers, which have little or no acute effect (Tables 4.11.1 through 4.11.4, Figure 4.11.1). In 24 groups of subjects in 15 studies, when guar gum was adequately mixed with a test meal, the blood glucose response was reduced by an average of 44% ($p < 0.001$). The addition of pectin or hemicellulose did not enhance the effect of guar alone (Table 4.11.1). By contrast, pectin reduced the glucose response by an average of 29% ($n = 10$, $p < 0.01$, Table 4.11.2), psyllium by 29% ($n = 13$, $p < 0.001$, Table 4.11.3), 6 other gelling agents by 23% ($n = 8$, $p < 0.01$, Table 4.11.3), wheat bran by 27% ($n = 6$, $p < 0.01$, Table 4.11.2), and 7 other nongelling fibers by only 17% ($n = 10$, ns, Table 4.11.4). The degree of flattening of the glycemic response does not appear to be related to the dose of guar or pectin, possibly due to differences in experimental design, but a linear dose-response relationship is seen with psyllium (Figure 4.11.2, Table 4.11.3).

Necessity of Adequate Mixing of Fiber with Food

To be effective, guar and other viscous fibers must be mixed with the carbohydrate in a hydrated form. Thus, when guar (4 studies, Table 4.11.1) or psyllium (1 study, Table 4.11.3) was sprinkled dry onto foods or taken before the main carbohydrate portion of the test meal, there was no effect on blood glucose responses. The necessity of adequate mixing of fiber with carbohydrate for

**Table 4.11.1 Effect of Adding Guar Gum (G) Alone or with Hemicellulose (H) or Pectin (P) on
Blood Glucose, and Insulin Responses to Single Test Meals**

Fiber (g)	Available Carbohydrate (g) Source		Sub[b]	% Change with Fiber[a]		Ref.
				Glucose	Insulin	
G 2.5	50	Glucose	N	−24% ns	−64%***	1
G 2.5	50	Glucose	N	−34%*	−65%**	2
G 5	50	Glucose	N	0% ns	−44% +	3
G 5	50	Glucose	N		−66%**	4
G 5	49	Guar bread and soup	N	−41% + + +	−37% + + +	5
G 5	49	Bread and guar soup	N	−54%***	−50%***	5
G10	85	Cornflakes, sucrose, milk, bread, and jam (guar sprinkled on cereal)	D	−2% ns	−20% ns	6
G 8	58	Biscuits	D	− 53%		7
G15	100	Glucose	N	−36% + +	−37%**	8
G15	100	Glucose	GD	− 32%*	−68% ns	8
G 7	42	Bread and cheese	D	−49%		9
G 7	42	Bread and soybeans	D	−58%		9
G 9	50	Glucose	N	−23%*		3
G10	52	Soup, bread, egg, and butter	N	−48%**	−48%**	10
G10	52	Soup, bread, egg, and butter	D	−58%**		10
G10	47	Soup and bread	N,D	−78%*	−59%**	10
G10	46	Guar bread and guar soup	N	−68%***	−65%***	5
G 5	23	Mashed potato (guar mixed with meal)	D	−42%**	−40% ns	11
G 5	23	Mashed potato (guar taken before meal)	D	−5% ns	0% ns	11
G16	66	Guar pasta, butter, cheese	N,D	−9%*		12
G20	83	Guar pasta, egg, cheese, butter, ham	N	−80%**	−45%**	12
G23	80	Sucrose	N	−29% ns	−55% + + +	13
G14.5	50	Glucose	N	−50%**	−54%**	2
G14.5	50	Glucose	N	−38%**	−60%**	14
G14.5	50	Glucose (mixed with guar)	N	−27%*		15
G14.5	50	Glucose (taken after guar)	N	−0% ns		15
G14.5	50	Glucose	N	−68%**	−58%***	16
G15	50	Glucose (taken after guar)	N	−2% ns	+28% ns	17
G10	20	Oatmeal porridge	D	−61%*		18
G 5,P 5	72	Bread, butter, honey, egg, and milk	N	−60%*	−6% ns	19
G 5,P 5	72	Bread, butter, honey, egg, and milk	D	−41%*	−16% ns	19
G 5,P 5	72	Bread, butter, honey, egg, and milk	AN	− 2% ns	0% ns	19
G16,P10	102	Bread, margarine, jam, and milk	N,D	−23%	−51%	20
G16,P10	106	Bread, butter, jam, and milk	D	−51%**	−50%**	21
G15,P10	50	Glucose (after fiber)	N	−7% ns	−1% ns	17
G 4,H 4	25	Bread	D	−22%	−71%	22

[a] % change in area under the curve (or peak rise) of blood glucose and insulin (lack of a figure means that the data is not available). * = $p < 0.05$; + = $p < 0.025$; ** = $p < 0.01$; + + = $p < 0.005$; + + + = $p < 0.002$; *** = $p < 0.001$; ns = not significant.
[b] Subjects: N = normal, D = diabetic, GD = gestational diabetes, AN = diabetes with autonomic neuropathy.

effectiveness is important because the mechanism of action of viscous fiber is related to its ability to reduce the rate of diffusion of nutrients from the lumen of the small intestine,[14,213–215] although delayed gastric emptying may also play a role.[26,30,77,216] Nevertheless, viscous fiber has not been demonstrated to cause carbohydrate malabsorption.[16,30]

Effect of Food Refining on Postprandial Glucose Responses

Removal of cereal fiber from foods by refining has no effect on the postprandial glucose and insulin responses (Table 4.11.5). This is consistent with the lack of effect of cereal fiber when added to carbohydrate test meals (Table 4.11.2). On the other hand, the consumption of fruit juice

Table 4.11.2 Effect of Adding Pectin (P) Alone or Wheat Bran (B) on Blood Glucose, and Insulin Responses to Single Test Meals

Fiber (g)	Available Carbohydrate (g) Source	Sub[b]	%Change with Fiber[a] Glucose	Insulin	Ref.
P10	100 Glucose and beef	N	−59%**	−22% ns	23
P10	100 Glucose	N	−4% ns	+11% ns	23
P10	85 Cornflakes, sucrose, milk, bread, and jam (pectin sprinkled on cereal)	N	−23% ns	−18% ns	6
P 7	60 Bread, cheese, rice, meat, and Peach	D	−12%*	−35%*	24
P15	105 Bread and jam	D	−44%		25
P10.5	75 Glucose	PGS	−23%**	−56% +	26
P10	50 Glucose (after pectin)	N	+5% ns	+6% ns	17
P 9	45 Glucose[c]	IGT	−25% +	−11% ns	27
P14.5	50 Glucose	N	−11% ns	−2% ns	16
P14.5	50 Glucose	PGS	−20%**		28
P14.5	50 Glucose	PGS	−40%***	−76%***	29
P14.5	50 Glucose	N	−55% +		30
B10	50 Glucose (after bran)	N	+7% ns	+11% ns	17
B0.2g/kg	1 g/kg Glucose	N	−37%**		31
B20	90 Beef, bread, rice, corn, tomato	D	−11% ns	+6% ns[d]	32
B36	50 Glucose, beef, lactulose	N	−54% ns	−16% ns	33
B41.5	50 Glucose	N	−27% ns	−8% ns	16
B50	50 Glucose	D/D	−13% ns	−34% ++	34
B50	50 Glucose	D/O	−21% +	0% ns	34

[a] % change in area under the curve (or peak rise) of blood glucose and insulin (lack of a figure means that the data is not available). * = $p < 0.05$; + = $p < 0.025$; ** = $p < 0.01$; + + = $p < 0.005$; + + + = $p < 0.002$; *** = $p < 0.001$; ns = not significant.

[b] Subjects: N = normal; D = diabetic; PGS = postgastric surgery: IGT = impaired glucose tolerance with reactive hypoglycemia; D/D = diabetic on diet alone; D/O = diabetic on oral agents.

[c] Grams pectin and glucose are per square meter of body surface.

[d] Represents change in insulin requirements of Type 1 diabetics on an artificial pancreas.

as opposed to whole fruit is associated with a somewhat greater blood glucose response and markedly enhanced peripheral insulin levels.[50–52] In these cases, disruption of food form, rather than removal of fiber *per se*, may be important.

LONGER-TERM EFFECTS OF DIETARY FIBER SUPPLEMENTS

Normal Volunteers

Nonviscous fibers have been added to the diets of normal individuals more often than viscous fibers (Table 4.11.6). These studies show, paradoxically, that nonviscous fibers have more effect than viscous fibers in improving fiber-free glucose tolerance tests given after a period of fiber supplementation (Table 4.11.6).

Treatment of Diabetes

There have been more than 20 studies using guar gum or other viscous fibers to treat diabetes and about half that number using various nonviscous fibers (Tables 4.11.7 and 4.11.8). The improvements in diabetic control after the addition of viscous fibers were larger and more consistent than after the addition of nonviscous fibers (Figure 4.11.3). In 18 studies where urinary glucose was measured, losses were reduced by 41% after guar ($p < 0.001$), but in seven studies with nonviscous fibers, there was a mean increase of 34% (ns). Fasting blood glucose was reduced by a mean of

Table 4.11.3　Effect of Adding Various Gelling Agents on Blood Glucose and Insulin Responses to Single Test Meals

Fiber[a] (g)		Available Carbohydrate (g) Source	Sub[c]	% Change with Fiber[b]		Ref.
				Glucose	Insulin	
T14.5	50	Glucose	N	−34%**	−10% ns	16
M14.5	50	Glucose	N	−29%*	−18% ns	16
L2.5	50	Glucose	N	−29% ns	−19% ns	1
L10	85	Cornflakes, sucrose, milk, bread, jam	D	−15% ns	−11% ns	6
X2.5	50	Glucose	N	−41%*	−37%**	1
X/L2.5	50	Glucose	N	−28% ns	−64%**	1
A10	85	Cornflakes, sucrose, milk, bread, jam	D	−7% ns	+17% ns	6
K5	80	Glucose	N	0% ns	−28%*	35
S3.5	50	Glucose (psyllium as Fibogel)	N	−33% ns	−39% ns	2
S3.6		Bread, butter, cheese, meat, milk	D	−33%*	−19%*d	36
S6.6	50	Bread, butter, cheese	D	−29%		37
S7	50	Glucose (psyllium as Fibogel)	N	−12% ns	−28% ns	2
S7	50	Glucose (psyllium as Fibogel)	D	−17% ns	−13% ns	2
S7	50	Glucose (psyllium as Metamucil)	N	0% ns		2
S3.9	50	Psyllium-enriched flaked bran cereal	N	−12% ns		38
S8.1	50	Psyllium-enriched flaked bran cereal	N	−24% ns		38
S12.7	50	Psyllium-enriched flaked bran cereal	N	−20% ns		38
S16.8	50	Psyllium-enriched flaked bran cereal	N	−46%**		38
S15.7	50	Psyllium-enriched flaked bran cereal	N	−46%**		38
S15.7	50	Psyllium-enriched flaked bran cereal	D	−51%*		38
S16.2	50	Psyllium sprinkled on bran flakes	N	−56%**		38
S16.2	50	Psyllium taken just before bran flakes	N	−4% ns		38

[a] T = Gum tragacanth; M = Methyl cellulose; L = Locust bean gum; A = agar; S = psyllium; K = Konjac mannan.
[b] % change in area under the curve (or peak rise) of blood glucose and insulin (lack of a figure means that the data is not available). * = $p < 0.05$; + = $p < 0.025$; ** = $p < 0.01$; + + = $p < 0.005$; + + + = $p < 0.002$; *** = $p < 0.001$; ns = not significant.
[c] Subjects: N = normal; D = diabetic.
[d] This figure represents the percent reduction of GIP response.

Table 4.11.4　Effect of Adding Various Nongelling Fibers on Blood Glucose and Insulin Responses to Single Test Meals

Fiber (g)	Available Carbohydrate (g) Source	Sub[c]	% Change with Fiber[b]		Ref.
			Glucose	Insulin	
Q14.5	50 Glucose	N	−26% ns	−24% ns	16
B15	105 Bread and jam	D	−6%		25
C 9	45 Glucose	IGT	−22% ns	0% ns	27
C 0.2g/kg	1 g/kg Glucose	N	+16% ns		31
G 0.2g/kg	1 g/kg Glucose	N	+24% ns		31
S20	86 50 g sucrose, 45 g flour	N	−14% ns	0% ns	39
S22	50 Glucose, beef, lactulose	N	−65%*	−24% ns	33
F30	50 Glucose, beef, lactulose	N	−39% ns	−19% ns	33
P10	58 Noodles, egg, milk, juice, margarine	DO	−21%	0% ns	40
P10	67,35 Liquid formula diet	D	−18% ns	−7% ns	41

[a] Q = cholestyramine; B = barley bran; C = cellulose; G = bagasse; S = sugar beet fiber; P = soy polysaccharide; F = pea fiber.
[b] % change in area under the curve (or peak rise) of blood glucose and insulin (lack of a figure means that the data is not available). * = $p < 0.05$; + = $p < 0.025$; ** = $p < 0.01$; + + = $p < 0.005$; +++ = $p < 0.002$; *** = $p < 0.001$; ns = not significant.
[c] Subjects: N = normal; D = diabetic; IGT = impaired glucose tolerance; DO = obese diabetic.

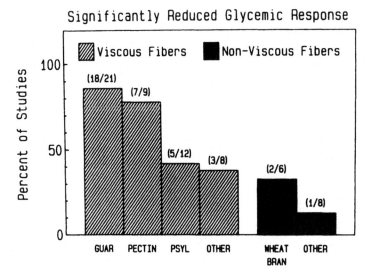

Figure 4.11.1   Effect of various types of purified dietary fiber on acute glycemic responses: proportion of studies with a statistically significant reduction (data from Tables 4.11.1 through 4.11.4).

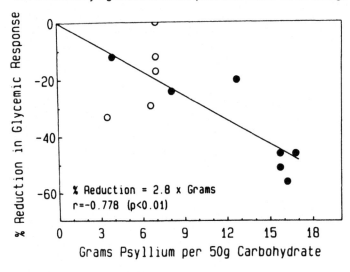

Figure 4.11.2   Effect of psyllium dose on acute glycemic responses (data from Table 4.11.3).

11% after guar ($p < 0.001$) and 3.8% after nonviscous fibers ($p < 0.02$). Glycosylated hemoglobin fell by a mean of 5.0% after guar ($p < 0.01$) and 3.4% (ns) after nonviscous fibers. Insulin doses tended to be reduced on guar (-11%, $p < 0.05$) but not after nonviscous fibers ($+1\%$, ns). Serum cholesterol fell by 11% after guar ($p < 0.001$) but not after nonviscous fibers (-1%, ns).

Summary — Long-Term Effects of Dietary Fiber Supplements

Those types of fiber with the most marked short-term effects also appear to have the greatest ability in the longer term to improve diabetic control. Viscous forms of dietary fiber such as guar gum are most able to alter events occurring within the gastrointestinal tract, such as the rate of absorption of glucose. These fibers are associated with short- and long-term beneficial changes in carbohydrate metabolism.

Table 4.11.5 Effect of Refining Food (i.e., Removal of Fiber) on Blood Glucose and Insulin Responses

Food	Available Carbohydrate	Dietary Fiber Whole	Dietary Fiber Refined	Sub[b]	% Change with Refining[a] Glucose	% Change with Refining[a] Insulin	Ref.
Wheat bread	50	10.2	2.8	N	− 6% ns		42
Wheat bread	50	10.2	2.8	D	− 2% ns		43
Wheat bread	58 and 60			N	−14% ns	−18% ns	44
Wheat bread	50			N	− 5% ns		45
Wheat bread	25			D	+ 7% ns		46
Rice	50	3.5	1.4	N	+11% ns		42
Rice	75			D	+ 6% ns	+14% ns	47
Spaghetti	50	7.3	2.0	N	+11% ns		42
Maize meal	50			N	+ 4% ns		48
Potato	50			N	+14% ns		49
Oranges	50			N	+15% ns		49
Oranges	50	16.0	0.0	N	ns	+50% + + +	50
Oranges	30	8.0	0.2	N	+6% ns	+32% +	51
Grapes	60	4.6	0.0	N	+28%*	+50% +	50
Apples	60			N	ns	+51%**	52

[a] % change in area under the curve (or peak rise) of blood glucose and insulin (lack of a figure means that the data is not available). * = $p < 0.05$; + = $p < 0.025$; ** = $p < 0.01$; + + = $p < 0.005$; + + + = $p < 0.002$; *** = $p < 0.001$; ns = not significant.
[b] Subjects: N = normal; D = diabetic.

Table 4.11.6 Effect of Dietary fiber on Fiber-Free Glucose Tolerance Tests[a]

Fiber Dose (g/day)	Study[b] Length	CHO	PRO	FAT	Comments	Change after Fiber[c] Glucose	Change after Fiber[c] Insulin	Ref.
Gum arabic, 25	21 D	39	15	42	FRD, all fiber in morning	+100% ns	ns	53
Pectin, 36	6 W				MD	+18% ns	+11% ns	54
Wheat bran, 12	4 W	47	14	36	FRD	ns	ns	55
Wheat bran, 20	7 W				MD	− 32%*	+36% +	56
Wheat bran, 24	6 M				FRD	−15%**		45
Wheat bran, 26	30 D				MD	− 17%	ns	57
Wheat bran, 26	30 D				MD	+24%	ns	57
Corn bran, 26	30 D				MD	− 56%*	ns	57
Soy hulls, 21	3 W	40	19	40	FRD undried DF	+5% ns	+10% ns	58
Soy hulls, 21	3 W	42	19	37	FRD dried DF	+59%*	−7% ns	58
Soy hulls, 26	30 D				MD	− 72%*	ns	57
Apple/carrot, 26	30 D				MD	− 28%*	ns	57
Xanthan gum, 12	6 W				FRD	− 25% ns[d]		59
Xanthan gum, 12	6 W(D)				FRD	− 31%*	−6% ns	59
Guar gum, 15	2 W				FRD	− 5% ns	− 4 % ns	60
Guar gum, 15	2 W(D)				FRD	−4% ns	+13% ns	60

[a] Subjects are normal except where indicated after study length (i.e., (D) = diabetic).
[b] Study length: D = days; W = weeks; M = months.
[c] % change in area under the curve (or peak rise) of blood glucose and insulin (lack of a figure means that the data is not available). * = $p < 0.05$; + = $p < 0.025$; ** = $p < 0.01$; + + = $p < 0.005$; + + + = $p < 0.002$; *** = $p < 0.001$; ns = not significant.
[d] 2-h postglucose blood glucose values.

Table 4.11.7 Treatment of Diabetes with Guar (G) or Guar plus Wheat Bran (B)

Dose (g)	Length	Subjects[a]	Comments[b] Diet	Form	% Change after Fiber Treatment[c] FBG	HbA1c	UG Loss	Insulin[d]	CHOL	TG	Ref.
G25	5D	6I,1N	MD	CB	-22%**		-50%**				61
G23	5D	6I,3N	MD	BI	-20%*		-38%++				62
G10	7D	2I,6N	FRD		-7%		-32%				7
G24	7D	12I	HD								63
G 9.2	2W	5I	FRD	BI	-8% ns	-11% ns	-80%**				7
G 9.2	2W	5N	FRD	BI	-18%***	-3%*	-62%***				7
G20	3W	6I,11N	FRD	GR	-10%*				-14%*		64
G15-25	4W	10N	FRD	GR	+13% ns		-51%***		-14%**		65
G.45g/kg	4W	10I,Child	FRD	BR			-8%				66
G20-25	4W	6I	FRD	SW	ns		-49% ns	-4% ns	-9%		67
G15	4W	41N,SU	FRD	MT	-11%*	-10%*	-50%*		-9%*	-12%*	68
G15	4W	38N,In	FRD	MT		+2% ns	-14%*	0%	-10%*	-2% ns	68
G15	4W	18N	FRD	GR					-10%*	+13% ns	69
G20	4W	9I	FRD	GR	-25%*	-7% ns		-5%+	-21%+	-25% ns	70
G15	4W	9N,O,PC	FRD	GR			-10% ns		-8% ns	0% ns	71
G8	6W	14N	FRD	BR	ns	ns			ns	ns	72
G12-19	6W	22I,Child	FRD	VF		-9%***	-15%***		-11%+		73
G10	8W	20N	FRD	GR	-3% ns	-9%***	-32% ns	-3% ns	0% ns	+5% ns	74
G 10-15	8W	2I,3N	MD	P	-24%**		-66%+		-16%*	-17%*	12
G15	8W	8N,ND,O	LOW	GR	-16% ns	-7% ns			-2% ns		75
G 15	8W	29N,EC	FRD	MT	0% ns	+2% ns			-10%***	+8% ns	76
G20,B10	8W	12N,O,PC	FRD	GR	-39%+		-73%*		-30%+	-40% ns	77
G21	3M	9N	FRD	GR	-17%+		-60%	-14%+	+11%+		78
G22	3M	10I,B	FRD	R	-19% ns	-3% ns			-18%***		79
G15	3M	6N,O,NC	FRD	CAP	0% ns	-5%ns			-9%***		80
G15	3M	20N,O,PC	FRD	GR	-10% ns				-10%*	-4% ns	81
G14-26	6M	8I,3N	FRD	CB	+4% ns		-7% ns	-28%***		+8% ns	82
G14-26	12M	6I,2N	FRD	CB			-44%*	-26%**			82

[a] Subjects: I = insulin–dependent; N = noninsulin–dependent; Child = children; SU = controlled on sulfonylureas; In = controlled on insulin; O = obese; PC = poorly controlled; ND = newly diagnosed; EC = excellent control; B = brittle; NC = poorly compliant.

[b] Diets: MD = metabolic diet; FRD = free-range diet; HD = hospital diet; LOW = weight-reducing, low-calorie (results for guar compared to a separate control group on a low-calorie diet not given guar). Form = type of guar formulation; CB = crispbread; BI = biscuits; P = pasta; GR = granulate; BR = bread; SW = snacks and sweets; MT = minitablets; FP = flavored powder taken in water before meals; VF = guar incorporated into various foods (bread, jelly, jam, fruit bar); R = rusks; CAP = capsules.

[c] FBG = fasting blood glucose; HbA1c = glycoylated hemoglobin; UG = urinary glucose; Insulin = daily insulin dose; CHOL = serum cholesterol; TG = serum triglycerides.
* = $p < 0.05$; + = $p < 0.025$; ** = $p < 0.01$; + + = $p < 0.002$; *** = $p < 0.001$.

[d] Represents fall in fasting serum insulin. In this study, guar increased peripheral insulin sensitivity by 70% ($p < 0.025$), insulin binding to monocytes by 28% ($p < 0.025$), and insulin receptor number by 50% ($p < 0.05$).

Table 4.11.8 Treatment of Diabetes with Miscellaneous Types of Dietary Fiber Nonviscous Fibers

Dose (g)	Length	Subjects[a]	Comments[b] Diet	Form	% Change after Fiber Treatment[c] FBG	HbA1c	UG Loss	Insulin[d]	CHOL	TG	Ref.
Apple Fiber											
26	4W	10N	FRD		−2% ns	+2% ns	+49% ns		−5% ns	+5% ns	83
52	4W	10N	FRD		−2% ns	+3% ns	+119% ns		+6%*	+2% ns	83
15	7W	12N	FRD		−8% ns	−8%**			−5% ns	0% ns	84
Corn Bran											
26	4W	10N	FRD		−6% ns	−2% ns	+26% ns		−2% ns	+1% ns	83
52	4W	10N	FRD		+2% ns	−8%*	+67% ns		+1% ns	−4% ns	83
Soy Hulls											
26	4W	10N	FRD		−10% ns	−2% ns	+5% ns		0% ns	+9% ns	83
52	4W	10N	FRD		−1% ns	−1% ns	+7% ns		+3% ns	+3% ns	83
Wheat Bran											
14	10–15D	17I	MD	BR	0% ns	−13% ns	−36%**	+2% ns	0% ns	+7% ns	85
15	4W	18N	FRD		−5% ns	−2% ns			−9%***	−10%*	69
20	4W	38IGT	FRD								86
Cellulose											
15	10D	8I	MD	BR	−6% ns			0%			87
Psyllium											
10.8	7D	9I	FRD	MM	+6% ns			0%			35
3.6	2M	20N	FRD	MM	−19%**	−6% ns			−5%*		88
7.2	2M	20N	FRD	MM	−18%***	−11% ns			−5%*		87
Konjac Mannan											
3.6–7	30D	13N	MD		−29%+			Reduced	−11%		89
Xanthan Gum											
12	6W	9N	FRD	MU	−38%*				−13%*	−25% ns	59

[a] Length: D = days; W = weeks; M = months. Subjects: N = noninsulin-dependent diabetes; I = insulin-dependent diabetes; IGT = impaired glucose tolerance.

[b] Diets: MD = metabolic diet; FRD = free-range diet. Form = type of fiber formulation; MM = "Metamucil"; BR = bread; MU = fiber in muffins.

[c] FBG = fasting blood glucose; HbA1c = glycoylated hemoglobin; UG = urinary glucose; Insulin = daily insulin dose; CHOL = serum cholesterol; TG = serum triglycerides. * = $p < 0.05$; + = $p < 0.025$; ** = $p < 0.01$; ++ = $p < 0.002$; *** = $p < 0.001$.

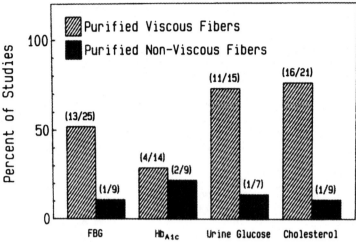

Figure 4.11.3 Effect of purified dietary fiber in the treatment of diabetes. Proportion of studies with statistically significant improvements in fasting blood glucose (FBG), glycosylated hemoglobin (HbA1c), urinary glucose excretion, and serum cholesterol concentration (data from Tables 4.11.7 and 4.11.8).

BLOOD GLUCOSE RESPONSE TO FOODS

In whole foods, many factors in addition to dietary fiber may alter digestion and absorption of nutrients and hence the glycemic response. Among these are antinutrients such as phytate,[105,217] lectins,[218] tannins,[219] and enzyme inhibitors,[220,221] macronutrient interactions such as protein-starch[222] and lipid-starch,[223] the nature of the starch (amylose vs. amylopectin),[224,225] gastric emptying rate[226] food form (e.g., bread as opposed to spaghetti), cooking, and particle size. It therefore becomes important in any discussion of glycemic response to be able to assess the collective interaction of all these factors in terms of the glycemic response to the whole food, and also to compare the full range of foods, so that the relative importance of each of the factors can be determined, again in the context of the whole food.

The Glycemic Index of Foods

The glycemic index (GI) of foods is an expression which permits the blood glucose response to different foods to be compared directly and so allows the relevance of their constituents (e.g., fiber) to be assessed. It is defined as the incremental blood glucose response following consumption of a 50-g-available carbohydrate portion of a food expressed as a percent of the response after a standard 50-g-available carbohydrate portion of white bread taken by the same individual. The methods used to determine the glycemic response and calculate the area under the curve can have a major influence on the results obtained;[227] exact GI methods are given elsewhere.[158]

$$\text{Glycemic Index} = \frac{\text{Area under the glucose curve after a food} \times 100\%}{\text{Area under the glucose curve after white bread}}$$

In this way, the GI makes it possible to compare the blood glucose responses of foods tested in different groups of subjects. Tables 4.11.9 and 4.11.10 show the wide range of GI values for different foods. The legumes, as a class, have the lowest GI of all starchy foods. Table 4.11.9 shows

Table 4.11.9   Glycemic Index Values of Foods Tested in Several Studies

Food	Individual GI Values[a]	Studies[b]	Mean ± SD	CV[c]
Breads				
Rye (crispbread)	90, 100	C, A	95	
Rye (whole meal)	82, 89, 97, 105, 119	Ti, G, Tn, #, #	98 ± 14	15%
Rye (whole grain-pumpernickel)	58, 78	C, G	68	
Wheat (white)	100 (Defined)	A–K, M	100	
Wheat (whole meal)	93, 95, 96, 96, 100, 104, 106, 106, 108	C, Tn, Ti, G, B, A, J, S, #	100 ± 6	6%
Pasta				
Spaghetti (white)	46, 59, 68, 72, 88	I, B, C, A, Z	67 ± 16	23%
Cereal grains				
Barley (pearled)	31, 41	F, Xi	36	
Buckwheat	70, 74, 90	Xn, A, Xi	78 ± 11	14%
Rice (polished)	68, 70, 73, 77, 78, 83, 92, 104	M, L, C, Z, B, H, W, A	81 ± 12	15%
Rice (parboiled)	58, 66, 72, 78	D, H, E, P	69 ± 9	12%
Sweet corn	66,67, 85, 86, 87, 90	E, L, P, A, J, D	80 ± 11	13%
Breakfast cereals				
"All Bran"	71, 74, 76	B, A, N	74 ± 3	3%
Cornflakes	107, 116, 121, 139	L, A, B, W	121 ± 13	11%
Porridge oats	71, 88, 93, 96, 96	A, C, K, B, W	89 ± 10	12%
Cookies				
Digestive	77, 86	B, A	82	
Plain crackers (water biscuits)	91, 108	A, S	100	
Root Vegetables				
Carrots	96, 131	¢, A	114	
Potato (instant mashed)	116, 119, 126	A, L, Y	120 ± 5	4%
Potato (mashed)	96, 100	Y, J	98	
Potato (new/white boiled)	67, 75, 77, 78, 101	C, B, Y, L, A	80 ± 13	16%
Potato (Russett, baked)	80, 112, 134, 137	Y, E, P, D	116 ± 26	23%
Legumes				
Baked beans (canned)	60, 69, 80	A, £, U	70 ± 10	14%
Bengal gram dal	7, 16	J, M	12	
Butter beans	39, 52	J, A	46	
Chick peas (dried)	44, 46, 52	U, B, A	47 ± 4	9%
Green peas (dried)	32, 68	C, A	50	
Green peas (frozen)	55, 74	C, A	65	
White beans (dried)	18, 27, 43, 44, 45, 46, 56, 84	@n, @h, U, O, A, £, Pn, Pi	45 ± 20	43%
Kidney beans (dried)	27, 31, 32, 42, 60, 65	M, W, Z, A, U, B	43 ± 16	38%
Lentils (green, dried)	31, 41	U, Z	36	
Lentils (red, dried)	25, 30, 42, 43, 43, 45, 45	R, Xn, A, B, β, Xi, W	39 ± 8	21%
Pinto beans (dried)	55, 65	U, B	60	
Peanuts	10, 19	J, A	15	
Fruit				
Apple	48, 52, 57	C, V, A	52 ± 5	9%
Banana	66, 75, 81, 90, 99	C, $, B, A, J	82 ± 13	16%
Orange	46, 58, 73	J, A, C	59 ± 14	23%
Orange juice	56, 67, 90	V, A, V	71 ± 17	24%
Sugars				
Fructose	9, 29, 30, 35	V, A, C, K	26 ± 11	45%
Glucose	122, 131, 132, 137, 140, 141, 145, 158	E, K, Q, C, D, W, J, A, M	138 ± 10	7%

Table 4.11.9 (Continued) Glycemic Index Values of Foods Tested in Several Studies

Food	Individual GI Values[a]	Studies[b]	Mean ± SD	CV[c]
Lactose	45, 69	V, K	57	
Sucrose	61, 85, 86, 87, 91, 92, 100	V, C, A @h, K, J, @n	86 ± 12	14%
Dairy Products				
Ice cream	52, 54, 84, 86	A, @h, @n, S	69 ± 19	27%
Whole milk	26, 29, 39, 49	@h, @n, S, A	36 ± 10	29%
Snack Foods				
Potato chips	74, 79	A, L	77	

[a] Individual mean values from groups of subjects. Values have been adjusted proportionately so that the glycemic index (GI) of white bread = 100. Values have also been adjusted proportionately (studies C, peas; T, breads; Z, instant potatoes) for unequal amounts of carbohydrate. Where glucose, but not white bread, was given, the GI values were multiplied by 1.38 (the GI of glucose/100).

[b] The studies are listed in the same order as the values: A(49), B(90), C(46), D(91), E(92), F(93), G(94), H(95), I(96), J(97), K(98), L(99), M(100), N(101), O(102), P(103), Q(104), R(105), S(106), T(107), U(108), V(109), W(110), X(111), Y(112), Z(113), β(114), $(115), £(116), ¢(117), #(118), @(119), &(120): h = healthy subjects; i = IDDM; n = NIDDM.

[c] CV = coefficient of variation (100 × SD/Mean).

the mean GI values for foods tested in different groups of subjects and by different investigators. In general, there is reasonable agreement between the values derived in different centers. For 27 foods tested by 3 or more groups of subjects, the mean SD of the mean GI values is 12 (Table 4.11.9), regardless of whether the subjects tested were normal or diabetic

Insulin-dependent diabetic subjects (IDDM) tend to show slightly higher GI values than subjects with noninsulin dependent diabetes.[111] This may be a reflection of the high degree of within-individual variability of blood glucose responses in IDDM to the same meal rather than to true differences between foods tested in these individuals.[111] In a recent study, 12 subjects with diabetes, including individuals with IDDM and NIDDM, tested 3 different foods 4 times each. Most of the variability in GI values was due to day-to-day variability within subjects with no significant difference in GI values between the different individuals. In all 12 subjects, the mean glycemic response to bread was greater than that to rice, which, in turn, was greater than that to spaghetti.[228]

The GI values of foods relate strongly to the rate of digestion of foods in vitro,[99,106,229–234] but only weakly to total fiber content, and not significantly to soluble fiber.[235] However, in one study, increasing the soluble fiber content of a meal with no change in its GI resulted in a major reduction of the postprandial glycemic response in subjects with NIDDM.[236] Surprisingly, the strongest correlation between food GI and components of fiber was with cellulose and the uronic acid fraction of insoluble fiber, major components of the cell wall (Figure 4.11.4). The lack of relationship between food GI and soluble fiber is probably due to the fact that many other factors in foods influence digestibility, and that soluble fibers have differing viscosities and hence variable effects in impeding glucose absorption.

The GI values of foods are related to their fat and protein contents.[49] Fat delays gastric emptying[237] and enhances GIP responses.[123,126] However, only in large amounts (45 to 65% of total test meal calories) does it significantly reduce postprandial glucose and insulin responses (Table 4.11.11). In addition, fat taken at one meal may impair carbohydrate tolerance in the subsequent meal.[238] Large amounts of protein enhance insulin secretion (Table 4.11.11) but have little effect on the blood glucose response in the smaller amounts normally eaten, e.g., bread with cheese.[49,90,103]

Particle size is particularly important in determining the responses of starchy foods (Table 4.11.12). The glycemic response to wheat and barley breads increases linearly as the proportion of flour, as opposed to whole grains, in the bread increases;[135] finely ground flour produces higher glycemic responses than coarse flour;[136] and the whole grain rye breads popular in Northern

Europe have relatively flat glycemic and insulinemic responses.[94] Increased particle size is probably related to the reduced glycemic effect after swallowing foods without adequate chewing.[239] In addition, cooking and processing of foods markedly affect their *in vitro* digestibility, and these changes are reflected in similar alterations of metabolic responses *in vivo* (Table 4.11.13). Differences in food form may also be of great importance in determining the glycemic index of a food, as exemplified by the similar composition but very different GI values of white bread and spaghetti (Table 4.11.9). Variables such as food variety (e.g., new vs. russet potato; Table 4.11.9), the degree of ripeness (e.g., banana; Tables 4.11.9, 4.11.10), and differences in cooking and processing (e.g., rice; Table 4.11.9) may therefore explain some of the differences in GI values obtained for the same food by different investigators.

Clinical Utility of the Glycemic Index

The GI of mixed meals can be estimated from the weighted mean of the GI values of the individual carbohydrate foods in the meal, with the weighting based on the proportion of the total carbohydrate contributed by each food (Table 4.11.14). In our hands, the GI value of mixed meals predicts almost exactly the relative differences between their mean glycemic responses (Figure 4.11.5). To be of predictive value, accurate GI values for the foods fed must be used, the calculation of meal GI must take into account all of the carbohydrate foods in the meal, and the method of calculation of area under the curve must be the same as that used for the GI.[160,240] In a meta-analysis of data from the literature (Table 4.11.14), the Stanford group has been unable to predict mixed meal glycemic responses using the GI of foods. However, data from 11 other groups worldwide (Lund, Melbourne, Morgantown, Minneapolis (2 different groups), Toronto, Naples, Aarhus, London (Canada), Bristol, and Sydney) are grouped around the line of identity (Figure 4.11.6). For small numbers of subjects, the most appropriate use of the GI is to help in determining which of two meals is likely to produce the greater glycemic response. The chance of a correct prediction depends upon the day-to-day variability of glycemic responses in the subjects being tested, the expected difference in meal GI, and the number of subjects or repeat tests done.[161,228] For a subject with NIDDM, there is a 95% chance of a correct prediction for a GI difference of 34 (i.e., 34 is the predictive difference); in subjects with IDDM, who have greater variability of glycemic responses, the predictive difference is 50. As the number of tests done increases, the predictive difference is reduced by a factor of $1/\sqrt{n}$.[161]

Treatment of Diabetes with High-Carbohydrate, High-Fiber Diets

High-carbohydrate diets, in the absence of increased fiber, are not consistently effective in reducing fasting blood glucose and serum cholesterol levels (mean reductions, $3.4 \pm 2.0\%$ and $3.4 \pm 2.2\%$, respectively [ns], Table 4.11.15) and may increase postprandial blood glucose and insulin responses, increase fasting triglyceride levels, and reduce HDL cholesterol, at least in the short term (2 to 6 weeks; Table 4.11.15, Figure 4.11.7). For these reasons, the safety of high-carbohydrate diets in diabetes has been questioned.[241] However, the use of foods rich in dietary fiber may offset the deleterious effects of high-carbohydrate diets on blood glucose, insulin, and triglycerides and enhance their cholesterol-lowering effects.

The use of high-fiber foods in the diet, where overall carbohydrate content is kept constant, improves diabetic blood glucose and lipid control, but only when the increase in fiber comes from low-glycemic-index foods (Table 4.11.16, Figure 4.11.8). In the limited number of studies done in this situation, fiber appears to be more effective at higher rather than lower carbohydrate intakes (Table 4.11.16). When guar gum was added to the diets of diabetic patients for 5 days, a similar phenomenon was observed.[242] Those patients whose diets contained more than 40% carbohydrates had a larger reduction of their urinary glucose output on guar than those patients whose diets contained less than 40% carbohydrates (64% compared with 33%, $p < 0.02$).

The combined use of high-carbohydrate/high-fiber diets has benefited both IDDM and NIDDM patients in terms of improved blood glucose control, reduced serum lipid levels, and lower insulin dosage, but only in those studies where the increase in carbohydrate and fiber was achieved with low-GI foods such as legumes and pasta (Table 4.11.16, Figure 4.11.8). In studies where the carbohydrate and fiber intakes were increased using high-GI, cereal products (e.g., whole meal bread), fasting blood glucose and cholesterol levels were improved, but this was achieved often at the expense of increased postprandial blood glucose and serum triglyceride levels (Table 4.11.16, Figure 4.11.8).

A number of dietary trials have been undertaken where the GI of the diet has been reduced without changing its overall macronutrient or fiber content (Table 4.11.17, Figure 4.11.7). In these studies, blood glucose and lipid lowering effects similar to those produced by high-carbohydrate/high-fiber diets were seen with no changes in carbohydrate or fiber intake. This suggests that the long-term metabolic effects of high-carbohydrate/high-fiber diets depend, at least in part, upon the ability to reduce the rate of carbohydrate absorption and hence reduce the acute postprandial blood glucose response. The mechanism for the lipid-lowering effect of slow absorption may relate to reduced insulin secretion and hence reduced stimulus to lipid synthesis. Recent studies where the rate of absorption was reduced by nibbling small meals at regular intervals throughout the day instead of consuming exactly the same food in three large meals indicate that nibbling reduces mean day-long insulin levels by about 30%[243,244] and is associated with significant reductions in serum total and LDL cholesterol and apolipoprotein B levels.[244]

CONCLUSIONS

Long-term benefits have been demonstrated using high-carbohydrate/high-fiber diets in both insulin- and noninsulin-dependent diabetes. These are associated with, and may be due to, slowing the rate of carbohydrate absorption within the gastrointestinal tract. Slow-release carbohydrate may be obtained by the addition of viscous types of dietary fiber, the use of low-glycemic-index foods, increased meal frequency, or pharmacologic intervention with amylase inhibitors such as Acarbose.[245,246] Fiber has been shown to alter gut morphology in experimental animals.[247-252] Increased starch consumption,[253,254] low-glycemic-index foods,[255-260] and dietary fiber[261-264] also increase the amount of fermentable carbohydrate which enters the colon. This will result in the formation and absorption of the short-chain fatty acids and acetic, propionic, and butyric acids,[265-268] which influence carbohydrate and lipid metabolism[269-271] and may be part of the mechanism of action of high-carbohydrate/high-fiber diets.[272-274] The long-term consequences of these morphologic and absorptive changes are likely to be important and remain to be explored.

Table 4.11.10   Glycemic Index (GI) of Foods Tested Only Once

Food	GI	Ref.[a]
Breads		
Wheat (French baguette)	131	Z
Wheat (puffed crispbread)	112	S
Pasta		
Fettuccine (nondurum)	44	#
Ravioli (durum)	54	#
Macaroni (white, boiled 5′)	64	I
Spaghetti (brown, boiled 15′)	61	I
Spaghetti (white, boiled 5′)	45	I
Spaghetti (protein-enriched)	38	I
Spirali (durum)	59	#
Star pasta (white, boiled 5′)	54	I
Vermicelli (nondurum)	48	#
Cereal Grains		
Bulgur (cracked wheat)	65	G
Millet	103	A
Rice (instant, boiled 1′)	65	H
Rice (instant, boiled 6′)	121	L
Rice (polished, boiled 5′)	58	H
Rice (parboiled, boiled 5′)	54	H
Rye kernels	47	6
Unrefined maize meal porridge	71	J
Refined maize meal porridge	74	J
Wheat kernels	63	G
Wheat kernels (quick-cooking)	75	S
Breakfast Cereals		
Muesli	96	A
Puffed rice	132	L
Puffed wheat	110	S
Shredded wheat	97	A
"Weetabix"	109	A
Cookies		
Oatmeal	78	A
"Rich Tea"	80	A
Shortbread	88	S
Miscellaneous		
Mars bar	99	A
Corn chips	99	L
Tomato soup	55	A
Root Vegetables		
Beetroot	93	A
Cassava (flakes)	113	&
Cassava (Eba)	99	&
Cassava (Lafun)	73	&
M'fino	68	J
Sweet potato	70	A
Yam	74	A
Pumpkin	75	J
Legumes		
Chick peas (canned)	60	U
Kidney beans (canned)	74	U
Lentils (green, canned)	74	U
Pinto beans (canned)	64	U
Black-eyed peas	48	A
Brown beans	24	J

Table 4.11.10 (Continued) Glycemic Index (GI) of Foods Tested Only Once

Food	GI	Ref.[a]
Soybeans (canned)	20	A
Soybeans (dried)	22	A
Fruit		
Apple juice	45	V
Banana (slightly underripe)	59	$
Banana (slight overripe)	90	$
Cherries (raw)	32	C
Grapefruit	36	C
Grapes	62	C
Peaches	40	C
Pears	47	C
Plums	34	C
Raisins	93	A
Sugars		
Honey	126	A
Maltose	152	A
Dairy Products		
Custard	59	S
Skim milk	46	A
Yogurt	52	A

[a] See legend for Table 4.11.9 for identification of references.

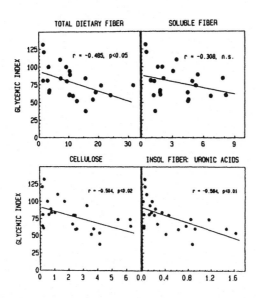

Figure 4.11.4 Relationship between the glycemic index values of 25 foods and their content of total dietary fiber, and selected fiber fractions (grams/50 g available carbohydrate portion; data from Reference 235).

Table 4.11.11   Effect of Fat and Protein on Metabolic Responses to Foods

Test Meal Constituents	CHO (g)	PRO	FAT	Sub[a]	Glucose	Insulin	GIP	Ref.
Effect of Adding Fat Alone								
Flummery ± fat	50	0	10	N	-49%*	-8% ns	+100% ns	121
Flummery ± fat	50	0	10	NID	0% ns	+5% ns	+400%***	121
Flummery ± fat	50	0	10	ID	0% ns		+700%*	121
Potatoes ± olive oil	50	0	18	N	+40%			122
Rice ± olive oil	50	0	18	N	+108%			122
Lentils ± olive oil	50	0	18	N	-27%			122
Bread ± butter	50	0	23	NID	-16% ns			103
Potato ± butter	75	0	38	N	-58%*	-9% ns	+640%**	123
Lentils ± butter	75	0	38	N	-52%*	-26% ns	+650%***	123
Potato ± corn oil	50	0	28	N	-85%**	-89%**		124
Glucose ± avocado oil	50	0	40	NID	-12% ns	+14% ns		125
Potato ± intralipid (ileum)[c]	50	0	41	N	-87%**	-79%***		125
Potato ± intralipid (duodenum)[c]	50	0	41	N	-85%	-63%		125
Potato ± butter	50	0	50	N	-52%++	-7% ns	+800%++	126
Effect of Adding Protein Alone								
Glucose ± lean hamburger	50	10	3	NID	+9% ns	+25% ns		127
Bread ± cottage cheese	50	12	2	NID	-2% ns			90
Bread ± skim milk cheese	50	12	2	NID	-21% ns			103
Potato ± tuna	25	25	1	NID	-8%*	+59%***		128
Spaghetti ± tuna	25	25	1	NID	+9% ns	+69%****		128
Glucose ± beef	50	25	8	NID	-10% ns	+230%*		129
Glucose ± turkey	50	25	3	NID	-20%*	+230%*		129
Glucose ± gelatin	50	25	0	NID	-33%*	+260%*		129
Glucose ± egg white	50	25	0	NID	0% ns	+190%*		129
Glucose ± cottage cheese	50	25	0	NID	-34%*	+360%*		129
Glucose ± fish	50	25	1	NID	-10% ns	+230%*		129
Glucose ± soy	50	25	0	NID	-33% ns	+220%*		129

	Sub			Subjects				
Glucose ± casein	50	30	0	NID	-37%	+99%**		125
Potatoes ± veal	50	42	1	N	+29%			122
Rice ± veal	50	42	1	N	+52%			122
Lentils ± veal	50	42	1	N	+12%			122
Glucose ± lean hamburger	50	30	9	NID	-9% ns	+100%*		127
Glucose ± lean hamburger	50	50	15	NID	-35%**	+207%***		127
Sugars ± milk/soy protein	58	16	tr	N	-40%**	+102%**		130
Sugars ± milk/soy protein	58	25	tr	N	-51%**	+117%**		130
Sugars ± milk/soy protein	58	34	tr	N	-70%**	+115%**		130
Sugars ± milk/soy protein	58	50	tr	N	-78%***	+129%***		130
Effect of Adding Fat and Protein								
Bread, rice, spaghetti, or barley ± cheddar cheese	50	8	11	NID	+3% ns			111
	50	8	11	ID	+25%*			111
Flummery ± fat and protein	50	21	10	N	-89%*	+70%*	+340%**	121
Flummery ± fat and protein	50	21	10	NID	0% ns	+185%***	+600%***	121
Flummery ± fat and protein	50	21	10	ID	+63%***		+1000%*	121
Bread, potato, rice, spaghetti, or beans ± cheese and butter	50	4–20	19	NID	-20% ns	+56%*		113
Bread ± skim cheese and butter	50	12	25	NID	-4% ns			103
Bread ± peanut butter	50	14	25	NID	-27%**			103
Bread ± peanut butter	50	14	25	ID	+2% ns			103
Potato ± tuna and margarine	25	25	26	NID	-27%***	+70%***		128
Spaghetti ± tuna and margarine	25	25	26	NID	-7% ns	+85%***		128
Glucose ± casein and avocado oil	50	30	40	NID	-60%***	+16% ns		125

a Sub = subjects; NID = noninsulin-dependent diabetes; ID = insulin-dependent diabetes; N = normal.
Change in incremental area under curve or peak rise compared to low protein/fat; * = $p < 0.05$; + = $p < 0.025$; ** = $p < 0.01$; + + = $p < 0.005$; *** = $p < 0.001$; ns = not significant.
c The fat was infused into the intestine and the potato taken by mouth.

Table 4.11.12   Effect of Grinding on Metabolic Responses

Carbohydrate (g) and Source	Degree of Grinding	Sub[a]	% Change[b]			Ref.
			Glucose	Insulin	GIP	
75, White rice	Fine	N	+38%**	+138%+ +		131
75, Brown rice	Fine	N	+46%***	+95%***		128
75, Brown rice	Fine	D	+67%*	+46%*	+60%+	132
75, Brown rice	Fine	N	+48%*	+54%**	+54%*	132
50, Cooked lentils	Fine	N	+6% ns			133
50, Lentils	Fine	N	+80%+	−11% ns		134
50, Cracked wheat[c]	25% Flour	D	+5% ns			135
50, Cracked wheat	50% Flour	D	+26%*			135
50, Cracked wheat	100% Flour	D	+39%*			135
50, Barley[c]	25% Flour	D	0% ns			135
50, Barley	50% Flour	D	+59%*			135
50, Barley	100% Flour	D	+146%*			135
50, Wheat kernels	100% Flour	D	+52%*			94
50, Wheat kernels	Cracked (bulgur)	D	+3% ns			94
50, Rye kernels	100% Flour	D	+89%*			94
50, Rye kernels	Pumpernickel[d]	D	+66%			94
50, Wheat[e]	Cracked grains	N	+7% ns	+16% ns		136
50, Wheat	Coarse flour	N	+34% ns	+42%*		136
50, Wheat	Fine flour	N	+32% ns	+95%***		136
50, Corn[e]	Cracked grains	N	−21% ns	+18% ns		136
50, Corn	Flour	N	−3% ns	+89%**		136
50, Oats[e]	Rolled oats	N	+29% ns	+53% ns		136
50, Oats	Flour	N	+75% ns	+19% ns		136

[a] Sub = subjects; D = diabetic; N = normal.

[b] Change in incremental area under the curve or peak rise; * = $p < 0.05$; + = $p < 0.025$; ** = $p < 0.01$; + + = $p < 0.005$; *** = $p < 0.001$; ns = not significant.

[c] Varied proportions of whole grain and flour in breads compared to whole grain alone. Wheat breads made with bulgur (cracked, parboiled wheat) plus various proportions of whole meal flour; barley bread vs. cooked pearled barley.

[d] Rye kernels vs. pumpernickel bread (bread containing whole kernels).

[e] Wheat: cracked, each kernel broken into 6 pieces; coarse, 17% retained on 2200-μm sieve, 52% retained on 710-μm sieve; fine, 0% retained on 710-μm sieve. Corn; cracked, each kernel broken into 23 pieces; flour, 0.2% retained on 710-μm sieve. Oats, flour, 0.2% retained on 710-μm sieve.

Table 4.11.13 Effect of Cooking/Processing on Metabolic Responses

Carbohydrate (g) and Source	Cooking/Processing Procedures	Sub[a]	% Change[b] Glucose	Insulin	Ref.
50, Red lentils	Boiled: 1 h vs. 20 min	N	+24% ns		133
50, Red lintils	Boiled 20 min, ground and dried 12 h at 250°F vs. boiled 20 min and ground	N	+78% +		133
1 g/kg, Corn starch	Heated in water at 68 to 70°C until gelled vs. raw	N	+160%**	+133%**	137
50, Yam[c]	Roasted vs. boiled	N	+15% ns		138
50, Plantain[c]	Roasted vs. boiled	N	−2% ns		138
50, Potatoes	Raw vs. boiled 20 min	D	+196% ++		139
25, Carrots	Raw vs. boiled 20 min	D	+3% ns		139
50, Polished rice	Boiled 5 min vs. boiled 15 rain	D	+43% **		95
50, Parboiled rice	Boiled 5 min vs. boiled 15 min	D	+24% ns		95
50, Parboiled rice	Boiled 5 min vs. boiled 25 min	D	+22% ns		95
50, Spaghetti	Boiled 5 min vs. boiled 15 min	D	+2% ns		96
50, Spaghetti	Boiled 11 min vs. boiled 16.5 min	N	+10% ns	+8%ns	140
50, Spaghetti	Boiled 11 min vs. boiled 22 min	N	−22% ns	0%ns	140
50, Baked beans	Home cooked vs. canned	N	+50% +	+100%**	116
50, White beans	Home cooked vs. canned	D	+86%*		108
50, Green lentils	Home cooked vs. canned	D	+139%**		108
50, Pinto beans	Home cooked vs. canned	D	+16%**		108
50, Chick peas	Home cooked vs. canned	D	+36% ns		108
50, Kidney beans	Home cooked vs. canned	D	+23% ns		108

[a] Sub = subjects; D = diabetic; N = normal.
[b] Change in incremental area under the curve or peak rise; * = $p < 0.05$; + = $p < 0.025$; ** = $p < 0.01$; + + = $p < 0.005$; *** = $p < 0.001$; ns = not significant.
[c] Tested in different groups of nonstandardized subjects.

Table 4.11.14 Utility of Glycemic Index of Foods in Predicting the Relative Blood Glucose Responses of Single Mixed Meals

Text Meal	Meal GI	% Difference[a] GI	BG–NIDDM	BG–Normal	BG–IDDM	Ref.
1. White bread	89					141
2. Whole grain bread	56	−38%	−39%* (8)			
1. Flummery	96					142
2. Salad and apple	100	+4%	0% ns (12)	+5% ns (13)		
1. Potato and sucrose	110					143
2. Rice and corn	85	−22%	−28% + (12)	−8% ns (22)		144
1. Formula	117					145
2. Brown rice and beans	74	−37%		−31%* (7)		
1. Low-fiber	84					146
2. High-fiber	85	+1%		0% ns (8)		
1. Cornflakes, banana	113					147
2. Cornflakes, juice	90	−21%	−31%* (8)			
3. Potato, bread, juice	88	−27%	−31%* (8)			
4. Griddle cakes, juice	99	−12%	−20% ns (8)			

Table 4.11.14 (Continued) Utility of Glycemic Index of Foods in Predicting the Relative Blood Glucose Responses of Single Mixed Meals

Text Meal	Meal GI	GI	BG–NIDDM	BG–Normal	BG–IDDM	Ref.
			% Difference[a]			
1. Glucose, rice	111					148
2. Fructose, rice	53	–52%	–46%* (12)	–78%* (10)	–55% ns (10)	
3. Sucrose, rice	82	–26%	–23% ns (12)	–60%* (10)	–16% ns (10)	
4. Potato starch, rice	92	–17%	–7% ns (12)	–56%* (10)	–6% ns (10)	
5. Wheat starch, rice	94	–16%	0% ns (12)	–25% ns (10)	–8% ns (10)	
1. Potato meal	123					149
2. Rice meal	89	–28%	–23%** (8)			
3. Spaghetti meal	77	–37%	–31%** (8)			
4. Lentils meal	62	–50%	–43%** (8)			
1. Potato meal	97					150
2. Bread meal	86	–10%	–13% ns (6)			
3. Rice meal	76	–22%	–26%** (6)			
4. Spaghetti meal	65	–33%	–44%** (6)			
5. Barley, lentils meal	47	–52%	–56%** (6)			
1. Mashed potato, bread	92					151
2. Sweet potato, orange	66	–29%	–5% ns (12)	–11% ns (13)		
3. Beans, cherries	53	–42%	–9% ns (12)	–44% ns (13)		
1. Bread meal	75					152
2. Potato meal	67	–11%	–12%			
3. Spaghetti meal	60	–20%	–41%** (7)			
1. Potato meal	80					153
2. Spaghetti meal	66	–17%			–49%***(7)	
1. Rice meal	71					154
2. Spaghetti meal	48	–32%	–13% ns (9)	–6% ns (6)		
3. Lentils meal	34	–52%	–19% ns (9)	–6% ns (6)		
1. Mashed potato meal	105					155
2. Lentils, barley meal	41	–61%		–61%* (5)		
1. Cornflakes, juice	95					156
2. "All Bran," juice	68	–28%		–24%* (11)		
1. Candy bar, tea	110					157
2. Cola, potato chips	105	–4%		–7% ns (10)		
3. Raisins, peanuts	87	–21%		–2% ns (10)		
4. Banana, peanuts	75	–32%		–51% ns (10)		
1. Lebanese meal	69					158
2. Western meal	69	0%		–27% (8)		
3. Chinese meal	65	–6%		–15% (8)		
4. Indian meal	60	–13%		–30% (8)		
5. Italian meal	40	–42%		–40% (8)		
6. Greek meal	38	–45%		–53% (8)		

[a] Percent difference from meal 1 for each study for GI = glycemic index, BG = blood glucose response incremental area, NIDDM = noninsulin-dependent diabetic subjects, IDDM = insulin-dependent diabetic subjects. GI values have been adjusted for unequal carbohydrate in meals. Figures in brackets = number of subjects. Meal GI for references 141 through 149, 152, 153, 156, and 157 were not reported in the original references. The meal GI calculations for studies 141 through 146 are presented in (159), for studies 147 and 148 in (102), for study 149 in (160), for studies 152 and 153 in (161), and for study 156 in (162). The GI values for the meals in study 157 have not been presented previously.

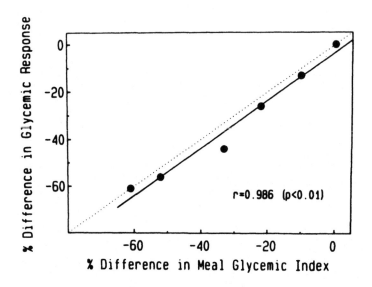

Figure 4.11.5 Prediction of mixed meal glycemic response using the glycemic index by Wolever et al.[150,155] Solid line = regression equation (% difference in glycemic response = 3.3 + 1.01 × % difference in GI); dotted line = line of identity.

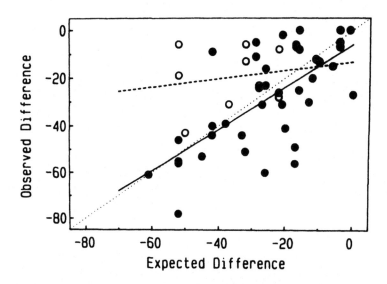

Figure 4.11.6 Prediction of mixed meal glycemic response using the glycemic index using the data from Table 4.11.14. Expected difference (ED) = percent difference of the glycemic index of each mixed meal from that of the meal with the highest glycemic index; observed difference (OD) = percent difference of glycemic response of each meal from that of the meal with the highest glycemic index. Dashed line, open circles = regression equation of data from the Stanford group (OD = −13 + 0.18 × ED, r = 0.168, n = 9, ns); solid line, closed circles = regression equation of data from 11 other groups worldwide (OD = −6 + 0.88 × ED, r = 0.690, n = 41, p < 0.001); dotted line = line of identity.

Table 4.11.15   Metabolic Effects of High-Carbohydrate, Low-Fiber Diets

Diet Composition[a]		Comment	LEN[c]	SUB[d]	% Change on High-Carbohydrate Diet[b]				Ref.
CARB	FAT				FBG	GTT	CHOL	TG	
44 → 77%	36 → 16%	MD,NF	7D	IGt	-15%*	G -7% ns		+36%**	163
40 → 55%	45 → 30%	FD	10D	N	-2% ns	D 0% ns	0% ns	+42%***	164
40 → 60%	41 → 21%	HD,NF	10D	N	0% ns	D 0% ns	-2% ns	+49%***	165
45 → 85%	40 → 0%	FD	7–10D	UD	+7% ns				166
45 → 85%	40 → 0%	FD	7–10	TD	-13%+				166
45 → 85%	40 → 0%	FD	10D	IGT	-10%***	G -8%*			167
42 → 53%	37 → 30%	MD,NF	10D	D	-2% ns	D +3% ns	+5% ns	ns	168
41 → 60%	41 → 20%	OPD	10D	ID	+6% ns	D +36%***	-2% ns	+19% ns	169
35 → 60%	47 → 22%	OPD	4W	NID	-10%*	D +11%+	0% ns	+11% ns	170
40 → 60%	40 → 20%	MD,NF	6W	NID	+2% ns	D +65%***	+2% ns	+25%***	171
42 → 55%	39 → 29%	OPD	6W	NID	-14% ns		-2% ns		172
41 → 56%	43 → 28%	OPD	40W	NID	0% ns		ns	ns	173
40 → 54%	40 → 26%	OPD	12M	NDN	+3% ns		-11%*	0% ns	174
53 → 58%	33 → 29%	OPD	12M	IDC	+1% ns[e]		-6%*	+33%*	175
41 → 64%	42 → 20%	OPD	13M	ID	0% ns		-21%***	-17% ns	176

[a] % of energy as carbohydrate (CARB) or fat on low → high carbohydrate diet. MD = metabolic diet, NF = normal foods, FD = formula diet, OPD = outpatient diets.

[b] % change of: FBG = fasting blood glucose; GTT = area under blood glucose curve after a standard oral glucose load (G) or while actually eating the diet (D); CHOL = serum cholesterol; TG = serum triglyceride. * = $p < 0.05$; + = $p < 0.025$; ** = $p < 0.01$; *** = $p < 0.001$.

[c] Study length: D = days; W = weeks; M = months.

[d] Subjects: N = normal; IGT = impaired glucose tolerance; UD = untreated diabetics; TD = treated diabetics; NID = noninsulin–dependent diabetes; NDN = newly diagnosed, noninsulin-requiring diabetes; ID = insulin-dependent diabetes; D = combined ID and NID; IDC = insulin-dependent diabetic children.

[e] Change in HbA1c.

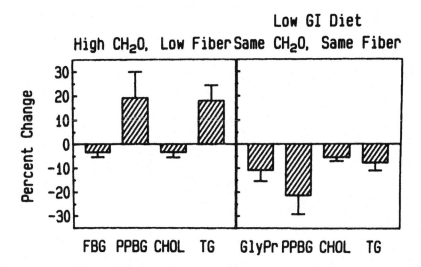

Figure 4.11.7 Left: effect of increasing dietary carbohydrate with no change in fiber on fasting (FBG) and postprandial (PPBG) blood glucose and serum cholesterol (CHOL) and triglyceride (TG) levels (mean ± SEM of data from Table 4.11.15). Right: effect of decreasing dietary glycemic index with no change in carbohydrate or fiber intake on glycosylated hemoglobin or albumin (GlyPr), postprandial blood glucose (PPBG), and serum cholesterol (CHOL) and triglyceride (TG) levels (mean ± SEM of data from Table 4.11.18).

Table 4.11.16 Metabolic Effects of Increasing Fiber Intake from Whole Foods with no Change in Available Carbohydrate

Diet Composition[a]				LEN[b]	SUB[c]	% Change on High-Fiber Diet[d]					Ref.
CHO	PRO	FAT	FIBER			FBG	PPBG	UGO	CHOL	TG	
Fiber Increased with LOW Glycemic Index Foods											
53	17	30	16 → 54	10D	8D	-34%*	-37%**	-82%+	-14%*	-12%*	177
53	17	30	16 → 54	10D	14D	-6% ns	-24%++		-20%**	ns	168
39	20	40	2 → 20[e]	15D	8D	-24%++	-18%++				178
55	15	30	19 → 56	6W	10C	-38%***	-30%***	-76%**			179
35	17	47	18 → 33	6W	16D		-20%*	-19% ns	0% ns		180
40	13	46	18 → 36	6W	10CSII		+1% ns		-5% ns	-26% ns	181
53		30	14 → 23	6W	25NID	-9% ns	-5%[h] ns		-13%*		172
Fiber Increased with HIGH Glycemic Index Foods											
47	21	34	19 → 42	3W	14NID	-6%*	-13%***	-37%*	+2% ns	+11% ns	182
59	17	23	11 → 27[f]	4W	6NID	+10% ns	ns	-10% ns	+5% ns	+8% ns	183
44	19	37	+ 14 → 24 g[g]	4W	12ID	-14%	-15%				184
44	23	33	16 → 44	8W	14NID	-6%**	+6% ns		-4%+	+10% ns	185
53	16	28	30 → 41	8W	42NID	-7%[h]			-6% ns	-7% ns	186

a Percent of calories from carbohydrate (CHO), protein (PRO), and fat, and increase in dietary fiber (FIBER) from low to high fiber diet.
b Study length: D = days; W = weeks.
c Subjects: D = diabetic; NID = noninsulin-dependent diabetic; C = diabetic children; CSII-ID = on continuous insulin infusion therapy.
d % change of: FBG = fasting blood glucose; PPBG = postprandial blood glucose levels; UGO = urinary glucose output; CHOL = serum cholesterol; TG = serum triglyceride. * = $p < 0.05$; + = $p < 0.025$; ** = $p < 0.01$; ++ = $p < 0.005$; *** = $p < 0.001$.
e Crude fiber.
f Grams dietary fiber per 1000 Kcal.
g Increase in fiber of 14 to 24 g/day.
h Change in HbA1c, ns.

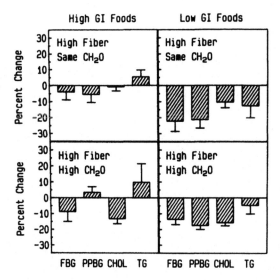

Figure 4.11.8 Effect of high-carbohydrate, high-fiber diets on fasting (FBG) and postprandial (PPBG) blood glucose and serum cholesterol (CHOL) and triglyceride (TG) levels. Left: increased fiber from foods with high glycemic index (GI). Right: increased fiber from foods with low GI. Top: effects of increasing fiber intake with no change in available carbohydrate intake (data from Table 4.11.16). Bottom: effects of increasing both fiber and available carbohydrate intakes (data from Table 4.11.17).

Table 4.11.17   Metabolic Effects of High-Carbohydrate, High-Fiber Diets

Diet Composition[a]			LEN[c]	SUB[d]	% Change on High-Carbohydrate Diet[b]					Ref.
CARB	FAT	FIBER			FBG	HbA1c	UGO/ID/BG	CHOL	TG	
Fiber and Carbohydrate Increased with LOW Glycemic Index Foods										
42 → 53%	37 → 37%	20 → 54 g	10D	D	− 13% ns		U−56% ns	− 19%***	+ 23% ns	177
42 → 53%	37 → 30%	20 → 54 g	10D	D	− 7% ns		B−15% +	− 16%***	ns	168
40 → 50%	51 → 38%	22 → 65 g	10D	D,R	0% ns		B−20%*	− 18%*	− 6% ns	187
43 → 75%	34 → 9%	5 → 14[e]	2W	NID	− 26% ++		I−56% +	− 24%***	− 15% ns	188
43 → 70%	37 → 9%	26 → 65 g	16D	NID	− 7% ns		I−58%***	− 29%***	− 2% ns	189
43 → 68%	42 → 14%	17 → 78 g	3–4W	H	− 5%*			− 22%*	+ 21% ns	190
43 → 65%	42 → 21%	9 → 19[f]	5W	NID	+ 5% ns		U−11% ns	− 10% ns	ns	191
40 → 61%	39 → 18%	18 → 97 g	6W	NID	− 15%***	− 10% +	U−94%*	− 14%*	− 14% ns	192
40 → 61%	39 → 18%	18 → 97 g	6W	ID	− 38% ns	− 2% ns	U−80%*	− 15%*	− 18% ns	192
42 → 50%	39 → 32%	8 → 23 g	6W	NID	− 23%*	− 19%*		− 15%*		172
40 → 58%	40 → 30%	30 → 70 g	2M	ID	− 5%	− 12%**	U−64% ns	− 4% ns	+ 11% ns	193
43 → 55%	34 → 27%	26 → 40 g	15M	NID	− 25%***		I−90%***	− 5% ns	− 43%+ +	194
? → 66%	? → 13%	? → 25 g	48M	NID	− 18%*			− 13%	− 15%*	195
Fiber and Carbohydrate Increased with HIGH Glycemic Index Foods										
46 → 60%	35 → 23%	22 → 64 g	14D	ID	− 11% ns		B− ns	− 10%***	+ 10% ns	196
28 → 60%	49 → 21%	21 → 57 g	3W	NID	− 18%**		U−33% ns	− 22%*	+ 20%**	197
45 → 65%	40 → 20%	28 → 50 g	4W	ID	− 1% ns		U−14% ns	− 14%***	− 6% ns	198
34 → 61%	50 → 23%	36 → 78 g	6W	NID	− 12%**	− 11%**	R+26% +	− 10%***	− 9% ns	199
34 → 61%	50 → 23%	36 → 78 g	6W	ID	− 36%**	+ 1% ns	I−6%**	− 10%***	+ 61%**	200
45 → 65%	40 → 20%	28 → 50 g	6W	ID	− 1% ns	+ 2% ns	I−0% ns	− 22%*	− 17%*	201
47 → 53%	40 → 25%	28 → 42 g	12W	NH		− 15%***		2% ns		202
38 → 45%	43 → 34%	20 → 32 g	4M	ID		+ 19%**				203
40 → 65%	40 → 15%	20 → 65 g	4M	D,P		− 30%	I−65%*			204
35 → 40%	45 → 41%	19 → 35 g	6M	PC	+ 17%**	+ 6% ns	B+7%			205

[a] % of energy as carbohydrate (CARB), fat, and dietary fiber (FIBER) on low → high carbohydrate diet.

[b] + change of: FBG = fasting blood glucose; HbA1c = glycosylated hemoglobin; UGO = urinary glucose output (U); ID = insulin dose (I) or rate of glucose disposal during euglycemic insulin clamp (R); mean blood glucose on the diet (B); CHOL = serum cholesterol; TG = serum triglyceride. * = $p < 0.05$; + = $p < 0.025$; ** = $p < 0.01$; *** = $p < 0.001$.

[c] Study length: D = days; W = weeks; M = months.

[d] Subjects: D = diabetic, unspecified or mixed types; R = chronic renal failure; NID = noninsulin-dependent diabetes; ID = insulin-dependent diabetes; H = healthy; NH = hypertensive NID; P = pregnant; PC = NID in poor control.

[e] Grams of crude fiber.

[f] Grams dietary fiber per 1000 Kcal.

Table 4.11.18 Long-Term Effects of Low-Glycemic-Index (GI) Diets

Diet Composition[a]						Diet GI	Change on Low GI Diet[b]					Ref.
CHO	FAT	PRO	DF	LEN	SUBJ		PPBG	GlyPr	Ins/CP	CHOL	TG	
61%	20%	19%	29 g	2W	6N	-41(39%)	-37%**	F - 2% ns	C -39%**	-11%*	-13% ns	206
50%	29%	21%	21 g	1M	12HT	-13(16%)				-9%***	-16%***	93
49%	29%	19%	22 g	1M	24HT	-11(13%)				-9%***	-19%***	207
49%	29%	19%	22 g	1M	6HC	-11(13%)				-3% ns	-1% ns	207
60%	20%			4W	24N + I	-7(12%)	-13%	H -0% ns				208
54%	25%	21%	31 g	2W	8NID	-23(26%)		H -3% ns	0% ns	-3% ns	0% ns	209
48%	35%	17%	32 g[c]	6W	7IDC	-12(15%)		F - 27%*	I -14% ns	-9%**	-3% ns	210
46%	36%	17%	31 g[d]	3W	8IDA	-14(23%)		F -22%	I -9%*	0% ns	-16%*	211
45%	31%	21%	26 g	3M	16NID	-13(14%)	-14%*	H -11%*		0% ns	+6% ns	212

[a] These studies were designed to have equivalent dietary composition during the high and low GI periods, but in some cases there were small differences in macronutrients. CHO = carbohydrate as % of energy; FAT = fat as % of energy; PRO = protein as percent of energy; DF = dietary fiber in grams per day; LEN = study length (W= weeks; M = months); SUBJ = subjects (N = normal; HT = hypertriglyceridemic; HC = type 2a hypercholesterolemia; NID = noninsulin-dependent diabetes; IDC = insulin-dependent diabetes, children; IDA = insulin-dependent diabetes, adults; N + I = NID and IDA.

[b] PPBG = postprandial blood glucose high-GI diet vs. low-GI diet; GlyPr = glycosylated protein (F = fructosamine; H = hemoglobin); Ins/CP = insulin dose (I) or urinary c-peptide output (C); CHOL = serum cholesterol; TG = serum triglycerides.

[c] Significant increase in dietary fiber on low-GI diet (39 vs. 24 g/d).

[d] Significant decrease in dietary fiber on low-GI diet (28 vs. 34 g/d).

REFERENCES

1. Edwards, C. A., Blackburn, N. A., Craigen, L., Davison, P., Tomlin, J., Sugden, K., Johnson, I. T., and Read, N. W., Viscosity of food gums determined in vitro related to their hypoglycemic actions, *Am. J. Clin. Nutr.*, 46, 72, 1987.

2. Jaris, H. A., Blackburn, N. A., Redfern, J. S., and Read, N. W., The effect of ispaghula (Fybogel and Metamucil) and guar gum on glucose tolerance in man, *Brit. J. Nutr.*, 51, 371, 1984.

3. O'Connor, N., Tredger, J., and Morgan, L., Viscosity differences between various guar gums, *Diabetologia*, 20, 612, 1981.

4. Morgan, L. M., Tredger, J. A., Madden, A., Kwasowski, P., and Marks, V., The effect of guar gum on carbohydrate-, fat- and protein-stimulated gut hormone secretion: modification of postprandial gastric inhibitory polypeptide and gastrin responses, *Brit. J. Nutr.*, 53, 467, 1985.

5. Wolever, T. M. S., Jenkins, D. J. A., Nineham, R., and Alberti, K. G. M. M., Guar gum and reduction of post-prandial glycaemia: effect of incorporation into solid food, liquid food and both, *Brit. J. Nurr.*, 41, 505, 1979,

6. Williams, D. R. R., James, W. P. T., and Evans, I. E., Dietary fibre supplementation of a normal breakfast administered to diabetics, *Diabetologia*, 18, 379, 1980.

7. Smith, C. J., Roseman, M. S., Levitt, N. S., and Jackson, W. P. U., Guar biscuits in the diabetic diet, *S. Afr. Med. J.*, 61, 196, 1982.

8. Gabbe, S. G., Cohen, A. W., Refhman, O. G., and Schwartz, S., Effect of dietary fiber on the oral glucose tolerance test in pregnancy, *Am. J. Obstet. Gynecol.*, 143, 514, 1982.

9. Jenkins, D. J. A., Wolever, T. M. S., Taylor, R. H., Barker, H. M., Fielden, H., and Jenkins, A. L., Effect of guar crispbread with cereal products and leguminous seeds on blood glucose concentrations of diabetics, *Brit. Med. J.*, 281, 1248, 1980.

10. Morgan, L. M., Gondler, T. J., Tsiolakis, D., Marks, V., and Alberti, K. G. M. M., The effects of unabsorbable carbohydrate on gut hormones: modification of postprandial GIP secretion by guar, *Diabetologia*, 17, 85, 1979.

11. Fuessl, S., Adrian, T. E., Bacarese-Hamilton, A. J., and Bloom, S. R., Guar in NIDD: effect of different modes of administration on plasma glucose and insulin responses to a starch meal, *Practical Diabetes*, 3(5), 258, 1986.

12. Gatti, E., Catenazzo, G., Camisasca, E., Torri, A., Denegri, E., and Sirtori, D. R., Effects of guar-enriched pasta in the treatment of diabetes and hyperlipidemia, *Annu. Nutr. Metab.*, 28, 1, 1984.

13. Nestler, J. E., Bariascini, C. O., Clore, J. N., and Blackard, W. G., Absorption characteristic of breakfast determines insulin sensitivity and carbohydrate tolerance for lunch, *Diabetes Care*, 11, 755, 1988.

14. Blackburn, N. A., Redfern, J. S., Jarjis, H., Holgate, A. M., Hanning, I, Scarpello, J. H. B., Johnson, I. T., and Read, N. W., The mechanism of action of guar gum in improving glucose tolerance in man, *Clin. Sci.*, 66, 329, 1984.

15. Jenkins, D. J. A., Nineham, R., Craddock, C., Craig-McFeely, P., Donaldson, K., Leigh, T., and Snook, J., Fibre and diabetes, *Lancet*, 1, 434, 1979.

16. Jenkins, D. J. A., Wolever, T. M. S., Leeds, A. R., Gassull, M. A., Dilawari, J. B., Goff, D. V., Metz, G. L., and Alberti, K. G. M. M., Dietary fibres, fibre analogues and glucose tolerance: importance of viscosity, *Brit. Med. J.*, 1, 1392, 1978.

17. Walquist, M. L., Morris, M. J., Littlejohn, G. O., Bond, A., and Jackson, R. V. J., The effect of dietary fiber on glucose tolerance in healthy males, *Aust. N.Z. J. Med.*, 9, 154, 1979.

18. Leatherdale, B. A., Green, D. J., Harding, L. K., Griffin, D., and Bailey, C. J., Guar and gastric emptying in non-insulin dependent diabetes, *Acta Diabetol. Lat.*, 19, 339, 1982.

19. Levitt, N. S., Vinik, A. I., Sive, A. A., Child, P. T., and Jackson, W. P. U., The effect of dietary fiber on glucose and hormone responses to a mixed meal in normal subjects and in diabetic subjects with and without autonomic neuropathy, *Diabetes Care*, 3, 515, 1980.

20. Kanter, Y., Eitan, N., Brook, G., and Barzilae, D., Improved glucose tolerance and insulin response in obese and diabetic patients on fiber-enriched diet, *Ist. J. Med. Sci.*, 16, 1, 1980.

21. Jenkins, D. J. A., Leeds, A. R., Gassull, M. A., Wolever, T. M. S., Goff, D. V., Alberti, K. G. M. M., and Hockaday, T. D. R., Unabsorbable carbohydrates and diabetes: decreased postprandial hyperglycaemia, *Lancet*, 2, 172, 1976.

22. Monnier, L. H., Colette, C., Aguirre, L., Orsetti, A., and Combeaux, D., Restored synergistic entro-hormonal response after addition of dietary fiber to patients with impaired glucose tolerance and reactive hypoglycemia, *Diabete Metab.*, 8, 217, 1982.
23. Gold, L. A., McCourt, J. P., and Merimee, T. J., Pectin: an examination in normal subjects, *Diabetes Care*, 3, 50, 1980.
24. Poynard, T., Slama, G., and Tchobroutsky, G., Reduction of post-prandial insulin needs by pectin as assessed by the artificial pancreas in insulin-dependent diabetics, *Diabete Metab.*, 8, 187, 1982.
25. Vaaler, S., Hanssen, K. F., and Aagenase, O., Effect of different kinds of fibre on postprandial blood glucose in insulin-dependent diabetics, *Acta Med. Scand.*, 208, 389, 1980.
26. Leeds, A. R., Ralphs, D. N. L., Ebied, F., Metz, G. L., and Dilawari, J., Pectin in the dumping syndrome: reduction of symptoms and plasma volume changes, *Lancet*, 1, 1075, 1981.
27. Monnier, L., Pham, T. C., Aguirre, L., Orsetti, A., and Mirouze, J., Influence of indigestible fibers on glucose tolerance, *Diabetes Care*, 1, 83, 1978.
28. Jenkins, D. J. A., Gassull, M. A., Leeds, A. R., Metz, G., Dilawari, J. B., Slavin, B., and Blendis, L. M., Effect of dietary fiber on complications of gastric surgery: prevention of postprandial hypoglycemia by pectin, *Gastroenterology*, 72, 215, 1977.
29. Jenkins, D. J. A., Leeds, A. R., Bloom, S. R., Sarson, D. L., Albuquerque, R. H., Metz, G. L., and Alberti, K. G. M. M., Pectin and post-gastric surgery complications: normalisation of postprandial glucose and insulin responses, *Gut*, 21, 574, 1980.
30. Holt, S., Heading, R. C., Carter, D. C., Prescott, L. F., and Tothill, P., Effect of gel fibre on gastric emptying and absorption of glucose and paracetomol, *Lancet*, 1, 636, 1979.
31. Jefferys, D. B., The effect of dietary fibre on the response to orally administered glucose, *Proc. Nutr. Soc.*, 33, 11A, 1974.
32. McMurry, J. F. and Baumgardner, B., A high-wheat bran diet in insulin-treated diabetes mellitus: assessment with the artificial pancreas, *Diabetes Care*, 7, 211, 1984.
33. Hamberg, O., Rumessen, J. J., and Gudmand-Høyer, E., Blood glucose response to pea fiber: comparisons with sugar beet fiber and wheat bran, *Am. J. Clin. Nutr.*, 50, 324, 1989.
34. Hall, S. E. H., Bolton, T. M., and Hetenyi, G., The effect of bran on glucose kinetics and plasma insulin in noninsulin-dependent diabetes mellitus, *Diabetes Care*, 3, 520, 1980.
35. Ebihara, K., Masuhara, R., and Kiriyama, S., Effect of Konjac mannan, a water-soluble dietary fiber on plasma glucose and insulin responses in young men undergone (sic) glucose tolerance test, *Nutr. Rep. Int.*, 23, 577, 1981.
36. Florholmen, J., Ardvidssonlenner, R., Jorde, R., and Burhol, P. G., The effect of Metamucil on postprandial blood glucose and plasma gastric inhibitory peptide in insulin-dependent diabetics, *Acta Med. Scand.*, 212, 237, 1982.
37. Sartor, G., Carlstrom, S., and Schersten, B., Dietary supplementation of fiber (lunelax) as a means to reduce postprandial glucose in diabetics, *Acta Med. Scand.*, 656 (Suppl.), 51, 1981.
38. Wolever, T. M. S., Vuksan, V., Eshuis, H., Spadafora, P., Peterson, R. D., Chao, E. S. M., Storey, M. L., and Jenkins, D. J. A., Effect of method of administration of psyllium on the glycemic response and carbohydrate digestibility, *J. Am. Col. Nutr.*, in press.
39. Tredger, J., Sheard, C., and Marks, V., Blood glucose and insulin levels in normal subjects following a meal with and without added sugar beet pulp, *Diabete Metab.*, 7, 169, 1981.
40. Tsai, A. C., Vinik, A. I., Lasichak, A., and Lo, G. S., Effects of soy polysaccharide on postprandial plasma glucose, insulin, glucagon, pancreatic polypeptide, somatostatin, and triglyceride in obese diabetic patients, *Am. J. Clin. Nutr.*, 45, 596, 1987.
41. Thomas, B. L., Laine, D. C., and Goetz, F. C., Glucose and insulin response in diabetic subjects: acute effect of carbohydrate level and the addition of soy polysaccharide in defined formula diets, *Am. J. Clin. Nutr.*, 48, 1048, 1988.
42. Jenkins, D. J. A., Wolever, T. M. S., Taylor, R. H., Barker, H. M., Fielden, H., and Gassull, M. A., Lack of effect of refining on the glycemic response to cereals, *Diabetes Care*, 4, 509, 1981.
43. Jenkins, D. J. A., Wolever, T. M. S., Jenkins, A. L., Lee, R., Wong, G. S., and Josse, R. G., Glycemic response to wheat products: reduced response to pasta but no effect of fiber, *Diabetes Care*, 6, 155, 1983.
44. Vaaler, S., Hanssen, K. F., and Aagenaes, O., Plasma glucose and insulin responses to orally administered carbohydrate-rich foodstuffs, *Nutr. Metab.*, 24, 168, 1980.

45. Brodribb, A. J. M. and Humphreys, D. M., Diverticular disease: three studies. Part III. Metabolic effect of bran in patients with diverticular disease, *Brit. Med. J.*, 1, 428, 1976.

46. Otto, H. and Niklas, L., Differences d'action sur la glycemie d'aliments contenant des hydrates de carbone. Consequences pour le traitment dietetique du diabete sucre, *Med. Hyg.*, 38, 3424, 1980.

47. O'Dea, K., Nestel, P. J., and Antonoff, L., Physical factors influencing postprandial glucose and insulin responses to starch, *Am. J. Clin. Nutr.*, 33, 760, 1980.

48. Walker, A. R. P. and Walker, B. R., Glycaemic index of South African foods determined in rural blacks — a population at low risk to diabetes, Hum. *Nutr. Clin. Nutr.*, 36C, 215, 1984.

49. Jenkins, D. J. A., Wolever, T. M. S., Taylor, R. H., Barker, H. M., Fielden, H., Baldwin, J. M., Bowling, A. C., Newman, H. C., Jenkins, A. L., and Goff, D. V., Glycemic index of foods: a Physiological basis for carbohydrate exchange, *Am. J. Clin. Nutr.*, 34, 362, 1981,

50. Bolton, R. P., Heaton, K. W., and Burroughs, L. F., The role of dietary fiber in satiety, glucose, and insulin: studies with fruit and fruit juice, *Am. J. Clin. Nutr.*, 34, 211, 1981.

51. Kay, R. M., Food form, post-prandial glycemia, and satiety, *Am. J. Clin. Nutr.*, 31, 738, 1978.

52. Haber, G. B., Heaton, K. W., Murphy, D., and Burroughs, L. F., Depletion and disruption of dietary fibre: effects on satiety, plasma-glucose, and insulin, *Lancet*, 2, 679, 1977.

53. McLean Ross, A. H., Eastwood, M. A., Brydon, W. G., Anderson, J. R., and Anderson, D. M. W., A study of the effects of dietary gum arabic in humans, *Am. J. Clin. Nutr.*, 37, 368, 1983.

54. Jenkins, D. J. A., Leeds, A. R., Houston, H., Hinks, L., Alberti, K. G. M. M., and Cummings, J. H., Carbohydrate tolerance in man after six weeks of pectin administration, *Proc. Nutr. Soc.*, 36, 60A, 1977.

55. Kestin, M., Moss, R., Clifton, P. M., and Nestel, P. J., Comparative effects of three cereal brans on plasma lipids, blood pressure, and glucose metabolism in mildly hypercholesterolemic men, *Am. J. Clin. Nutr.*, 52, 661, 1990.

56. Villaume, C., Beck, B., Gariot, P., Desalme, A., and Debry, G., Long-term evolution of the effect of bran ingestion on meal-induced glucose and insulin response in healthy man, *Am. J. Clin. Nutr.*, 40, 1023, 1984.

57. Munoz, J. A., Sandstead, H. H., Jacob, L. K., Johnson, L., and Mako, M. E., Effects of dietary fiber on glucose tolerance of normal men, *Diabetes*, 28, 496, 1979.

58. Schweizer, T. F., Bekhechi, A. R., Koellreutter, B., Reimann, S., Pometta, D., and Bron, B. A., Metabolic effects of dietary fiber from dehulled soybeans in humans, *Am. J. Clin. Nutr.*, 38, 1–11, 1983.

59. Osilesi, O., Trout, D. L., Glover, E. E., Harper, S. M., Koh, E. T., Behall, K. M., O'Dorisio, T. M., and Tartt, J., Use of xanthan gum in dietary management of diabetes mellitus, *Am. J. Clin. Nut.*, 42, 597, 1985.

60. Groop, P. H., Groop, L., Totterman, K. J., and Fyhrquist, F., Relationship between changes in GIP concentrations and changes in insulin and c-peptide concentrations after guar gum therapy, *Scand. J. Clin. Lab. Invest.*, 46, 505, 1986.

61. Jenkins, D. J. A., Wolever, T. M. S., Hockaday, T. D. R., Leeds, A. R., Haworth, R., Bacon, S., Apling, E. C., and Dilawari, J., Treatment of diabetes with guar gum, *Lancet*, 2, 779, 1977.

62. Jenkins, D. J. A., Wolever, T. M. S., Nineham, R., Taylor, R. H., Metz, G. L., Bacon, S., and Hockaday, T. D. R., Guar crispbread in the diabetic diet, *Brit. Med. J.*, 2, 1744, 1978.

63. Kuhl, C., Molsted-Pedersen, L., and Hornnes, P. J., Guar gum and glycemic control of pregnant insulin-dependent diabetic patients, *Diabetes Care*, 6, 152, 1983.

64. Smith, U. and Holm, G., Effect of a modified guar gum preparation on glucose and lipid levels in diabetics and healthy volunteers, *Atherosclerosis*, 45, 1, 1982.

65. Johansen, K., Decreased urinary glucose excretion and plasma cholesterol level in non-insulin-dependent diabetic patients with guar, *Diabete Metab.*, 7, 87, 1981.

66. Koepp, P. and Hegewisch, S., Effects of guar on plasma viscosity and related parameters in diabetic children, *Eur. J. Pediatr.*, 137, 31, 1981.

67. Carroll, D. G., Dykes, V., and Hodgson, W., Guar gum is not a panacea in diabetes management, *NZ Med. J.*, 93, 292, 1981.

68. Najemnik, C., Kritz, H., Irsigler, K., Laube, H., Knick, B., Klimm, H. D., Wahl, P., Vollmar, J., and Brauning, C., Guar and its effects on metabolic control in type II diabetic subjects, *Diabetes Care*, 7, 215, 1984.

69. Fuessl, H. S., Williams, G., Adrian, T. E., and Bloom, S. R., Guar sprinkled on food: effect on glycaemic control, plasma lipids and gut hormones in non-insulin dependent diabetic patients, *Diabetic Med.*, 4, 463, 1987.

70. Eberling, P., Yki-Jarvinen, H., Aro, A., Helve, E., Sinisalo, M., and Kiovisto, V., Glucose and lipid metabolism and insulin sensitivity in type I diabetes: the effect of guar gum, *Am. J. Clin. Nutr.*, 48, 98, 1988.

71. Atkins, T. W., Al-Hussary, N. A. J., and Taylor, K. G., The treatment of poorly controlled non-insulin-dependent diabetic subjects with granulated guar gum, *Diabetes Res. Clin. Practice*, 3, 153, 1987.

72. Sels, J. P., Flendrig, J. A., and Postmes, T. H. J., The influence of guar-gum brerad on the regulation of diabetes mellitus type 11 in elderly patients, *Brit. J. Nutr.*, 57, 177, 1987.

73. Paganus, A., Maenpaa, J., Akerblom, H. K., Stenman, U. H., Knip, M., and Simell, O., Beneficial effects of palatable guar and guar plus fructose diets in diabetic children, *Acta Paediatr. Scand.*, 76, 76, 1987.

74. Jones, D. B., Slaughter, P., Lousley, S., Carter, R. D., Jelfs, R., and Mann, J. I., Low-dose guar improves diabetic control, *J. Roy. Soc. Med.*, 78, 546, 1985.

75. Beattie, V. A., Edwards, C. A., Hosker, J. P., Cullen, D. R., Ward, J. D., and Read, N. W., Does adding fibre to a low energy, high carbohydrate, low fat diet confer any benefit to the management of newly diagnosed overweight type II diabetics?, *Brit. Med. J.*, 296, 1147, 1988.

76. Holman, R. R., Steemson, J., Darling, P., and Turner, R. C., No glycemic benefit from guar administration in NIDDM, *Diabetes Care*, 10, 68, 1987.

77. Ray, T. K., Mansell, K. M., Knight, L. C., Malmud, L. S., Owen, O. E., and Boden, G., Longterm effects of dietary fiber on glucose tolerance and gastric emptying in noninsulin-dependent diabetic patients, *Am. J. Clin. Nutr.*, 37, 376, 1983.

78. Aro, A., Uusitupa, M., Vontilainen, E., Hersio, K., Korhonen, T., and Siitonen, O., Improved diabetic control and hypocholesterolemic effect induced by long-term dietary supplementation with guar gum in type 2 (insulin-independent) diabetes, *Diabetologia*, 21, 29, 1981.

79. Botha., A. P. J., Steyn, A. F., Esterhuysen, A. J., and Slabbert, M., Glycosylated haemoglobin, blood glucose and serum cholesterol levels in diabetics treated with guar gum, *S. Afr. Med. J.*, 59, 333, 1981.

80. Cohen, M., Leong, V. W., Salmon, E., and Martin, F. I. R., The role of guar and dietary fibre in the management of diabetes mellitus, *Med. J. Aust.*, 1, 59, 1980.

81. Uusitupa, M., Siitonen, O., Savolainen, K., Silvasti, M., Penttila, I., and Parviainen, M., Metabolic and nutritional effects of long-term use of guar gum in treatment of noninsulin-dependent diabetes of poor metabolic control, *Am. J. Clin. Nutr.*, 49, 345, 1989.

82. Jenkins, D. J. A., Wolever, T. M. S., Taylor, R. H., Reynolds, D., Nineham, R., and Hockaday, T. D. R., Diabetic glucose control, lipids, and trace elements on long term guar, *Brit. Med. J.*, 1, 1353, 1980.

83. Mahalko, J. R., Sandstead, H. H., Johnson, L. K., Inman, L. F., Milne, D. B., Warner, R. C., and Haunz, E. A., Effect of consuming fiber from corn bran, soy hulls, or apple powder on glucose tolerance and plasma lipids in type II diabetes, *Am. J. Clin. Nutr.*, 39, 25, 1984.

84. Mayne, P. D., McGill, A. R., Gormley, T. R., Tomplin, G. H., Julian, T. R., and O'Moore, R. R., The effect of apple fibre on diabetic control and plasma lipids, *Ir. J. Med. Sci.*, 151, 36, 1982.

85. Monnier, L. H., Blotman, M. J., Colette, C., Monnier, M. P., and Mirouze, J., Effects of dietary fibre supplementation in stable and labile insulin-independent diabetics, *Diabetologia*, 20, 12, 1981.

86. Bosello, O., Ostuzzi, R., Aimellini, F., Micciolo, R. M., and Ludovico, A. S., Glucose tolerance and blood lipids in bran fed patients with impaired glucose tolerance, *Diabetes Care*, 3, 46, 1980.

87. Miranda, P. M. and Horwitz, D. L., High fiber diets in the treatment of diabetes mellitus, *Ann. Intern. Med.*, 88, 482, 1978.

88. Fagerberg, S. E., The effects of a bulk laxative (metamucil) on fasting blood glucose, serum lipids, and other variables in constipated patients with noninsulin-dependent diabetes, *Current Therapeutic Res.*, 31, 166, 1992.

89. Doi, K., Matsuura, M., Kawara, A., and Baba, S., Treatment of diabetes with glucomannan (Konjac mannan), *Lancet*, 1, 987, 1979.

90. Jenkins, D. J. A., Wolever, T. M. S., Jenkins, A. L., Thorne, M. J., Lee, R., Kalmusky, J., Reichert, R., and Wong, G. S., The glycaemic index of foods tested in diabetic patients: a new basis for carbohydrate exchange favouring the use of legumes, *Diabetologia*, 24, 257, 1983.

91. Crapo, P. A., Reaven, G., and Olevsky, J., Post-prandial plasma-glucose and -insulin responses to different complex carbohydrates, *Diabetes*, 26, 1178, 1977.
92. Crapo, P. A., Insel, J., Sperling, M., and Kolterman, O. G., Comparison of serum glucose, insulin and glucagon responses to different types of complex carbohydrate in noninsulin-dependent diabetic patients, *Am. J. Clin. Nutr.*, 34, 184, 1981.
93. Jenkins, D. J. A., Wolever, T. M. S., Kalmusky, J., Giudici, S., Giordano, C., Wong, G. S., Bird, J. H., Patten, R., Hall, M., Buckley, G. C., and Little, J. A., Low glycemic index food in the management of hyperlipidemia, *Am. J. Clin. Nutr.*, 42, 604, 1985.
94. Jenkins, D. J. A., Wolever, T. M. S., Jenkins, A. L., Giordano, C., Giudici, S., Thompson, L. U., Kalmusky, J., Josse, R. G., and Wong, G. S., Low glycemic response to traditionally processed wheat and rye products: bulgur and pumpernickel bread, *Am. J. Clin. Nutr.*, 43, 516, 1986.
95. Wolever, T. M. S., Jenkins, D. J. A., Kalmusky, J., Jenkins, A. L., Giordano, C., Giudici, S., Josse, R. G., and Wong, G. S., Comparison of regular and parboiled rices: explanation of discrepancies between reported glycemic responses to rice, *Nutr. Res.*, 6, 349, 1986.
96. Wolever, T. M. S., Jenkins, D. J. A., Kalmusky, J., Giordano, C., Giudici, S., Jenkins, A. L., Josse, R. G., and Wong, G. S., Glycemic response to pasta: effect of food form, cooking and protein enrichment, *Diabetes Care*, 9, 401, 1986.
97. Walker, A. R. P. and Walker, B. R., Glycaemic index of South African foods determined in rural blacks — a population at low risk to diabetes, *Hum. Nutr. Clin. Nutr.*, 36C, 215, 1984.
98. Wolever, T. M. S., Wong, G. S., Kenshole, A., Josse, R. G., Thompson, L. U., Lam, K. Y., and Jenkins, D. J. A., Lactose in the diabetic diet: a comparison with other carbohydrates, *Nutr. Res.*, 5, 1335, 1985.
99. Brand, J. C., Nicholson, P. L., Thorburn, A. W., and Truswell, A. S., Food processing and the glycemic index, *Am. J. Clin. Nutr.*, 42, 1192, 1985.
100. Dilawari, J. B., Kamath, P. S., Batta, R. P., Mukewar, S., and Raghavan, S., Reduction of postprandial plasma glucose by bengal gram dal *(Cicer arietnum)* and rajmah *(Phaseolus vulgaris)*, *Am. J. Clin. Nutr.*, 34, 2450, 1981.
101. Potter, J. G., Coffman, K. P., Reid, R. L., Krall, J. M., and Albrink, M. J., Effect of test meals of varying dietary fiber content on plasma insulin and glucose response, *Am. J. Clin. Nutr.*, 34, 328, 1981.
102. Wolever, T. M. S., Nuttall, F. Q., Lee, R., Wong, G. S., Josse, R. G., Csima, A., and Jenkins, D. J. A., Prediction of the relative blood glucose response of mixed meals using the white bread glycemic index, *Diabetes Care*, 8, 418, 1985.
103. Jenkins, D. J. A., Wolever, T. M. S., Wong, G. S., Kenshole, A., Josse, R. G., Thompson, L. U., and Lam, K. Y., Glycemic responses to foods: possible differences between insulin-dependent and noninsulin-dependent diabetics, *Am. J. Clin. Nutr.*, 40, 971, 1984.
104. Crapo, P. A., Kolterman, O. G., Waldeck, N., Reaven, G. M., and Olefsky, J. M., Postprandial hormonal responses to different types of complex carbohydrate in individuals with impaired glucose tolerance, *Am. J. Clin. Nutr.*, 33, 1723, 1980.
105. Yoon, J. H., Thompson, L. U., and Jenkins, D. J. A., The effect of phytic acid on in vitro rate of starch digestibility and blood glucose response, *Am. J. Clin. Nutr.*, 38, 835, 1983.
106. Ross, S. W., Brand, J. C., Thorburn, A. W., and Truswell, A. S., Glycemic index of processed wheat products, *Am. J. Clin. Nutr.*, 46, 631, 1987.
107. Heinonen, L., Korpela, R., and Mantere, S., The effect of different types of Finnish bread on postprandial glucose responses in diabetic patients, *Hum. Nutr. Appl. Nutr.*, 39A, 108, 1985.
108. Wolever, T. M. S., Jenkins, D. J. A., Thompson, L. U., Wong, G. S., and Josse, R. G., Effect of canning on the blood glucose response to beans in patients with type 2 diabetes, *Hum. Nutr. Clin. Nutr.*, 41C, 135, 1987.
109. Gannon, M. C., Nuttall, F. Q., Krezowski, P. A., Billington, C. J., and Parker, S., The serum insulin and plasma glucose responses to milk and fruit products in Type 2 (non-insulin-dependent) diabetic patients, *Diabetologia*, 29, 784, 1986.
110. Krezowski, P. A., Nuttall, F. Q., Gannon, M. C., Billington, C. J., and Parker, S., Insulin and glucose responses to various starch-containing foods in type II diabetic subjects, *Diabetes Care*, 10, 205, 1987.
111. Wolever, T. M. S., Jenkins, D. J. A., Josse, R. G., Wong, G. S., and Lee, R., The glycemic index: similarity of values derived in insulin-dependent and non-insulin-dependent diabetic patients, *J. Am. Col. Nutr.*, 6, 295, 1987.

112. Wolever, T. M. S., Kalmusky, J., Giudici, S., Giordano, C., and Jenkins, D. J. A., Effect of processing/preparation on the blood glucose response to potatoes, *Can. Inst. Food. Sci. Technol. J.*, 18, xxxv, 1985.

113. Bornet, F. R. J., Costagliola, D., Blayo, A., Fontvielle, A., Haardt, M. J., Letanoux, M., Tchobroutsky, G., and Slama, G., Insulinogenic and glycemic indexes of six starch-rich foods taken alone and in a mixed meal by type 2 diabetics, *Am. J. Clin. Nutr.*, 45, 588, 1987.

114. Wolever, T. M. S., Jenkins, D. J. A., Collier, G. R., Ehrlich, R. M., Josse, R. G., Wong, G. S., and Lee, R., The glycaemic index: effect of age in insulin dependent diabetes mellitus, *Diabetes Res.*, 7, 71, 1988.

115. Wolever, T. M. S., Jenkins, D. J. A., Vuksan, V., Wong, G. S., and Josse, R. G., Effect of ripeness on the glycaemic response to banana, *J. Clin. Nutr. Gastroenterol.*, 3, 85, 1988.

116. Traianedes, K. and O'Dea, K., Commercial canning increases the digestibility of beans in vitro and postprandial metabolic responses to them in vivo, *Am. J. Clin. Nutr.*, 44, 390, 1986.

117. Philippides, P., Katsilambros, N., Galanopoulos, A., Peppas, T., Kofotzouli, L., Frangaki, D., Siskoudis, P., and Sfikakis, P., Glycaemic response to carrot in Type II diabetic patients, *Diab. Nutr. Metab.*, 1, 363, 1988.

118. Brand, J. C., Foster, K. A. F., Crossman, S., and Truswell, A. S., The glycaemic and insulin indices of realistic meals and rye breads tested in healthy subjects, *Diab. Nutr. Metab.*, 3, 137, 1990.

119. Bucalossi, A., Conti, A., Lombardo, S., Marsilii, A., Petruzzi, E., Piazza, E., and Pulini, M., Glycaemic and insulinaemic responses to different carbohydrates in Type II (NIDD) diabetic patients, *Diab. Nutr. Metab.*, 3, 143, 1990.

120. Akanji, A. O., Adeyefa, I., Charles-Davies, M., and Osotimehin, B. O., Plasma glucose and thiocyanate responses to different mixed cassava meals in non-diabetic Nigerians, *Eur. J. Clin. Nutr.*, 44, 71, 1990.

121. Simpson, R. W., McDonald, J., Walqvist, M. L., Atley, L., and Outch, K., Macronutrients have different metabolic effects in nondiabetics and diabetics, *Am. J. Clin. Nutr.*, 42, 449, 1985.

122. Calle-Pascual, A. L., Bordiu, E., Romeo, S., Romero, C., Martin-Alvarez, P. J., and Maranes, J. P., Food glycaemic index or meal glycaemic response?, *Hum. Nutr. Appl. Nutr.*, 40A, 282, 1986 and 41A, 435(letter), 1987.

123. Collier, G., McLean, A., and O'Dea, K., Effect of co-ingestion of fat on the metabolic responses to slowly and rapidly absorbed carbohydrates, *Diabetologia*, 26, 50, 1984.

124. Welch, I., Bruce, C., Hill, S. E., and Read, N. W., Duodenal and ileal lipid suppresses postprandial blood glucose and insulin responses in man: possible implications for the dietary management of diabetes mellitus, *Clin. Sci.*, 72, 209, 1987.

125. Estrich, D., Ravnick, A., Schlierf, G., Fukayama, G., and Kinsell, L., Effects of co-ingestion of fat and protein upon carbohydrate-induced hyperglycemia, *Diabetes*, 16, 232, 1967.

126. Collier, G. and O'Dea, K., The effect of coingestion of fat on the glucose, insulin and gastric inhibitory polypeptide responses to carbohydrate and protein, *Am. J. Clin. Nutr.*, 37, 941, 1983.

127. Nuttall, F. Q., Mooradian, A. D., Gannon, M. C., Billington, C., and Krezowski, P., Effect of protein ingestion on the glucose and insulin response to a standardized oral glucose load, *Diabetes Care*, 7, 465, 1984.

128. Guilliford, M. C., Bicknell, E. J., and Scarpello, J. H., Differential effect of protein and fat ingestion on blood glucose responses to high- and low-glycemic-index carbohydrates in noninsulin-dependent diabetic subjects, *Am. J. Clin. Nutr.*, 50, 773, 1989.

129. Gannon, M. C., Nuttall, F. Q., Neil, B. J., and Westphal, S. A., The insulin and glucose responses to meals of glucose plus various proteins in type II diabetic subjects, *Metabolism*, 37, 1081, 1988.

130. Spiller, G. A., Jensen, C. D., Pattison, T. S., Chuck, C. S., Whittam, J. H., and Scala, J., Effect of protein dose on serum glucose and insulin response to sugars, *Am. J. Clin. Nutr.*, 46, 474, 1987.

131. O'Dea, K., Nestel, P. J., and Antonoff, L., Physical factors influencing postprandial glucose and insulin responses to starch, *Am. J. Clin. Nutr.*, 33, 760, 1980.

132. Collier, G. and O'Dea, K., Effect of physical form of carbohydrate on the post-prandial glucose, insulin and gastric inhibitory polypeptide responses in type 2 diabetes, *Am. J. Clin. Nutr.*, 36, 10, 1982.

133. Jenkins, D. J. A., Thorne, M. J., Camelon, K., Jenkins, A. L., Rao, A. V., Taylor, R. H., Thompson, L. U., Kalmusky, J., Reichert, R., and Francis, T., Effect of processing on digestibility and the blood glucose response: a study of lentils, *Am. J. Clin. Nutr.*, 36, 1093, 1982.

134. O'Dea, K. and Wong, S., The rate of starch hydrolysis in vitro does not predict the metabolic responses to legumes in vivo, *Am. J. Clin. Nutr.*, 38, 382, 1983.

135. Jenkins, D. J. A., Wesson, V., Wolever, T. M. S., Jenkins, A. L., Kalmusky, J., Giudici, S., Csima, A., Josse, R. G., and Wong, G. S., Wholemeal versus wholegrain breads: proportion of whole or cracked grain and the glycaemic response, *Brit. Med. J.*, 297, 958, 1988.

136. Heaton, K. W., Marcus, S. N., Emmett, P. M., and Bolton, C. H., Particle size of wheat, maize, and oat test meals: effects on plasma glucose and insulin responses and on the rate of starch digestion in vitro, *Am. J. Clin. Nutr.*, 47, 675, 1988.

137. Collings, P., Williams, C., and MacDonald, I, Effect of cooking on serum glucose and insulin responses to starch, *Br. Med. J.*, 282, 1032, 1981.

138. Oli, J. M., Ikeakor, I P., and Onwuameze, I. C., Blood glucose responses to common Nigerian foods, *Trop. Geog. Med.*, 34, 317, 1982.

139. Vaaler, S., Hanssen, K. F. and Aagenaes, O., The effect of cooking upon the blood glucose response to ingested carrots and potatoes, *Diabetes Care*, 7, 221, 1984.

140. Bornet, F. R. J., Cloarec, D., Barry, J., Colonna, P., Gouilloud, S., Laval, J. D., and Calmiche, J., Pasta cooking time: influence on starch digestion and plasma glucose and insulin responses in healthy subjects, *Am. J. Clin. Nutr.*, 51, 421, 1990.

141. Asp, N.G., Agardh, C.-D., Ahren, B., Dencker, L, Johansson, C.-G., and Lundquist, I., Nyman, M., Sartor, G., and Schersten, B., Dietary fiber in type II diabetes, *Acta Med. Scand.*, 656 (Suppl.), 47, 1981.

142. Simpson, R. W., McDonald, J., Wahlqvist, M., Balaza, N., and Dunlop, M., Effect of naturally occurring dietary fibre in Western foods on blood glucose, *Aust. NZ J. Med.*, 11, 484, 1981.

143. Coulston, A. M., Greenfield, M. S., Enger, F., Tokay, T., and Reaven, G. M., Effect of source of dietary carbohydrate on plasma glucose and insulin responses to test meals in normal subjects, *Am. J. Clin. Nutr.*, 33, 1279, 1980.

144. Coulston, A. M., Greenfield, M. S., Kraemer, F. B., Tobey, R. A., and Reaven, G. M., Effect of differences in source of dietary carbohydrate on plasma glucose and insulin responses to meals in patients with impaired carbohydrate tolerance, *Am. J. Clin. Nutr.*, 34, 2716, 1981.

145. Albrink, M. J., Newman, T., and Davidson, P. C., Effect of high- and low-fiber diets on plasma lipids and insulin, *Am. J. Clin. Nutr.*, 32, 1486, 1979.

146. Ulirich, I. H. and Albrink, M. J., Lack of effect of dietary fiber on serum lipids, glucose, and insulin in healthy young men fed high starch diets, *Am. J. Clin. Nutr.*, 36, 1, 1982.

147. Nuttall, F. Q., Mooradian, A. D., DeMarais, R., and Parker, S., The glycemic effect of different meals approximately isocaloric and similar in protein, carbohydrate, and fat content as calculated using the ADA exchange lists, *Diabetes Care*, 6, 432, 1983.

148. Bantle, J. P., Laine, D. C., Castle, G. W., Thomas, J. W., Hoogwerf, B. J., and Goetz, F. C., PostPrandial glucose and insulin responses to meals containing different carbohydrates in normal and diabetic subjects, *New Engl. J. Med.*, 309, 7, 1983.

149. Coulston, A. M., Hollenbeck, C. B., Liu, G. C., Williams, R. A., Starich, G. H., Mazzaferri, E. L., and Reaven, G. M., Effect of source of dietary carbohydrate on plasma glucose, insulin, and gastric inhibitory polypeptide responses to test meals in subjects with noninsulin-dependent diabetes mellitus, *Am. J. Clin, Nutr.*, 40, 965, 1984.

150. Collier, G. R., Wolever, T. M. S., Wong, G. S., and Josse, R. G., Prediction of glycemic response to mixed meals in non-insulin dependent diabetic subjects, *Am. J. Clin. Nutr.*, 44, 349, 1986.

151. Laine, D. C., Thomas, W., Levitt, M. D., and Bantle, J. P., Comparison of predictive capabilities of diabetic exchange lists and glycemic index of foods, *Diabetes Care*, 10, 387, 1987.

152. Parillo, M., Giacco, R., Riccardi, G., Pacioni, D., and Rivellese, A., Different glycaemic responses to pasta, bread, and potatoes in diabetic patients, *Diabetic Med.*, 2, 374, 1985.

153. Hermansen, K., Rasmussen, O., Arnfred, J., Winther, E., and Schmitz, O., Glycemic effects of spaghetti and potato consumed as part of mixed meal on IDDM patients, *Diabetes Care*, 10, 401, 1987.

154. Coulston, A. M., Hollenbeck, C. B., Swislocki, A. L. M., and Reaven, G. M., Effect of source of dietary carbohydrate on plasma glucose and insulin responses to mixed meals in subjects with NIDDM, *Diabetes Care*, 10, 395, 1997.

155. Wolever, T. M. S., Jenkins, D. J. A., Ocana, A. M., Rao, A. V., and Collier, G. R., Second-meal effect: low-glycemic-index foods eaten at dinner improve subsequent breakfast glycemic response, *Am. J. Clin. Nutr.*, 48, 1041, 1988.

156. Behme, M. T. and Dupre, J., All bran vs. corn flakes: plasma glucose and insulin responses in young females, *Am. J. Clin. Nutr.*, 50, 1240, 1989.
157. Oettle, G. J., Emmett, P. M., and Heaton, K. W., Glucose and insulin responses to manufactured and whole-food snacks, *Am. J. Clin. Nutr.*, 45, 86, 1987.
158. Chew, I., Brand, J. C., Thorburn, A. W., and Truswell, A. S., Application of glycemic index to mixed meals, *Am. J. Clin. Nutr.*, 47, 53, 1988.
159. Wolever, T. M. S. and Jenkins, D. J. A., Effect of dietary fiber and foods on carbohydrate metabolism, in *CRC Handbook of Dietary Fiber in Human Nutrition*, Spiller, G. A., Ed., CRC Press, Boca Raton, FL, 1986, 87.
160. Wolever, T. M. S. and Jenkins, D. J. A., Use of the glycemic index in predicting the blood glucose response to mixed meals; *Am. J. Clin. Nutr.*, 43, 167, 1986.
161. Wolever, T. M. S., Csima, A., Jenkins, D. J. A., Wong, G. S., and Josse, R. G., The glycemic index: variation between subjects and predictive difference, *J. Am. Col. Nutr.*, 8, 235, 1989.
162. Wolever, T. M. S., Glycemic index and mixed meals, *Am. J. Clin. Nutr.*, 51, 1113, 1990.
163. Anderson, J. W., Effect of carbohydrate restriction and high carbohydrate diets in men with chemical diabetes, *Am. J. Clin. Nutr.*, 30, 402, 1977.
164. Ginsberg, H., Olefsky, J. M., Kimmerling, G., Crapo, P. A., and Reaven, G. M., Induction of hypertriglyceridemia by a low fat diet, *J. Clin. Endocrinol. Metab.*, 42, 729, 1976.
165. Coulston, A. M., Liu, G. C., and Reaven, G. M., Plasma glucose, insulin and lipid responses to high carbohydrate low fat diets in normal humans, *Metabolism*, 32, 52, 1983.
166. Brunzell, J. D., Lerner, R. L., Porte, D., and Bierman, E. L., Effect of a fat free, high carbohydrate diet on diabetic subjects with fasting hyperglycemia, *Diabetes*, 23, 138, 1974.
167. Brunzell, J. D., Lerner, R. L., Hazard, W. R., Porte, D., and Bierman, E. L., Improved glucose tolerance with high carbohydrate feeding in mild diabetes, *New Engl. J. Med.*, 284, 521, 1971.
168. Riccardi, G., Rivellese, A., Pacioni, D., Genovese, S., Mastranzo, P., and Mancini, M., Separate influence of dietary carbohydrate and fibre on the metabolic control in diabetes, *Diabetologia*, 26, 116, 1984.
169. Perrotti, N., Santoro, D., Genovese, S., Giacco, A., Rivellese, A., and Riccardi, G., Effect of digestible carbohydrates on glucose control in insulin-dependent diabetic patients, *Diabetes Care*, 7, 354, 1984.
170. Simpson, H. C. R., Carter, R. D., Lousley, S., and Mann, J. I., Digestible carbohydrate—an independent effect on diabetic control in type II (non-insulin-dependent) diabetic patients?, *Diabetologia*, 23, 235, 1982.
171. Coulston, A. M., Hollenbeck, C. B., Swislocki, A. L. M., and Reaven, G. M., Persistence of hypertriglyceridemic effect of low-fat high-carbohydrate diets in NIDDM patients, *Diabetes Care*, 12, 94, 1989.
172. Stevens, J., Burgess, M. B., Kaiser, D. L., and Sheppa, C. M., Outpatient management of diabetes mellitus with patient education to increase dietary carbohydrate and fiber, *Diabetes Care*, 8, 359, 1985.
173. Weinsier, R. L., Seeman, A., Henera, M. G., Assal, J. P., Soeldner, J. S., and Gleason, R. E., High and low carbohydrate diets in diabetes mellitus. Study of effects on diabetic control, insulin secretion and blood lipids, *Ann. Intern. Med.*, 80, 332, 1974.
174. Hockaday, T. D. R., Hockaday, J. M., Mann, J. I., and Turner, R. C., Prospective comparison of modified-fat-high-carbohydrate with standard low-carbohydrate dietary advice in the treatment of diabetes: one year follow-up study, *Brit. J. Nutr.*, 39, 357, 1978.
175. Chiarelli, F., Verrotti, A., Tumini, S., and Morgese, G., Effects of normal carbohydrate/low fat diet on lipid metabolism in insulin-dependent diabetes mellitus in childhood, *Diab. Nutr. Metab.*, 2, 285, 1989.
176. Stone, D. B. and Connor, W. E., Prolonged effects of a low cholesterol, high carbohydrate diet upon the serum lipids in diabetic patients, *Diabetes*, 12, 127, 1965.
177. Rivellese, A., Riccardi, G., Giacco, A., Pancioni, D., Genovese, S., Mattioli, P. L., and Mancini, M., Effect of dietary fibre on glucose control and serum lipoproteins in diabetic patients, *Lancet*, 2, 447, 1980.
178. Garcia, R., Garza, S., De La Garza, S., Espinosa-Campos, J., and Ovalle-Berumen, F., Dieta alta in fibras preparada con alimentos regionales como complemento in il control de la diabetes, *Rev. Invest. Clin. (Mex.)*, 34, 105, 1982.
179. Kinmonth, A-L., Angus, R. M., Jenkins, P. A., Smith, M. A., and Baum, D., Whole foods and increased dietary fibre improve blood glucose control in diabetic children, *Arch. Dis. Child.*, 57, 187, 1982.

180. Manhire, A., Henry, C. L., Hartog, M., and Heaton, K. W., Unrefined carbohydrate and dietary fibre in treatment of diabetes mellitus, *J. Hum. Nutr.*, 35, 99, 1981.
181. Venhous, A. and Chantelau, E., Self-selected unrefined and refined carbohydrate diets do not affect metabolic control in pump-treated diabetic patients, *Diabetologia*, 31, 153, 1988.
182. Karlström, B., Vessby, B., Asp, N. G., Boberg, M., Gustafsson, I. B., Lithell, H., and Werner, I., Effects of an increased content of cereal fibre in the diet of Type 2 (non-insulin-dependent) diabetic patients, *Diabetologia*, 26, 272, 1984.
183. Hollenbeck, C. B., Coulston, A. M., and Reaven, G. M., To what extent does increased dietary fiber improve glucose and lipid metabolism in patients with non-insulin-dependent diabetes mellitus (NIDDM)?, *Am. J. Clin. Nutr.*, 43, 16, 1986.
184. Nygren, C., Hallmans, G., and Lithner, F., Effects of high-bran bread on blood glucose control in insulin-dependent diabetic patients, *Diabete Meiab. (Paris)*, 10, 39, 1984.
185. Hagander, B., Asp, N. G., Efendic, Nilsson-Ehle, P., and Scherstén, B., Dietary fiber decreases fasting blood glucose levels and plasma LDL concentration in non-insulin-dependent diabetes mellitus patients, *Am. J. Clin. Nutr.*, 47, 852, 1988.
186. Silvis, N., Vorster, H. H., Mollentzer, W. F., de Jager, J., and Huisman, H. W., Metabolic and haemostatic consequences of dietary fibre and n-3 fatty acids in black type 2 (NIDDM) diabetic subjects: a placebo controlled study, *Int. Clin. Nutr. Rev.*, 10, 362, 1990.
187. Parillo, M., Riccardi, G., Pacioni, D., Iovine, C., Contaldo, F., Isernia, C., DeMarco, F., Perrotti, N., and Rivellese, A., Metabolic consequences of feeding a high-carbohydrate, high-fiber diet to diabetic patients with chronic kidney failure, *Am. J. Clin. Nutr.*, 48, 255, 1988.
188. Kiehm, T. G., Anderson, J. W., and Ward, K., Beneficial effects of a high carbohydrate high fiber diet in hyperglycemic men, *Am. J. Clin. Nutr.*, 29, 895, 1976.
189. Anderson, J. W. and Ward, K., High carbohydrate, high fiber diets for insulin treated men with diabetes mellitus, *Am. J. Clin. Nutr.*, 32, 2312, 1979.
190. Fukagawa, N. K., Anderson, J. W., Hageman, G., Young, V. R., and Minaker, K. L., High-carbohydrate, high-fiber diets increase peripheral insulin sensitivity in healthy young and old adults, *Am. J. Clin. Nutr.*, 52, 524, 1990.
191. Abbott, W. G. H., Boyce, V. L., Grundy, S. M., and Howard, B. V., Effects of replacing saturated fat with complex carbohydrate in diets of subjects with NIDDM, *Diabetes Care*, 12, 102, 1989.
192. Simpson, H. R. C., Simpson, R. W., Lousley, S., Carter, R. D., Geekie, M., Hockaday, T. D. R., and Mann, J. I., A high carbohydrate leguminous fibre diet improves all aspects of diabetic control, *Lancet*, 1, 1, 1981.
193. Bruttomesso, D., Briani, G., Bilardo, G., Vitale, E., Lavagnini, T., Marescotti, C., Duner, E., Giorato, C., and Tiengo, A., The medium-term effect of natural or extractive dietary fibers on plasma amino acids and lipids in type 1 diabetes, *Diab. Res. Clin. Prac.*, 6, 149, 1989.
194. Anderson, J. W. and Ward, K., Long-term effects of high carbohydrate, high fiber diets on glucose and lipid metabolism: a preliminary report in patients with diabetes, *Diabetes Care*, 1, 77, 1978.
195. Barnard, R. J., Massey, M. R., Cherny, S., O'Brien, L. T., and Pritikin, N., Long-term use of a high-complex-carbohydrate, high-fiber, low-fat diet and exercise in the gratement of NIDDM patients, *Diabetes Care*, 6, 268, 1983.
196. Lindsay, A. N., Hardy, S., Jarrett, L., and Rallinson, M. L., High-carbohydrate, high-fiber diet in children with type I diabetes mellitus, *Diabetes Care*, 7, 63, 1984.
197. Simpson, R. W., McDonald, J., Wahlqvist, M. L., Balasz, N., Sissons, M., and Atley, L., Temporal study of metabolic change when poorly controlled non insulin-dependent diabetics change from low to high carbohydrate and fiber diet, *Am. J. Clin. Nutr.*, 48, 104, 1988.
198. Hollenbeck, C. B., Connor, W. E., Riddle, M. C., Alaupovic, P., and Leklem, J. E., The effects of a high-carbohydrate low-fat cholesterol-restricted diet on plasma lipid, lipoprotein, and apoprotein concentrations in insulin-dependent (Type I) diabetes mellitus, *Metabolism*, 34, 559, 1985.
199. Simpson, R. W., Mann, J. I., Eaton, J., Moore, R. A., Carter, R., and Hockaday, T. D. R., Improved glucose control in maturity onset diabetes treated with high carbohydrate-modified fat diet, *Brit. Med. J.*, 1, 1752, 1979.
200. Simpson, R. W., Mann, J. I., Eaton, J., Carter, R. D., and Hockaday, T. D. R., High carbohydrate diets in insulin-dependent diabetes, *Brit. Med. J.*, 2, 523, 1979.

201. Hollenbeck, C. B., Riddle, M. C., Connor, W. E., and Leklem, J. E., The effects of subject-selected high carbohydrate, low fat diets on glycemic control in insulin dependent diabetes mellitus, *Am. J. Clin. Nutr.*, 41, 293, 1985.

202. Dodson, P. M., Pacy, P. J., Bal, P., Kubicki, A. J., Fletcher, R. F., and Taylor, K. G., A controlled trial of a high fibre, low fat and low sodium diet for mild hypertension in Type 2 (non-insulin-dependent) diabetic patients, *Diabetologia*, 27, 522, 1984.

203. McCulloch, D. K., Mitchell, R. D., Ambler, J., and Tattersall, R. B., A prospective comparison of I conventional and high carbohydrate/high fiber/low fat diets in adults with established Type 1 (insulin dependent) diabetes, *Diabetologia*, 28, 208, 1985.

204. Ney, D., Hollingsworth, D. R., and Cousins, L., Decreased insulin requirement and improved control of diabetes in pregnant women given a high-carbohydrate, high-fiber, low-fat diet, *Diabetes Care*, 5, 529, 1982.

205. Scott, A. R., Attenborough, Y., Peacock, I., Fletcher, E., Jeffcoate, W. J., and Tattersall, R. B., Comparison of high fibre diets, basal insulin supplements, and flexible insulin treatment for non-insulin dependent (type II) diabetics poorly controlled with sulphonylureas, *Brit. Med. J.*, 297, 707, 1988.

206. Jenkins, D. J. A., Wolever, T. M. S., Collier, G. R., Ocana, A., Rao, A. V., Buckley, G., Lam, K. Y., Meyer, A., and Thompson, L. U., The metabolic effects of a low glycemic index diet, *Am. J. Clin. Nutr.*, 46, 968, 1987.

207. Jenkins, D. J. A., Wolever, T. M. S., Kalmusky, J., Giudici, S., Giordano, C., Patten, R., Wong, G. S., Bird, J. N., Hall, M., Buckley, G., Csima, A., and Little, J. A., Low-glycemic index diet in hyperlipidemia: use of traditional starchy foods, *Am. J. Clin. Nutr.*, 46, 66, 1987.

208. Calle-Pascual, A. L., Gomez, V., Leon, E., and Bordiu, E., Foods with a low glycemic index do not improve glycemic control of both type I and type 2 diabetic patients after one month of therapy, *Diabete Metab. (Paris)*, 14, 629, 1988.

209. Jenkins, D. J. A., Wolever, T. M. S., Buckley, G., Lam, K. Y., Giudici, S., Kalmusky, J., Jenkins, A. L., Patten, R. L., Bird, J., Wong, G. S., and Josse, R. G., Low glycemic-index starchy food in the diabetic diet, *Am. J. Clin. Nutr*, 48, 248, 1988.

210. Collier, G. R., Giudici, S., Kalmusky, J., Wolever, T. M. S., Heiman, G., Wesson, V., Ehrlich, R. M., and Jenkins, D. J. A., Low glycaemic index starchy foods improve glucose control and lower serum cholesterol in diabetic children, *Diab. Nutr. Metab.*, 1, 11, 1988.

211. Fontvieille, A. M., Acosta, M., Rizkalla, S. W., Bornet, F., David, P., Letanoux, M., Tchobroutsky, G., and Slama, G., A moderate switch from high to low glycaemic-index foods for 3 weeks improves metabolic control of Type I (IDDM) diabetic subjects, *Diab. Nutr. Metab.*, 1, 139, 1988.

212. Brand, J. C., Colagiuri, S., Crossman, S., Allen, A., Roberts, D. C. K., and Truswell, A. S., Low glycemic index foods improve long term glycemic control in non-insulin-dependent diabetes mellitus, *Diabetes Care*, 14, 95, 1991.

213. Elsenhaus, B., Sufke, U., Blume, R., and Caspary, W. F., The influence of carbohydrate gelling agents on rat intestinal transport of monosaccharides and neutral amino acids in vitro, *Clin. Sci.*, 59, 373, 1980.

214. Rainbird, A. L., Low, A. G., and Zebrowska, T., Effect of guar gum on glucose absorption from isolated loops of jejunum in conscious growing pigs, *Proc. Nutr. Soc.*, 39, 48A, 1982.

215. Isaksson, G., Lundquist, I., and Ihse, I., Effect of dietary fiber on pancreatic enzyme activity in vitro: the importance of viscosity, pH, ionic strength, adsorption, and time of incubation, *Gastroenterology*, 82, 918, 1982.

216. Leatherdale, B. A., Green, D. J., Harding, L. K., Griffin, D., and Bailey, C. J., Guar and gastric emptying in non-insulin dependent diabetes, *Acta Diabet. Lat.*, 19, 339, 1982.

217. Thompson, L. U., Button, C. L., and Jenkins, D. J. A., Phytic acid and calcium affect the in vitro rate of navy bean starch digestion and blood glucose response in humans, *Am. J. Clin. Nutr.*, 46, 467, 1987.

218. Rea, R. L., Thompson, L. U., and Jenkins, D. J. A., Lectins in foods and their relation to starch digestibility, *Nutr. Res.*, 5, 919, 1985.

219. Thompson, L. U., Yoon, J. H., Jenkins, D. J. A., Wolever, T. M. S., and Jenkins, A. L., Relationship between polyphenol intake and blood glucose response of normal and diabetic individuals, *Am. J. Clin. Nutr.*, 39, 745, 1984.

220. Marshall, J. J. and Lauda, C. M., Purification and properties of phaseolamin, an inhibitor of alpha-amylase from the kidney bean *phaseolus vuloaris*, *J. Biol. Chem.*, 250, 8030, 1975.

221. Wolever, T. M. S., Chan, C., Law, C., Bird, L., Ramdath, D., Moran, J. J., and Jenkins, D. J. A., The in vitro and in vivo anti-amylase activity of starch blockers, *J. Plant Foods*, 5, 23, 1983.

222. Jenkins, D. J. A., Thorne, M. J., Wolever, T. M. S., Jenkins, A. L., Rao, A. V., and Thompson, L. U., The effect of starch-protein interaction in wheat on the glycemic response and rate of in vitro digestion, *Am. J. Clin. Nutr.*, 45, 946, 1987.

223. Holm, J., Bjork, I., Ostrowska, S., Eliasson, A. C., Asp, N. G., Larsson, K., and Lundquist, I., Digestibility of amylose-lipid complexes in-vitro and in-vivo, *Starch/Starke*, 35, 294, 1983.

224. Behall, K. M., Scholfield, D. J., and Canary, J., Effect of starch structure on glucose and insulin responses in adults, *Am. J. Clin. Nutr.*, 47, 428, 1988.

225. Goddard, M. S., Young, G., and Marcus, R., The effect of amylose content on insulin and glucose responses to ingested rice, *Am. J. Clin. Nutr.*, 39, 388, 1984.

226. Mourot, J., Thouvenot, P., Couet, C., Antoine, J. M., Krobicka, A., and Debry, G., Relationship between the rate of gastric emptying and glucose and insulin responses to starchy foods in young healthy adults, *Am. J. Clin. Nutr.*, 48, 1035, 1988.

227. Gannon, M. C. and Nuttall, F. Q., Factors affecting interpretation of postprandial glucose and insulin areas, *Diabetes Care*, 10, 759, 1987.

228. Wolever, T. M. S., Jenkins, D. J. A., Vuksan, V., Josse, R. G., Wong, G. S., and Jenkins, A. L., Glycemic index in individual subjects, *Diabetes Care*, 13, 126, 1990.

229. Jenkins, D. J. A., Wolever, T. M. S., Taylor, R. H., Ghafari, H., Jenkins, A. L., Barker, H., and Jenkins, M. J. A., Rate of digestion of foods and postprandial glycaemia in normal and diabetic subjects, *Brit. Med. J.*, 2, 14, 1980.

230. Jenkins, D. J. A., Ghafari, H., Wolever, T. M. S., Taylor, R. H., Barker, H. M., Fielden, H., Jenkins, A. L., and Bowling, A. C., Relationship between the rate of digestion of foods and postprandial glycaemia, *Diabetologia*, 22, 450, 1982.

231. O'Dea, K., Snow, P., and Nestel, P., Rate of starch hydrolysis in vitro as a predictor of metabolic responses to complex carbohydrate in vivo, *Am. J. Clin. Nutr.*, 34, 1991, 1981.

232. Jenkins, D. J. A., Wolever, T. M. S., Thorne, M. J., Jenkins, A. L., Wong, G. S., Josse, R. G., and Csima, A., The relationship between glycemic response, digestibility, and factors influencing the dietary habits of diabetics, *Am. J. Clin. Nutr.*, 40, 1175, 1984.

233. Thorburn, A. W., Brand, J. C., and Truswell, A. S., Slowly digested and absorbed carbohydrate in traditional bushfoods: a protective factor against diabetes?, *Am. J. Clin. Nutr.*, 45, 98, 1987.

234. Bornet, F. R. J., Fontvieille, A. M., Rizkalla, S., Colonna, P., Blayo, A., Mercier, C., and Slama, G., Insulin and glycemic responses in healthy humans to native starches processed in different ways: correlation with in vitro alpha-amylase hydrolysis, *Am. J. Clin. Nutr.*, 50, 315, 1989.

235. Wolever, T. M. S., Relationship between dietary fiber content and composition in foods and the glycemic index, *Am. J. Clin. Nutr.*, 51, 72, 1990.

236. Del Toma, E., Clementi, A., Marcelli, M., Cappelloni, M., and Lintas, C., Food fiber choices for diabetic diets, *Am. J. Clin. Nutr.*, 37, 667, 1988.

237. Thomas, E. J., Mechanics and regulation of gastric emptying, *Physiol. Rev.*, 37, 453, 1957.

238. Collier, G. R., Wolever, T. M. S., and Jenkins, D. J. A., Concurrent ingestion of fat and reduction in starch content impairs carbohydrate tolerance to subsequent meals, *Am. J. Clin. Nutr.*, 45, 963, 1987.

239. Read, N. W., Welch, I. M. L., Austen, C. J., et al., Swallowing food without chewing; a simple way to reduce postpranidal glycaemia, *Brit. J. Nutr.*, 55, 43, 1986.

240. Jenkins, D. J. A., Wolever, T. M. S., and Jenkins, A. L., Starchy foods and the glycemic index, *Diabetes Care*, 11, 149, 1988.

241. Reaven, G. M., Dietary therapy for non-insulin-dependent diabetes mellitus, *New Engl. J. Med.*, 319, 862, 1980.

242. Jenkins, D. J. A., Wolever, T. M. S., Bacon, S., Nineham, R., Lees, R., Rowden, R., Love, M., and Hockaday, T. D. R., Diabetic diets: high carbohydrate combined with high fiber, *Am. J. Clin. Nutr.*, 33, 1729, 1980.

243. Wolever, T. M. S., Metabolic effects of continuous feeding, *Metabolism*, 39, 947, 1990.

244. Jenkins, D. J. A., Wolever, T. M. S., Vuksan, V., Brighenti, F., Cunnane, S. C., Rao, A. V., Jenkins, A., Buckley, G., Patten, R., Singer, W., Corey, P., and Josse, R. G., "Nibbling versus gorging": Metabolic advantages of increased meal frequency, *New Engl. J. Med.*, 321, 929, 1989.

245. Creutzfeldt, W., Ed., Proceedings of first international symposium on acarbose, Montreux, Oct. 1981, *Excerpta Med.*, Amsterdam, 1982.

246. Hanefeld, M., Fischer, S., Schulze, J., Lüthke, C., and Spengler, M., Potential use of acarbose as first line drug in non-insulin dependent diabetes mellitus insufficiently treated with diet alone, *Diab. Nutr. Metab.*, 3 (Suppl. 1), 51, 1990.

247. Tasman-Jones, C., Effects of dietary fiber on the structure and function of the small intestine, in *Medical Aspects of Dietary Fiber*, Spiller, G. A. and Kay, R. M., Eds., Plenum Medical Books, New York, 1980, 67.

248. Cassidy, M. M., Lightfoot, F. G., Gray, L. E., Story, J. A., Kritchevsky, D., and Vahouny, G. V., Effect of chronic intake of dietary fibers on the ultrastructural topography of rat jejunum and colon: a scanning electron microscopy study, *Am. J. Clin. Nutr.*, 34, 218, 1981.

249. Tasman-Jones, C., Owen, R. L., and Jones, A. L., Semipurified dietary fiber and small bowel morphology in rats, *Dig. Dis. Sci.*, 27, 519, 1982.

250. Jacobs, L. R. and Schneeman, B. O., Effects of dietary wheat bran on rat colonic structure and mucosal cell growth, *J. Nutr.*, 111, 798, 1981.

251. Jacobs, L. R. and White, F. A., Modulation of mucosal cell proliferation in the intestine of rats fed a wheat bran diet, *Am. J. Clin. Nutr.*, 37, 945, 1983.

252. Jacobs, L. R., Effects of dietary fiber on mucosal growth and cell proliferation in the small intestine of the rat: a comparison of oat bran, pectin, and guar with total fiber derpivation, *Am. J. Clin. Nutr.*, 37, 954, 1983.

253. Shetty, P. S. and Kurpad, A. V., Increased starch intake in the human diet increases fecal bulking, *Am. J. Clin. Nutr.*, 43, 210, 1986.

254. Flourié, B., Leblond, A., Florent, Ch., Rautureau, M., Bisalli, A., and Rambaud, J.-C., Starch malabsorption and breath gas excretion in healthy humans consuming low- and high-starch diets, *Gastroenterology*, 95, 356, 1988.

255. Stephen, A. M., Haddad, A. C., and Phillips, S. F., Passage of carbohydrate into the colon: direct measurements in humans, *Gastroenterology*, 85, 589, 1983.

256. Wolever, T. M. S., Cohen, Z., Thompson, L. U., Thorne, M. J., Jenkins, M. J. A., Prokipchuk, E. J., and Jenkins, D. J. A., Ileal loss of available carbohydrate in man: comparison of a breath hydrogen method with direct measurement using a human ileostomy model, *Am. J. Gastroenterol.*, 81, 115, 1986.

257. Jenkins, D. J. A., Cuff, D., Wolever, T. M. S., Knowland, D., Thompson, L. U., Cohen, Z., and Prokipchuk, E., Digestibility of carbohydrate foods in an ileostomate: relationship to dietary fiber, in vitro digestibility, and glycemic response, *Am. J. Gastroenterol.*, 82, 709, 1987.

258. Levitt, M. D., Hirsh, P., Fetzer, C. A., Sheahan, M., and Levine, A. S., H2 excretion after ingestion of complex carbohydrates, *Gastroenterology*, 92, 383, 1987.

259. McBurney, M. I., Thompson, L. U., Cuff, D. J., and Jenkins, D. J. A., Comparison of ileal effluents, dietary fibers, and whole foods in predicting the physiological importance of colonic fermentation, *Am. J. Gastroenterol.*, 83, 536, 1988.

260. McBurney, M. I., Thompson, L. U., and Jenkins, D. J. A., Colonic fermentation of some breads and its implication for energy availability in man, *Nutr. Res.*, 7, 1229, 1987.

261. Cummings, J. H., Southgate, D. A. T., Branch, W. J., Wiggins, H. S., Houston, H., Jenkins, D. J. A., Jivraj, T., and Hill, M. J., The digestion of pectin in the human gut and its effect on calcium absorption and large bowel function, *Brit. J. Nutr.*, 41, 477, 1979.

262. Holloway, W. D., Tasman-Jones, C., and Lee, S. P., Digestion of certain fractions of dietary fiber in humans, *Am. J. Clin. Nutr.*, 31, 927, 1978.

263. Holloway, W. D., Tasman-Jones, C., and Maher, K., Pectin digestion in humans, *Am. J. Clin. Nutr.*, 37, 253, 1983.

264. McBurney, M. I. and Thompson, L. U., In vitro fermentabilities of purified fiber supplements, *J. Food Sci.*, 54, 347, 1989.

265. Bond, J. H. and Levitt, M. D., Fate of soluble carbohydrate in the colon of rats and man, *J. Clin. Invest.*, 57, 1158, 1976.

266. Bond, J. A., Currier, B. E., Buchwald, H., and Levitt, M. D., Colonic conservation of malabsorbed carbohydrate, *Gastroenterology*, 78, 444, 1980.

267. Cummings, J. H., Short chain fatty acids in the human colon, *Gut*, 22, 763, 1981.

268. Cummings, J. H., Pomare, E. W., Branch, W. J., Naylor, C. P. E., and MacFarlane, G. T., Short chain fatty acids in human large intestine, portal, hepatic and venous blood, *Gut*, 28, 1221, 1987.
269. Wolever, T. M. S., Brighenti, F., Royall, D., Jenkins, A. L., and Jenkins, D. J. A., Effect of rectal infusion of short chain fatty acids in human subjects, *Am. J. Gastroenterol.*, 84, 1027, 1989.
270. Royall, D., Wolever, T. M. S., and Jeejeebhoy, K. N., Clinical significance of colonic fermentation, *Am. J. Gastroenterol.*, 85, 1307, 1990.
271. Wolever, T. M. S., Spadafora, P., and Eshuis, H., Interaction between colonic acetate and propionate in man, *Am. J. Clin. Nutr.*, 53, 681, 1991.
272. Chen, W.-J. L., Anderson, J. W., and Jennings, D., Propionate may mediate the hypocholesterolemic effects of certain soluble plant fibers in cholesterol fed rats, *Proc. Soc. Exp. Biol. Med.*, 175, 215, 1984.
273. Illman, R. J., Topping, D. L., McIntosh, G. H., Trimble, R. P., Storer, G. B., Taylor, M. N., and Cheng, B. Q., Hypocholesterolaemic effects of dietary propionate: studies in whole animals and perfused rat liver, *Ann. Nutr. Metab.*, 32, 97, 1988.
274. Thacker, P. A., Salomons, M. O., Aherne, F. X., Milligan, L. P., and Bowland, J. P., Influence of propionic acid on the cholesterol metabolism of pigs fed hypercholesterolemic diets, *Can. J. Anim. Sci.*, 61, 969, 1981.

Dietary Fiber in the Prevention and Treatment of Disease

Disease Patterns in South Africa as Related to Dietary Fiber Intake

Alexander R. P. Walker

In South Africa there are four ethnic populations: blacks (25 million), coloreds (Euro-Africa-Malay) (3 million), Indians (1 million), and whites (5 million). These populations exhibit considerable differences in patterns of diseases. Indeed, between them they afford probably greater contrasts, as juxtaposed populations, than are encountered elsewhere in the world. The Asian population exhibits high frequencies of obesity, hypertension, diabetes, and coronary heart disease (CHD).[1-3] Among rural blacks, there are very low frequencies of dental caries, hypertension, CHD, noninfective bowel diseases, e.g., appendicitis and certain cancers (e.g., colon, breast).[5-9] Among urban blacks, Asians, and coloreds, rises are occurring in all these disorders and diseases. To exemplify the magnitude of changes, the teeth of urban black children are now *inferior* to those of white children.[10] Among urban black adults, the frequency of hypertension (WHO criteria) now exceeds that in whites[11] (Tables 5.1.1 through 5.1.3).

Most of the differences, although not all, are related to differences in environmental factors, especially diet. In this respect there are great contrasts in the patterns consumed by the different populations and their segments. At the one extreme, the diet of rural blacks[12] (which in pattern resembles that of ancestors of Western populations[13,14]) is characterized by a relatively low intake of energy, of total protein (especially of animal protein), and of total fat (especially of animal fat), yet their diet is high in fiber intake. In contrast, the diet of whites,[15] and that of the more privileged segments of the other populations, is high in energy, total protein, and fat, especially the respective moieties of animal origin; however, dietary fiber intake is low. The first pattern of diet, in contexts of indigence, is well nigh invariably associated with very low or low frequencies of degenerative disorders and diseases (although high frequencies of infections); conversely, the second is associated with very high or high frequencies of diseases of prosperity (Table 5.1.4).

As to the precise assessment of the protective role of dietary fiber intake, first it must be appreciated that patterns of health and disease are determined not only by diet but also by genetic and by nondietary factors. The latter include degree of physical activity,[16] extent of smoking practice,[17] stresses (particularly those linked with urbanization and rise in income), and the availability and utilization of medical services. Each of these components has a variable although often powerful influence in the regulation of the frequencies of the diseases mentioned. Next, it must be appreciated that the levels of a number of dietary components are powerfully correlated with level of fiber. Thus, the latter is inversely correlated with level of fat intake (especially of animal fat), of protein intake (especially animal protein), and with animal foods as a whole. Thus, with changes

Table 5.1.1   Frequencies of Some Diseases of Prosperity in South African Populations

	Rural Blacks	Urban Blacks	Coloreds	Indians	Whites
Dental caries	+	+ + +	+ + +	+ + + +	+ + +
Femoral fractures	+	+	+ +	+ +	+ + + + +
Obesity	+	+ + +	+ + +	+ + +	+ + +
Hypertension	+	+ + + +	+ + + +	+ + +	+ + +
Diabetes	+	+ + +	+ + + +	+ + + + +	+ + +
CHD	—[a]	+ +	+ + +	+ + + + +	+ + + + +
Stroke	+	+ +	+ + +	+ + +	+ +

[a] Implies that occurrence is rare.

Table 5.1.2   Cancer Patterns in South African Populations

	Rural Blacks	Urban Blacks	Coloreds	Indians	Whites
Lung	—[a]	+ +	+ + +	+ +	+ + + +
Breast	—[a]	+ +	+ + +	+ + +	+ + + + +
Colon	—	+	+ +	+ +	+ + + + +
Stomach	—	+	+ + +	+ +	+ +
Pancreas	—	+	+ +	+	+ + +
Liver	+ +[b]	+ +	+ +	+	+
Esophagus	+ + + +[b]	+ + +	+ +	+	+
Cervix	+ +	+ + + +	+ + +	+	+

[a] Implies that occurrence is rare.
[b] Frequency of occurrence related to some regional but not nationwide populations.

Table 5.1.3   Frequencies of Noninfective Bowel Diseases in South African Populations

	Rural Blacks	Urban Blacks	Coloreds	Indians	Whites
Hemorrhoids	—[a]	+ +	+ +	+ +	+ + +
Appendicitis	+	+ +	+ +	+ +	+ + + + +
Ulcerative colitis	—	+	+	+	+ + + + +
Irritable bowel syndrome	—	+ +	+ +	+	+ + + +
Diverticular disease	—	+	+ +	+ +	+ + + + +
Colon cancer	—	+	+ +	+ +	+ + + + +

[a] Implies that occurrence is rare.

Table 5.1.4   Dietary Patterns Respecting Fat, Total Carbohydrate, and Fiber Intakes

	Rural Blacks	Urban Blacks	Coloreds	Indians	Whites
Energy from fat (%)	10–15	20–30	30–35	35–40	35–45
Energy from carbohydrate (%)	70–75	65–75	60	60	55
Dietary fiber (g)	20–25[a]	10–20	15–20	15–20	15–20

[a] Intake depends on the season; seasonal fruits and "spinaches" are high in dietary fiber.

in diet, such as those which took place from the time of our ancestors to the present, and also which occurred when such changes became somewhat reversed as prevailed in certain wartime populations,[18,19] propounders of etiological hypotheses must be on their guard against overclaiming and overblaming. Account must be taken of changes and of contexts, holistically, rather than the focusing of attention and explanations almost exclusively on the changes that occurred in one or more food components. However, having said this, there is little doubt that changes in intakes of fat and of fiber are particularly influential.

Understandably, therefore, the *extent* of the specific involvement of dietary fiber remains a subject of uncertainty,[20-22] which does not lend itself to ready resolution. On the positive side, experimental studies on animals support the validity of a relationship,[23] as do many short-term studies on humans.[24-26] Probably the epidemiological evidence of the character already referred to provides the most persuasive support for a relationship. Briefly, there are similarities in the patterns of diet and disease exhibited by ancestors of Western populations and the patterns displayed by rural third-world dwellers, such as South African blacks. Moreover, in World War II, circumstances caused diets in certain countries to change, involving, *inter alia,* reductions in fat intake and increase in fiber intake.[18,19] There were associated changes in disease pattern; e.g., there were falls in dental caries, obesity, diabetes, atherosclerotic lesions of aorta and coronary vessels, constipation, and appendicitis.[18,19,27-29] Additionally, among church groups such as Seventh-Day Adventists,[30,31] and among vegetarians whose diet usually contains much more dietary fiber than the diet of omnivorous eaters, there are lower frequencies of a number of diseases[32] — obesity,[33] hypertension,[34] diabetes,[35] CHD,[36] appendicitis,[37] diverticular diseases,[38] cancers of the breast[39] and colon,[30,31] and osteoporosis.[40]

In fairness, it must be stressed that although ameliorative decreases in degenerative diseases *can* be accomplished by changes in diet, the magnitude of the alterations required is too great to win widespread public acceptance. As evidence of this, prosperous Western populations are having enormous difficulties in seeking to reduce their energy intake from fat to that level recommended of 30%. Equally great problems are latent in endeavors to, say, double intake of dietary fiber. Only a very small proportion of populations have changed their eating habits and adopted a "prudent diet."[41]

A perplexing fact in the present local situation in South Africa is that among urban blacks, while their frequencies of chronic bowel diseases have risen slightly, they are still far lower than those in the white population, despite the fact of the now relatively low fiber intake of urban dwellers.[42] Can this be explained? In his recent review, Heaton[22] noted that there are many ways in which a high fiber intake "ought to" protect against colorectal cancer;[43] yet low fiber intakes are not a consistent feature of populations prone to this cancer, nor of people who actually have it.[44,45] He suggested that fiber is only a part of the story, and that if fiber exerts its anticancer effect by being fermented into short-chain fatty acids, then any carbohydrate that enters the colon and is similarly fermented could be protective, since a considerable amount of the starch consumed escapes digestion and enters the colon, where it is rapidly fermented.[46] Perhaps starch intake matters as much as fiber intake in terms of protection from cancer. How much starch reaches the colon? This varies enormously, tenfold, from person to person.[47] According to one small study, people with colonic polyps are unusually efficient at digesting starch.[48] Should this be confirmed, then possibly cancer might be prevented by people eating more starch and by eating it in a less digestible form.[49] In South Africa, evidence indicates that maize, the staple food of the black population, is malabsorbed.[50] This implies that a variable, indeed, possibly a large proportion of "resistant" starch enters the colon and is therefore available for fermentation. Conceivably, therefore, it is this phenomenon which contributes to maintaining blacks' still faster transit time[51] and lower fecal pH value[52] and so protects them in measure against the development of chronic bowel diseases. In this type of context, it is important to keep in mind that while different sources of fiber have different physiological actions, it must be recognized that in rural Africa, *irrespective* of the source of fiber (cereals, legumes, vegetables, or fruit), chronic bowel diseases are uniformly rare or very uncommon.

REFERENCES

1. Seedat, Y. K., Lifestyle and disease: hypertension and ischaemic heart disease in Indian people in South African and in India, *S. Afr. Med. J.*, 61, 965, 1982.
2. Omar, M. A. K., Seedat, M. A., Dyer, R. B., Rajput, M. C., Motala, A. A., and Joubert, S. M., The prevalence of diabetes mellitus in a large group of South African Indians, *S. Afr. Med. J.*, 67, 924, 1985.
3. Seedat, Y. K., Mayet, F. G. H., Khan, S., Somers, S. R., and Joubert, G., Risk factors for coronary heart disease in the Indians of Durban, *S. Afr. Med. J.*, 78, 447, 1990.
4. Walker, A. R. P., Walker, B. F., Dison, E., and Walker, C., Dental caries and malnutrition in rural South African Black ten to twelve-year-olds, *J. Dent. Assoc. S. Afr.*, 43, 581, 1988.
5. Seedat, Y. K. and Hackland, D. B. T., The prevalence of hypertension in 4,993 rural Zulus, *Trans. R. Soc. Trop. Med. Hyg.*, 78, 785, 1984.
6. Walker, A. R. P. and Walker, B. F., Appendicectomy in South African inter-ethnic school pupils, *Am. J. Gastroenterol.*, 82, 219, 1987.
7. Walker, A. R. P. and Segal, I., Colorectal cancer. Some aspects of epidemiology, risk factors, treatment, screening and survival, *S. Aft. Med. J.*, 73, 653, 1988.
8. Walker, A. R. P., Walker, B. F., Funani, S., and Walker, A. J., Characteristics of black women with breast cancer in Soweto, South Africa, *The Cancer J.*, 2, 316, 1989.
9. Walker, A. R. P. and Walker, B. F., Coronary heart disease in blacks in underdeveloped populations, *Am. Heart J.*, 109, 1410, 1985.
10. Steyn, N. P. and Albertse, E. C., Sucrose consumption and dental caries in twelve-year-old children residing in Cape Town, *J. Dent. Assoc. S. Afr.*, 42, 43, 1987.
11. Seedat, Y. K. and Seedat, M. A., An inter-racial study of the prevalence of hypertension in an urban South African population, *Trans. R. Soc. Trop. Med. Hyg.*, 76, 62, 1982.
12. Richter, M. J. C., Langenhoven, M. L., Du Plessis, J. P., Ferreira, J. J., Swanepoel, A. S. P., and Jordaan, P. C. J., Nutritional value of diets of blacks in Ciskei, *S. Afr. Med. J.*, 65, 338, 1984.
13. Steven, M., Food and longevity in 18th century Scotland, *Nutr. Health*, 7, 3, 1990.
14. Hollingsworth, D., Changing patterns of food consumption in Britain, *Nutr. Rev.*, 32, 353, 1974.
15. Rossouw, D. J., Fourie, J. J., van Heerden, L. E., and Engelbrecht, F. M., A dietary survey of free-living middle-aged white males in the Western Cape, *S. Afr. Med. J.*, 48, 2528, 1974.
16. Blair, S. N., Kohl, H. W., Paffenbarger, R. S., Clark, D. G., Cooper, K. H., and Gibbons, L. W., Physical fitness and all-cause mortality: a prospective study of healthy men and women, *JAMA*, 262, 2395, 1989.
17. Stokes, J., III and Rigotti, N. A., The health consequences of cigarette smoking and the internist's role in smoking cessation, *Adv. Intern. Med.*, 33, 431, 1988.
18. Banks, A. L. and Magee, H. E., Effect of enemy occupation on the state of health and nutrition in the Channel Islands, *Mon. Bull. Min. Health Publ. Lab. Serv.*, 16, 184, 1945.
19. Fleisch, A., Nutrition in Switzerland during the war, *Schweiz. Med. Wochenschr.*, 16, 889, 1946.
20. Council on Scientific Affairs, Dietary fiber and health, *JAMA*, 118, 1591, 1988.
21. Nestel, P. J., Dietary fibre, *Med. J. Aust.*, 153, 123, 1990.
22. Heaton, K. W., Dietary fibre: After 21 years of study the verdict remains one of fruition and frustration, *Br. Med. J.*, 300, 1479, 1990.
23. Bianchini, F., Caderni, G., Dolara, P., Fanetti, L., and Kriebel, D., Effect of dietary fat, starch and cellulose on fecal bile acids in mice, *J. Nutr.*, 119, 1617, 1989.
24. Malinow, M. R., Regression of atherosclerosis in humans, *Postgrad. Med.*, 73, 232, 1983.
25. DeCosse, J. J., Miller, H. H., and Lesser, M. L., Effect of wheat fiber and vitamins C and E on rectal polyps in patients with familial adenomatous polyposis, *J. Nat. Cancer Inst.*, 81, 1290, 1989.
26. Ornish, D., Brown, S. E., Scherwitz, L. W., Billings, J. H., Armstrong, W. T., Ports, T. A., McLanahan, S. M., Kirkeeide, R. L., Brand, R. J., and Gould, K. L., Can lifestyle changes reverse coronary heart disease?, *Lancet*, 336, 129, 1990.
27. Pezold, F. A., *Arteriosclerose and Ernahrung*, Steinkopf, Darmstadt, 1959, 162.
28. Trowell, H., Diabetes mellitus death-rates in England and Wales 1920–70 and food supplies, *Lancet*, ii, 998, 1974.
29. Schettler, G., Cardiovascular disease during and after World War II: a comparison of the Federal Republic of Germany with other European countries, *Prev. Med.*, 8, 581, 1979.

30. Phillips, R. I., Role of life-style and dietary habits in risk of cancer among Seventh-Day Adventists, *Cancer Res.*, 35, 3513, 1975.
31. Snowdon, D. A., Animal product consumption and mortality because of all causes combined, coronary heart disease, stroke, diabetes, and cancer in Seventh-Day Adventists, *Am. J. Clin. Nutr.*, 48, 739, 1988.
32. Dwyer, J. T., Health aspects of vegetarian diets, *Am. J. Clin. Nutr.*, 48, 712, 1988.
33. Barbosa, J. C., Shultz, T. D., Filley, S. J., and Nieman, D. C., The relationship among adiposity, diet, and hormone concentrations in vegetarian and nonvegetarian postmenopausal women, *Am. J. Clin. Nutr.*, 51, 798, 1990.
34. Beillin, L. J., Rouse, I. L., Armstrong, B. K., Margetts, B. M., and Vandongen, R., Vegetarian diet and blood pressure levels: incidental or causal association?, *Am. J. Clin. Nutr.*, 48, 806, 1988.
35. Anderson, J. W., The role of dietary carbohydrate and fibre in the control of diabetes, *Adv. Intern. Med.*, 26, 67, 1980.
36. Burr, M. L. and Butland, B. K., Heart disease in British vegetarians, *Am. J. Clin. Nutr.*, 48, 830, 1988.
37. Westlake, C. A., St. Leger, A. S., and Burr, M. L., Appendicectomy and dietary fibre, *J. Hum. Nutr.*, 34, 267, 1980.
38. Gear, J. S. S., Fursdon, P., Nolan, D. J., Ware, A., Mann, J. I., Vessey, M. P., and Brodribb, A. K. M., Symptomless diverticular disease and intake of dietary fibre, *Lancet*, i, 511, 1979.
39. Adlercreutz, H., Hämäläinen, E., Gorbach, S. L., Goldin, B. R., Woods, M. N., and Dwyer, J. T., Diet and plasma androgens in postmenopausal vegetarian and omnivorous women and postmenopausal women with breast cancer, *Am. J. Clin. Nutr.*, 49, 433, 1989.
40. Marsh, A. G., Sanchez, T. V., Michelsen, O., Chaffee, F. L., and Fagal, S. M., Vegetarian lifestyle and bone mineral density, *Am. J. Clin. Nutr.*, 48, 837, 1988.
41. Anonymous, Nutrition and cancer, facts, fallacies, and ACS activities, *Cancer News*, Summer, 18, 1987.
42. Segal, I. and Walker, A. R. P., Low-fat intake with falling fiber intake commensurate with rarity of noninfective bowel diseases in Blacks in Soweto, Johannesburg, South Africa, *Nutr. Cancer*, 8, 185, 1986.
43. Cummings, J. H. and Bingham, S. A., Dietary fibre, fermentation and large bowel cancer, *Cancer Surv.*, 6, 601, 1987.
44. Jacobs, L. R., Fiber and colon cancer, *Gastroenterol. Clin. North Am.*, 17, 747, 1988.
45. Rozen, P., Horwitz, C., and Tabenkin, C., Dietary habits and colorectal cancer incidence in a second-defined kibbutz population, *Nutr. Cancer*, 9, 177, 1987.
46. Cummings, J. H. and Englyst, H. N., Fermentation in the human large intestine and the available substrates, *Am. J. Clin. Nutr.*, 45, 1243, 1987.
47. Stephen, A. M., Haddad, A. C., and Phillips, S. F., Passage of carbohydrate into the colon. Direct measurements in humans, *Gastroenterology*, 85, 589, 1983.
48. Thornton, J. R., Dryden, A., Kelleher, J., and Losowsky, M. S., Super-efficient starch absorption. A risk factor for colonic neoplasia?, *Dig. Dis. Sci.*, 32, 1088, 1987.
49. Heaton, K. W., Marcus, S. N., Emmett, P. M., and Bolton, C. H., Particle size of wheat, maize and oat test meals: effects on plasma glucose and insulin responses and on the rate of starch digestion in vitro, *Am. J. Clin. Nutr.*, 47, 675, 1988.
50. Segal, I., Walker, A. R. P., Naik, I., Riedel, L., Daya, B., and De Beer, M., Malabsorption of carbohydrate foods by blacks in Soweto, South Africa, *S. Afr. Med. J.*, 80, 543, 1991.
51 Walker, A. R. P., Walker, B. F., Lelake, A., Manetsi, B., Tlotetsi, G. N., Verardi, M. M., and Walker, A. J., Transit time and fibre intake in black and white adolescents in South Africa, *S. Aft. J. Food Science Nutr.*, in press.
52. Walker, A. R. P. and Walker, B. F., Intra- and inter-individual variations in serial faecal pH values in South African interethnic schoolchildren, *S. Afr. J. Food Science Nutr.*, 4(1), 10, 1992.

Development of the Dietary Fiber Hypothesis of Diabetes Mellitus*

Hugh C. Trowell

DIABETES AND OBESITY BECAME COMMON IN EAST AFRICAN BLACKS (1930–1960)

Diabetes mellitus and obesity were extremely rare diseases in East African blacks when I started treating medical patients in Nairobi Hospital, Kenya, in 1930. After teaching medicine for nearly 30 years in East Africa, I reviewed the rising incidence of diabetes in sub-Saharan urban blacks and suggested that "their high-carbohydrate low-fat diets are protective and that low-carbohydrate high-fat diets predispose. African diets are usually high in their fiber content but in towns refined flours, sugar, and fats form a large part of the diet which may contain little fiber."[1] No earlier reference has been traced to any connection between fiber and diabetes. On returning to East Africa in 1970 I was amazed to see two new phenomena: first, many grossly obese African blacks in urban streets and second, large diabetes clinics in all towns.[2]

HIGH FIBER BRITISH NATIONAL FLOUR

In 1948, Himsworth published diabetes mortality death rates in British women during the period of the Second World War (1940 to 1945) and the postwar food rations; he attributed falling death rates to reduced fat intakes.[3] In 1966, Cleave and Campbell republished these mortality and food data but concluded that reduced sugar intakes caused the falling death rates.[4] Postwar food regulations, however, lasted until 1953. A comprehensive British government report on human food supplies from 1938 through 1958 allowed a more detailed reexamination of this problem. This reported that diabetes death rates started falling not in 1940, but in 1942, and fell until 1953, not only until 1948, 55% in men and 54% in women, mainly in middle-aged and elderly groups. Diabetes death rates started to rise again in 1954. Fat and sugar supplies, however, rose in 1949 to prewar levels and continued thus thereafter, but death rates continued falling for another 5 years. High fiber high extraction national flour became mandatory for the entire British population from 1942 until 1953, then ceased and low fiber white bread was eaten. During the years of the national

---

* Dr. Trowell passed away in 1989. This historical chapter is unchanged from the 1986 edition of this handbook.

flour, bread consumption rose about 25%. Total energy intakes rarely decreased below 3000 kcal/day per head and were stationary during all these years.[5]

This provided the basis of the hypothesis that high fiber high *starchy* carbohydrate diets are protective against maturity-onset noninsulin-dependent Type II diabetes mellitus.[6] This protective diet, which resembles the ancient tranditional diet of most peasants, is *not* the same as a high carbohydrate high fiber diet because the latter might be a diet containing much white flour and sucrose supplemented by much wheat bran. The original hypothesis carries a corollary that low fiber starchy carbohydrates, such as white wheat flour and white rice, are the main causative factors in the production of Type II diabetes mellitus. High energy diets, containing much fat and sucrose, both of which contain no fiber, encourage overweight and obesity; they are probably contributory etiological factors.

GENETIC AND AUTOIMMUNE FACTORS

Genetic factors predispose strongly to Type II diabetes but are weak in Type I diabetes. Possibly viral infection or other noxious agents damage the pancreatic cells in Type I diabetes. This variety is an autoimmune disease. Many autoimmune diseases are certainly very rare in African blacks: multiple sclerosis has not yet been definitely reported; pernicious anemia and Hashimoto's thyroiditis are extremely rare; rheumatoid arthritis is certainly uncommon.[7] Unknown dietary factors or lifestyle protect sub-Saharan blacks from all or almost all autoimmune diseases.

NEW HIGH FIBER HIGH STARCH DIETS

In the U.S., Anderson and colleagues pioneered high fiber high starch carbohydrates in the treatment of diabetes.[8] In Britain, Mann and colleagues treated both Type I diabetes and Type II diabetes with a comparable diet; they reported improved diabetic control.[9] Jenkins studied purified fiber supplements such as pectin and guar gum; these slowed digestion and absorption, reduced GIP, and lowered enteroglucagon responses.[10]

IMPROVED DIABETIC DIETS

In 1979, the American Diabetes Association recommended that carbohydrate intakes of Type I diabetic patients be increased to 50 to 60% of total calories.[11] In 1981, the British Diabetic Association made similar recommendations.[12] These also recommended that simple sugar intakes be restricted and that carbohydrate, wherever possible, should be fiber-rich unprocessed starchy foods. One overall aim was to reduce fat consumption and hopefully in the long term to reduce the risk of cardiovascular disease.

IMPROVED DIETS FOR THE WHOLE COMMUNITY

In 1983, the (British National) Health Council recommended guidelines for nutritional changes in the whole population to decrease the incidence of modern metabolic diseases such as overweight and obesity, diabetes, coronary heart disease, and gallstones. They recommended increasing starch carbohydrates to 50% total calories by increased consumption of fiber-rich whole wheat and brown bread and potatoes, thereby increasing dietary fiber intake by 25%; they recommended that sugar intake be decreased to 50% and fat decreased by 25%.[13]

A consensus of opinion is emerging about desirable changes in modem Western diets in order to decrease the incidence of many diseases characteristic of modern affluent communities. Uncertainty about the degree of change and the desirable rate of change will continue for a decade or more.[14]

REFERENCES

1. Trowell, H. C., *Non-Infective Disease in Africa,* Edward Arnold, London, 1960, 217, 218, 303.
2. Trowell, H., Diabetes mellitus and dietary fiber of starchy foods, *Am. J. Clin. Nutr.,* 31, S53, 1978.
3. Himsworth H. P., Diet in the aetiology of human diabetes, *Proc. R. Soc. Med.,* 42, 323, 1949.
4. Cleave, T. L., Campbell, G. D., and Painter, N. S., *Diabetes, Coronary Thrombosis, and the Saccharine Disease,* John Wright, Bristol, 1969, chap 3.
5. Trowell, H., Diabetes mellitus death rates in England and Wales 1920–70 and food supplies, *Lancet,* 2, 998, 1974.
6. Trowell, H., Dietary-fiber hypothesis of the etiology of diabetes mellitus, *Diabetes,* 24, 762, 1975.
7. Trowell, H. C. and Burkitt, D. P., Eds., *Western Diseases, Their Emergence and Prevention,* Harvard University Press, Cambridge, MA, 1981, 439.
8. Anderson, J. W. and Ward, K., Long-term effects of high carbohydrate, high fiber diets on glucose and lipid metabolism, *Diabetes Care,* 1, 77, 1982.
9. Mann, J. L., Diet and diabetes, *Diabetologia,* 18, 89, 1980.
10. Jenkins, D. J. A., Taylor, R. H., and Wolever, T. M. S., The diabetic diet, dietary carbohydrates and differences in digestibility, *Diabetologia,* 23, 477, 1982.
11. Committee of the American Diabetes Association on Food and Nutrition Special Report, Principles of nutrition and dietary recommendations for individuals with diabetes mellitus, *Diabetes Care,* 2, 520, 1979.
12. British Diabetic Association Medical Advisory Committee, Dietary recommendations for diabetes for the 1980s, *Hum. Nutr. Appl. Nutr.,* 36A, 378, 1982.
13. National Advisory Committee on Nutrition Education, Proposals for nutritional guidelines for health education in Britain, *Lancet,* ii, 719, 782, 835, 902, 1983.
14. Do, R., Prospects for prevention, *Lancet,* i, 445, 1983.

Treatment of Diabetes with High-Fiber Diets

James W. Anderson, Abayomi O. Akanji, and Kim M. Randles

INTRODUCTION

Diabetes mellitus is emerging as a major health problem throughout the world, and current evidence suggests that increased fat intake and decreased fiber intake may contribute.[1,226] These and other observations led Trowell[1] to postulate that diabetes was a fiber deficiency disorder. Since 1976,[3,4] many basic and clinical investigators have documented the therapeutic benefits of fiber in diabetes and its complications.

While the clinical utility of dietary fiber in the treatment of diabetes is well established,[2] the role of fiber in the prevention of diabetes and reduction of risk for atherosclerotic complications is not established and data are still emerging. Some studies, however, report that

1. The frequency of post-meal hypoglycemica is reduced in "chemical diabetes" on a high-fiber diet.[12,25]
2. High-fiber diets have favorable effects on blood rheology and hemostatic variables in diabetic subjects.[44,63,121]
3. High-fiber diets may reduce risk factors for atherosclerotic cardiovascular disease — serum lipids (see tables), blood pressure,[125,134,143,219] and obesity.[229]
4. High-fiber diets may ameliorate the frequency of discomfort associated with intermittent claudication in diabetic subjects.[144]
5. High-fiber diets may specifically prevent the "carbohydrate-induced hypertriglyceridemia" associated with low-fiber, high-carbohydrate intakes for diabetic subjects.[215,226]
6. High-fiber diets may decrease the emergence of obesity and resultant diabetes.[115,134,143,144,156,159,229]

The tables summarize the clinical studies of diabetic subjects using either fiber supplements or diets generous in high-fiber foods (herein termed "high-fiber diets"). The tables are an extension of our earlier report[225] and include material in the medical literature between 1976 and 2000, drawn from the following sources: (1) computer (Medline) search on diabetes and fiber, including Scientific Citation Indexes, Nutritional Abstracts, and Index Medicus; (2) an excellent bibliographic survey of dietary fiber, up to and including the year 1986;[10] and (3) review of references in cited articles and reviews.

CLINICAL STUDIES

Fiber-Supplemented Meals

Table 5.3.1 summarizes the reported responses of diabetic subjects to glucose loads or meals with or without fiber supplements of high-fiber foods. The responses of normal subjects to similar test meals are described in a separate chapter. Water-soluble fibers such as guar, pectin, and psyllium extract clearly have greater effects on the glycemic response than do water-insoluble fibers such as cellulose and wheat bran. Other fiber supplements investigated in this context include cottonseed fiber,[99] soy fiber,[40,76,190] apple powder,[68,76] Mexican nopal leaves,[70] Indian fenugreek seeds,[88] Japanese glucomannan,[48,206] and xanthan gum.[83] High-fiber foods with a low glycemic index — oat bran, legumes, or barley — had greater effects than high-glycemic foods such as white bread or potatoes.[19,39] The glucose loads or meals supplemented with these soluble fibers are followed by lower glycemic responses than are control loads without fiber. These findings could be interpreted to suggest that fiber supplements may improve long-term glycemic control.

Fiber-Supplemented Diets

To extend the meal studies, many investigators examined the response of diabetic subjects to fiber-supplemented diets (Table 5.3.2). Most investigators used guar or another fiber source rich in soluble fiber such as glucomannan, psyllium, or apple fiber. To improve palatability, and hence acceptability, these fiber supplements, especially guar, were incorporated into everyday foods such as bread,[15,46,95,199] biscuits,[27] and chocolate bars.[90] Most studies suggest that fiber supplements lower average blood glucose and cholesterol (especially LDL) levels and reduce requirements for insulin or oral hypoglycemic agents. Many of the studies[78,79,89,92,100] were adequately controlled and used random allocation, random order, or crossover techniques. The controlled studies of Uusitupa et al.[102] in NIDDM and Vaaler et al.[89] in IDDM demonstrate the effects of guar supplementation on long-term (3-month) glycemic control and blood cholesterol levels. Several studies suggest that wheat bran supplements[11,57,89] also improve glycemic control and reduce the requirements for insulin and/or oral hypoglycemic agents. Corn bran hemicellulose[198] and oat bran[199] were also shown to lower the serum insulin response.

High-Fiber Diets

Table 5.3.3 summarizes the responses of diabetic subjects to high-fiber diets developed from high-fiber foods rather than fiber supplements. Most investigators used high-carbohydrate, high-fiber (HCHF) diets, although some tested high-fiber (HF) diets that were similar in carbohydrate content to the control diets. Our initial studies[3,105] with HCHF diets documented that these diets improved glycemic control, lowered insulin requirements, and reduced blood lipid levels. We have extended these studies[106,109,110,212] and they have been confirmed by many other groups (Table 5.3.3). Many of the more recent studies were well controlled using random allocation and crossover techniques, and it is now generally accepted that diabetic subjects derive distinct advantages from both HCHF and HF diets, the former probably being more beneficial. A particularly useful study is that reported by O'Dea et al.,[156] which investigated the effects of varying proportion of carbohydrate, fiber, and fat on metabolic control in NIDDM and concluded that high-carbohydrate diets for diabetic patients should select carbohydrates that are unrefined and high in fiber. It should be noted that one study[217] found that a high-carbohydrate, moderately high-fiber diet does not improve glycemic control in patients with mild NIDDM as compared to a low-carbohydrate, moderately high-fiber diet. In fact, the high-carbohydrate, moderately high-fiber diet actually increased plasma triglyceride and VLDL cholesterol concentrations. Another study[216] indicated that a high-carbohydrate diet without a concomitant increase in fiber intake results in deterioration of glycemic control and increased plasma triglyceride and VLDL levels. High-carbohydrate, high-fiber diets have also been shown to improve peripheral insulin sensitivity in healthy individuals.[218]

Use of Dietary Fiber in Distinct Diabetic Groups

The various investigators (Tables 5.3.1, 5.3.2, and 5.3.3) confirm that fiber confers distinct advantages to both IDDM and NIDDM subjects, including patients on the insulin pump and artificial pancreas treatment,[26,28,52] improving glycemic and lipidemic control, irrespective of body weight (lean or obese), state of diabetic control, or degree of compliance to treatment. Special groups such as children,[22,63,94,118,132] pregnant women,[23,71,75,119] and geriatric subjects[61,95] also benefit from fiber supplementation. Dietary fiber confers additional benefits in the management of diabetic patients who are hypertensive,[101,130,134,143,196] have chronic renal failure,[139,150] or have hepatic encephalopathy from liver cirrhosis.[85]

Mechanism of Effect of Dietary Fiber

High-fiber diets, especially those with a high carbohydrate content, probably exert their effect on glycemic control by improving insulin sensitivity. This is obvious from the reduced need for antidiabetic medication or insulin in subjects on these diets. However, reports on insulin clamp studies to assess insulin sensitivity in these subjects are not consistent, being variously reported as unchanged[98,117,162] or improved.[164,212] However, various studies[120,123,126] report increased insulin binding to monocytes and adipocytes in subjects on HF diets. It has also been reported in both normal subjects and diabetics[165–167,193] that fiber taken at a meal could improve glycemic response to subsequent meals. Other possible mechanisms of action of fiber may be via modulation of the secretion of gut hormones[13,25,30,40,86,101,140,194] or the intermediary metabolic effects of short-chain fatty acids — acetate, propionate, and butyrate — derived from the colonic fermentation of fiber in the diet.[174,175] High-fiber foods also are rich in phytochemicals and phytoestrogens that may favorably affect glucose metabolism and insulin sensitivity.[222]

Long-Term Safety of Fiber Preparations

Many investigators have reported on the long-term efficacy and safety of high-fiber diets.[90,100,102,157] The consensus is that there are no significant long-term nutritional risks for patients on these diets. Vitamin, mineral, and trace element levels were generally unaffected, as was absorption of simultaneously administered drugs.[168,169] A potential problem is with acceptability and palatability of the diets, especially in light of abdominal discomfort routinely experienced by many patients. This has partially been obviated by the use of low-dose guar preparations,[80,93] impregnation of guar with fructose for children,[94] and incorporation of natural high-fiber foods rather than fiber-enriched supplements. The major potential problems with prolonged fiber intake remain hypertriglyceridemia, especially in high-carbohydrate, low-fiber diets,[155] and small bowel obstruction,[170] although the latter appears quite rare.

High-Fiber Diets and Lipid Levels

Many studies have shown a clear correlation between a high-fiber diet and reduced plasma lipid levels. Plantago psyllium has been shown to reduce both total and LDL cholesterol levels while raising HDL cholesterol levels.[197] Wheat bran,[30,89,91] oat bran,[199] apple fiber,[68] xantham gum,[83] beet fiber,[101] fenugreek seeds,[88] guar and glucomannan[48,196,206] also demonstrate cholesterol- and triglyceride-reducing properties. In the long term, both high-fiber and high-fiber, high-carbohydrate diets reduce plasma cholesterol and triglyceride levels.[96,152,213]

Table 5.3.1 Effects of Dietary Fiber on Glycemic Responses to Single Meals for Diabetic Subjects

No. of Subjects	Special Group	Nature of Meal	Type of Fiber	Glycemic Response	Comments	Ref.
11 3 IDDM 8 NIDDM	—	Breakfast	Guar and pectin	Lower	Serum insulin lower after test than after control meal	4
6 IDDM	—	Breakfast	Guar	Lower	Serum alanine, lactate, and pyruvate similar after control and test meals	11
6 IGT	"Chemical" diabetes	Breakfast	Guar and hemicellulose	Lower	Fiber decreased reactive hypoglycemia	12
6 IDDM	—	Mixed	Guar	Lower	Serum GIP lower, glucagon unchanged after test compared to control meal	13
14 NIDDM		Glucose solution	Wheat bran	Lower or unchanged	Metabolic clearance of radioactive glucose unaffected by bran	14
6 1 IDDM 5 NIDDM		Breakfast	Guar or lentils or soybeans	All lower	High-fiber foods used	15
12 NIDDM	Autonomic neuropathy	Breakfast	Guar and pectin	Lower or unchanged	Fiber did not affect response of patients with autonomic neuropathy; serum insulin, glucagon, GIP unchanged	16
13 NIDDM	—	Breakfast	Guar or pectin or agar or locust bean gum	All unchanged	These fiber-supplemented meals were unpalatable	17
8 NIDDM	—	Breakfast	High-fiber foods	Lower	Whole grain bread and apples compared to white bread and apple juice	19
12 NIDDM 12 NIDDM	— —	Mixed meal Mixed	Psyllium High-fiber	Lower Unchanged	Blood glucose and insulin response similar after control and test meals —	20 21
21 IDDM 4 GDM 10 DM	Children Gestational diabetes	Mixed Glucose solution Oatmeal	High-fiber foods Guar Guar	Lower Lower Lower	Exercise did not affect blood glucose Glucose tolerance normalized Gastric emptying time similar after control and test meals	22 23 24
8 IGT	"Chemical" diabetes	Glucose	Pectin or cellulose phosphate or cellulose	Lower for pectin and cellulose phosphate; unchanged for cellulose	Variable changes in serum insulin	25

Subjects		Test/meal	Fiber	Effect	Comments	Ref.
4 IDDM	—	Mixed meal	Pectin	—	Insulin needs with artificial pancreas lower after test than control meals	26
9 — 3 IDDM, 6 NIDDM	—	Glucose solution	Guar	Lower	Guar biscuit used	27
6 IDDM	—	Breakfast and lunch	Guar	Lower	HF breakfast had no effect on glucose tolerance to lunch (insulin pump treatment)	28
5 — 2 IDDM, 3 NIDDM	—	Pasta breakfast	Guar	Lower	—	29
8 NIDDM	—	Breakfast	Mixed and rye	Lower	Postprandial C-peptide, GIP response reduced	30
14 NIDDM	—	OGTT	Psyllium	Unchanged	Insulin response unchanged	31
7 IDDM	—	Lunch or supper	Wheat bran	Unchanged	Insulin requirement unchanged with artificial pancreas	32
5 NIDDM	Lean	Breakfast	Wheat bran	Lower	Xylose absorption reduced; insulin levels unchanged	33
10 NIDDM	—	Breakfast	Guar	Lower	Absorption of lactose from milk-containing foods reduced	34
9 NIDDM	—	Breakfast	Wheat flour: extrusion vs. baking	Lowest with whole grain bread	Insulin response lowest with conventional whole grain bread	35
37 — 16 IDDM, 21 NIDDM	—	Breakfast	Rye bread	Lower	—	36
22 — 20 NIDDM, 2 IGT	—	Breakfast or lunch	Guar	Lower	Glycemic effect persisted through late postprandial period	37
19 — 8 IDDM, 11 NIDDM	—	Breakfast	Mixed (and beans)	Lower with beans	Postprandial insulin reponse lowest with beans; effect of processed food may be different in diabetic vs. non-diabetic subjects	38
4 NIDDM	Obese subjects	Breakfast	Beans vs. potato	Lower with beans	Glucose oxidation rates, insulin, and GIP reponses reduced after beans despite similar fiber content to potato	39
7 NIDDM	Obese subjects	Mixed breakfast	Soy polysaccharide	Lower	Insulin unchanged, serum triglycerides, glucagon, pancreatic polypeptide, somatostatin reduced	40

Table 5.3.1 (Continued) Effects of Dietary Fiber on Glycemic Responses to Single Meals for Diabetic Subjects

No. of Subjects	Special Group	Nature of Meal	Type of Fiber	Glycemic Response	Comments	Ref.
5 IGT	North Indians	OGTT	Mixed high-fiber	Lower	Typical North Indian diet improves glucose tolerance	41
13 NIDDM	—	Breakfast	Mixed high-fiber	Lower	Postprandial insulin responses lower	42
22	—	Breakfast	Mixed high-fiber	Unchanged	Insulin requirement with artificial pancreas reduced in IDDM but not in NIDDM	43
10 IDDM 12 NIDDM						
55 DM	Indian population	OGTT	Bran	Lower	Platelet adhesiveness reduced when fiber was given with glucose	44
12 NIDDM	—	Breakfast	Plantago psyllium	Lower	Lower AUC-glucose, AUC-insulin, and insulinic index	180
4 NIDDM	Obese	Breakfast and lunch	Fiber + lactulose	Lower	Lower glucose and insulin responses to meals	181
14 NIDDM	—	Breakfast	Guar	Lower	Lower postprandial rise in blood glucose, lower plasma insulin and plasma GIP; no reduction in postprandial plasma C-peptide levels	182
8 NIDDM	Mildly hypertriglyceridemic	Breakfast	Oat bran, wheat bran, fruit	Lower	Lower area under curve for glucose and insulin; soluble:insoluble ratio did not affect glycemic response	183
8 NIDDM	—	Breakfast	Oat bran enriched with β-glucans	Lower	Lower AUC-glucose and postprandial insulin level	184
14 NIDDM	—	Breakfast	Locust bean	Lower	Decreased glucose response; lower insulin response in patients with BMI > 30	185
14 NIDDM	—	Breakfast	Lupin	No change	Glucose and insulin levels unchanged	185
14 NIDDM	—	Breakfast	Insoluble maize-cob	No change	Glucose and insulin levels unchanged	185
10 NIDDM	—	Breakfast	Oat bran	Lower	Reduced postprandial plasma glucose and insulin	186

10 NIDDM	—	Breakfast	Wheat farina + oat gum	Lower	Reduced postprandial plasma glucose and insulin	186
8 NIDDM	—	Dinner	Food fiber	Higher	Greater postprandial glycemic response compared to equicaloric higher-fat and lower-fiber meal	187
6 NIDDM	—	Breakfast	Vegetable	Lower	Blood glucose levels inversely related to quantity of vegetable fiber in test diet	188
6 NIDDM	—	Spaghetti	Guar	No change	No change in integrated postprandial glucose or C-peptide response	189
8 NIDDM	—	Breakfast	Soya	Lower	Lower glycemic profile as compared to that produced by equivalent weight of cellulose	190
6 NIDDM	—	Breakfast	Psyllium flake cereal	Lower	Lower blood glucose; no effect on blood glucose when psyllium taken in water before the cereal	192
18 NIDDM	—	Breakfast and dinner	Psyllium	Lower	Reduced postprandial glucose elevation and serum insulin concentration; reduced postprandial glucose elevation after lunch, categorized as second-meal effect	193
7 NIDDM	Well-controlled	Breakfast	Algae-isolate	Lower	Lower postprandial rises in blood glucose, serum insulin, and plasma C-peptide; slower gastric emptying	194
30 IDDM	Youths	Pasta	Guar	No change	No change in blood sugar levels	195
10 NIDDM	Excellent metabolic control	Pasta	Beet fiber	Lower	Lower AUC-glucose vs. pasta, rice, and barley	214
10 NIDDM	Excellent metabolic control	Pasta	Barley	Lower	Lower AUC-glucose vs. pasta or rice	214

Note: DM, diabetes mellitus (type not indicated); IDDM, insulin-dependent (type I) diabetes mellitus; NIDDM, noninsulin-dependent (type II) diabetes mellitus; GDM, gestational diabetes mellitus; IGT, impaired glucose tolerance (formerly called chemical or latent diabetes); OGTT, oral glucose tolerance test; HF, high-fiber; MFLC, moderate-fiber, low-carbohydrate; HCHF, high-fiber, high-carbohydrate; LFHC, low-fiber, high-carbohydrate.

Table 5.3.2 Response of Diabetic Subjects to Fiber-Supplemented Diets

No. of Subjects	Special Group	Type of Fiber	Duration (days)	Glycemic Response	Comments	Ref.
9 DM	—	Guar	7	—	Glycosuria with guar supplements less than half of control values	45
9	—	Guar	5	—	Glycosuria 38% lower with guar crispbread than with control diet	46, 49
7 IDDM 2 NIDDM						
8 IDDM	—	Cellulose in bread	10	Lower	—	47
13 NIDDM	—	Glucomannan	90	Lower	Insulin requirements, cholesterol lower	48
6 DM	—	Guar	56		Insulin requirements lower	50
38 IGT	—	Wheat bran	30	Lower	Serum cholesterol, triglycerides lower	51
7 IDDM	—	Guar	1	Unchanged	Insulin needs with artificial pancreas lower in 5 out of 7 patients	52
22 NIDDM	Poorly controlled, poorly compliant	Guar or wheat bran	91	Unchanged	No beneficial effects	53
19 IDDM	—	Guar	5	—	Glycosuria reduced more with higher than lower carbohydrate intake	54
11	—	Guar + pectin	3	Lower	Glucose and insulin responses lower	55
5 IGT 6 NIDDM						
11	—	Guar	183–365	Unchanged	Insulin requirements, serum cholesterol lower	56
8 IDDM 3 NIDDM						
14 IDDM	—	Wheat bran	14–28	Lower	Insulin requirements lower	57
10 IDDM	—	Guar	91	Unchanged	Serum cholesterol lower	59
6 IDDM	—	Guar	28	Lower	Serum cholesterol 9% lower	60

Subjects	Condition	Fiber	Amount	Effect	Results	Ref.
8 IDDM	—	Guar	91	Unchanged	Body weight, insulin requirements, cholesterol lower	61
8 NIDDM	—	Wheat bran	91	Unchanged	Oral hypoglycemic agent doses and cholesterol decreased	61
10 NIDDM	—	Guar	28	—	Glycosuria and cholesterol decreased	62
10 NIDDM	Children	Guar	28	—	Insulin requirements decreased	63
14 NIDDM	Geriatric subjects	Guar	61	Lower	Serum cholesterol lower	64
17 IDDM	Stable and labile diabetic subjects	Wheat bran	10–15	Lower	Improved glycemic control	65
10 NIDDM	Subjects taken off all drugs	Guar		Lower	Urine glucose excretion 31% lower	66
40 NIDDM	Constipated patients	Psyllium	122	Lower	Glycohemoglobin and serum cholesterol lower	67
12 NIDDM	—	Apple fiber	49	Lower	Serum cholesterol lower	68
17 (6 IDDM, 11 NIDDM)	—	Guar	7–21	Lower	Serum cholesterol lower	69
7 DM	—	Boiled nopal leaves (Mex.)	10	Lower	Body weight, total, LDL cholesterol, triglycerides reduced	70
12 IDDM	Pregnant	Guar	7	Unchanged	Improvements with guar persisted after guar was stopped	71
12 NIDDM	Obese, poorly controlled subjects	Guar + wheat bran	61	Lower	Plasma cholesterol lower on guar	72
28 IDDM	—	Guar or wheat bran	91	Lower	Guar lowered glycohemoglobin, cholesterol; bran increased cholesterol	73
17 IDDM	—	Pectin	91	Unchanged	Glycohemoglobin, glycated albumin unchanged	74
5 (2 IDDM, 3 NIDDM)	—	Guar	14	Lower	Total cholesterol, triglyceride, drug requirements reduced	29

Table 5.3.2 (Continued) Response of Diabetic Subjects to Fiber-Supplemented Diets

No. of Subjects	Special Group	Type of Fiber	Duration (days)	Glycemic Response	Comments	Ref.
8 NIDDM	—	Soy hull	28	Lower	Glycosuria, glycohemoglobin unchanged, HDL cholesterol increased	76
		Corn bran	28	Unchanged	VLDL cholesterol, triglyceride, glycohemoglobin lower	
79 38 IDDM 41 NIDDM	—	Apple powder Guar	28 14	Unchanged Lower	Total, LDL cholesterol higher Serum cholesterol, glycosuria reduced, blood/urine chemistry unchanged	77
12 IDDM	—	Rye bran	28	Lower	Insulin requirements lower	78
4 IDDM	—	Cellulose	42	Lower	Total, HDL cholesterol lower, insulin need greater with cellulose	79
	—	Wheat bran	42	Lower	Glycohemoglobin, insulin need lower with wheat bran	
20 8 IDDM 12 NIDDM	—	Guar (low dose)	61	Unchanged	Glycohemoglobin, antidiabetic medication reduced	80
8 NIDDM	—	Guar	112	Unchanged	Hematologic parameters, blood chemistry, trace elements unaffected	81
13 8 IDDM 5 NIDDM	—	Guar	98	—	Serum cholesterol lower, triglyceride unchanged	82
9 NIDDM	—	Xanthan gum	42	Lower	Total, VLDL, LDL cholesterol, total, VLDL triglyceride, gastrin, and GIP responses lower	83
10 NIDDM	—	Guar	42	Lower	Insulin response, glycohemoglobin, total, HDL cholesterol lower, insulin sensitivity and receptor binding greater, HDL, phospholipids, triglycerides, hepatic glucose production unchanged	84

8 NIDDM	Subjects with portal systemic encephalopathy (PSE) from liver cirrhosis	Vegetable protein and psyllium	15	Lower	Tolbutamide dose reduced, bowel movements greater, PSE parameters unchanged	85
11 NIDDM	—	Guar	14	Unchanged	Serum cholesterol, GIP response lower, insulin, C-peptide responses unchanged	86
8 NIDDM	Obese	Guar	183	—	Serum triglyceride higher, LDL lower in men, effect not maintained over 6 months	87
5 NIDDM	Asian Indians	Fenugreek seeds	21	Lower	Glycosuria, serum cholesterol, insulin response lower	88
28 IDDM	—	Guar	91	Lower	Glycohemoglobin, total, LDL cholesterol lower	89
		Wheat bran	91	Lower	HDL cholesterol total cholesterol ratio higher	
16 NIDDM	—	Guar	183	—	Nutritional parameters unchanged	90
7 NIDDM	Poorly controlled, non-compliant subjects	Guar	30	Lower	Glycosuria, fasting insulin lower, erythrocyte insulin binding, serum calcium, cholesterol triglyceride, OGTT and glycohemoglobin unchanged	91
29 NIDDM	Subjects with near normal fasting plasma glucose levels	Guar	56	Unchanged	Glycohemoglobin, C-peptide, HDL cholesterol, triglyceride unchanged, LDL cholesterol lower	92
16 NIDDM	—	Guar	42	Unchanged	Glycohemoglobin, LDL, total cholesterol, triglyceride reduced	93
22 IDDM	Children	Guar	42	—	Glycosuria, glycohemoglobin, total cholesterol reduced	94
14 NIDDM	Geriatric	Guar	183	Lower	C-peptide lower, glycohemoglobin increased, HDL cholesterol, triglycerides unchanged	95
17 NIDDM	Obese	Guar gum	112	Unchanged	No additional benefit	97
9 IDDM	Lean patients on insulin pump treatment	Guar	28	Lower	Glycohemoglobin, insulin sensitivity unchanged, insulin needs, LDL cholesterol lower	98

Table 5.3.2 (Continued) Response of Diabetic Subjects to Fiber-Supplemented Diets

No. of Subjects	Special Group	Type of Fiber	Duration (days)	Glycemic Response	Comments	Ref.
12 NIDDM	—	Cotton seed fiber	30	Lower	Insulin response to test meal, serum lipids unchanged	99
8 NIDDM	—	Guar	183	—	Mineral (Fe, Cu, Zn, Ca, Mn, Mg) balance unchanged	100
12 NIDDM	—	Beet fiber	56	Unchanged	Systolic BP, cholesterol, triglycerides lower, HDL increased, postprandial insulin, pancreatic polypeptide and motilin lower in obese, glycohemoglobin unchanged	101
33 NIDDM	Poorly controlled obese	Guar	396	Unchanged	Serum total cholesterol, vitamins A and E lower, plasma Zn higher	102
19 NIDDM	Obese	Guar	91	Lower	Total, LDL cholesterol lower (if serum cholesterol > 6.5 mmol/l)	103
12 NIDDM	—	Guar	14	Lower	Serum cholesterol, triglyceride lower, insulin enteroglucagon, glucagon, GIP, PYY unchanged, neurotensin higher	104
11 NIDDM	Hyperlipidemic, hypertensive	Glucomannan	21	Lower	Lower fructosamine, cholesterol, and blood pressure; glucose and insulin unchanged	196
125 IDDM	—	Plantago psyllium	42	Lower	Lower fasting plasma glucose, total cholesterol, LDL, and triglycerides; higher HDL	197
28 NIDDM	Mild IGT, 20 obese, 8 non-obese	Soluble corn bran hemicellulose	180	Lower	Lower serum insulin response, decreased HbA$_{1c}$, and fasting glucose	198
8 NIDDM	Free-living men	Oat bran	84	Lower	Lower mean glycemic and insulin responses, lower total cholesterol, LDL, and LDL:HDL	199
100 NIDDM	Hyperlipidemic	Wheat bran	28	Lower	Hypoglycemic effect	200
100 NIDDM	Hyperlipidemic	Lignin-enriched bran	28	No change	No change in basal or aftermeal glycemia	200
100 NIDDM	Hyperlipidemic	Cellulose pulp	28	No change	No change in basal or aftermeal glycemia	200

						Ref.
100 NIDDM	Hyperlipidemic	Citrus pectin	28	No change	No change in basal or aftermeal glycemia	200
15 NIDDM	—	Guar	336	Lower	Improved long-term glycemic control, postprandial glucose tolerance, and lipid concentrations; C-peptide response increased; insulin response unchanged	201
16 NIDDM	—	Guar	56	Lower	Lower fasting insulin and HbA_{1c} concentrations	202
7 IDDM	Moderately poor metabolic control	Guar	90	No change	Lower cholesterol; concentrations of all other substrates unchanged	203
13 NIDDM	—	Beet fiber	42	No change	No change in fasting blood glucose, HbA_{1c}, serum triglycerides, or body weight	204
16 NIDDM	—	Sweet lupine hull	60	No change	Blood glucose increased and cholesterol decreased during first month of supplementation; blood glucose decreased to control levels during second month	205
72 NIDDM	—	Konjac food	65	Lower	Reduced fasting blood glucose, postprandial blood glucose, and HbA_{1c}; decreased triglyceride levels in hypertriglyceridemic subjects	206
10 NIDDM	—	Wheat bran	90	Lower	Lower postprandial plasma insulin; no change in blood glucose or HbA_{1c}	207
10 NIDDM	—	Guar	90	Lower	Lower postprandial plasma insulin; no change in blood glucose or HbA_{1c}	207
17 IDDM	Mildly hypercholesterolemic	Guar	42	Lower	Decreased fasting blood glucose and HbA_{1c}	208
40 33 NIDDM 7 IDDM	—	Guar	90	Lower	Lower HbA_{1c} and cholesterol	191

Note: See Table 5.3.1 for definition of abbreviations.

Table 5.3.3   Response of Diabetic Subjects to High-Fiber Diets Developed from High-Fiber Foods

No. of Subjects	Special Group	Nature of Diet	Duration (Days)	Glycemic Response	Comments	Ref.
13 8 IDDM 5 NIDDM	—	HCHF	12–28	Lower	Insulin or oral hypoglycemic agent needs, blood lipids reduced	3
14 3 IDDM 11 NIDDM	—	HCHF	1478	Lower	Insulin dose, serum cholesterol, triglycerides lower; good long-term outpatient compliance	96
10 7 IDDM 3 NIDDM	—	HCHF	182–1095	Lower	Insulin requirements, serum lipids lower	105
20 IDDM	Lean	HCHF	16	Lower	Insulin requirements, blood lipids reduced	106
14 NIDDM	—	HCHF	42	Lower	Glycohemoglobin, cholesterol lower	107
11 IDDM	—	HCHF	42	Unchanged	Insulin requirements, serum cholesterol lower	108
21 12 IDDM 9 NIDDM	Obese	HCHF	12–42	Lower	Insulin requirements, blood lipids lower	109
11 4 IDDM 7 NIDDM	—	HCHF	18–26	Lower	HCHF and LFHC diets had equivalent insulin dose-reducing effects	110
8 4 IDDM 4 NIDDM	—	HCHF	10	Lower	Serum cholesterol lower	111
5 NIDDM	Geriatric nursing home residents	HF	14	Lower	Diabetic control improved	112
16 10 IDDM 6 NIDDM	—	MFLC	42	Slightly lower	With low carbohydrate, increasing fiber from 18 to 33 g/day did not change glycemic control	113
27 9 IDDM 18 NIDDM	—	HCHF	42	Lower	Serum cholesterol lower, HDL:LDL ratio higher	114

Subjects	Notes	Diet	Duration		Results	Ref
60 NIDDM	Pritikin program with exercise	HCHF	26	Lower	Insulin or oral hypoglycemic agent needs, blood lipids, body weight lower	115
8 NIDDM	Obese	HF	2	Lower	Urinary C-peptide excretion lower on high-bean diet than on high-bran diet	116
7 NIDDM	Very obese	HCHF	7	Unchanged	Insulin sensitivity unchanged	117
10 IDDM	Children	HF	42	Lower	Glycosuria decreased	118
20 (10 IDDM, 10 NIDDM)	Pregnant	HCHF	28–210	Lower	Insulin requirements decreased	119
20 IDDM	—	HCHF	28	Unchanged	Insulin requirements lower, insulin binding to circulating monocytes increased	120
21 (10 IDDM, 11 NIDDM)	—	HCHF	42	Slightly lower	Plasma-clotting factors reduced	121
7 NIDDM	—	HCHF	42	—	Insulin binding to circulating monocytes increased	123
69 NIDDM	Pritikin program and exercise	HCHF	730–1095	Lower	Diet and exercise sustained lower serum lipids	124
35 (1 IDDM, 34 NIDDM)	16 white, 10 black, 9 Asian, hypertensives	HCHF (low sodium)	30	—	Blood pressure lower in whites and blacks, but not in Asians	125
9 NIDDM	—	HCHF	21	Lower	Glycosuria reduced; fasting insulin unchanged; improved insulin receptor binding and sensitivity	126
10 (2 IDDM, 8 NIDDM)	Long-term outpatient study	HF	91	Lower	Serum triglycerides lower	127
10 IDDM	—	HCHF	42	—	Serum cholesterol lower by 15%; postheparin plasma lipoprotein lipase activity unchanged	128
14 (6 IDDM, 8 NIDDM)	—	HCHF	10	Lower	Total, LDL, VLDL cholesterol lower	129
25 NIDDM	Mild hypertension	HF	91	—	Glycohemoglobin, triglyceride, mean blood pressure lower	130

Table 5.3.3 (Continued) Response of Diabetic Subjects to High-Fiber Diets Developed from High-Fiber Foods

No. of Subjects	Special Group	Nature of Diet	Duration (Days)	Glycemic Response	Comments	Ref.
14 NIDDM	—	HF	21	Lower	Insulin sensitivity improved; glycosuria, HDL, total cholesterol reduced; lipase activity in muscle or adipose tissue, i.v. fat tolerance, fecal fat, trace elements (K, Zn), hematologic variables unchanged	131
12 IDDM	Children	HCHF	14	Unchanged	Frequency of hypoglycemic reactions and insulin dose unchanged	132
25 5 IDDM 20 NIDDM	Mild hypertension	HCHF (low-fat, low-sodium)	91	—	Triglyceride, glycohemoglobin, body weight lower; same blood pressure reduction as bendrofluazide; HDL higher	134
14 6 IDDM 8 NIDDM	—	HCHF	10	Lower	LDL, HDL, total cholesterol lower, body weight higher	135
4 IDDM	—	HF	42	Lower	Glycohemoglobin, insulin requirement, total, HDL cholesterol lower	136
6 IDDM	Self-selected foods used	HCHF	42	Unchanged	Glycosuria, insulin need, glycohemoglobin unchanged compared to MCLF (high-fat) diet	137
13 IDDM	Poorly controlled	HCHF	580	Worsened	Health education is probably the best method for achieving optimal control in IDDM subjects	138
5 IDDM	Chronic renal failure (hospitalized)	HF	10	Lower	No deleterious effect on blood urea and nutritional status; plasma creatinine reduced	139
22 NIDDM	—	HCHF	42	Lower	Total, HDL cholesterol lower when diet complements intensive patient education	141
6 NIDDM	Lean	HCHF	28	Unchanged	Insulin, triglycerides, LDL, HDL, total cholesterol unchanged	142
7 NIDDM	Moderate hypertension; no drug treatment	HCHF	91	—	Glycohemoglobin, LDL cholesterol, blood pressure, body weight lower	143

Subjects	Condition/Study	Diet	Days	Result	Findings	Ref.
17 6 IDDM 11 NIDDM	Intermittent claudication	HF (low-fat, low-sodium)	91	—	Blood pressure, LDL cholesterol, triglyceride, glycohemoglobin, body weight lower; symptom frequency reduced; Doppler ankle/arm ratios unchanged	144
35 15 IDDM 20 NIDDM	—	HCHF	365	Unchanged	Glycohemoglobin, cholesterol, body weight unchanged	145
15 NIDDM	Poorly controlled in metabolic ward study	HF (legumes)	21	Lower	Glycosuria lower, insulin, insulin sensitivity unchanged	146
1 GDM	—	Mixed HF	30	Lower	Control throughout pregnancy with high-cereal, -legumes, and -fiber diet without need for insulin	147
14 NIDDM	Obese, geriatric	HF	56	Lower	Total, LDL cholesterol, LDL:HDL ratio lower; glycohemoglobin, insulin, C-peptide, glucagon, somatostatin unchanged	149
6 IDDM	Chronic renal failure, moderate protein restriction	HCHF	10	Lower	Total cholesterol lower, triglycerides, renal function, nitrogen balance, nutritional status unchanged; serum phosphate increased	150
28 NIDDM	Poorly controlled	HF	183	Elevated	Glycohemoglobin, total, and HDL unchanged	151
13 NIDDM	Poorly controlled	HCHF	21	Lower	Glycosuria, total, HDL cholesterol, tri-glyceride, glucagon reduced; insulin, fatty acids, insulin receptor binding unchanged	152
10 IDDM	Patients on insulin pump treatment	HF	42	Unchanged	Body weight, insulin needs, blood lipids unchanged	153
40 19 IDDM 21 NIDDM	Retrospective evaluation of three studies	HCHF	700	—	Subjects complied best to fiber recommendation; least compliance was to carbohydrate recommendation	154
10 NIDDM	Outpatient study	HCHF	14	Lower	Body weight, body mass index, total, LDL cholesterol, insulin responses reduced, OGTT improved	156
16 NIDDM	To compare low glycemic index (GI) with high-GI foods	About 45% carbohydrate	84	Lower on low-GI diet	Glycohemoglobin, glycosuria reduced on low-GI diet; lipoproteins unchanged	158

Table 5.3.3 (Continued) Response of Diabetic Subjects to High-Fiber Diets Developed from High-Fiber Foods

No. of Subjects	Special Group	Nature of Diet	Duration (Days)	Glycemic Response	Comments	Ref.
9 IDDM	Well controlled, highly motivated	HF	12	Lower	Lower postprandial capillary blood glucose	209
NIDDM	Early NIDDM	HF	—	Lower	Lower basal insulin and body weight; amelioration of clinical symptoms; increase in insulin immediate pool; reduction of insulinemia and hyperglycemia in glucose tolerance test	210
70 NIDDM	—	HCHF	540	No change	Improvement in glycemic control during recruitment phase	211
10 IDDM	—	HCHF	28	Lower	Reduced basal insulin requirements; lower total cholesterol and HDL; glycemic control and other lipid fractions unchanged	212
84 NIDDM	Obese	HCHF	30	Lower	Better glycemic control, lower blood glucose, HbA$_{1c}$, and fructosamine; decreased total cholesterol and triglycerides with no effect on HDL	213
13 NIDDM	—	HF	42	Lower	Lower preprandial plasma glucose, glucose excretion, AUC-glucose, and AUC-insulin; lower total cholesterol, triglyceride, and VLDL	215

Note: See Table 5.3.1 for definition of abbreviations.

High-Fiber Diets and Epidemiological Studies

High fiber intakes appear to reduce risk for developing diabetes. Two independent studies have confirmed an inverse correlation between a high-fiber diet and the risk for NIDDM in both men and women.[223,224] Insulin resistance appears to be a forerunner or risk factor for development of diabetes.[222] In non-diabetic subjects, a high-fiber diet is associated with a lower fasting insulin concentration.[220] A high fasting insulin concentration has been linked to an increased incidence of heart disease.[221] Several epidemiological studies have indicated a strong link between a high-fiber diet, especially a generous intake of whole grains, and the prevention of coronary heart disease.[222,227,228] High fiber intakes also appear to protect from development of hypertension.[219] Further observational studies suggest that high fiber intakes may protect from development of obesity.[229]

CONCLUSIONS

High-fiber diets provide many benefits for diabetic patients, by lowering blood glucose concentration, reducing postprandial insulin levels and antidiabetic drug requirements, and decreasing blood lipid concentrations. For lean individuals with type 1 diabetes, these diets can reduce insulin requirements by 25 to 50% and improve glycemic control.[171] For lean individuals with type 2 diabetes, these diets can lower antidiabetic drug needs by 50 to 100% and often eliminate the need for insulin.[171] For obese persons with diabetes, these diets associated with high satiety promote weight loss and usually provide reasonable glycemic control without specific antidiabetic medication. These diets also lower blood glycohemoglobin levels, plasma cholesterol levels (20 to 30%), triglycerides (slightly to moderately), and blood pressure (average of 10%).

We routinely recommend a prudent diabetic diet containing the following:[7,161,226]

1. 55 to 60% of energy from carbohydrate (two-thirds derived from polysaccharides).
2. 12 to 16% of total calories from protein (or daily intake of 0.8–1.2 g/kg desirable body weight to a maximum of 90 g/day). This amount should be reduced in individuals with nephropathy.[176,226]
3. Less than 30% of total calories from fat, consistent with the American Heart Association recommendations,[177] with less than 10% saturated fat and daily cholesterol intake of less than 200 mg. When increased carbohydrate intake cannot be tolerated or is impractical, total fat intake could be increased to 30 to 40% energy, with the increase mainly from monounsaturated fats. While still controversial with yet unclear long-term effects,[179] a high–monounsaturated fat diet has been shown to increase HDL cholesterol levels and reduce the risk of hypertriglyceridemia associated with high-carbohydrate, fiber-deficient diets.[135,148,155,178]
4. Dietary fiber of about 35 g/d (or 15 to 25 g/1000 kcal), to include soluble and insoluble fibers from commonly available foods. Diets high in carbohydrate but not fiber content, as indicated above, may adversely affect blood lipid levels.
5. The specific benefits of whole grain intake deserve special mention. Whole grains appear to increase insulin sensitivity and reduce risk for developing diabetes and coronary heart disease. The bran layer of cereal fibers is rich in fiber and phytochemicals that may have specific antioxidant, anti-inflammatory, phytoestrogen, and other effects that provide these benefits.[222,227] We recommend three servings daily.

Other features of the diabetes diet, especially in relation to total caloric intake, use of alternative sweeteners, intake of salt and vitamin and mineral supplements, as well as alcohol ingestion, have been reviewed elsewhere.[7,226] Because of the cardioprotective and anti-inflammatory effects of vitamin E, we recommend an intake of 800 IU daily for adults with diabetes.[230]

REFERENCES

1. Trowell, H. C., Dietary fiber hypothesis of the etiology of diabetes mellitus, *Diabetes*, 24, 762, 1975.
2. Anderson, J. W., The role of dietary carbohydrate and fiber in the control of diabetes, *Adv. Intern. Med.*, 26, 67, 1980.
3. Kiehm, T. G., Anderson, J. W., and Ward, K., Beneficial effects of a high carbohydrate, high fiber diet on hyperglycemic diabetic men, *Am. J. Clin. Nutr.*, 29, 895, 1976.
4. Jenkins, D. J. A. et al., Unabsorbable carbohydrates and diabetes: decreased postprandial hyperglycaemia, *Lancet*, 2, 172, 1976.
5. Wahlquist, M. L., Dietary fiber and carbohydrate metabolism, *Am. J. Clin. Nutr.*, 45, 1232, 1987.
6. Vinik, A. I. and Jenkins, D. J. A., Dietary fiber in management of diabetes, *Diabetes Care*, 11, 160, 1988.
7. Anderson, J. W. and Geil, P. B., New perspectives in nutrition management of diabetes mellitus, *Am. J. Med.*, 85, 159, 1988.
8. Council on Scientific Affairs, American Medical Association, Dietary fiber and health, *JAMA*, 262, 542, 1989.
9. Anderson, J. W., Treatment of diabetes with high fiber diets, in *CRC Handbook of Dietary Fiber in Human Nutrition*, Spiller, G. A., Ed., CRC Press, Boca Raton, FL, 1984, 349.
10. Leeds, A. R. and Burley, V. J., Eds., *Dietary Fibre Perspectives. Reviews and Bibliography*, vol. 2, John Libbey, London, 1990.
11. Goulder, T. J., Alberti, K. G. M. M., and Jenkins, D. A., Effect of added fiber on the glucose and metabolic response to a mixed meal in normal and diabetic subjects, *Diabetes Care*, 1, 351, 1978.
12. Monnier, L. et al., Influence of indigestible fibers on glucose tolerance, *Diabetes Care*, 1, 83, 1978.
13. Morgan, L. M. et al., The effect of unabsorbable carbohydrate on gut hormones, *Diabetologia*, 17, 85, 1979.
14. Hall, S. E. H., Bolton, T. M., and Hetenyi, G., The effect of bran on glucose kinetics and plasma insulin in noninsulin-dependent diabetes mellitus, *Diabetes Care*, 3, 520, 1980.
15. Jenkins, D. J. et al., Effect of guar crispbread with cereal products and leguminous seeds on blood glucose concentrations of diabetics, *Br. Med. J.*, 281, 1248, 1980.
16. Levitt, N. S. et al., The effect of dietary fiber on glucose and hormone responses to a mixed meal in normal subjects and in diabetic subjects with and without autonomic neuropathy, *Diabetes Care*, 3, 515, 1980.
17. Williams, D. A. R., James, W. P. T., and Evans, I. E., Dietary fiber supplementation of a "normal" breakfast administered to diabetics, *Diabetologia*, 18, 379, 1980.
18. Vaaler, S., Hanssen, K. F., and Aagenase, O., Effect of different kinds of fiber on postprandial blood glucose in insulin-dependent diabetics, *Acta Med. Scand.*, 208, 389, 1980.
19. Asp, N. G. et al., Dietary fiber in type II diabetes, *Acta Med. Scand.*, 656 (suppl.), 47, 1981.
20. Sartos, G., Carlstrom, S., and Schersten, B., Dietary supplementation of fibre (Lunelax) as a means to reduce postprandial glucose in diabetics, *Acta Med. Scand.*, 656 (suppl.), 51, 1981.
21. Simpson, R. W. et al., Effect of naturally occurring dietary fiber in Western foods on blood glucose, *Aust. N.Z. J. Med.*, 11, 484, 1981.
22. Baumer, J. H. et al., Effects of dietary fiber and exercise in mid-morning diabetic control — a controlled study, *Arch Dis. Child.*, 57, 905, 1982.
23. Gabbe, S. G. et al., Effect of dietary fiber on the oral glucose tolerance test in pregnancy, *Am. J. Obstet. Gynecol.*, 143, 514, 1982.
24. Leatherdale, B. A. et al., Guar and gastric emptying in noninsulin dependent diabetes, *Acta Diabetol. Lat.*, 19, 339, 1982.
25. Monnier, L. H. et al., Restored synergistic enterohormonal response after addition of dietary fiber to patients with impaired glucose tolerance and reactive hypoglycaemia, *Diabetes Metab.*, 8, 217, 1982.
26. Poynard, T., Slama, G., and Tchobroutsky, G., Reduction of postprandial insulin needs by pectin as assessed by the artificial pancreas in insulin-dependent diabetics, *Diabetes Metab.*, 8, 187, 1982.
27. Smith, J. et al., Guar biscuits in the diabetic diet, *S. Afr. Med. J.*, 61, 196, 1982.
28. Chenon, D. et al., Effects of dietary fiber on postprandial glycemic profiles in diabetic patients subjected to continuous programmed insulin infusion, *Am. J. Clin. Nutr.*, 40, 58, 1984.
29. Gatti, E. et al., Effects of guar-enriched pasta in the treatment of diabetes and hyperlipidemia, *Ann. Nutr. Metab.*, 28, 1, 1984.

30. Hagander, B. et al., Effect of dietary fiber on blood glucose, plasma immunoreactive insulin, C-peptide and GIP responses in non-insulin-dependent (type II) diabetics and controls, *Acta Med. Scand.*, 215, 205, 1984.

31. Jarjis, H. A. et al., The effect of ispaghula (Fybogel and Metamucil) and guar gum or glucose tolerance in man, *Br. J. Nutr.*, 51, 371, 1984.

32. McMurry, J. F. and Baumgardner, B., A high wheat bran diet in insulin treated diabetes mellitus: assessment with the artificial pancreas, *Diabetes Care*, 7, 211, 1984.

33. Parsons, S. R., Effects of high fiber breakfasts on glucose metabolism in non-insulin-dependent diabetics, *Am. J. Clin. Nutr.*, 40, 66, 1984.

34. Uusitupa, M. et al., Blood glucose and serum insulin responses to breakfast including guar gum and cooked or uncooked milk in type 2 (non-insulin-dependent) diabetic patients, *Diabetologia*, 26, 453, 1984.

35. Hagander, B. et al., Hormonal and metabolic responses to breakfast meals in NIDDM: comparison of white and whole-grain wheat bread and corresponding extruded products, *Hum. Nutr. Appl. Nutr.*, 39A, 114, 1985.

36. Heinonen, L., Korpela, R., and Mantere, S., The effect of different types of Finnish bread on postprandial glucose response in diabetic patients, *Hum. Nutr. Appl. Nutr.*, 39A, 108, 1985.

37. McIvor, M. E. et al., Flattening postprandial blood glucose responses with guar gum: acute effects, *Diabetes Care*, 8, 274, 1985.

38. Simpson, R. W. et al., Food physical factors have different metabolic effects in nondiabetics and diabetics, *Am. J. Clin. Nutr.*, 42, 462, 1985.

39. Tappy, L. et al., Metabolic effect of pre-cooked instant preparations of bean and potato in normal and in diabetic subjects, *Am. J. Clin. Nutr.*, 43, 30, 1986.

40. Tsai, A. C. et al., Effects of soy polysaccharide on postprandial plasma glucose, insulin, glucagon, pancreatic polypeptide, somatostatin, and triglyceride in obese diabetic patients, *Am. J. Clin. Nutr.*, 45, 596, 1987.

41. Bhatnagar, D., Glucose tolerance in North Indians taking a high fibre diet, *Eur. J. Clin. Nutr.*, 42, 1023, 1988.

42. Karlstrom, B. et al., Effects of four meals with different kinds of dietary fiber on glucose metabolism in healthy subjects and non-insulin-dependent diabetic subjects, *Eur. J. Clin. Nutr.*, 42, 519, 1988.

43. Schrezenmeir, J. et al., Comparison of glycaemic response and insulin requirements after mixed meals of equal carbohydrate content in healthy, type 1 and type 2 diabetic man, *Klin. Wochenschr.*, 67, 985, 1989.

44. Khan, H. S. et al., Role of dietary fiber on platelet adhesiveness, *J. Assoc. Phys. India*, 38, 219, 1990.

45. Jenkins, D. J. A. et al., Treatment of diabetes with guar gum. Reduction of urinary glucose loss in diabetics, *Lancet*, ii, 779, 1977.

46. Jenkins, D. J. A. et al., Guar crispbread in the diabetic diet, *Br. Med. J.*, 2, 1744, 1978.

47. Miranda, P. M. and Horwitz, D. L., High fiber diets in the treatment of diabetes mellitus, *Ann. Intern. Med.*, 88, 482, 1978.

48. Doi, K. et al., Treatment of diabetes with glucomannan (Konjac mannan), *Lancet*, 1, 987, 1979.

49. Jenkins, D. J. A. et al., Dietary fiber and ketone bodies: reduced urinary 3-hydroxybutyrate excretion in diabetics on guar, *Br. Med. J.*, 2, 1555, 1979.

50. Jenkins, D. J. A. et al., Dietary fiber and diabetic therapy: a progressive effect with time, *Adv. Exp. Med. Biol.*, 119, 275, 1979.

51. Bosello, O. et al., Glucose tolerance and blood lipids in bran-fed patients with impaired glucose tolerance, *Diabetes Care*, 3, 46, 1980.

52. Christiansen, J. S. et al., Effect of guar gum on 24-hour insulin requirements of insulin-dependent diabetic subjects as assessed by the artificial pancreas, *Diabetes Care*, 3, 659, 1980.

53. Cohen, M. et al., Role of guar and dietary fibre in the management of diabetes mellitus, *Med. J. Aust.*, 1, 59, 1980.

54. Jenkins, D. J. A. et al., Diabetic diets: high carbohydrate combined with high fiber, *Am. J. Clin. Nutr.*, 33, 1729, 1980.

55. Kanter, Y. et al., Improved glucose tolerance and insulin response in obese and diabetic patients on a fiber-enriched diet, *Isr. J. Med. Sci.*, 16, 1, 1980.

56. Jenkins, D. J. A. et al., Diabetic glucose control, lipids, and trace elements on long-term guar, *Br. Med. J.*, 1, 1353, 1980.

57. Nygren, C. et al., The effect of a high bran diet on diabetes in mice and humans, *Acta Endocrinol.*, 94 (S 237), 66, 1980.

58. Aro, A. et al., Improved diabetic control and hypocholesterolaemic effect induced by long-term dietary supplementation with guar gum in type II (non-insulin-dependent) diabetes, *Diabetologia*, 21, 29, 1981.

59. Botha, A. P. J. et al., Glycosylated hemoglobin, blood glucose and serum cholesterol levels in diabetics treated with guar gum, *S. Afr. Med. J.*, 59, 333, 1981.

60. Carroll, D. G., Dykes, A., and Hodgson, W., Guar gum is not a panacea in diabetes management, *N.Z. Med. J.*, 93, 292, 1981.

61. Dodson, P. M. et al., High fiber and low fat diets in diabetes mellitus, *Br. J. Nutr.*, 46, 289, 1981.

62. Johansen, K., Decreased urinary glucose excretion and plasma cholesterol level in non-insulin-dependent diabetic patients with guar, *Diabetes Metab.*, 7, 87, 1981.

63. Koepp, P. and Hegewisch, S., Effect of guar on plasma viscosity and related parameters in diabetic children, *Eur. J. Pediatr.*, 137, 31, 1981.

64. Kyllastinen, M. and Lahikainen, T., Long-term dietary supplementation with a fiber product (guar gum) in elderly diabetics, *Curr. Ther. Res.*, 30, 872, 1981.

65. Monnier, L. H. et al., Effects of dietary fiber supplementation in stable and labile insulin-dependent diabetics, *Diabetologia*, 20, 12, 1981.

66. Stokholm, K. H., Laursten, H. B., and Larsen, H., Reduced glycosuria during guar gum supplementation in non-insulin-dependent diabetes, *Dan. Med. Bull.*, 28, 41, 1981.

67. Fagerberg, S. E., The effects of a bulk laxative (metamucil) on fasting blood glucose, serum lipids, and other variables in constipated patients with non-insulin dependent adult diabetes, *Curr. Ther. Res.*, 31, 166, 1982.

68. Mayne, P. D. et al., The effect of apple fiber on diabetic control and blood lipids, *Ir. J. Med. Sci.*, 151, 36, 1982.

69. Smith, U. and Holm, G., Effect of a modified guar gum preparation on glucose and lipid levels in diabetics and healthy volunteers, *Atherosclerosis*, 45, 1, 1982.

70. Frati-Munari, A. C. et al., Effects of nopal (*Opuntia sp.*) on serum lipids, glycemia and body weight, *Arch. Invest. Med. (Mex.)*, 14, 117, 1983.

71. Kuhl, C., Molsted-Pederson, L., and Hornnes, P. J., Guar gum and glycemic control of pregnant insulin dependent diabetic patients, *Diabetes Care*, 6, 152, 1983.

72. Ray, T. K. et al., Long-term effects of dietary fiber on glucose tolerance and gastric emptying in non-insulin-dependent diabetic patients, *Am. J. Clin. Nutr.*, 37, 376, 1983.

73. Vaaler, S. et al., Improvement in long-term diabetic control after high fibre (bran and guar) diets, *Diabetologia*, 25, 200, 1983.

74. Gardner, D. F. et al., Dietary pectin and glycemic control in diabetes, *Diabetes Care*, 7, 143, 1984.

75. Fraser, R. B., Ford, F. A., and Milner, R. D. G., A controlled trial of a high dietary fiber intake in pregnancy — effects on plasma glucose and insulin levels, *Diabetologia*, 25, 238, 19X3.

76. Mahalko, J. R. et al., Effect of consuming fiber from corn bran, soy hulls of apple powder on glucose tolerance and plasma lipids in type II diabetes, *Am. J. Clin. Nutr.*, 39, 25, 1984.

77. Najemnik, C. et al., Guar and its effects on metabolic control in type II diabetic subjects, *Diabetes Care*, 7, 215, 1984.

78. Nygren, C., Hallmans, G., and Lithner, F., Effects of high bran bread on blood glucose control in insulin-dependent diabetic patients, *Diabete Metab.*, 10, 39, 1984.

79. Harold, M. R. et al., Effect of dietary fiber in insulin-dependent diabetics: insulin requirements and serum lipids, *J. Am Diet. Assoc.*, 85, 1455, 1985.

80. Jones, D. B. et al., Low dose guar improves diabetic control, *J. R. Soc. Med.*, 78, 546, 1985.

81. McIvor, M. E., Cummings, C. C., and Mendeloff, A. I., Long-term ingestion of guar gum is not toxic in patients with non-insulin-dependent diabetes mellitus, *Am. J. Clin. Nutr.*, 41, 891, 1985.

82. McNaughton, J. P. et al., Changes in total serum cholesterol levels of diabetics fed five grams guar gum daily, *Nutr. Rep. Int.*, 31, 505, 1985.

83. Osilesi, O. et al., Use of xantham gum in dietary management of diabetes mellitus, *Am. J. Clin. Nutr.*, 42, 597, 1985.

84. Tagliaferro, V. et al., Moderate guar gum addition to usual diet improves peripheral sensitivity to insulin and lipaemic profile in NIDDM, *Diabetes Metab.*, 11, 380, 1985.

85. Uribe, M. et al., Beneficial effect of vegetable protein diet supplemented with psyllium plantago in patients with hepatic encephalopathy and diabetes mellitus, *Gastroenterology*, 88, 901, 1985.

86. Groop, P.-H. et al., Relationship between changes in GIP concentrations and changes in insulin and C-peptide concentrations after guar gum therapy, *Scand. J. Clin. Lab. Invest.*, 46, 505, 1986.

87. McIvor, M. E. et al., Long-term effects of guar gum on blood lipids, *Atherosclerosis*, 60, 7, 1986.

88. Sharma, R. D., Effect of fenugreek seeds and leaves on blood glucose and serum insulin responses in human subjects, *Nutr. Res.*, 6, 1353, 1986.

89. Vaaler, S. et al., Diabetic control is improved by guar gum and wheat bran supplementation, *Diab. Med.*, 3, 230, 1986.

90. Van Duyn, M. A. S. et al., Nutritional risk of high-carbohydrate, guar gum dietary supplementation in non-insulin-dependent diabetes mellitus, *Diabetes Care*, 9, 497, 1986.

91. Atkins, T. W., Al-Hussary, N. A. J., and Taylor, K. G., The treatment of poorly controlled non-insulin dependent diabetic subjects with granulated guar gum, *Diab. Res. Clin. Pract.*, 3, 153, 1987.

92. Holman, R. R. et al., No glycemic benefit from guar administration in NIDDM, *Diabetes Care*, 10, 68, 1987.

93. Peterson, D. B. et al., Low dose guar in a novel food product: improved metabolic control in non-insulin-dependent diabetes, *Diab. Med.*, 4, 111, 1987.

94. Paganus, A. et al., Beneficial effects of palatable guar and guar plus fructose diets in diabetic children, *Acta Paediatr. Scand.*, 76, 76, 1987.

95. Sels, J. P., Flendrig, J. A., and Postmes, T. J., The influence of guar gum bread on the regulation of diabetes mellitus type II in elderly patients, *Br. J. Nutr.*, 57, 177, 1987.

96. Story, L. et al., Adherence to high carbohydrate, high fiber diets: long-term studies of non-obese diabetic men, *J. Am. Diet. Assoc.*, 85, 1105, 1985.

97. Beattie, A. et al., Does adding fiber to a low energy, high carbohydrate, low fat diet confer any benefit to the management of newly diagnosed and overweight type II diabetics?, *Br. Med. J.*, 296, 1147, 1988.

98. Ebeling, P. et al., Glucose and lipid metabolism and insulin sensitivity in type I diabetes: the effect of guar gum, *Am. J. Clin. Nutr.*, 48, 98, 1988.

99. Madar, Z. et al., Effects of cottonseed dietary fiber on metabolic parameters in diabetic rats and non-insulin-dependent diabetic humans, *J. Nutr.*, 118, 1143, 1988.

100. Behall, K. M. et al., Effect of guar gum on mineral balances in NIDDM adults, *Diabetes Care*, 12, 357, 1989.

101. Hagander, B. et al., Dietary fiber enrichment, blood pressure, lipoprotein profile and gut hormones in NIDDM patients, *Eur. J. Clin. Nutr.*, 43, 35, 1989.

102. Uusitupa, M. et al., Metabolic and nutritional effects of long-term use of guar gum in the treatment of non-insulin-dependent diabetes of poor metabolic control, *Am. J. Clin. Nutr.*, 49, 345, 1989.

103. Lalor, B. C. et al., Placebo-controlled trial of the effects of guar gum and metformin on fasting blood glucose and serum lipids in obese, type 2 diabetic patients, *Diab. Med.*, 7, 242, 1990.

104. Requejo, F., Uttenhal, L. O., and Bloom, S. R., Effects of alpha-glucosidase inhibition and viscous fiber on diabetic control and postprandial gut hormone responses, *Diab. Med.*, 7, 515, 1990.

105. Anderson, J. W. and Ward, K., Long-term effects of high carbohydrate, high fiber diets on glucose and lipid metabolism: a preliminary report on patients with diabetes, *Diabetes Care*, 1, 77, 1978.

106. Anderson, J. W. and Ward, K., High carbohydrate, high fiber diets for insulin-treated men with diabetes mellitus, *Am. J. Clin. Nutr.*, 32, 2312, 1979.

107. Simpson, R. W. et al., Improved glucose control in maturity onset diabetes treated with high carbohydrate, modified fat diet, *Br. Med. J.*, 1, 1753, 1979.

108. Simpson, R. W. et al., High carbohydrate diets and insulin dependent diabetes, *Br. Med. J.*, 2, 523, 1979.

109. Anderson, J. W. and Sieling, B., High fiber diets for obese diabetic patients, *Obesity/Bariatric Med.*, 9, 109, 1980.

110. Anderson, J. W., Chen, W. L., and Sieling, B., Hypolipidemic effects of high-carbohydrate, high fiber diets, *Metabolism*, 29, 551, 1980.

111. Rivellese, A. et al., Effect of dietary fiber on glucose control and serum lipoproteins in diabetic patients, *Lancet*, ii, 447, 1980.

112. Kay, R. M., Grobin, W., and Track, N. S., Diets rich in natural fibre improve carbohydrate tolerance in maturity-onset, non-insulin dependent diabetics, *Diabetologia*, 20, 18, 1981.
113. Manhire, A. et al., Unrefined carbohydrate and dietary fibre in the treatment of diabetes mellitus, *J. Hum. Nutr.*, 35, 99, 1981.
114. Simpson, H. C. et al., A high carbohydrate leguminous fibre diet improves all aspects of diabetic control, *Lancet*, i, 1, 1981.
115. Barnard, R. J. et al., Response of non-insulin dependent diabetic patients to an intensive program of diet and exercising, *Diabetes Care*, 5, 370, 1982.
116. Burke, B. J. et al., Assessment of the metabolic effects of dietary carbohydrate and fiber by measuring urinary excretion of C-peptide, *Hum. Nutr. Clin. Nutr.*, 36C, 373, 1982.
117. Hoffman, C. R. et al., Short-term effects of a high fiber, high carbohydrate diet in very obese diabetic individuals, *Diabetes Care*, 5, 605, 1982.
118. Kinmonth, A. L. et al., Whole foods and increased dietary fiber improve blood glucose control in diabetic children, *Arch. Dis. Child.*, 57, 187, 1982.
119. Ney, D., Hollingsworth, D. R., and Cousins, L., Decreased insulin requirement and improved control of diabetes in pregnant women given a high carbohydrate, high fiber, low fat diet, *Diabetes Care*, 5, 529, 1982.
120. Pedersen, O. et al., Increased insulin receptor binding to monocytes from insulin dependent diabetic patients after a low fat, high starch, high fiber diet, *Diabetes Care*, 5, 284, 1982.
121. Simpson, H. C. et al., Effect of high fiber diet on haemostatic variables in diabetes, *Br. Med. J.*, 284, 1608, 1982.
122. Simpson, H. C. R. et al., Digestible carbohydrate — an independent effect on diabetic control in type 2 (non-insulin-dependent) diabetic patients?, *Diabetologia*, 23, 235, 1982.
123. Ward, G. M. et al., Insulin receptor binding increased by high carbohydrate low fat diet in non-insulin-dependent diabetics, *Eur. J. Clin. Invest.*, 12, 93, 1982.
124. Barnard, R. J. et al., Long term use of a high complex carbohydrate, high fiber, low fat diet and exercise in the treatment of NIDDM patients, *Diabetes Care*, 6, 268, 1983.
125. Dodson, P. M. et al., The effects of a high fiber, low fat and low sodium dietary regime on diabetic hypertensive patients of different ethnic groups, *Postgrad. Med. J.*, 59, 641, 1983.
126. Hjollund, E. et al., Increased insulin binding to adipocytes and monocytes and increased insulin sensitivity off glucose transport and metabolism in adipocytes from non-insulin-dependent diabetics after a low-fat/high starch/high fiber diet, *Metabolism*, 32, 1067, 1983.
127. Rosman, M. S., Smith, C. J., and Jackson, W. P. U., The effect of long-term high fiber diets in diabetic outpatients, *S. Afr. Med. J.*, 63, 310, 1983.
128. Taskinen, M., Nikkila, E. A., and Allus, A., Serum lipids and lipoproteins in insulin dependent diabetic subjects during high carbohydrate, high fiber diet, *Diabetes Care*, 6, 224, 1983.
129. Rivellese, A. et al., Reduction of risk factors for atherosclerosis in diabetic patients treated with a high-fiber diet, *Prev. Med.*, 12, 128, 1983.
130. Dodson, P. M. et al., A controlled trial of a high fiber, low fat and low sodium diet for mild hypertension in type 2 (non-insulin-dependent) diabetic patients, *Diabetologia*, 27, 522, 1984.
131. Karlstrom, B. et al., Effects of an increased content of cereal fiber in the diet of type II (non-insulin-dependent) diabetic patients, *Diabetologia*, 26, 272, 1984.
132. Lindsay, A. N. et al., High carbohydrate, high fiber diet in children with type I diabetes, *Diabetes Care*, 7, 63, 1984.
133. Anderson, J. W., Physiologic and metabolic effects of dietary fiber, *Fed. Proc.*, 44, 2902, 1985.
134. Pacy, P. J. et al., Comparison of the hypotensive and metabolic effects of bendrofluazide therapy and a high fiber, low fat, low sodium diet in diabetic subjects with mild hypertension, *J. Hypertension*, 2, 215, 1984.
135. Riccardi, G. et al., Separate influence of dietary carbohydrate and fiber on the metabolic control of diabetes, *Diabetologia*, 26, 116, 1984.
136. Anderson, J. W., Fiber and health: an overview, *Am. J. Gastroenterol.*, 81, 892, 1986.
137. Hollenbeck, C. B. et al., The effects of subject-selected high carbohydrate, low fat diets on glycaemic control in insulin-dependent diabetes mellitus, *Am. J. Clin. Nutr.*, 41, 293, 1985.

138. McCulloch, D. K. et al., A prospective comparison of "conventional" and high carbohydrate/high fiber/low fat diets in adults with established type I (insulin dependent) diabetes, *Diabetologia*, 28, 208, 1985.

139. Rivellese, A. et al., A fiber-rich diet for the treatment of diabetic patients with chronic renal failure, *Diabetes Care*, 8, 620, 1985.

140. Sestoft, L. et al., High carbohydrate, low fat diet: effect on lipid and carbohydrate metabolism, GIP and insulin secretion in diabetics, *Dan. Med. Bull.*, 32, 64, 1985.

141. Stevens, J. et al., Outpatient management of diabetes mellitus with patient education to increase dietary carbohydrate and fiber, *Diabetes Care*, 8, 359, 1985.

142. Hollenbeck, C. B., Coulston, A. M., and Reaven, G. M., To what extent does increased dietary fiber improve glucose and lipid metabolism in patients with noninsulin-dependent diabetes mellitus (NIDDM), *Am. J. Clin. Nutr.*, 43, 16, 1986.

143. Pacy, P. J., Dodson, P. M., and Fletcher, R. F., Effect of a high carbohydrate, low sodium and low fat diet in type 2 diabetics with moderate hypertension, *Int. J. Obesity*, 10, 43, 1986.

144. Pacy, P. J., Dodson, P. M., and Taylor, K. G., The effect of a high fiber, low fat, low sodium diet on diabetics with intermittent claudication, *Br. J. Clin. Pract.*, 46, 313, 1986.

145. Teuscher, A., Die kohlenhydrate und nahrungsfasern in der diabetesdiat, *Schweiz, Med. Wechenschr.*, 116, 282, 1986.

146. Karlstrom, B. et al., Effects of leguminous seeds in a mixed diet in NIDDM (non-insulin-dependent) diabetic patients, *Diab. Res.*, 5, 199, 1987.

147. Paisley, R. B., Hartog, M., and Savage, P., A high fiber diet in gestational diabetes-wheat fiber, leguminous fiber or both?, *Hum. Nutr. Appl. Nutr.*, 41A, 146, 1987.

148. Garg, A. et al., Comparison of a high carbohydrate diet with a high monounsaturated fat diet in patients with non-insulin-dependent diabetes mellitus, *N. Engl. J. Med.*, 319, 829, 1988.

149. Hagander, B. et al., Dietary fiber decreases fasting blood glucose levels and plasma LDL concentration in noninsulin-dependent diabetes mellitus patients, *Am. J. Clin. Nutr.*, 47, 852, 1988.

150. Parillo, M. et al., Metabolic consequences of feeding a high-carbohydrate, high-fiber diet to diabetic patients with chronic kidney failure, *Am. J. Clin. Nutr.*, 48, 255, 1988.

151. Scott, A. R. et al., Comparison of high fiber diets, basal insulin supplements, and flexible insulin treatment for non-insulin dependent (type II) diabetics poorly controlled with sulphonylureas, *Br. Med. J.*, 297, 707, 1988.

152. Simpson, R. W. et al., Temporal study of metabolic change when poorly controlled noninsulin-dependent diabetics change from low to high carbohydrate and fiber diet, *Am. J. Clin. Nutr.*, 48, 104, 1988.

153. Venhaus, A. and Chantelau, E., Self-selected unrefined and refined carbohydrate diets do not affect metabolic control in pump-treated diabetic patients, *Diabetologia*, 31, 153, 1988.

154. Anderson, J. W. and Gustafson, N. J., Adherence to high carbohydrate, high fiber diets, *Diabetes Educator*, 15, 429, 1989.

155. Coulston, A. M. et al., Persistence of hypertriglyceridemic effect of low-fat high-carbohydrate diets in NIDDM patients, *Diabetes Care*, 12, 94, 1989.

156. O'Dea, K. et al., The effects of diet differing in fat, carbohydrate, and fiber on carbohydrate and lipid metabolism in type II diabetes, *J. Am. Diet. Assoc.*, 89, 1076, 1989.

157. Garg, A. et al., Effects of dietary carbohydrates on metabolism of calcium and other minerals in normal subjects and patients with non-insulin-dependent diabetes mellitus, *J. Clin. Endocrinol. Metab.*, 70, 1007, 1990.

158. Brand, J. C. et al., Low glycemic index foods improve long-term glycemic control in NIDDM, *Diabetes Care*, 14, 95, 1991.

159. Anderson, J. W. and Bryant, C. A., Dietary fiber: diabetes and obesity, *Am. J. Gastroenterol.*, 81, 898, 1986.

160. Anderson, J. W., Dietary fiber in nutrition management of diabetes, in *Dietary Fiber (Basic and Clinical Aspects)*, Vahouny, G. V. and Kritchevsky, D., Eds., Plenum Press, New York, 1986, 343.

161. Anderson, J. W., Nutrition management of diabetes mellitus, in *Modern Nutrition in Health and Disease*, 3rd ed., Shils, M. E. and Young, V. R., Eds., Lea and Febiger, Philadelphia, 1988.

162. Nestel, P. J. et al., Effects of a high-starch diet with low or high fiber content on postabsorptive glucose utilization and glucose production in normal subjects, *Diabetes Care*, 7, 207, 1984.

163. Anderson, J. W. et al., Dietary fiber and coronary heart disease, *CRC Crit. Rev. Food Sci. Nutr.*, 29, 95, 1990.

164. Fukagawa, N. K. et al., High carbohydrate, high fiber diets increase peripheral insulin sensitivity in healthy young and old adults, *Am. J. Clin. Nutr.*, 52, 524, 1990.

165. Nestler, J. E. et al., Absorption characteristic of breakfast determines insulin sensitivity and carbohydrate tolerance for lunch, *Diabetes Care*, 11, 755, 1988.

166. Trinick, T. R. et al., Effect of guar on second-meal glucose tolerance in normal man, *Clin. Sci.*, 71, 49, 1986.

167. Sundell, I. B. et al., Plasma glucose and insulin, urinary catecholamine and cortisol responses to test breakfasts with high or low fiber content: the importance of the previous diet, *Ann. Nutr. Metab.*, 33, 333, 1989.

168. Hunpponen, R., Karhuvaara, S., and Seppala, P., Effect of guar gum on glipizide absorption in man, *Eur. J. Clin. Pharmacol.*, 28, 717, 1985.

169. Hunpponen, R., The effect of guar gum on the acute metabolic response to glyburide, *Res. Commun. Chem. Pathol. Pharmacol.*, 54, 137, 1986.

170. Miller, D. L., Miller, P. F., and Dekker, J. J., Small bowel obstruction from bran cereal, *JAMA*, 263, 813, 1990.

171. Anderson, J. W., *Nutrition Management of Metabolic Conditions*, HCF Diabetes Research Foundation, Lexington, KY, 1981.

172. Hockaday, T. D. R., Fibre in the management of diabetes. I. Natural fibre useful as part of total dietary prescription, *Br. Med. J.*, 300, 1334, 1990.

173. Tattersall, R. and Mansell, P., Fibre in the management of diabetes. II. Benefits of fibre itself are uncertain, *Br. Med. J.*, 300, 1336, 1990.

174. Anderson, J. W. and Bridges, S. R., Short-chain fatty acid fermentation products of plant fiber affect glucose metabolism of isolated rat hepatocytes, *Proc. Soc. Exp. Biol. Med.*, 177, 372, 1984.

175. Akanji, A. O. et al., Change in plasma acetate levels in diabetic subjects on mixed high fiber diets, *Am. J. Gastroenterol.*, 84, 1365, 1989.

176. Ciavarella, A. et al., Reduced albuminuria after dietary protein restriction in insulin-dependent diabetic patients with clinical nephropathy, *Diabetes Care*, 10, 407, 1987.

177. American Heart Association, Position statement. Dietary guidelines for healthy American adults, *Circulation*, 77, 721A, 1988.

178. Rivellese, A. A. et al., Effects of changing amount of carbohydrate in diet on plasma lipoproteins and apoproteins in type II diabetic patients, *Diabetes Care*, 13, 446, 1990.

179. Anderson, J. W. and Akanji, A. O., Dietary fiber — an overview, *Diabetes Care*, 14, 1126, 1991.

180. Frati-Munari, A. C. et al., Lowering glycemic index of food by acarbose and Plantago psyllium mucilage, *Arch. Med. Res.*, 29, 137, 1998.

181. Blanchi, G., Ronchi, M., and Marchesini, G., Effect of lactulose on carbohydrate metabolism and diabetes mellitus, *Scand. J. Gastroenterol.*, (suppl.), 222, 62, 1997.

182. Gatenby, S. J. et al., Effect of partially depolymerized guar gum on acute metabolic variables in patients with non-insulin-dependent diabetes, *Diabetic Medicine*, 13, 358, 1996.

183. Guevin, N. et al., Postprandial glucose, insulin, and lipid responses to four meals containing unpurified dietary fiber in non-insulin dependent diabetes mellitus (NIDDM), hypertriglyceridemic subjects, *J. Am. Coll. Nutr.*, 15, 289, 1996.

184. Tappy, L., Gugolz, E., and Wursch, P., Effects of breakfast cereals containing various amounts of beta-glucan fibers on plasma glucose and insulin responses in NIDDM subjects, *Diabetes Care*, 19, 831, 1996.

185. Feldman, N. et al., Enrichment of an Israeli ethnic food with fibres and their effects on the glycaemic and insulinaemic responses in subjects with non-insulin-dependent diabetes mellitus, *Brit. J. Nutr.*, 74, 681, 1995.

186. Braaten, J. T. et al., High beta-glucan oat bran and oat gum reduce postprandial blood glucose and insulin in subjects with and without type 2 diabetes, *Diabetic Medicine*, 11, 312, 1994.

187. Harnden, K. E., Judd, P. A., and Hockaday, T. D., Glycaemic responses in type 2 diabetic patients to various mixed meals taken at home, *Diabetic Medicine*, 10, 654, 1993.

188. Chaturvedi, S. and Chaturvedi, A., Effect of vegetable fibre on postprandial glycemia, *Plant Foods Human Nutr.*, 44, 71, 1993.

189. Sels, J. P. et al., Absence of guar efficacy in complex spaghetti meals on postprandial glucose and C-peptide levels in healthy control and non-insulin-dependent diabetes mellitus subjects, *Hormone Metab. Res.*, (suppl.), 26, 52, 1992.

190. Librenti, M. C. et al., Effect of soya and cellulose fibers on postprandial glycemic response in type II diabetic patients, *Diabetes Care*, 15, 111, 1992.

191. Kirsten, R. et al., Influence of two guar preparations on glycosylated hemoglobin, total cholesterol and triglycerides in patients with diabetes mellitus, *Int. J. Clin. Pharm. Ther. Tox.*, 30, 582, 1992.

192. Wolever, T. M. et al., Effect of method of administration of psyllium on glycemic response and carbohydrate digestibility, *J. Am. Coll. Nutr.*, 10, 362, 1991.

193. Pastors, J. G. et al., Psyllium fiber reduces rise in postprandial glucose and insulin concentrations in patients with non-insulin-dependent diabetes, *Am. J. Clin. Nutr.*, 53, 1431, 1991.

194. Torsdottir, I. et al., A small dose of soluble alginate-fiber affects postprandial glycemia and gastric emptying in humans with diabetes, *J. Nutr.*, 121, 795, 1991.

195. Carra, M. et al., Blood sugar response to administration of bran or guar added to pasta in children with type I diabetes, *Minerva Pediatrica*, 42, 333, 1990.

196. Vuksan, V. et al., Konjac-mannan (glucomannan) improves glycemia and other associated risk factors for coronary heart disease in type 2 diabetes. A randomized controlled metabolic trial, *Diabetes Care*, 22, 913, 1999.

197. Rodriquez-Moran, M., Guerrero-Romero, F., and Lazcano-Burciaga, G., Lipid- and glucose-lowering efficacy of Plantago psyllium in type II diabetes, *J. Diabetes Complications*, 12, 273, 1998.

198. Hanai, H. et al., Long-term effects of water-soluble corn bran hemicellulose on glucose tolerance in obese and non-obese patients: improved insulin sensitivity and glucose metabolism in obese subjects, *Biosci. Biotech. Biochem.*, 61, 1358, 1997.

199. Pick, M. E. et al., Oat bran concentrate bread products improve long-term control of diabetes: a pilot study, *J. Am. Diet. Assoc.*, 96, 1254, 1996.

200. Sharafetdinov, Kh., Plotnikova, O. A., and Tsagikian, T. A., Comparative efficiency of various food fibers in the correction of carbohydrate and lipid metabolism in patients with type II diabetes mellitus, *Voprosy Pitaniia*, 3, 9, 1993.

201. Groop, P. H. et al., Long-term effects of guar gum in subjects with non-insulin-dependent diabetes mellitus, *Am. J. Clin. Nutr.*, 58, 513, 1993.

202. Chuang, L. M. et al., Therapeutic effect of guar gum in patients with non-insulin-dependent diabetes mellitus, *J. Formosan Med. Assoc.*, 91, 15, 1992.

203. Bruttomesso, D. et al., No effects of high-fiber diets on metabolic control and insulin-sensitivity in type 1 diabetic subjects, *Diabetes Res. Clin. Prac.*, 13, 15, 1991.

204. Karlander, S., Armyr, I., and Efendic, S., Metabolic effects and clinical value of beet fiber treatment in NIDDM patients, *Diabetes Res. Clin. Prac.*, 11, 65, 1991.

205. Diaz, J. et al., The effects of a dietary fiber (white lupine bran) in the treatment of non-insulin-dependent diabetes, *Rev. Med. Chile*, 118, 24, 1990.

206. Huang, C. Y. et al., Effect of Konjac food on blood glucose level in patients with diabetes, *Biomed. Env. Sci.*, 3, 123, 1990.

207. Stahl, M. and Berger, W., Comparison of guar gum, wheat bran and placebo on carbohydrate and lipid metabolism in type II diabetics, *Schweiz. Med. Wschr.*, 24, 402, 1990.

208. Vuorinen-Markkola, H., Sinisalo, M., and Koivisto, V., Guar gum in insulin-dependent diabetes: effects on glycemic control and serum lipoproteins, *Am. J. Clin. Nutr.*, 56, 1056, 1992.

209. Lafrance, L. et al., Effects of different glycaemic index foods and dietary fibre intake on glycaemic control in type I diabetic patients on intensive insulin therapy, *Diabetic Medicine*, 15, 972, 1998.

210. Krashenitsa, G. M., Botvineva, L. A., and Mogila, A. V., Effectiveness of increased contents of dietary fiber in early stages of non-insulin dependent diabetes mellitus, *Voprosy Pitaniia*, 4, 35, 1994.

211. Milne, R. M. et al., Long-term comparison of three dietary prescription in the treatment of NIDDM, *Diabetes Care*, 17, 74, 1994.

212. Anderson, J. W. et al., Metabolic effects of high-carbohydrate, high-fiber diets for insulin-dependent diabetic individuals, *Am. J. Clin. Nutr.*, 54, 936, 1991.

213. Comi, D., Brugnani, M., and Gianino, A., Metabolic effects of hypocaloric high-carbohydrate/high-fibre diet in non-insulin dependent diabetic patients, *Eur. J. Clin. Nutr.*, 49 (suppl. 3), S242, 1995.

214. Lintas, C. et al., Dietary fibre, resistant starch and in vitro starch digestibility of cereal meals. Glycaemic and insulinaemic responses in NIDDM patients, *Eur. J. Clin. Nutr.*, 49 (suppl. 3), S264, 1995.

215. Chandalia, M. et al., Beneficial effects of high dietary fiber intake in patients with Type 2 diabetes mellitus, *New Engl. J. Med.*, 342, 1392, 2000.

216. Garg, A. et al., Effects of varying carbohydrate content of diet in patients with non-insulin-dependent diabetes mellitus, *J. Am. Med. Assoc.*, 271, 1421, 1994.

217. Garg, A., Grundy, S. M., and Unger, R. H., Comparison of effects of high and low carbohydrate diets on plasma lipoproteins and insulin sensitivity in patients with mild NIDDM, *Diabetes*, 41, 1278, 1992.

218. Fukagawa, N. K. et al., High-carbohydrate, high-fiber diets increase peripheral insulin sensitivity in healthy young and old adults, *Am. J. Clin. Nutr.*, 52, 524, 1990.

219. He, J. and Whelton, P. K., Effect of dietary fiber and protein intake on blood pressure: a review of epidemiologic evidence, *Clin. Exp. Hypertension*, 21, 785, 1999.

220. Marshall, J. A., Bessesen, D. H., and Hamman, R. F., High saturated fat and low starch and fibre are associated with hyperinsulinaemia in a non-diabetic population: the San Luis Valley Diabetes Study, *Diabetologia*, 40, 430, 1997.

221. Despres, J.-P. et al., Hyperinsulinemia as an independent risk factor for ischemic heart disease, *N. Engl. J. Med.*, 334, 952, 1996.

222. Anderson, J. W., and Hanna, T. J., Whole grains and protection against coronary heart disease: what are the active components and mechanisms?, *Am. J. Clin. Nutr.*, 70, 307, 1999.

223. Salmeron, J. et al., Dietary fiber, glycemic load and risk of NIDDM in men, *Diabetes Care*, 20, 545, 1997.

224. Salmeron, J. et al., Dietary fiber, glycemic load, and risk of non-insulin-dependent diabetes mellitus in women, *J. Am. Med. Assoc.*, 277, 472, 1997.

225. Anderson, J. W. and Akanji, A. O., Treatment of diabetes with high fiber diets, in *CRC Handbook of Dietary Fiber in Human Nutrition*, Spiller, G. A., Ed., CRC Press, Boca Raton, FL, 1993, 443.

226. Anderson, J. W., Nutritional management of diabetes mellitus, in *Modern Nutrition in Health and Disease*, Shils, M. E., Olson, J. A., Shike, M. et al., Eds., Williams & Wilkins, Baltimore, 1999, 1365.

227. Anderson, J. W. et al., Whole grain foods and CHD risk, *J. Am. Coll. Nutr.*, 19, 291S, 2000.

228. Stampfer, M. et al., Primary prevention of coronary heart disease in women through diet and lifestyle, *N. Engl. J. Med.*, 343, 16, 2000.

229. Lugwig, D. et al., Dietary fiber, weight gain, and cardiovascular risk factors in young adults, *J. Am. Med. Assoc.*, 282, 1539, 1999.

230. Anderson, J. W. et al., Antioxidant supplementation effects on low-density lipoprotein oxidation for individuals with type 2 diabetes, *J. Am. Coll. Nutr.*, 18, 451, 1999.

Fiber in the Treatment of Hyperlipidemia

Alexandra L. Jenkins, Vladimir Vuksan, and David J. A. Jenkins

INTRODUCTION

It is now well accepted that viscous types of fiber may lower serum cholesterol levels, and national agencies concerned with cardiovascular health also endorse the use of soluble fiber foods (oats, barley, and legumes) as part of the strategies to reduce the risk of CHD.[1] Indeed, the U.S. Food and Drug Administration (FDA) has allowed two viscous fiber health claims, one for oats and the other for psyllium, for cholesterol lowering and cardiovascular risk reduction. These two fiber sources were the first of the four food components to be permitted by FDA to make health claims. The others include soy proteins and most recently plant sterols.[2,3] One is tempted to speculate that studies of viscous fibers opened the way for the systematic assessment of food components with cholesterol-lowering properties. Furthermore, a combination of these four elements — viscous fibers, vegetable protein, low-glycemic-index foods, and plant sterols — into a "cholesterol-lowering diet portfolio" may permit a diet to reduce serum lipids to a similar extent to a starting dose of a statin, the currently preferred treatment for cholesterol reduction (Table 5.4.1).

Table 5.4.1 Dietary Factors Portfolio for Cholesterol Reduction

Dietary Strategy	Amount	Reductions in LDL (approx. % reduction)
Viscous fibers: Psyllium Guar Konjac Beta-glucan, etc.	5–10 g/day	5
Soy protein	25 g/day	5
Plant sterols[a]	1–3 g/day	5
Dietary cholesterol	<200 mg/day	5
Saturated fat[b]	<7% of calories	10
Body weight	Lose 10 lb	5
Low-glycemic-index diet	Reduce by 10 GI units	5
Total	Full portfolio[c]	40%

[a] Depending on the sterol and stanol.
[b] Reduce trans-fatty acids to as close to zero as possible.
[c] Assuming the effects are additive.

Source: Adapted from Jenkins et al.[151]

META-ANALYSIS

There are a number of meta-analyses of the effects of viscous fibers in lowering serum cholesterol.[4-6] The meta-analysis by Brown et al. looked at four viscous fibers: pectin, oat bran, guar, and psyllium. The authors emphasized the smallness of the reduction of LDL-cholesterol (0.57 mmol/l/g fiber) with no major differences between the fibers.[6] However, this meta-analysis did not include all the studies which were used by the FDA in determining health claims. Other meta-analyses on psyllium[4,5] alone found reductions in LDL-cholesterol of 0.7 mmol/l/g of psyllium. Although this reduction is not equivalent to reductions seen with standard drug therapies, it represents a potential building block for a dietary portfolio (Table 5.4.1). Implementing a range of dietary strategies, such as incorporating viscous fibers, soy protein, plant sterols, and low-glycemic-index foods together with a National Cholesterol Education Program (NCEP) step 2 diet,[7] may result in clinically significant reductions in serum cholesterol (Table 5.4.1).

DIETARY FIBER AND POSSIBLE MECHANISMS OF ACTION

A number of possible mechanisms are likely to be involved in the hypocholesterolemic effect of dietary fiber, and different mechanisms are likely to predominate depending on the fiber. The pioneer studies of Kritchevsky and colleagues demonstrated that a number of fiber sources were capable of binding bile acids *in vitro*[8-10] and provided a rationale for the increased bile acid losses seen *in vivo*. Together with this mechanism of action, there are possibly three other broad reasons why fiber lowers serum cholesterol levels, none of which are mutually exclusive in providing an explanation of the mechanism for an individual food. Indeed, it is likely that for a given food, more than one mechanism is operative.

Increased Fecal Sterol Losses

From the beginning, it was recognized that increased fecal sterol losses provided one explanation for the lipid-lowering effect of fiber.[8] There is general agreement that purified viscous fiber[11] administration increases bile acid outputs by 20 to 80%,[12,13] but the effect of fiber in foods is less clear.[14,15] Studies have been limited in number due to the unsavory nature of this line of work, and further data are therefore urgently required.

Increased Short-Chain Fatty Acid Generation

Bacterial fermentation of fiber in the colon gives rise to short-chain fatty acids (SCFA), which are absorbed. One of the SCFAs, propionate, has been shown in pigs[16] and rats[17] to reduce serum cholesterol levels and to inhibit cholesterol synthesis in liver *in vitro*. Propionate has also been demonstrated in humans to inhibit, acutely, the acetate-induced rise in serum cholesterol after rectal infusion.[19] However, human-feeding studies of propionate[20,21] have not demonstrated a clear effect in reducing LDL-cholesterol levels. On the other hand, when colonic fermentation is increased using the non-absorbable sugar lactulose, LDL-cholesterol levels appear to rise rather than fall.[22] Another mechanism through which SCFAs may reduce cardiovascular risk factors is through their effects on clotting factors.[23] Increasing acetate levels by feeding either pectin or acetate increases permeability and lysability of fibrin networks while at the same decreasing the tensile strength.[23] This effect is seen despite total plasma fibrinogen levels remaining unchanged.[23] The nature of the fermentation and the type of fiber may therefore be important in determining the final outcome. This area also requires further studies for its definition.

Reduced Insulin Levels

Increased insulin levels have been linked with CHD.[24–27] A common effect of the viscous fibers and high-fiber foods which reduce serum cholesterol levels is that they produce relatively flat postprandial glucose and insulin responses.[28,29] Early studies demonstrated that hepatic cholesterol synthesis in the rat increased during periods of maximum insulin secretion.[30] The explanation was that insulin induced an increase in activity of hepatic HMG-COA reductase, a rate-limiting step in cholesterol synthesis.[30] The cholesterol-lowering effect associated with reduced insulin levels has been confirmed using a model of altered food frequency ("nibbling")[31] to mimic slow absorption. Finally, fiber consumption predicted insulin levels and other cardiovascular risk factors more strongly than did total or saturated fat consumption in a 10-year, multicenter population-based cohort study.[32]

Altered Lipid Absorption and Genetic Factors

Fiber delays the rate of nutrient absorption[29] and, in the longer term, may alter small intestinal morphology and lipid absorption.[33,34] Alteration in the rate and site of lipid absorption may alter the pattern of lipoprotein secretion[35] and catabolism. Vitamin A tolerance tests with added fiber indicate that some fibers appear to enhance chylomicronemia.[36,37] Added to this are the genetic differences which may make fiber more or less effective. Among genetic variants which influence serum lipids, differences in the apo E genotype and dietary change, including a prudent diet, dietary cholesterol, and vegetable protein[39,40] have attracted much attention and may influence the response to drugs such as gemfibrozil.[38] In view of the association of E genotype with differences in remnant particle uptake, cholesterol absorption, and bile acid excretion,[41–46] this genetic classification may be particularly useful in predicting responses to altered fat and fiber intakes. Viscous fiber seems to equally effective in lowering serum cholesterol in both E3 and E4 phenotype; however, only those with the E3 phenotype have shown an increase in apparent fat absorption, presumably due to an increase in the bile acid pool and chylomicron formation.[37] Insoluble fiber does not seem to alter fat absorption, irrespective of phenotype.[37] Other genetic markers have not, as yet, received this degree of scrutiny. No detailed studies have been carried out at different levels of dietary fat to assess the effect on the different possible mechanisms of action of dietary fiber, i.e., whether some mechanisms are more or less effective at different levels of dietary fat intake. Hypothetically, fiber foods which induce a bile salt loss might be more effective if the bile salt pool is expanded through greater intakes of dietary fat. On the other hand, reduction in carbohydrate intake may minimize differences in glycemic response and, hence, mechanisms which relate to altered insulin secretion. In the absence of studies, however, these are simply speculations to be explored.

EXPERIENCE WITH SPECIFIC FIBERS

The early studies described the hypolipidemic effects of fibers in healthy volunteers before they were tested on patient groups. The literature relating to healthy volunteers has already been reviewed. The present discussion will therefore focus on the therapeutic use of fiber. In general, viscous fibers have proved useful in lowering serum lipids,[47–52] while nonviscous fibers have for the most part been without effect.[53–57] There are exceptions to this generalization.[58]

Lignin and Cellulose

Early on, the suggestion that lignin may be hypocholesterolemic by virtue of its bile acid–binding ability resulted in two conflicting clinical studies.[54,59] The dosages were small (Table 5.4.2), and

Table 5.4.2 Effects of Lignin and Cellulose on Serum Lipid Concentrations

Fiber	Dose (g/day)	Control	Duration	Subjects	Cholesterol (% change)				TG (% change)	Comments	Ref.
					Total	LDL	VLDL	HDL			
Lignin	4	Cholestyramine	2–5 mo	6 hyperlipidemia	−21				0	Celluline duplicated effect or maintained effect of cholestyramine	59
	2	Normal diet	4 wk	7 hyperlipidemia	+8						53
	12	Normal diet	4 wk	10 healthy	NC			6.3 NS	−2.6 NS		56
Cellulose	60			60 healthy	NC				NC	−22% change in total-C on test and control	54
		Soyhull	3 mo	14 hyperlipidemia	+8 NS				+6 NS		55
	15	Normal diet	12 wk	Type 2 diabetes	1.6 NS			NC	NC	NC in FBG, or HbA1c	55
	15	Normal diet	4 wk	10 healthy	−5.6 NS			−11.8 NS	−10.7 NS		56

Note: Abbreviations: TG, triglycerides; HLP, hyperlipoproteinemia; HC, hypercholesterolemia; NC, no change; LDL-C, low-density lipoprotein cholesterol; total-C, total cholesterol; HDL-C, high-density lipoprotein cholesterol.

the work has not been repeated. Similarly, the particulate fiber,[54,55] cellulose, was without effect on serum cholesterol or triglyceride levels (Table 5.4.2).

Psyllium

Psyllium is a concentrated source of soluble fiber derived from the husks of blonde psyllium seed. Psyllium has long been accepted as a safe and reliable bulk laxative. Many studies have been conducted to explore the lipid-lowering effects of psyllium,[52,60–82] including three meta-analyses[4,5,6] (Table 5.4.3). Psyllium consumption of 9.1–10.2 g/day is associated with reductions in LDL-cholesterol of 6–7.2%, with no change in HDL-cholesterol level.[4,5,6] Improvements in the ratio of Apo B to Apo A-1 are also observed. Consistent with the postulated mechanism of action that fiber delays the rate of nutrient absorption, and hence needs to be mixed intimately with the food, psyllium too seems to exerts its greatest effect only when mixed with foods.[83]

Table 5.4.3 Meta-Analysis on LDL Reduction by Psyllium

No. of Subjects Taking Psyllium	Average Dose (g/day)	Mean LDL Starting Value (mmol/l)	LDL Reduction (%)	Reduction per Gram Psyllium	Ref.
479	9.1	4.37	6.0	0.66	6
209	9.4	4.33	7.4	0.79	4
384	10.2	4.19	7.2	0.70	5

Source: Adapted from Jenkins et al.[151]

Pectin

The early studies of Palmer and Dixon[84] in normal volunteers were followed by those of Miettinen and colleagues[85] on hyperlipidemic patients who consumed relatively large doses of pectin (40 to 50 g/d) (Table 5.4.4). The observation that the resulting falls in serum cholesterol levels were associated with only modest increases in fecal sterol loss suggested that increased sterol excretion was likely to be only one of a number of mechanisms responsible. No changes were seen in serum triglycerides. Palmer and Dixon demonstrated that little cholesterol-lowering effect could be seen in healthy individuals taking 6 g or less of pectin daily.[84] Subsequent studies in hyperlipidemic patients confirmed this observation.[86] However, a substantial lowering of serum total and LDL-cholesterol levels was observed even when as little as 12 g of pectin daily were taken.[48] A clear dose–response is not evident from these studies. The interest in pectin has continued, in general, to support the earlier work[87] (Table 5.4.4).

Guar

Again following observations in healthy volunteers, studies testing the effects of guar were undertaken in hyperlipidemic patients.[47,49,88–93] The cholesterol-lowering results with guar were materially the same as those observed with pectin. The effect was predominantly reflected in the LDL-cholesterol fraction, with much less or no change in the HDL-cholesterol fraction. Triglyceride levels were reduced, but the reduction was significant only when the guar was incorporated into very low fat, starchy carbohydrate foods, such as crisp bread or spaghetti.[47,89]

The physicochemical nature of the guar and the formulation in which it is provided may be very important factors, since greatly differing effects were reported by different investigators when doses of guar of the order of 15 g/d were given.[47,49,88–93] Nevertheless, in a study in which the same guar was added in powder form to fruit juices and soup, baked into conventional breads, or incorporated into a dry crisp bread or melba toast-type formulation, all were equally effective.[89] These findings suggested that prehydration was not a prerequisite for the hypolipidemic action

Table 5.4.4 Effects of Soluble, Purified Fibers on Lipid Concentrations in Normal and Hyperlipidemic Subjects

Fiber	Dose (g/day)	Duration	Subjects	Cholesterol (% change)				TG (% change)	Comments	Ref.
				Total	LDL	VLDL	HDL			
Pectin										
	40–50	2 wk	7 hyperlipidemia 2 healthy	-13			-5 NS			85
Lemon	6	6 wk	33 hyperlipidemia	+5				+0.7 NS		86
Apple	6	6 wk	33 hyperlipidemia	-4 NS				+36 NS		86
Citrus	15	3 wk	10 healthy	18						51
Grapefruit	15	4 wk	27 hyperlipidemia	-7.6	-10.7	2.4 NS	-1.2 NS	2.7 NS	9.8% decline in LDL:HDL	56
Cereal	57	6 wk	58 hyperlipidemia	-2.1 NS	-3.8 NS		2.5 NS	3.7 NS		73
Citrus	12	4 wk	10 healthy	NC			NC	4.1 NS		56
K-Pectin + Gum Arabic	5–15	8 wk	110 hyperlipidemic	3.5				28.5	Fiber was incorporated into apple juice	149
Psyllium										
Granules	9–12	5 wk	9 healthy	-14.4 NS	-26.6		22.1 NS	-11.7 NS	Weight loss with psyllium	60
Metamucil	11	8 wk	14 HC	-14.8	-20.1		-6.5 NS	-12.7 NS		63
Ground husk	21	3 wk	7 healthy	-16	-18		-8.2			52
Cereal	57	6 wk	58 HC males	-5.9	-5.7		-1.6 NS	-10.9		73
Vi-Siblin	30	11 d	9 HLP	-6.0	-9.2		20.0	-6 NS		64
Metamucil	20.4	13 wk	27 HC	-7.1	-8.6		6.2	-10.9 NS	LDL:HDL decreased 13.3%	74
Metamucil	10.2	8 wk	20 HC	-4.2	-7.7		1.9 NS	2.6 NS	8.8% fall in Apo B on psyllium	62
Plantago	15	6 wk	125 type 2 diabetes	-9	-15		45	-25		75
Seed husk	10.2	24 wk	70 HLP	-5.3			NC	NC		76
Cereal	1.4 g/MJ	4 wk	32 HLP		-12.3			NS	-6% MUFA diet	77
Cereal	1.4 g/MJ	4 wk	27 HLP		15.3			-16.6	-12% MUFA diet	
Husk	7	90 d	24 HC type 2 diabetes	-19.7	-23.7		-23.7	-27.2		78
Cereal	6.4	12 wk	50 healthy children (6–11 y)		-63					79
Cereal	6.7	2 wk	42 HLP	-6.4	-7.8		-3.5	NC	LDL:HDL decrease by 4.8%	80
Metamucil	10.2	26 wk	250 HLP	-4.7	-6.7		NC	NC	50 subjects acted as control group	81
Metamucil	10.2	8 wk	34 type 2 diabetes, male	-8.9	-13		NC	NC		82

Guar

Preparation		Duration	Subjects						Comments	
Crispbread	15	2 wk	10 type 2 diabetes	-11			-26 NS	13 NS		88
Granules	13	8 wk	11 HLP	-14	-16			-13 NS		89
Granules	15	4 mo	32 HLP, females	-3 NS			0	-3 NS		90
Granules	16	2 mo	12 HLP	-7	-14	NC	-13 NS	28 NS	Apo B decreased by 20%	91
In pasta	18	3–12 mo	17 HLP	-13	-18	17 NS	-0.4 NS	8 NS	Preparation with gel inhibitor	49
	14–19	2 wk	8 HLP	-32				-40		47
		8 wk	5 HLP	-6				-27		
Granulate	15	12 wk	14 HC, males	-8 NS	-14 NS	-21 NS	-6 NS	-4 NS	Significant changes seen at 6 weeks, but not sustained	92
Powder	16	60 d	12 HLP	-10	-10	-23	2	-22		93
Gel	16	6 wk	10 type 2 diabetes	-11	-18	17.9 NS	-1.8 NS	-10.8 NS	FBG decreased 9.6%	94
Guar bars	26–40	24 wk	8 type 2 diabetes	3 NS		-16 NS	-9 NS	9		95
Crispbread	11.4	2 wk	6 healthy, male	-16				1.8 NS		106
Pasta	10	4 d	10 obese women	-11.9			2.2 NS	-6 NS	Diabetes control improved	107
Granules	20–30	50 wk	23 HC	-10	-14.9	-23.5 NS	17.9 NS	-9.9 NS	Increase in ApoA1/ApoB by 11.8%	96
Cracker	15	8 wk	32 HLP	-5.8	-9.8		-2.2 NS	12 NS		97
	15	12 wk	22 type 2 diabetes	-10.6			NC	NC		57
Gel	40	11 d	8 diverticular disease	-9.6	-13.2	-3.7 NS	-1.1 NS	-2.1 NS		64
Powder	15	21 d	13 HLP	-10	-17	-3	1.6	-1.4		127
Granules	15	24 mo	20 with carotid stenosis	-17	NC		-26	NC		98
Minolest (guar + psyllium)	16.5	3 mo	83 healthy/HLP	-3.2			-5.4	NC		99
	20	14 mo	20 obese, females	NC	NC			NC	Weight gain same in control and test	100
Guarita		8 wk	16 type 2 diabetes	NC	NC		NC	NC	FBG + HbA₁c decreased significantly	102
Guar, pectin, soy, pea, corn bran	20	36 wk	58 HLP	-8.5	-12.1					103

Table 5.4.4 (Continued) Effects of Soluble, Purified Fibers on Lipid Concentrations in Normal and Hyperlipidemic Subjects

Fiber	Dose (g/day)	Duration	Subjects	Cholesterol (% change)				TG (% change)	Comments	Ref.
				Total	LDL	VLDL	HDL			
Locust Bean Gum										
	18–30	8 wk	18 HC adults/children, 10 healthy	–6 to 19	–10 to 19	–10 to 19	0 to –17	–10		50
Locust, psyllium, pectin, guar	15	4–12 wk		–8.3	–12.4		NC	NC		58
Locust, psyllium, pectin, guar	15	6 mo		–6.4	–10.5		NC	NC		99

Note: Abbreviations: TG, triglycerides; HLP, hyperlipoproteinemia; HC, hypercholesterolemia; NC, no change; LDL-C, low-density lipoprotein cholesterol; total-C, total cholesterol; HDL-C, high-density lipoprotein cholesterol.

of this viscous fiber. In 2-week studies in which the maximum acceptable dose of guar given in crisp bread form was compared with the maximum acceptable dose of cholestyramine in the same patients, the falls in total and LDL-cholesterol were comparable.[89] This indicates that, in pharmacological terms, the effects of viscous fiber on lipid metabolism might have significant clinical utility.

Results from long-term studies of guar have been conflicting,[49,57,89,94–103] possibly because of differences in dietary formulations of the guar supplement, study design, etc. However, of the 13 studies cited, 9 reported a sustained, positive effect of guar.[49,89,94,95,98,100–103] In the majority of the guar and pectin studies, fiber was added to the patients' preexisting diet and/or drug therapy, which was then maintained constant. This included low-fat, low-cholesterol diets, with or without cholestyramine, clofibrate, or their analogs. It is not possible at present to say whether the mechanism or action of fiber overlaps with those of the established hypolipidemic drugs and whether specific combinations might bestow an advantage. In view of the relatively small bile acid losses seen with pectin[85,104,105] and guar[104] compared with specific drugs, it is likely that the mechanisms of fiber will complement those of the bile salt–binding (anion exchange) resins (e.g., cholestyramine). On the other hand, when the maximum effect has been achieved with clofibrate, it is possible that any further effect of the fiber may be reduced.[91] Further work has contributed support to previous evidence (Table 5.4.4).[57,64, 65,94–97,106,107]

Locust Bean Gum

This viscous fiber has also been used successfully in a range of hyperlipidemic patients to lower serum cholesterol[50] (Table 5.4.4). Its advantage has been claimed to be its superior taste (or lack of taste) in comparison with guar. However, the taste of guar depends on its purity and, since both substances are galactomannans, direct comparative studies must be undertaken before any statement about their relative efficacy can be made.

Konjac Mannan

Konjac-mannan fiber is obtained from the tuber of the perennial *Amorphophallus Konjac k* and has been known in Japan for over 1000 years. Traditionally, Konjac mannan is made into a rubbery jelly and has been used as a food and a remedy. The purified powder (Konjac mannan) from the tuber is a viscous, water-soluble fiber which has been shown to lower blood lipids,[108–111] systolic blood pressure,[112] and glycemia[112–114] when taken as a supplement. The physiologically active component is a high-molecular-weight glucomannan polymer. After 3 weeks of Konjac supplementation, subjects with insulin resistance syndrome showed decreases in total and LDL-cholesterol by 12 and 22%, respectively.[114] Improvements in the ratio of Apo B to Apo A were also observed. These results were accompanied by a 5% reduction in serum fructosamine levels, a marker of glycemic control.[114] Konjac also reduced serum fructosamine (5.7%), the ratio of total to HDL cholesterol (10%), and systolic blood pressure (6.9%) in subjects with diabetes, following a 3-week Konjac-supplemented diet compared to the control.[112]

Wheat Bran

Wheat fiber appears to protect from cardiovascular disease despite[115,116] its lack of consistent effects on serum lipids.[63,117–121] Of the different wheat brans, only hard red spring wheat bran has been convincingly shown to lower serum cholesterol levels in normal humans.[117] As with normal volunteers, almost all studies which have used other wheat bran preparations have failed to show significant reductions in blood lipid levels of hyperlipidemic individuals[118,119,122] (Table 5.4.5), although there is one report of a significant rise in HDL-cholesterol.[120] The lack of consistent effect of wheat bran on blood lipids is of interest from the standpoint of mechanisms, since the bile acid losses in the stool following bran consumption have been shown to be comparable to those following pectin,[104] which consistently lowers serum cholesterol. It has been suggested that perhaps the displacement of carbohydrate by wheat gluten on a high–wheat bran diet[122] may be responsible for the positive relationship of wheat bran and cardiovascular disease. Further studies are required to explore this relationship.

Oat Bran

Since the early studies of DeGroot et al.,[123] it was realized that oat constituents may have hypocholesterolemic effects. Unlike wheat bran, oat fiber contains an appreciable proportion of viscous fiber (beta glucan), and it is likely that this constituent may be one of its active hypolipidemic ingredients. Studies of Anderson and co-workers have demonstrated the lipid-lowering effect of oat bran given to hyperlipidemic patients (predominantly Types IIa and IIb) for 10 days to 2 years[124–126] (Table 5.4.5). Although there were highly significant falls in all cholesterol fractions together with serum triglyceride during the initial 3 weeks of fiber treatment, the HDL-cholesterol level increased slowly to almost approximately the starting value by 24 weeks. The other fractions remained low throughout the maintenance treatment period and for the four patients who were followed for 2 years.[126] Again, the increase in fecal acidic steroids was small, in proportion to the increase in fecal bulk, and unlikely to provide more than a small part of the explanation of the hypocholesterolemic action of oat bran. In this respect, it has been proposed that the volatile fatty acids from oat bran and other viscous fibers, which arise from colonic fermentation of fiber and are subsequently absorbed, may produce metabolic changes which favor reduced cholesterol synthesis.[124] Despite early enthusiasm, then apparent despair, the body of evidence supports that oat bran will have a significant, although small, beneficial effect on serum lipids (Table 5.4.5).[63,65,69,127–129]

Dried Legumes

Cooked, dried legumes have been shown to lower serum cholesterol levels of middle-aged men,[130] although not of young student volunteers.[131] More recently, with interest in their effect of improving glucose tolerance[132] and other aspects of diabetic control,[133] high-legume diets have been studied in types IIa and IV hyperlipidemic patients[124,126,134,135](Table 5.4.5). All studies have shown falls in serum cholesterol irrespective of the class of hyperlipidemia studied. One investigator also recorded falls in serum triglyceride comparable to those seen with oat bran of equivalent soluble fiber content (20 g/day).[126] As with oat bran, the effects on blood lipids appear to be sustained for 4 months to 2 years.[126] Diets which increased the total fiber intake by increasing not only the intake of legumes but also of whole grains, vegetables and fruits, and nuts and seeds have also been shown to be effective in reducing cardiovascular risk factors.[136,137] The reasons for the effects, however, are not clear. Increases in fecal output on 115 g of beans are small and not significant in hyper-lipidemic individuals.[124] In addition, where recorded, increases in fecal acidic steroid losses were not noted. Nevertheless, the falls in blood lipids, especially triglycerides, may be related to the flatter postprandial glucose and insulin responses elicited by legumes.[132] These may result in a chronically reduced stimulus to hepatic triglyceride synthesis and hepatic lipid synthesis in general. Evidence for this hypothesis has been drawn together in the studies of Albrink et al.[138] in healthy volunteers and is supported by the observation, also in healthy volunteers, that 24-h urinary C-peptide outputs were reduced on high-legume diets.[139]

Legume Protein

In addition to legume fibers (e.g., guar and locust bean gum), some legume proteins, notably soy protein, have been shown to reduce cholesterol levels of hyperlipidemic patients (total and LDL)[140–146] (Table 5.4.6). The effect does not appear to be related to associated fiber or saponins,

Table 5.4.5 Effects of Fiber-Rich Whole Foods and Supplements on Serum Lipids

Fiber	Dose (g/day)	Duration	Subjects	Cholesterol (% change)				TG (% change)	Comments	Ref.
				Total	LDL	VLDL	HDL			
Wheat bran	50	3 mo	5 HLP	3	-2 NS	20 NS	30 NS	0		118
	50	2 mo	8 HLP, male	-2 NS				5 NS		119
Fiberform	10.5	8 wk	12 HC, male	0.7 NS	-2 NS	-30 NS	23	-24		120
Bread, muffins	35	4 wk	24 HC males	0.8	0.2		3.8	3.1	NC insulin, glucose, BP	63
Oat bran	100	3 mo	8 HLP, healthy	-13	-14		-2 NS	-9 NS		125
Flakes	25	2 wk	12 HC, male	-5.4	-8.5		-3.3 NS	8.7	Apo B decreased by 9.8%	69
Bread, muffins	17	28 d	19 Healthy	-5 NS	-9 NS		2 NS	-8 NS		66
	95	4 wk	24 HC, male	-4.9	-6.8		2.9	-3.1		63
Powder	77	21 d	13 moderate HLP	-3.3	-5.9	3.3	NC	5.5		127
	100	3 wk	10 HLP	-19	-23		-6 NS	-18		124
Mixed	52	5–11 mo	31 HLP, 6 Healthy	-22	-25	-37	-4	-24		150
Cookies	2.6	8 wk	30 HLP, males		-26		NC	-28		128
Instant oats	56.7	8 wk	42 HC	-6.3	-9.2	1.4	0.8	1.3		65
Oatmeal	56	8 wk	113 Healthy	-3 NS	NS		NS	NS		67
	84	6 wk	13 HLP	-13	-17.1		NC	NC		129
Beans	50 (100 g dried)	3–6 mo	136 HLP	-17				13–32 NS		134
			106	-9						
Baked beans	110 dried	2 wk	17 HLP	-8			-15 NS	-25 NS		135
	140 dried	4 mo	7 HLP	-7	-5		-25	-25		135
	115	3 wk	10 HLP	-10	-24		-12	-3 NS		124
	450	2 wk	13 Healthy, male	-12			-14.8	7.5 NS		68
	120–162	3 wk	24 HLP	-10.4	-8.4		-6.9	-10.8		70
Beans/oat bran	100 beans or oats	3 wk	10 HLP, male	-23	-23		-20	-21		126
	50 oats or 134 beans	24 wk	10 HLP, male	-4	-2		17 NS	-6	4 subjects were followed for 99 weeks	126

Note: Abbreviations: TG, triglycerides; HLP, hyperlipoproteinemia; HC, hypercholesterolemia; NC, no change; LDL-C, low-density lipoprotein cholesterol, total-C, total cholesterol; HDL-C, high-density lipoprotein cholesterol.

since it is also found after administration of soy isolate. The effects of soy protein in lowering serum cholesterol are well recognized. A large meta-analysis of studies up to 1997 by Anderson et al. demonstrated a 13% reduction in LDL cholesterol for a soy protein intake of 43g/d.[147] In a study with hyperlipidemic subjects where both the soy protein and the soluble fiber intake were increased, the total-to-HDL cholesterol ratio was reduced by 6.3%.[136] However, the capacity to lower blood lipids may not be a universal property of all legume proteins, since fava protein isolate failed to achieve the desired effect.[145]

The mechanisms for the hypolipidemic action of soy protein remain obscure but may relate to the amino acid profile[148] or the presence of specific pharmacologically active peptides liberated during digestion. With respect to the whole bean, although specific fiber and protein effects may be relevant to the action of some beans, other factors will have to be uncovered to explain the general hypolipidemic effect of legumes in hyperlipidemic individuals. Data continue to accumulate supporting the lipid-lowering effect of legume protein (Table 5.4.6).[71,72]

Effective Fiber Dosage and Formulation

In general, the effective dose of the viscous fibers required to lower serum cholesterol levels has been of the order of 12 to 30 g/d. Interestingly, the levels of fiber in the oat bran– and bean–containing diets have also been of this order of magnitude, since soluble fiber composes approximately 20% of the dry weight of both beans and oat bran. However, the effectiveness of the supplement in hyperlipidemia may be determined by its formulation, in addition to the background diet. The viscosity of viscous fibers is responsible for the slowing of absorption in the small intestine; therefore, reducing or destroying the viscosity will eliminate its beneficial effects. Incorporation of a small quantity of pectin into apple juice failed to reduce cholesterol levels, presumably because of the low viscosity of the apple juice mixture.[149] On the other hand, when Gatti and colleagues enriched spaghetti with guar, the greatest lowering of cholesterol and triglyceride levels of all the studies to date was seen.[47] Spaghetti is already recognized as a slowly digested carbohydrate form which causes an unexpectedly low rise in blood glucose.[150] This effect is likely to have been greatly enhanced by the addition of guar, resulting in the creation of a very effective sustained release carbohydrate source. The addition of guar would likely not only have enhanced the reduction of glycemic and insulinemic responses to the pasta but may, in effect, have resulted in a proportion of the pasta starch being converted to "fiber," i.e., carbohydrate which is unavailable for small intestinal absorption but which acts as an additional source for synthesis of SCFAs in the colon. The choice by Gatti and co-workers of spaghetti as the vehicle for delivery of the fiber may have been in large measure the reason for the success of their trial, since it encompassed many of the mechanisms responsible for reducing blood lipids. One of the important directions for future development in this field would, therefore, appear to lie in finding the most effective food vehicles in which to incorporate fiber.

CONCLUSION

Viscous fibers such as pectin, guar, locust bean gum, Konjac mannan, and high-fiber foods such as oat bran and dried beans, all providing 12 to 30 g fiber daily, have been shown to reduce serum total and LDL-cholesterol levels by 10 to 20% and with a lesser fall in HDL-cholesterol levels. When the fiber was provided in a starchy food such as pasta, crisp bread, oat bran, or beans, significant falls in serum triglyceride levels have also been observed. The mechanisms of action of fiber are likely to be complex and possibly include increased bile salt loss, altered site and rate of absorption, reduced hepatic lipogenesis secondary to reduced postprandial glucose and insulin responses, and enhanced colonic synthesis and uptake of SCFAs.

Table 5.4.6 Effects of Legume Protein (± Saponins) on Serum Lipid Concentrations of Hyperlipidemic Subjects

Fiber	Dose (g/day)	Duration	Subjects	Cholesterol (% change)				TG (% change)	Comments	Ref.
				Total	LDL	VLDL	HDL			
Textured soybean protein										
Granules		3 wk	20 HLP	−19	−18			−17		140
Granules		6 wk	8 HLP	−23				NC	500 mg cholesterol added	140
Granules	60–100	8 wk	127 HLP	−20			NC			141
"Cholsoy"	60–100	4 wk (18 mo)	27 HLP	−26	−33	15 NS		−11	Changes sustained over 18 months	153
"Cholsoy"	60–100	4 wk	19 HLP	−21	−26		13			144
Mixed food		2 wk	6 HLP	−10	−9	−17	0	11 NS		143
Mixed meals		4 wk	21 HLP, 1 healthy	−3 NS	−0.8 NS	3 NS	−12 NS	3 NS		144
"Cholsoy"	70–80	4 wk	21 HC	−20.8	−25.8	32.6 NS	−7.2 NS	−69 NS		71

Note: Abbreviations: TG, triglycerides; HLP, hyperlipoprotemia; HC, hypercholesterolemia; NC, no change; LDL-C, low-density lipoprotein cholesterol, total-C, total cholesterol; HDL-C, high-density lipoprotein cholesterol.

Further developments to enhance the clinical utility of this approach should include not only a search for effective fiber types but also the appropriate vehicles in which to deliver them.

REFERENCES

1. Krauss, R. M. et al., AHA dietary guidelines. Revision 200: A statement for healthcare professionals from the nutrition committee of the American Heart Association, *Circulation*, 102, 2284-2299, 2000.
2. Food and Drug Administration, Final rule for food labeling: health claims: soy protein and coronary heart disease, *The Federal Register* 64 (October 26), 57699-57733, 1999.
3. Food and Drug Administration, Interim final rule for food labeling: health claims; plant sterol/stanol esters and coronary heart disease, *Federal Register*, 65 (September 8), 175, 54685-54739, 2000.
4. Olson, B. H., Anderson, S. M., Becker, M. P., Anderson, J. W., Hunninghake, D. B., Jenkins, D. J., LaRosa, J. C., Rippe, J. M., Roberts, D. C., Stoy, D. B., Summerbell, C. D., Truswell, A. S., Wolever, T. M., Morris, D. H., Fulgoni, V. L., Psyllium enriched cereals lower blood total cholesterol and LDL cholesterol, but not HDL cholesterol, in hypercholesterolemic adults: results of a meta-analysis, *J. Nutr.*, 127, 1973–80, 1997.
5. Anderson, J. W., Allgood, L. D., Lawrence, A., Altringer, L., Jerdack, G. R., and Hengehold, D. A., Cholesterol-lowering effects of psyllium intake adjunctive to diet therapy in men and women with hypercholesterolemia: meta-analysis of 8 controlled trials, *Am. J. Clin. Nutr.*, 71, 472–9, 2000.
6. Brown, L., Rosner, B., Willett, W. W., and Sacks, F. M., Cholesterol-lowering effects of dietary fiber: a meta analysis, *Am. J. Clin. Nutr.*, 69, 30–42, 1999.
7. Summary of the Second Report of the National Cholesterol Education Program (NCEP) Expert Panel on Detection, Evaluation and Treatment of High Blood Cholesterol in Adults, (Adult Treatment Panel II), *JAMA*, 269, 3015–3023, 1993.
8. Kritchevsky, D. and Story, J. A., Binding of bile salts in vitro by nonnutritive fiber, *J. Nutr.*, 104, 458, 1974.
9. Kritchevsky, D. and Story, J. A., *In vitro* binding of bile acids and bile salts, *Am. J. Clin. Nutr.*, 28, 305, 1975.
10. Vahouny, G. V., Tombes, R., Cassidy, M. M., Kritchevsky, D., and Gallo, L. L., Dietary fibers. V. Binding of bile salts, phospholipids and cholesterol from mixed micelles by bile sequestrants and dietary fibers, *Lipids*, 15, 1012, 1980.
11. Jenkins, D. J. A., Wolever, T. M. S., Leeds, A. R., Gassull, M. A., Haisman, P., Dilawari, J., Goff, D. V., Metz, G. L., and Alberti, K. G. M. M., Dietary fibres, fibre analogues and glucose tolerance: importance of viscosity, *Br. Med. J.*, 1, 1372, 1978.
12. Kay, R. M. and Truswell, A. S., Effect of citrus pectin on blood lipids and fecal steroid excretion in man, *Am. J. Clin. Nutr.*, 30, 171, 1977.
13. Jenkins, D. J. A., Leeds, A. R., Gassull, M. A., Houston, H., Goff, D. V., and Hill, M. J., The cholesterol lowering properties of guar and pectin, *Clin. Sci. Mol. Med.*, 51, 8, 1976.
14. Raymond, T. L., Conner, W. E., Lin, D. S., Warner, S., Fry, M. M., and Connor, S. L., The interaction of dietary fibers and cholesterol upon the plasma lipids and lipoproteins, sterol balance and bowel function in human subjects, *J. Clin. Invest.*, 60, 1429, 1977.
15. Anderson, J. W., Story, L., Sieling, B., Chen, W. J. L., Petro, M. S., and Story, J., Hypocholesterolemic effects of oat-bran or bean intake for hypercholesterolemic men, *Am. J. Clin. Nutr.*, 40(b), 1146, 1984.
16. Thacker, P. A., Salomons, M. O., Aherne, F. X. et al., Influence of propionic acid on the cholesterol metabolism of pigs fed hypercholesterolemic diets, *Can. J. Anim. Sci.*, 61, 969, 1981.
17. Chen, W. L., Anderson, J. W., and Jennings, D., Propionate may mediate the hypocholesterolemic effects of certain soluble plant fibers in cholesterol-fed rats (41791), *Proc. Soc. Exp. Biol. Med.*, 175, 215, 1984.
18. Chen, W. J. L. and Anderson, J. W., Hypercholesterolemic effects of soluble fibers, in *Dietary Fiber: Basic and Clinical Aspects*, Kritchevsky, D. and Vahouny, G. V., Eds., Plenum Press, New York, 1986, 275.
19. Wolever, T. M. S., Brighenti, F., and Jenkins, D. J. A., Serum short chain fatty acids after rectal infusion of acetate and propionate in man, *J. Clin. Nutr. Gastroenterol.*, 3, 42, 1988.

20. Venter, C. S., Vorster, H. H., and Cummings, J. H., Effects of dietary propionate on carbohydrate and lipid metabolism in healthy volunteers, *Am. J. Gastroenterol.*, 85(5), 549, 1990.

21. Todesco, T., Rao, A. V., Bosello, O., and Jenkins, D. J. A., Propionate lowers blood glucose and alters lipid metabolism in healthy subjects, *Am. J. Clin. Nutr.*, 54, 1991.

22. Jenkins, D. J. A., Wolever, T. M. S., Jenkins, A. L., Brighenti, F., Vuksan, V., Rao, A. V., Cunnane, S., Ocana, A. M., Corey, P., Vezina, C., Connelly, P., Buckley, G., and Patten, R., Specific types of colonic fermentation may raise low-density-lipoprotein-cholesterol concentrations, *Am. J. Clin. Nutr.*, 54, 141, 1991.

23. Veldman, F. J., Nair, C. H., Vorster, H. H., Vermaak, W. J., Jerling, J. C., Osthuizen, W., and Venter, C. S., Possible mechanisms through which dietary pectin influences fibrin network architecture in hypercholesterolemic subjects, *Thromb. Res.*, 93, 253–64, 1999.

24. Reaven, G. M., Banting Lecture 1988. Role of insulin resistance in human disease, *Diabetes*, 37, 1595, 1988.

25. Ducimetiere, P., Eschwege, E., Papoz, L., Richard, J. L., Claude, J. R., and Rosselin, G., Relationship of plasma insulin levels to the incidence of myocardial infarction and coronary heart disease mortality in a middle-aged population, *Diabetologia*, 19, 205, 1980.

26. Welborn, T. A. and Wearne, K., Coronary heart disease incidence and cardiovascular mortality in Busselton with reference to glucose and insulin concentrations, *Diabetes Care*, 2, 154, 1979.

27. Pyorala, K., Relationship of glucose tolerance and plasma insulin to incidence of coronary heart disease: results from two population studies in Finland, *Diabetes Care*, 2, 131, 1979.

28. Jenkins, D. J. A., Leeds, A. R., Gmull, M. A., Cochet, B., and Alberti, K. G. M. M., Decrease in postprandial insulin and glucose concentrations by guar and pectin, *Ann. Int. Med.*, 86, 20, 1977.

29. Jenkins, D. J. A., Wolever, T. M. S., Leeds, A. R., Gassull, M. A., Dilawari, J. B., Goff, D. V., Metz, G. L., and Alberti, K. G. M. M., Dietary fibers, fiber analogues and glucose tolerance: importance of viscosity, *Br. Med. J.*, 1, 1392, 1978.

30. Lakeshmanan, M. R., Nepokroeff, C. M., Ness, G. C., Dugan, R. E., and Porter, J. W., Stimulation by insulin of rat liver Beta-hydroxy-Beta-methylglutaryl coenzyme A reductase and cholesterol-synthesizing activities, *Biochem. Biophys. Res. Commun.*, 50, 704, 1973.

31. Jenkins, D. J. A., Wolever, T. M. S., Ocana, A. M., Vuksan, V. et al., Metabolic effects of reducing rate of glucose ingestion by single bolus versus continuous sipping, *Diabetes*, 39, 775, 1990.

32. Ludwig, D. S., Pereira, M. A., Kroenke, C. H., Van Horn, L., Slattery, M. L., and Jacobs, D. R., Jr., Dietary fiber, weight gain, and cardiovascular disease risk factors in young adults, *JAMA*, 27, 282, 1539–46, 1999.

33. Vahouny, G. V. and Cassidy, M. M., Dietary fiber and intestinal adaptation, in *Dietary Fiber: Basic and Clinical Aspects*, Vahouny, G. V. and Kritchevsky, D., Eds., Plenum Press, New York, 1986, 181.

34. Story, J. A., Modification of steroid excretion in response to dietary fiber, in *Dietary Fiber: Basic and Clinical Aspects*, Vahouny, G. V. and Kritchevsky, D., Eds., Plenum Press, New York, 1986, 253.

35. Schneeman, B. O., Cimmarusti, J., Cohen, W., Downes, L., and Lefevre, M., Composition of high density lipoproteins in rats, *J. Nutr.*, 45, 564, 1976.

36. Kasper, H., Rabast, U., Fassi, H., and Fehle, F., The effect of dietary fiber on the postprandial serum vitamin A concentration in man, *Am. J. Clin. Nutr.*, 32, 1847, 1979.

37. Wolever, T. M. S., Hegele, R. A., Connelly, P. W., Ransom, T. P., Story, J. A., and Furumoto, E. J., Long-term effect of soluble-fiber foods on postprandial fat metabolism in dyslipidemic subjects with apo E3 and apo E4 genotypes, *Am. J. Clin. Nutr.*, 66, 584–90, 1997.

38. Manttani, M., Koskinen, P., Ehnholm, C., Hutlunen, J. K., and Manninen, V., Apolipoprotein E polymorphism influences the serum cholesterol response to dietary intervention, *Metabolism*, 40, 217, 1991.

39. Kesaniemi, Y. A., Ehnholm, C., and Miettinen, T. A., Intestinal cholesterol absorption efficiency in man is related to Apoprotein E phenotype, *J. Clin. Invest.*, 80, 578, 1987.

40. Gatti, A., Clanocchi, A., Matteucci, A., Rimondi, S., Ravalia, G., Descovich, G. C., and Sirtori, C. R., Dietary treatment of familial hypercholesterolemia — differential effects of soy protein according to the Apolipoprotein E phenotypes, *Am. J. Clin. Nutr.*, 53, 1191, 1991.

41. Gregg, R. E., Zech, L. A., Schaefer, E. J., and Brewer, H. B., Apolipoprotein E metabolism in normolipoproteinemic human subject, *J. Lipid Res.*, 25, 1167, 1984.

42. Gregg, R. E., Zech, L. A., Cabelli, C., and Brewer, H. B., Apo E modulates the metabolism of apo B containing lipoproteins by multiple mechanisms, in *Cholesterol Transport Systems and Their Relation to Atherosclerosis,* Steimetz, A., Kalparik, H., and Schneider, J., Eds., Springer Verlag, Berlin, 1989, II.

43. Breslow, J. L., Genetic basis of lipoprotein disorders, *J. Clin. Invest.,* 84, 373, 1989.

44. Gotto, A. M., Cholesterol intake and serum cholesterol level, *New Engl. J. Med.,* 324, 912, 1991.

45. Kern, F., Normal plasma cholesterol in an 88-year old man who eats 25 eggs a day. Mechanisms of adaptation, *New Engl. J. Med.,* 324, 896, 1991.

46. Miettinen, T. A. and Kesaniemi, Y. A., Cholesterol absorption: regulation of cholesterol synthesis and elimination and within-population variations of serum cholesterol levels, *Am. J. Clin. Nutr.,* 49, 629, 1989.

47. Gatti, E., Catenazzo, G., Camisasca, E., Torri, A., Denegri, E., and Sirtori, C. R., Effects of guar-enriched pasta in the treatment of diabetes and hyperlipidemia, *Ann. Nutr. Metab.,* 28, 1, 1984.

48. Schwandt, P., Richter, W. O., Weisweiler, P., and Neureuther, G., Cholestyramine plus pectin in treatment of patients with familial hypercholesterolemia, *Atherosclerosis,* 44, 379, 1982.

49. Simons, L. A., Gayst, S., Balasubramaniam, S., and Ruys, J., Long-term treatment of hypercholester-olaemia with a new palatable formulation of guar gum, *Atherosclerosis,* 45, 101, 1982.

50. Zavoral, J. H., Hannan, P., Fields, D. J., Hanson, M. N., Frantz, I. D., Kuba, K., Elmer, P., and Jacobs, D. R., The hypocholesterolemic effect of locust bean food products in hypercholesterolemic adults and children, *Am. J. Clin. Nutr.,* 38, 285, 1983.

51. Vargo, D., Doyle, R., and Floch, M. H., Colonic bacterial flora and serum cholesterol: alterations induced by dietary citrus pectin, *Am. J. Gastroenterol.,* 80(5), 361, 1985.

52. Abraham, Z. D. and Mehfa, T., Three-week psyllium-husk supplementation: effect on plasma choles-terol concentrations fecal steroid excretion, and carbohydrate absorption in men, *Am. J. Clin. Nutr.,* 47, 67, 1988.

53. Lindner, P. and Moller, B., Lignin: a cholesterol-lowering agent?, *Lancet,* 2, 1259, 1973.

54. Huth, K. and Fettel, M., Bran and blood lipids, *Lancet,* 2, 456, 1975.

55. Palumbo, P. J., Briones, E. R., and Nelson, R. A., High fiber diet in hyperlipidemia. Comparison with cholestyramine treatment in Type IIa hyperlipoproteinemia, *JAMA,* 240, 223, 1978.

56. Hillman, L. C., Peters, S. G., Fisher, C. A., and Pomare, E. W., The effects of the fiber components pectin, cellulose and lignin on serum cholesterol levels, *Am. J. Clin. Nutr.,* 42, 207, 1985.

57. Niemi, M. K., Keinanen-Kiukaanniemi, S. M., and Salmela, P. I., Long-term effects of guar gum and microcrystalline cellulose on glycemic control and serum lipids in type II diabetes, *Eur. J. Clin. Pharmacol.,* 34, 427, 1988.

58. Haskell, W. L., Spiller, G. A., Gates, J., Jensen, C., Ellis, B. K., and Gates, J. E., Role of water-soluble dietary fiber in the management of elevated plasma cholesterol in healthy subjects, *Am. J. Cardiol.,* 15, 433–9, 1992.

59. Thiffault, C., Belanger, M., and Pouliot, M., Traitement de l'hyperlipoproteinemie essentielle de type II par un nouvel agent pierapeutique, la celluline, *Can. Med. Assoc. J.,* 103, 165, 1970.

60. Nakamura, H., Ishikawa, T., Tada, N., Kagami, A., Kondo, K., Miyazima, E., and Takeyama, S., Effect of several kinds of dietary fibers on serum and lipoprotein lipids, *Nutr. Rep. Int.,* 26(2), 215, 1982.

61. Anderson, J. W., Zettwoch, N., Feldman, T., Tietyen-Clark, J., Oeltgen, P., and Bishop, C. W., Cholesterol lowering effects of psyllium hydrophilic mucilloid for hypercholesterolemic men, *Arch. Int. Med.,* 148, 292, 1988.

62. Bell, L. P., Hectorne, K., Reynolds, H., Balm, T. K., and Huninghake, D. B., Cholesterol-lowering effects of psyllium hydrophilic mucilloid, *JAMA,* 261(23), 3419, 1989.

63. Kestin, M., Moss, R., Clifton, P. M., and Nestel, P. J., Comparative effects of three cereal brans on plasma lipids, blood pressure and glucose metabolism in mildly hypercholesterolemic men, *Am. J. Clin. Nutr.,* 52, 661, 1990.

64. Miettinen, T. A. and Tarpila, S., Serum lipids and cholesterol metabolism during guar gum, plantago ovata and high fiber treatments, *Clinica Chim. Acta,* 183, 253, 1989.

65. Van Horn, L., Moag-Stahlberg, A., Liu, K., Ballew, C., Ruth, K., Hughes, R., and Stamler, J., Effects on serum lipids of adding instant oats to usual American diets, *Am. J. Public Health,* 81(2), 183, 1991.

66. Gold, K. V. and Davidson, D. M., Oat bran as a cholesterol-reducing dietary adjunct in a young, healthy population, *West J. Med.,* 148, 299, 1988.

67. Van Horn, L., Emidy, L. A., Liu, K., Liao, V., Baliew, C., King, J., and Stamler, J., Serum lipid response to a fat-modified oatmeal-enhanced diet, *Prev. Med.*, 17, 377, 1988.

68. Shutler, S. M., Bircher, G. M., Tredger, J. A., Morgan, L. M., Walker, A. F., and Low, A. G., The effect of daily baked bean (*Phaseolus vulgaris*) consumption on the plasma lipid levels of young, normo-cholesterolemic men, *Br. J. Nutr.*, 61, 257, 1988.

69. Anderson, J. W., Spencer, D. B., Hamilton, C. C., Smith, S. F., Tietyen, J., Bryant, C. A., and Oeltgen, P., Oat-bran cereal lowers serum total and LDL cholesterol in hypercholesterolemic men, *Am. J. Clin. Nutr.*, 52, 495, 1990.

70. Anderson, J. W., Gustafson, N. J., Spencer, D. B., Tietyen, J., and Bryant, C. A., Serum lipid response of hypercholesterolemic men to single and divided doses of canned beans, *Am. J. Clin. Nutr.*, 51, 1013, 1990.

71. Gaddi, A., Ciarrocchi, A., Matteucci, A., Rimondi, S., Ravaglia, G., Descovich, G. C., and Sirtori, C. R., Dietary treatment for familial hypercholesterolemia — differential effects of dietary soy protein according to the apolipoprotein E phenotypes, *Am. J. Clin. Nutr.*, 53, 1191, 1991.

72. Laurin, D., Jacques, H., Moorjani, S., Steinke, F. H., Gagne, C., Brun, D., and Lupien, F.-J., Effects of a soy-protein beverage on plasma lipoproteins in children with familial hypercholesterolernia, *Am. J. Clin. Nutr.*, 54, 98, 1991.

73. Bell, L. P., Hectorn, K. J., Reynolds, H., and Hunninghake, D. B., Cholesterol lowering effects of soluble fiber cereals as part of a prudent diet for patients with mild to moderate hypercholesterolemia, *Am. J. Clin. Nutr.*, 52, 1020, 1990

74. Neal, G. W. and Balm, T. K., Synergistic effects of psyllium in the dietary treatment of hypercholesterolemia, *South Med. J.*, 83(10), 1131, 1990.

75. Rodriguez-Moran, M., Guerrero-Romero, F., and Lazcano-Burciaga, G., Lipid- and glucose-lowering efficacy of Plantago psyllium in type II diabetes, *J. Diabetes Complications*, 12, 272–8, 1998.

76. Davidson, M. H., Maki, K. C., Kong, J. C., Dugan, L. D., Torri, S. A., Hall, H. A., Drennan, K. B., Anderson, S. M., Fulgoni, V. L., Saldanha, L. G., and Olson, B. H., Long-term effects of consuming foods containing psyllium seed husk on serum lipids in subjects with hypercholesterolemia, *Am. J. Clin. Nutr.*, 67, 367–76, 1998.

77. Jenkins, D. J., Wolever, T. M. S., Vidgen, E., Kendall, C. W., Ransom, T. P., Mehling, C. C., Mueller, S., Cunnane, S. C., O'Conell, N. C., Setchell, K. D., Lau, H., Teitel, J. M., Garvey, M. B., Fulgoni, V., Conelly, P. W., Patten, R., and Crey, P. N., Effect of psyllium in hypercholesterolemia at two monounsaturated fatty acid intakes, *Am. J. Clin. Nutr.*, 65, 1524–33, 1997.

78. Gupta, R. R., Agrawal, C. G., Singh, G. P., and Ghatak, A., Lipid-lowering efficacy of psyllium hydrophilic mucilloid in non insulin dependent diabetes mellitus with hyperlipidaemia, *Indian J. Med. Res.*, 100, 237–41, 1994.

79. Williams, C. L., Bollella, M., Spark, A., and Puder, D., Soluble fiber enhances the hypercholesterolemic effect of step 1 diet in childhood, *J. Am. Coll. Nutr.*, 14, 251–7, 1995.

80. Wolever, T. M., Jenkins, D. J., Mueller, S., Patten, R., Relle, L. K., Boctor, D., Ransom, T. P., Chao, E. S., McMillan, K., and Fulgoni, V., Psyllium reduces blood lipids in men and women with hyperlipidemia, *Am. J. Med. Sci.*, 307, 269–73, 1994.

81. Anderson, J. W., Davidson, M. H., Blonde, L., Brown, W. V., Howard, W. J., Ginsberg, H., Allgood, L. D., and Weingand, K. W., Long-term cholesterol-lowering effects of psyllium as an adjunct to diet therapy in the treatment of hypercholesterolemia, *Am. J. Clin. Nutr.*, 71, 1433–8, 2000.

82. Anderson, J. W., Allgood, L. D., Turner, J., Oeltgen, P. R., and Daggy, B. P., Effects of psyllium on glucose and serum lipid responses in men with type 2 diabetes and hypercholesterolemia, *Am. J. Clin. Nutr.*, 70, 466–73, 1999.

83. Wolever, T. M., Jenkins, D. J., Mueller, S., Boctor, D. L., Ranson, T. P., Patten, R., Chao, E. S., McMillan, K., and Fulgoni, V., Method of administration influences the serum cholesterol-lowering effect of psyllium, *Am. J. Clin. Nutr.*, 59, 1055–9, 1994.

84. Palmer, G. H. and Dixon, D. G., Effect of pectin dose on serum-cholesterol levels, *Am. J. Clin. Nutr.*, 18, 437, 1966.

85. Miettinen, T. A. and Tarpila, S., Effect of pectin on serum cholesterol, fecal bile acids and biliary lipids in normolipidemic and hyperlipidemic individuals, *Clin. Chim. Acta*, 79, 471, 1977.

86. Delbarre, F., Rondier, J., and de Gery, A., Lack of effect of two pectins in ideopathic or gout-associated hyperdyslipidemia hypercholesterolemia, *Am. J. Clin. Nutr.*, 30, 463, 1977.

87. Gruveda-Popova, J., Krachanova, M., Djurdjev, A., and Krachanov, C.. Application of soluble dietary fibres in treatment of hyperlipoproteinemias, *Folia Med.* (Plovdiv), 39, 39–43, 1997.
88. Jenkins, D. J. A., Leeds, A. R., Slavin, B., Mann, J., and Jepson, E. M., Dietary fiber and blood lipids: reduction of serum cholesterol in type II hyperlipidemia by guar gum, *Am. J. Clin. Nutr.*, 32, 16, 1979.
89. Jenkins, D. J. A., Reynolds, D., Slavin, B., Leeds, A. R., Jenkins, A. L., and Jepson, E. M., Dietary fiber and blood lipids: treatment of hypercholesterolemia with guar crispbread, *Am. J. Clin. Nutr.*, 33, 575, 1980.
90. Tuomilehto, J., Voutilainen, E., Huttunen, J., Vinni, S., and Homan, K., Effect of guar gum on body weight and serum lipids in hypercholesterolemic females, *Acta Med. Scand.*, 208, 45, 1980.
91. Wirth, A., Middlehoff, G., Brauning, C. H., and Schlierf, G., Treatment of familial hypercholesterolemia with a combination of bezafibrate and guar, *Atherosclerosis*, 45, 291, 1982.
92. Aro, A., Uusitupa, M., Voutilainen, E. V., and Korhonen, T., Effects of guar gum in male subjects with hypercholesterolemia, *Am. J. Clin. Nutr.*, 39, 911, 1984.
93. Bosello, O., Cominacini, L., Zocca, I., Garbin, U., Ferrari, F., and Davoli, A., Effects of guar gum on plasma lipoproteins and apolypoproteins C-II and C-III in patients affected by familial combined hyperlypoproteinemia, *Am. J. Clin. Nutr.*, 40(b), 1165, 1984.
94. Tagliaferro, V., Cassader, M., Bozzo, C., Pisu, E., Bruno, A., Marena, S., Cavallo-Perin, P., Cravero, L., and Pagano, G., Moderate guar-gum addition to usual diet improves peripheral sensitivity to insulin and lipemic profile in NIDDM, *Diab. Metabot.*, 11, 380, 1985.
95. Melvor, M. E., Cummings, C. C., Van Duyn, M. A., Leo, T. A., Margolis, S., Behall, K. M., Michnowski, J. E., and Mendeloff, A. I., Long-term effects of guar gum on blood lipids, *Atherosclerosis*, 60, 7, 1986.
96. Tuomilehto, J., Silvasti, M., Aro, A., Koistinen, A., Karttunen, P., Gref, C.-G., Ehnholm, C., and Uusitupa, M., Long term treatment of severe hypercholesterolemia with guar gum, *Atherosclerosis*, 72, 157, 1988.
97. Superko, H. R., Haskell, W. L., Sawrey-Kubicek, L., and Farquhar, J. W., Effects of solid and liquid guar gum on plasma cholesterol and triglyceride concentrations in moderate hypercholesterolemia, *Am. J. Cardiol.*, 62, 51, 1988.
98. Salenius, J. P., Harju, E., Jokela, H., Riekkinen, H., and Silvasti, M., Long term effects of guar gum on lipid metabolism after carotid endarterectomy, *BMJ*, 310, 95–96, 1995.
99. Jensen C. D., Haskell W., and Whittam, J. H., Long-term effects of water-soluble dietary fiber in the management of hypercholesterolemia in healthy men and women, *Am. J. Cardiol.*, 79, 34–7, 1997.
100. Pasman W. J., Westerterp-Plantenga, M. S., Muls, E., Vansant, G., van Ree, J., and Saris, W. H., The effectiveness of long-term fibre supplementation on weight maintenance in weight-reduced women, *Int. J. Obes. Relat. Metab. Disord.*, 21, 548–55, 1997.
101. Groop P. H., Aro A., Stenman S., and Groop L., Long-term effects of guar gum in subjects with non-insulin-dependent diabetes mellitus, *Am. J. Clin. Nutr.*, 58, 513–8, 1993.
102. Chuang, L. M., Jou, T. S., Yang, W. S., Wu, H. P., Huang, S. H., Tai, T. Y., and Lin, B.J., Therapeutic effect of guar gum in patients with non-insulin-dependant diabetes mellitus, *J. Formos. Med. Assoc.*, 91, 15–9, 1992.
103. Knopp, R. H., Superko, H. R., Davidson, M., Insull, W., Dujovne, C. A., Kwiterovich, P. O. , Zavoral, J. H., Graham, K., O'Connor, R. R., and Edelman, D. A., Long-term blood cholesterol-lowering effects of a dietary fiber supplement, *Am. J. Prev. Med.*, 17, 18–23, 1999.
104. Jenkins, D. J. A., Dietary fibre, diabetes and hyperlipidemia, *Lancet*, ii, 1287, 1979.
105. Kay, R. M., Dietary fiber, *J. Lipid Res.*, 23, 221, 1982.
106. Penagial, R., Velio, F., Rozzani, A., Castagnone, D., Ranzi, T., Bianchi, P. A., and Vigorelli, R., The effect of dietary guar on serum cholesterol, intestinal transit and fecal output in man, *Am. J. Gastroenterol.*, 81(2), 123, 1986.
107. Tognarelli, M., Miccoli, R., Giampietro, O., Cerri, M., and Navalesi, R., Guar-pasta: a new diet for obese subjects, *Acta Diabetol.*, 23, 77, 1986.
108. Kiriyama S., Enishi, A., Yoshida, A., Suhiama, N., and Shimahara, H., Hypercholesterolemic activity and molecular weight of Konjac-mannan, *Nutr. Rep. Intl.*, 6, 231–36, 1972.
109. Arvill, A. and Bodin L., Effect of short-term ingestion of Konjac glucomannan on serum cholesterol in healthy men, *Am. J. Clin. Nutr.*, 61, 585–89, 1995.

110. Terasawa, F., Tsuji, K., Tsuji, E., Oshima, S., Suzuki, S., and Seki, M., The effects of Konjac flour on blood lipids in elderly subjects, *J. Nutr.*, 37, 23–28, 1979.

111. Venter, C. S., Kruger, H. S., Vorster, H. H., Serfonrein, W. J., Ubbinik, J. B., and DeVilliers, L. S., The effects of dietary fiber component Konjac-glucomannan on serum cholesterol levels of hypocholesterolemic subject, *Hum. Nutr. Food Sci. Nutr.*, 41F, 55–61, 1987.

112. Vuksan, V., Jenkins, D. J. A., Spadafora, P., Sievenpiper, J., Owen, R., Vidgen, E., Brighenti, F., Josse, R., Leiter, L., and Bruce-Thompson, C., Konjac-mannan (glucomannan) improves glycemia and other associated risk factors for coronary heart disease in Type 2 diabetes: a randomized controlled metabolic trial, *Diabetes Care*, 22, 913–919, 1999.

113. Doi, K., Matsuura, M., Kawara, A., and Baba, S., Treatment of diabetes with glucomannan Konjacmanna, *Lancet*, 1, 987–988, 1979.

114. Vuksan, V., Sievenpiper, J. L., Owen, R., Swilley, J., Spadafora, P., Jenkins, D. J. A., Vidgen, E., Brighenti, F., Josse, R. G., Leiter, L., Xu, Z., and Novokmet, R., Beneficial effects of viscous dietary fiber from Konjac-mannan in subjects with the insulin resistance syndrome: result of a controlled metabolic trial, *Diabetes Care*, 23, 9–14, 2000.

115. Wolk, A., Manson, J. E., Stampfer, M. J., Colditz Hu, F. B., Speizer, F. E., Hennekens, C. H., and Willett, W. C., Long-term intake of dietary fiber and decreased risk of coronary heart disease among women, *JAMA*, 2, 281(21), 1998–2004, 1999.

116. Erkilla, A. T., Sarkkinen, E. S., Lehto, S., Pyorala, K., and Uusitupa, M. I., Dietary associates of serum total, LDL and HDL cholesterol and triglycerides in patients with coronary heart disease, *Prev. Med.*, 28, 558–565, 1999.

117. Munoz, J. M., Sandstead, H. H., Jacob, R. A., Logan, G. M., Jr., Reck, S. J., Klevay, L. M., Dintzis, F. R., Inglett, G. E., and Shuey, W. C., Effects of some cereal brans and textured vegetable protein on plasma lipids, *Am. J. Clin. Nutr.*, 35, 580, 1979.

118. Bremner, W. F., Brooks, P. M., Third, J. L. H. C., and Lawrie, T. D. V., Bran in hypertriglyceridaemia: a failure of response, *Br. Med. J.*, 3, 574, 1975.

119. Brooks, P. M., Bremner, W. F., and Third, J. L. H. C., Bran, hypertriglyceridaemia and urate clearance, *Med. J. Aust.*, 2, 753, 1976.

120. Lindegarde, F. and Larsson, L., Effects of a concentrated bran fibre preparation on HDL-cholesterol in hypercholesterolaemic men, *Hum. Nutr. Clin. Nutr.*, 38C, 39, 1984.

121. Vuksan, V., Jenkins, D. J., Vidgen, E., Ransom, T. P., Ng, M. K., Culhane, C. T., and O'Connor D., A novel source of wheat fiber and protein: effects on fecal bulk and serum lipids, *Am. J. Clin. Nutr.*, 69, 226–30, 1999.

122. Jenkins, D. J., Kendall, C. W., Vuksan, V., Augustin, L. S., Mehling, C., Parker, T., Vidgen, E., Lee, B., Faulkner, D., Seyler, H., Josse, R. G., Leiter, L. A., Connelly, P. W., and Fulgoni, V., Effect of wheat bran on serum lipids: influence of particle size and wheat protein, *J. Am. Coll. Nutr.*, 18, 159–65, 1999.

123. DeGroot, A. P., Luyken, R., and Pikaar, N. A., Cholesterol-lowering effect of rolled oats, *Lancet*, 2, 303, 1963.

124. Anderson, J. W., Story, L., Sieling, B., Chen, W.-J. L., Petro, M. S., and Story, J., Hypocholesterolemic effects of oat-bran or bean intake for hypercholesterolemic men, *Am. J. Clin. Nutr.*, 40(b), 1146, 1984.

125. Kirby, R. W., Anderson, J. W., Sieling, B., Rees, E. D., Chen, W. L., Miller, R. E., and Kay, R. M., Oat-bran intake selectively lowers serum low-density lipoprotein cholesterol concentrations of hypercholesterolemic men, *Am. J. Clin. Nutr.*, 34, 824, 1981.

126. Anderson, J. W., Story, L., Sieling, B., and Chen, W. L., Hypocholesterolemic effects of high-fibre diets rich in water-soluble plant fibres, *J. Can. Dietet. Assoc.*, 45, 2, 140, 1984.

127. Spiller, G. A., Farquhar, J. W., Gates, J. E., and Nichols, S. F., Guar gum and plasma cholesterol. Effect of guar gum and oat fiber source on plasma lipoproteins and cholesterol in hypercholesterolemic adults, *Arteriosclerosis Thrombosis*, 11, 1204, 1991.

128. Romero, A. L., Romero, J. E., Galaviz, S., and Fernandez, M. L., Cookies enriched with psyllium or oat bran lower plasma LDL cholesterol in normal and hypercholesterolemic men in Northern Mexico, *J. Am. Coll. Nutr.*, 17, 601–8, 1998.

129. Gerhardt, A. L. and Gallo, N. B., Full-fat rice bran and oat bran similarly reduce hypercholesterolemia in humans, *J. Nutr.*, 128, 865–9, 1998.

130. Grande, F., Anderson, J. T., and Keys, A., Effect of carbohydrates and leguminal seeds, wheat and potatoes on serum cholesterol concentration in man, *J. Nutr.*, 86, 313, 1965.

131. Grande, F., Anderson, J. T., and Keys, A., Sucrose and various carbohydrate containing foods and serum lipids in man, *Am. J. Clin. Nutr.*, 27, 1043, 1974.

132. Jenkins, D. J. A., Wolever, T. M. S., Jenkins, A. L., Thorne, M. J., Lee, R., Kalmusky, J., Reichert, R., and Wong, G. S., The glycemic index of foods tested in diabetic patients: a new basis for carbohydrate exchange favouring the use of legumes, *Diabetologia*, 24, 257, 1983.

133. Simpson, H. C. R., Simpson, R. W., Lonsley, S., Carter, R. D., Geekie, M., Hockaday, T. D. R., and Mann, J. I., A high carbohydrate leguminous fibre diet improves all aspects of diabetic control, *Lancet*, 1, 1, 1981.

134. Bingwen, L., Zhaofeng, W., Wanzhen, L., and Rongjue, Z., Effects of bean meal on serum cholesterol and triglycerides, *Chinese Med. J.*, 94, 7, 455, 1981.

135. Jenkins, D. J. A., Wong, G. S., Patten, R. P., Bird, J., Hall, M., Buckley, G. C., McGuire, V., Reichert, R., and Little, J. A., Leguminous seeds in the dietary management of hyperlipidemia, *Am. J. Clin. Nutr.*, 38, 567, 1983.

136. Jenkins, D. J., Kendall, C. W., Vidgen, E., Mehling, C.C., Parker, T., Seyler, H., Faulkner, D., Garsetti, M., Griffin, L. C., Agarwal, S., Rao A.V., Cunnane, S. C., Ryan, M. A., Connelly, P. W., Leiter, L. A., Vuksan, V., and Josse, R., The effect on serum lipids and oxidized low-density lipoprotein of supplementing self-selected low-fat diets with soluble-fiber, soy and vegetable protein foods, *Metabolism*, 49, 67–72, 2000.

137. Jenkins, D. J. et al., Combined effect of vegetable protein (soy) and soluble fiber added to a standard cholesterol-lowering diet, *Metabolism*, 48, 809–816, 1999.

138. Albrink, M. J., Newman, T., and Davidson, P. C., Effect of high- and low-fiber diets on plasma lipids and insulin, *Am. J. Clin. Nutr.*, 32, 1486, 1979.

139. Burke, B. J., Hartog, M., Heston, K. W., and Hooper, S., Assessment of the metabolic effects of dietary carbohydrate and fibre by measuring urinary excretion of C-peptide, *Hum. Nutr. Clin. Nutr.*, 36C, 373, 1982.

140. Sirtori, C. R., Agradi, E., Conti, F., Mantero, O., and Gatti, E., Soybean-protein diet in the treatment of Type II hyperlipoproteinemia, *Lancet*, i, 275, 1977.

141. Descovich, G. C., Ceredi, C., Gaddi, A. et al., Multicentre study of soybean protein diet for out-patient hypercholesterolemic patients, *Lancet*, ii, 709, 1980.

142. Descovich, G. C., Benassi, M. S., Cappelli, M., Gaddi, A., Grossi, G., Piazzi, S., Songiorgi, Z., Mannino, G., and Lenzi, S., Metabolic effects of lecithinated and non-lecithinated textured soy protein treatment in hypercholesterolemia, in *Lipoproteins and Coronary Atherosclerosis*, Noseda, G., Fragiacomo, C., Fumagalli, R., and Paoletti, R., Eds., Elsevier, Amsterdam, 1982, 279.

143. Vessby, B., Karlstrom, B., Lithell, H., Gustafsson, I. B., and Werner, I., The effects on lipid and carbohydrate metabolism of replacing some animal protein by soy-protein in a lipid-lowering diet for hypercholesterolemic patients, *Hum. Nutr. Appl. Nutr.*, 36Z, 179, 1982.

144. Holmes, W. L., Rubel, G. B., and Hood, S. S., Comparison of the effect of dietary meat versus dietary soybean protein on plasma lipids of hyperlipidemic individuals, *Atherosclerosis*, 36, 379, 1980.

145. Contaldo, F., DiBiase, G., Giacco, A., Pacioni, D., Moro, L. O., Grasso, L., Mancini, M., and Fidanza, F., Evaluation of the hypocholesterolemic effect of vegetable proteins, *Prevent. Med.*, 12, 138, 1983.

146. Calvert, G. D. and Blight, L., A trial of the effects of soya-bean flour and soya-bean saponins on plasma lipids, fecal bile acids and neutral sterols in hypercholesterolemic men, *Br. J. Nutr.*, 45, 277, 1981.

147. Anderson, J. W., Johnstone, B. M., and Cook-Newell, M. E., Meta-analysis of the effects of soy protein intake on serum lipids, *New Engl. J. Med.*, 333, 276–82, 1995.

148. Kritchevsky, D., Tepper, S. A., and Story, J. A., Influences of soy protein and cascin on atherosclerosis in rabbits, *Fed. Proc. Fed. Am. Soc. Exp. Biol.*, 37, 747, 1978.

149. Davidson, M. H., Dugan, L. D., Stocki, J., Dicklin, M. R., Maki, K. C., Coletta, F., Cotter, R., McLeod, M., and Hoersten K., A low-viscosity soluble fiber fruit juice supplement fails to lower cholesterol in hypercholesterolemic men and women, *J. Nutr.*, 128, 1927–1932, 1998.

150. Jenkins, D. J. A., Wolever, T. M. S., Jenkins, A. L., Lee, R., Wong, G. S., and Josse, R., Glycemic response to wheat product: reduced response to pasta but no effect of fiber, *Diabetes Care*, 6, 155, 1983.

151. Jenkins D. J., Kendall C. W., and Vuksan V., Viscous fibers, health claims and strategies to reduce cardiovascular disease risk, *Am. J. Clin. Nutr.*, 71, 401–2, 2000.

152. Jenkins, D. J. A. and Jepson, E. M., Leguminous seeds and their constituents in the treatment of hyperlipidemia and diabetes, in *Lipoproteins and Coronary Atherosclerosis*, Noseda, G., Fragiacomo, C., Fumagalli, R., and Paoletti, R., Eds., Elsevier, Amsterdam, 1982, 247.

153. Choudhury, S., Jackson, P., Katon, M. B., Marenah, C. B., Cortese, C., Miller, N. E., and Lewis, B., A multifactorical diet in the management of hyperlipidemia, *Atherosclerosis*, 50, 93, 1984.

Human Studies on Dietary Fiber and Colon Neoplasia

Hugh J. Freeman

ORIGIN OF THE FIBER HYPOTHESIS IN COLON CANCER

The possible role of dietary fiber in human colon cancer pathogenesis became of particular interest following epidemiologic studies in different populations; colon cancer was observed to be uncommon in many developing countries but relatively common among age-matched inhabitants of most Western nations. In large part, the hypothesis that fiber consumption may prevent subsequent colon cancer development appears to have emerged subsequent to the report by Higginson and Oettle[1] on studies in the Bantu of rural South Africa. Malhotra[2] subsequently found a low incidence of colon cancer in northern India, where the usual diet apparently contains large amounts of dietary fiber, and a high incidence of colon cancer in southern India, where the usual diet contains less cellulose. Later, the fiber hypothesis was widely popularized by Burkitt and colleagues,[3-5] and the possible role of fiber in prevention of the disease was emphasized.

EARLY FIBER STUDIES IN HUMANS

Following the development of the fiber hypothesis, a number of epidemiologic reports appeared, either supporting or refuting the importance of dietary fiber in colon cancer pathogenesis. A case-control study from Israel[6] described a highly significant inverse correlation between colon cancer and ingestion of certain fiber-containing foods. Interviewers were not aware of which patients had histologically confirmed malignant disease of the large bowel. Black patients from the San Francisco Bay area reported less frequent consumption of foods containing 0.5% fiber, although methods used to determine fiber content were not indicated.[7] A report by Graham and associates[8] suggested that the frequency of ingestion of certain vegetables, especially cabbage, sprouts, and broccoli, but not beef or other meats, was lower in white males with an increased colon cancer incidence.

Certain groups of Inuit in the Canadian Arctic, however, are not unusually prone to colon cancer, despite a diet low in plant fiber,[9] yet the Inuit eat large amounts of animal connective tissues composed of apparently nondigestible aminopolysaccharides.[10] Although this dietary characteristic is thought to be shared with certain African tribes, the role of these dietary substances, if any, in the pathogenesis of colon cancer has not been defined. Seventh-Day Adventists in Loma Linda, California, are reported to eat vegetarian diets[11] and have a low incidence of colon cancer.[12] However, other malignant diseases also occur at a low incidence in this group, and precise measurements of the content of individual fiber polymers in their diets have not been performed.

Some international and in-country studies were also done soon after this hypothesis was developed. In one, no correlation between crude dietary fiber consumption and colon cancer mortality was observed.[13] In another, cereal consumption appeared to be negatively correlated with colon cancer incidence data.[14] In a report from the U.K., differences in dietary fiber consumption within that country were correlated with its apparent protective role in colon carcinogenesis.[15]

Haenszel and colleagues[16] found a significant positive association between colon cancer and the frequency of ingestion of fiber containing legumes in Hawaiian Japanese. However, no other quantitative data were provided. In another study from Japan, cabbage was reported to be protective.[17] Graham and Mettlin,[18] on the other hand, drew attention to studies showing a protective role for vegetable intake, especially cruciferous vegetables rich in indoles. Similar observations supporting a possible protective role for vegetables were also previously noted.[19] While it was difficult to conduct studies on the basis of retrospective dietary histories dependent on respondent recall, discrepancies that emerged may have also reflected inadequate definition of the precise dietary fiber composition of foods ingested by the different groups.

Other earlier studies from Europe[20,21] further attempted to examine the fiber question from this perspective. Using the Southgate method of fiber measurement, diets from population samples in an area with a low incidence of colon cancer (Kuopio, Finland) and an area with a high incidence (Copenhagen) were analyzed. Although the proportions of dietary fiber polymers were similar, the mean intakes of total dietary fiber as well as specific fiber polymers (cellulose and lignin) were significantly less in Copenhagen. Although preliminary, measured intakes of specific fiber polymers were documented for the first time and differed in human populations with different incidence rates of colon carcinoma.

RECENT STUDIES AND FUTURE DIRECTIONS

These early studies served to stimulate considerable interest in the role of dietary fiber in colon cancer pathogenesis. Indeed, several epidemiologic studies appeared (Table 5.5.1); these included case-control studies, international and within-country correlation studies, cohort studies, and time-trend studies concerning colon cancer and fiber, vegetables, grains, or fruit. Most provided evidence for a protective effect, while some revealed only equivocal results or no evidence of a protective effect for fiber in colon cancer.

In the past decade, several studies have been published. Some of these have attracted significant media publicity. Review is critical to further refine the direction of future research. All of these recent studies have aided in definition of critical variables (Table 5.5.2) for subsequent studies important in further definition of dietary fiber in colon cancer. Particular emphasis may be needed for prevention studies in those with colonic disorders, such as inflammatory bowel disease (see Chapter 5.7) and colon polyps, both conditions that predispose to colon cancer. Clearly, there may be individual genetic factors that influence the potential benefits of dietary fiber and other environmental factors in risk reduction. In a recent study,[64] the effective risk reduction was less for those with a family history of colon cancer; in other words, genetic factors may be so significant in some highly predisposed individuals that it may be difficult to define any potential beneficial role for dietary fiber.

In a recent study by Fuchs et al.,[65] nurses who completed a retrospective dietary semiquantitative food frequency questionnaire in 1980 were evaluated. Over 16 years, follow-up studies included questions related to specific dietary constituents. Although 121,700 nurses were initially enrolled, almost 33,000 were excluded from the final analysis because of recognition of a potential high risk factor, such as familial polyposis, or loss of follow-up. In total, 787 cases of invasive adenocarcinoma and 1012 cases of adenoma in the distal colorectum were detected. Nurses were

Table 5.5.1 Studies on Fiber in Colon Neoplasia

Author, Year	Ref.
Evidence for Protective Effect	
Tuyns, 1986	22
Manousos et al., 1983	23
Macquart-Moulin et al., 1986	24
Kune et al., 1987	25
Slattery et al., 1988	26
Young and Wolf, 1988	27
La Vecchia et al., 1988	28
Graham et al., 1988	29
Lyon et al., 1987	30
Bristol et al., 1985	31
McKeown-Eyssen and Bright-See, 1984	32
Bingham et al., 1985	33
Rosen et al., 1988	34
Helms et al., 1982	35
Hirayama, 1981	36
Tuyns et al., 1988	37
Heilbrun et al., 1989	38
West et al., 1989	39
Lee et al., 1989	40
Freudenheim et al., 1990	41
Trock et al., 1990	42[a]
Olsen et al., 1994	55
Steinmetz et al., 1994	56
McKeown-Eyssen et al., 1994	57
Tsuji et al., 1996	59
Hardman et al., 1997	61
Ghadirian et al., 1997	62
Franceschi et al., 1998	63
Sellers et al., 1998	64
Macrae, 1999	66
Equivocal or Lack of Protective Effect	
Martinez et al., 1981	43
Pickle et al., 1984	44
Rozen et al., 1981	45
Jensen, 1983	46
Boing et al., 1985	47
Phillips and Snowdon, 1985	48
Tajima et al., 1985	49
Powles et al., 1984	50
Tajima and Tominaga, 1985	51
Potter and McMichael, 1986	52
Miller et al., 1983	53
Willett et al., 1990	54
Giovannucci et al., 1994	58
Alberts et al., 1997	60
Fuchs et al., 1999	65

[a] Meta-analyses of other published studies.

categorized into quintiles depending on computed fiber intake from the retrospective dietary data. The highest fiber diet was about 25 g per day. No difference in colon cancers or polyps was detected between different fiber groups. Several issues were not addressed in this highly publicized study. First, the measures used to collect data were imprecise and based on retrospective diet recall. Food-frequency questionnaires often fail to provide a true estimate of dietary macronutrient or

Table 5.5.2   Variables for Fiber Studies

Dietary Factors

- Individual fiber components (cellulose, hemicellulose, pectin, lignin, etc.)
- Fiber–macronutrient interactions (fat, protein, etc.)
- Fiber–micronutrient interactions (trace elements, vitamins, etc.)
- Digestion products of fiber (short-chain fatty acids, etc.)
- Source of dietary fiber components (grains, vegetables, etc.)
- Food preparation methods

Patient or Population Factors

- Sex and age
- Geographic locale
- Genetic variables (blood type, HLA type, etc.)
- Environmental variables (smoking, etc.)
- Medications for treatment (antibiotics, ulcer drugs)
- Medications for prophylaxis

Colonic Factors

- Colonic site-specific effects (e.g., cecal vs. rectosigmoid)
- Preneoplastic disorders (ulcerative colitis, Crohn's disease)
- Other colonic neoplastic disorders (colon polyps, polyposis syndrome)
- Underlying gastrointestinal or other diseases (diabetes, etc.)

micronutrient intakes, including dietary fiber. Second, high-fiber foods may not be equivalent, particularly in relation to individual fiber components, such as cellulose. Total dietary fiber measurements are of interest, but specific components of fiber in animal fiber studies have been shown to be critical for cancer prevention. Moreover, there was only a 2.5-fold difference in estimated total dietary fiber between the highest and lowest quintile, likely not sufficient to detect any differences. Finally, other important concerns have been subsequently raised, including the methods used to measure the endpoints of data collection; i.e., endoscopic evaluations and pathology reports may differ depending on levels of expertise. Moreover, important differences, even if present, may be missed because of the reported time-lag effects of dietary fiber in colon cancer, estimated to demonstrate a maximal negative correlation after a 15- to 27-year delay, with a maximum 23-year lag.[59] Clearly, the evaluation of this study raised many criticisms that need to be considered in the design of future, more definitive studies.[67,68]

REFERENCES

1. Higginson, J. and Oettle, A. G., Cancer incidence in Bantu and "Cape coloured" races of South Africa. Report of a cancer survey of the Transvaal (1953-1955), *J. Natl. Cancer Inst.*, 24, 589, 1960.
2. Malhotra, S. L., Geographical distribution of gastrointestinal cancers in India with special reference to causation, *Gut*, 8, 361, 1967.
3. Burkitt, D. P., Epidemiology of cancer of the colon and rectum, *Cancer*, 28, 1971.
4. Burkitt, D. P., Walker, A. R. P., and Painter, N. S., Effect of dietary fiber on stools and transit-times, and its role in the causation of disease, *Lancet*, 2, 1408, 1972.
5. Walker, A. R. P. and Burkitt, D. P., Colonic cancer — hypothesis of causation, dietary prophylaxis, an future research, *Am. J. Dig. Dis.*, 21, 910, 1976.
6. Modan, B., Barell, V., Lubin, F., Modan, M., Greenberg, R. A., and Graham, S., Low-fiber intake as an etiologic factor in cancer of the colon, *J. Natl. Cancer Inst.*, 55, 15, 1975.
7. Dales, L. G., Friedman, G. D., Ury, H. K., Grossman, S., and Williams, S. R., A case-control study of relationships of diet and other traits to colorectal cancer in American blacks, *Am. J. Epidemiol.*, 10, 132, 1979.

8. Graham, S., Dayal, H., Swanson, M., Mittelman, A., and Wilkinson, G., Diet in the epidemiology of cancer of the colon and rectum, *J. Natl. Cancer Inst.*, 61, 709, 1978.
9. Schaefer, O., Medical observations and problems of the Canadian Arctic. II. Nutrition and nutritional deficiencies, *Can. Med. Assoc. J.*, 81, 396, 1959.
10. Trowell, H., Godding, E., and Spiller, G., Fiber bibliographies and terminology, *Am. J. Clin. Nutr.*, 31, 1489, 1978.
11. Goldin, B. and Gorbach, S. L., Colon cancer connection: beef, bran, bile and bacteria, *Viewpoints Dig. Dis.*, 10, 3, 1978.
12. Lemon, F. R., Walden, R. T., and Woods, R. W., Cancer of the lung and mouth in Seventh-Day Adventists. Preliminary report of a population study, *Cancer*, 17, 486, 1964.
13. Draser, B. S. and Irving, D., Environmental factors in cancer of the colon and breast, *Br. J. Cancer*, 27, 167, 1973.
14. Armstrong, B. and Doll, R., Environmental factors in cancer incidence and mortality in different countries with special reference to dietary practices, *Int. J. Cancer*, 15, 617, 1975.
15. Bingham, S., Williams, D. R. R., Cole, T. F., and James, W. P. T., Dietary fibre and regional large bowel cancer mortality in Britain, *Br. J. Cancer*, 40, 456, 1979.
16. Haenszel, W., Berg, J. W., Segi, M., Kurihara, M., and Locke, F. B., Large bowel cancer in Hawaiian Japanese, *J. Natl. Cancer Inst.*, 51, 1765, 1973.
17. Haenszel, W., Locke, F. B., and Segi, M., A case control study of large bowel cancer in Japan, *J. Natl. Cancer Inst.*, 64, 17, 1980.
18. Graham, S. M. and Mettlin, C., Diet and colon cancer, *Am. J. Epidemiol.*, 109, 1, 1979.
19. Stocks, P. and Karn, M. K., A cooperative study of the habits, home life, dietary and family histories of 450 cancer patients and an equal number of control patients, *Ann. Eugen.*, 5, 237, 1933.
20. International Agency for Research on Cancer, Intestinal Microecology Group, Dietary fibre, transit time, faecal bacteria, steroids, and colon cancer in two Scandinavian populations, *Lancet*, 2, 207, 1977.
21. Jensen, O. M., MacLennan, R., Wahrendorff, J., and IARC, Large Bowel Cancer Group, Large bowel cancer in Scandinavia in relation to diet and faecal characteristics, *Nutr. Cancer*, 4, 5, 1982.
22. Tuyns, A. J., A case-control study on colorectal cancer in Belgium, *Soz. Praventivemed.*, 31, 81, 1986.
23. Manousos, O., Day, N. E., and Trichopoulos, D., Diet and colorectal cancer: a case control study in Greece, *Int. J. Cancer*, 32, 1, 1983.
24. Mcquart-Moulin, G., Riboli, E., Cornee, J., Charnay, B., Berthezene, P., and Day, N., Case-control study on colorectal cancer and diet in Marseilles, *Int. J. Cancer*, 38, 183, 1986.
25. Kune, S., Kune, G. A., and Watson, L. F., Case control study of dietary etiological factors: the Melbourne colorectal cancer study, *Nutr. Cancer*, 9, 21, 1987.
26. Slattery, M. L., Sorenson, A. W., Mahoney, A. W., French, T. K., Kritchevsky, D., and Street, J. C., Diet and colon cancer: assessment of risk by fiber type and food source (published erratum appears in *J. Natl. Cancer Inst.*, 81, 1042, 1989), *J. Natl. Cancer Inst.*, 80, 1474, 1988.
27. Young, T. B. and Wolf, D. A., Case control study of proximal and distal colon cancer and diet in Wisconsin, *Int. J. Cancer*, 42, 167, 1988.
28. La Vecchia, C., Negri, E., and Decarli, A., A case-control study of diet and colorectal cancer in northern Italy, *Int. J. Cancer*, 41, 492, 1988.
29. Graham, S., Marshall, J., Haughey, B., Mittelmann, A., Swanson, M., Zielezny, M., Byers, T., Wilkinson, G., and West, D., Dietary epidemiology of cancer of the colon in western New York, *Am. J. Epidemiol.*, 128, 490, 1988.
30. Lyon, J. L., Mahoney, A. W., West, D. W., Gardner, J. W., Smith, K. R., Sorenson, A. W., and Stanish, W., Energy intake: its relationship to colon cancer risk, *J. Natl. Cancer Inst.*, 78, 853, 1987.
31. Bristol, J. B., Emmett, P. M., and Heaton, K. W., Sugar, fat and the risk of colorectal cancer, *Br. Med. J.*, 291, 1467, 1985.
32. McKeown-Eyssen, G. E. and Bright-See, E., Dietary factors in colon cancer: international relationships. An update, *Nutr. Cancer*, 6, 160, 1984.
33. Bingham, S. A., Williams, D. R. R., and Cummings, J. H., Dietary fibre consumption in Britain: new estimates and their relation to large bowel cancer mortality, *Br. J. Cancer*, 52, 399, 1985.
34. Rosen, M., Nystrom, L., and Wall, S., Diet and cancer mortality in the counties of Sweden, *Am. J. Epidemiol.*, 127, 42, 1988.

35. Helms, P., Jorgensen, I. M., and Paerregaard, A., Dietary patterns in Them and Copenhagen, Denmark, *Nutr. Cancer*, 4, 34, 1982.

36. Hirayama, T., A large-scale cohort study on the relationship between diet and selected cancers of the digestive organs, in *Gastrointestinal Cancer: Endogenous Factors*, Bruce, W. R., Correa, P., and Lipkin, M., Eds., Cold Spring Harbor Laboratory, Cold Spring Harbor, NY, 1981, 409.

37. Tuyns, A. J., Kaaks, R., and Haelterman, M., Colorectal cancer and the consumption of foods: a case control study in Belgium, *Nutr. Cancer*, 11, 189, 1988.

38. Heilbrun, L. K., Nomura, A., Hankin, J. H., and Stemmermann, D. N., Diet and colorectal cancer with special reference to fiber intake, *Int. J. Cancer*, 44, 1, 1989.

39. West, D. W., Slattery, M. L., Robison, L. M., Schuman, K. L., Ford, M. H., Mahoney, A. W., Lyon, J. L., and Sorensen, A. W., Dietary intake and colon cancer: sex- and anatomic site-specific associations, *Am. J. Epidemiol.*, 130, 883, 1989.

40. Lee, H. P., Gourley, L., Duffy, S. W., Estieve, J., Lee, J., and Day, N. E., Colorectal cancer and diet in an Asian population — a case-control study among Singapore Chinese, *Int. J. Cancer*, 43, 1007, 1989.

41. Freudenheim, J. L., Graham, S., Horvath, P. J., Marshall, J. R., Haughey, B. P., and Wilkinson, G., Risks associated with source of fiber and fiber components in cancer of the colon and rectum. *Cancer Res.*, 50, 3295, 1990.

42. Trock, B., Lanza, E., and Greenwald, P., Dietary fiber, vegetables, and colon cancer: critical review and meta-analyses of the epidemiologic evidence, *J. Natl. Cancer Inst.*, 82, 650, 1990.

43. Martinez, I., Torres, R., and Frias, Z., Factors associated with adenocarcinomas of the large bowel in Puerto Rico, *Rev. Latinoam. Oncol. Clin.*, 13, 13, 1981.

44. Pickle, L. W., Greene, M. H., and Ziegler, R. G., Colorectal cancer in rural Nebraska, *Cancer Res.*, 44, 363, 1984.

45. Rozen, P., Hellerstein, S. M., and Horwitz, C., The low incidence of colorectal cancer in a "high risk" population: its correlation with dietary habits, *Cancer*, 48, 2692, 1981.

46. Jensen, O. M., Cancer risk among Danish male Seventh-Day Adventists and other temperance society members, *J. Natl. Cancer Inst.*, 70, 1011, 1983.

47. Boing, H., Martinez, L., and Frentzel-Beyme, R., Regional nutritional pattern of cancer mortality in the Federal Republic of Germany, relationships with fatal colorectal cancer among Seventh-Day Adventists, *J. Natl. Cancer Inst.*, 74, 307, 1985.

48. Phillips, R. L. and Snowdon, D. A., Dietary relationships with fatal colorectal cancer among Seventh-Day Adventists, *J. Natl. Cancer Inst.*, 74, 307, 1985.

49. Tajima, K., Hirose, K., and Nakagawa, N., Urban-rural difference in the trend of colo-rectal cancer mortality with special reference to the subsites of colon cancer in Japan, *Jpn. J. Cancer Res.*, 76, 717, 1985.

50. Powles, J. W. and Williams, D. R., Trends in bowel cancer in selected countries in relation to wartime changes in flour milling, *Nutr. Cancer*, 6, 40, 1984.

51. Tajima, K. and Tominaga, S., Dietary habits and gastro-intestinal cancers: a comparative case-control study of stomach and large intestinal cancers in Nagoya, Japan, *Jpn. J. Cancer Res.*, 76, 705, 1985.

52. Potter, J. D. and McMichael, A. J., Diet and cancer of the colon and rectum: a case-control study, *J. Natl. Cancer Inst.*, 76, 557, 1986.

53. Miller, A. B., Howe, G. R., Jain, M., Craib, K. J., and Harrison, L., Food items and food groups as risk factors in a case-control study of diet and colo-rectal cancer, *Int. J. Cancer*, 32, 155, 1983.

54. Willett, W. C., Stampfer, M. J., Colditz, G. A., Rosner, B. A., and Speizer, F. E., Relation of meat, fat, and fiber intake to the risk of colon cancer in a prospective study among women, *N. Engl. J. Med.*, 323, 1664, 1990.

55. Olsen, J., Kronborg, O., Lynggaard, J., and Ewertz, M., Dietary risk factors for cancer and adenomas of the large intestine. A case-control study within a screening trial in Denmark, *Eur. J. Cancer*, 30A, 53, 1994.

56. Steinmetz, K. A., Kushi, L. H., Bostick, R. M., Folsom, A. R., and Potter, J. D., Vegetables, fruit, and colon cancer in the Iowa Women's Health Study, *Am. J. Epidemiol.*, 139, 1, 1994.

57. McKeown-Eyssen, G. E., Bright-See, E., Bruce, W. R., Jazmaji, V., Cohen, L. B., Pappas, S. C., and Saibil, F. G., A randomized trial of a low fat high fibre diet in the recurrence of colorectal polyps. Toronto Polyp Prevention Group (published erratum appears in *J. Clin Epidemiol.*, 48, 1, 1995), *J. Clin. Epidemiol.*, 47, 525, 1994.

58. Giovannucci, E., Rimm, E. B., Stampfer, M. J., Colditz, G. A., Ascherio, A., and Willett, W. C., Intake of fat, meat, and fiber in relation to risk of colon cancer in men, *Cancer Res.*, 54, 2390, 1994.

59. Tsuji, K., Harashima, E., Nakagawa, Y., Urata, G., and Shirataka, M., Time-lag effect of dietary fiber and fat intake ratio on Japanese colon cancer mortality, *Biomed. Environ. Sci.*, 9, 223, 1996.

60. Alberts, D. S., Einspahr, J., Ritenbaugh, C., Aickin, M., Rees-McGee, S., Atwood, J., Emerson, S., Mason-Liddil, N., Bettinger, L., Patel, J., Bellapravalu, S., Ramanujam, P. S., Phelps, J., and Clark, L., The effect of wheat bran fiber and calcium supplementation on rectal mucosal proliferation rates in patients with resected adenomatous colorectal polyps, *Cancer Epidemiol. Biomarkers Prev.*, 6, 161, 1997.

61. Hardman, W. E., Cameron, I. L., Beer, W. H., Speeg, K. V., Kadakia, S. C., and Lang, K. A., Transforming growth factor alpha distribution in rectal crypts as a biomarker of decreased colon cancer risk in patients consuming cellulose, *Cancer Epidemiol. Biomarkers Prev.*, 6, 633, 1997.

62. Ghadirian, P., Lacroix, A., Maisonneuve, P., Perret, C., Potvin, C., Gravel, D., Bernard, D., and Boyle, P., Nutritional factors and colon carcinoma: a case-control study involving French Canadians in Montreal, Quebec, Canada, *Cancer*, 80, 858, 1997.

63. Franceschi, S., Favero, A., Parpinel, M., Giacosa, A., and La Vecchia, C., Italian study on colorectal cancer with emphasis on influence of cereals, *Eur. J. Cancer Prev.*, 7 (suppl. 2), S19, 1998.

64. Sellers, T. A., Bazyk, A. E., Bostick, R. M., Kushi, L. H., Olson, J. E., Anderson, K. E., Lazovich, D., and Folsom, A. R., Diet and risk of colon cancer in a large prospective study of older women: an analysis stratified on family history (Iowa, United States), *Cancer Causes Control*, 9, 357, 1998.

65. Fuchs, C. S., Giovannucci, E. L., Colditz, G. A., Hunter D. J., Stampfer, M. J., Rosner, B., Speizer, F. E., and Willett, W. C., Dietary fiber and the risk of colorectal cancer and adenoma in women, *N. Engl. J. Med.*, 340, 169, 1999.

66. Macrae, F., Wheat bran fiber and development of adenomatous polyps: evidence from randomized controlled clinical trials, *Am. J. Med.*, 106 (1A), 38S, 1999.

67. Ravin, N. D., Mohandras, K. M., Cummings, J. H., Southgate, D. A. T., Heaton, K. W., Lewis, S. J., Madar, Z., Stark, A., and Camire, M. E., Dietary fiber and colorectal cancer, *N. Engl. J. Med.*, 340, 1924, 1999.

68. Freeman, H. J., Role of high fibre foods in the prevention of colorectal neoplasia, *Canad. J. Gastroenterol.*, 13, 379, 1999.

Fiber and Colonic Diverticulosis

Hugh J. Freeman

Colonic diverticular disease is an acquired deformity of the colon that is generally irreversible but usually asymptomatic.[1] In developed nations, the disorder is extremely common and prevalence correlates well with increasing age.[2] Although there are different anatomical forms of colonic diverticulosis, the basic abnormality observed in most North American and European populations is the pseudodiverticulum; this is a herniation of mucosa and submucosa through the colonic muscle wall. Most often, these are multiple and involve the left side of the colon, especially the sigmoid colon. While precise figures are not available, it has been estimated that about 20% of patients with diverticulosis will develop symptoms and signs of illness, but only a small minority will endure more serious complications including diverticulitis, sepsis, obstruction, and hemorrhage.[1,3]

Dietary fiber was recommended for symptomatic diverticular disease as early as 1929 by Spriggs.[4] Subsequently, Painter and Burkitt published their hypothesis that diverticular disease was caused by a reduced intake of dietary fiber.[5] Later, this "fiber hypothesis" was examined in carefully matched population groups from Oxford; diverticulosis was observed to be significantly more frequent in non-vegetarians compared to vegetarians.[6]

A variety of epidemiologic studies on the relationship between dietary fiber consumption and diverticular disease have been done both from a historical as well as a geographic perspective. Although it has been suggested that the prevalence of diverticular disease has increased over the past century,[7] precise analyses are not available. Barium enema and colonoscopy are the most common current methods of diagnosis, but these techniques were not available to earlier clinicians; indeed, radiographic appearances were not described in detail until 1925.[8] Interestingly, Brodribb has cited several autopsy studies reporting very high prevalences of diverticular disease (Graser in 1899, 64%; Sudsuki in 1900, 37.5%; and Mourges in 1931, 30%).[9] To date, therefore, historical data providing strong support for an increased prevalence of colonic diverticulosis at the present time are limited and controversial.

More interesting information comes from geographic studies. Painter and Burkitt, using a variety of anecdotal sources,[7] suggested that diverticulosis is rare in many parts of Africa, except among Europeans, and uncommon in the Indian subcontinent, Middle East, Far East, and South America; all are economically developing areas with cereal-based diets typically high in fiber. This contrasts with the well-developed countries in Europe and North America where diets tend to be highly refined and fiber-depleted and where a high prevalence of diverticular disease is observed.

This relationship between decreasing dietary fiber and increasing prevalence of diverticular disease has also been reported in urban South African blacks[10] and Hawaiian Japanese,[11] but not in the Orient, including Japan.[12] Indeed, recent studies on the distributional pattern of diverticular disease contrast with the increased frequency in the left colon in Western communities compared to the right colon in Oriental populations.[13] Similar observations have been reported from Europe.[14-16] Although intriguing, the true incidence of diverticular disease in these populations is not known, in part because of variable diagnostic methods and availability of accurate postmortem studies. In those populations with available data, it is unknown how accurately these reflect the true frequency in the population as a whole. Finally, a major weakness of such correlative studies relates to the dietary component of the equation and, specifically, methods used to precisely calculate the fiber content of the diet or specific fiber components.

Although a definitive role for fiber-deficient diets in the pathogenesis of colonic diverticulosis has not been proven, a number of uncontrolled trials suggested that added fiber in the form of bran supplements may be therapeutically beneficial.[17-19] In addition, some supportive evidence for a role for deficient dietary fiber in the pathogenesis of diverticulosis comes from animal studies. As early as 1937, Lubbock et al.[20] fed low-fiber diets to rats and showed the development of diverticulae. Carlson and Hoelzel[21] found that about 57% of a colony of Wistar rats more than 100 weeks old had diverticulae in the proximal colon, while only 4% of rats fed a psyllium seed supplement developed diverticulae. Similar observations have been reported in rats and rabbits, but the presence of a large cecum in these animals raises doubts regarding the applicability of these results to humans; indeed, many dietary fibers are more extensively degraded in these animals than in humans. Brodribb et al.[22] chose the stub-tailed monkey with a gastrointestinal anatomy more similar to humans as a model for colonic studies. He found that colonic intraluminal pressure increased as the amount of fiber in the diet decreased gradually from 20 to 15, 10, 5, and 0 g per day. More recent studies in adult female vervet monkeys revealed that diverticulosis frequently developed in those administered a Western-type high-fat, low-fiber diet compared to diets with low fat and higher fiber content.[23] Using an experimental model, some studies[24,25] have also explored factors that may influence the appearance of increased numbers of colonic diverticulae in rats administered a fiber-deficient diet. In one report,[24] a high-fiber diet appeared to protect against collagen cross-linking with a resultant reduction in appearance of diverticulae. Later, the same investigators noted that maternal diet during gestation, including fiber intake, and subsequent nutrition of progeny may play a critical role in development of diverticulae.[25] Subsequently, the role of bran was examined in five controlled trials (Table 5.6.1).[26-30] In addition, ispaghula alone[31] and methylcellulose alone[32] have been studied in controlled trials; subjective improvement was reported with ispaghula but no effect was noted with methylcellulose. It appears that a high-fiber diet may be effective treatment for symptoms in some patients with uncomplicated diverticular disease, especially if symptoms are severe, but the data remain limited. Moreover, the most comprehensive and best-conducted study,[29] largely using patients with mild symptoms, showed no major benefit in pain scores but there was improvement in constipation.

Additional studies, especially in humans, are still required to determine if high-fiber diets can alter the natural history of diverticular disease over the long term or prevent its complications. In one interesting report, Hyland and Taylor[33] described 100 patients that had been retrospectively reviewed after 5 to 7 years on a high-fiber diet — over 90% remained symptom-free. In one prospective study in American males, the incidence of symptomatic colonic diverticular disease was lowest in those with high-fiber diets.[34] In a subsequent report of a prospective study of different dietary fiber types, this inverse relationship with measurable insoluble fiber was confirmed, especially for cellulose fiber.[35]

Table 5.6.1 Controlled Clinical Trials of Bran in Colonic Diverticular Disease

Fiber Type and Form	No. patients	Study Protocol	Results	Comments	Ref.
Wheat vs. bran crispbread	18 with X-ray diagnosis	Double-blind control trial × 12 wk	Reduced symptom pain scores, early placebo effect noted	Symptoms moderate to severe; pain scores subjective	26
Wheat bran (coarse) vs. isphagula vs. lactulose	31 with X-ray diagnosis	Control trial × 4 wk	Symptoms relieved to an equivalent extent in all groups; only bran reduced colon motility and pressures		27
Coarse bran vs. sterculia with or without antispasmotic	20, but diagnostic method not defined	Sterculia or bran × 4 wk	Equivalent improvement in constipation, but bran or sterculia with antispasmotic better than sterculia alone for pain relief		28
Bran crispbread vs. isphagula vs. placebo (either wheat crispbread or refined wheat)	58 with X-ray diagnosis controlled trial × 16 wk	Double-blind randomized crossover	Pain score not improved but improvement in constipation	Pain symptoms mild in degree; near normal stool weights and transit times	29
Coarse bran vs. hyoscyamine vs. placebo	105 with X-ray diagnosis	Control trial up to 52 wk	Improved symptom scale for bran and hyoscyamine	Symptom scale based on ability to work	30

REFERENCES

1. Almy, T. P. and Howell, D. A., Diverticular disease of the colon, *N. Engl. J. Med.*, 302, 324, 1980.
2. Parks, T. G., Natural history of diverticular disease of the colon, *Clin. Gastroenterol.*, 4, 53, 1975.
3. Hughes, L. E., Complications of diverticular disease: inflammation, obstruction and bleeding, *Clin. Gastroenterol.*, 4, 147, 1975.
4. Spriggs, E. I., Diverticulitis, *Br. Med. J.*, 2, 569, 1929.
5. Painter, N. G. and Burkitt, D. P., Diverticular disease of the colon: a deficiency disease of western civilization, *Br. Med. J.*, 2, 450, 1971.
6. Gear, J. S. S., Ware, A., Fursdon, P., Mann, J. L., Nolan, D. J., Brodribb, A. J. M., and Vessey, M. P., Symptomless diverticular disease and intake of dietary fiber, *Lancet*, 1, 511, 1979.
7. Painter, N. S. and Burkitt, D. P., Diverticular disease of the colon, a 20th century problem, *Clin. Gastroenterol.*, 4, 3, 75.
8. Spriggs, E. I. and Marxer, O. A., Intestinal diverticula, *Q. J. Med.*, 19, 1, 1925.
9. Brodribb, J. M., Dietary fiber in diverticular disease of the colon, in *Medical Aspects of Dietary Fiber*, Spiller, G. A. and Kay, R. M., Eds., Plenum Press, New York, 1980, 43.
10. Segal, I., Solomon, A., and Hunt, J. A., Emergence of diverticular disease in the urban South African black, *Gastroenterology*, 72, 215, 1977.
11. Stemmermann, G. N. and Yatani, R., Diverticulosis and polyps of the large intestine: a necropsy study of Hawaii Japanese, *Cancer*, 31, 1260, 1973.
12. Narasaka, T., Watanabe, H., Yamagata, S., Munakata, A., Tajima, T., and Matatsunaga, F., Statistical analysis of diverticulosis of the colon, *Tohoku J. Exp. Med.*, 115, 271, 1975.
13. Segal, I. and Leibowitz, B., The distributional pattern of diverticular disease, *Dis. Colon Rectum*, 32, 227, 1989.

14. Kohler, R., The incidence of colonic diverticulosis in Finland and Sweden, *Acta. Chir. Scand.*, 126, 148, 1963.

15. Havia, T., Diverticulosis of the colon, *Acta. Chir. Scand.*, 137, 167, 1971.

16. Hughes, L. E., Post-mortem survey of diverticular disease of the colon, *Gut*, 10, 336, 1969.

17. Painter, N. S., Almeida, A. Z., and Colebourne, K. W., Unprocessed bran in treatment of diverticular disease of the colon, *Br. Med. J.*, 2, 137, 1972.

18. Brodribb, A. J. M. and Humphreys, D. M., Diverticular disease: three studies, *Br. Med. J.*, 1, 424, 1976.

19. Plumley, P. F. and Francis, B., Dietary management of diverticular disease, *J. Am. Dietet. Assoc.*, 63, 527, 1973.

20. Lubbock, D. M., Thomson, W., and Garry, R. C., Epithelial overgrowth and diverticula of the gut, *Br. Med. J.*, 1, 1252, 1937.

21. Carlson, A. J. and Hoelzel, F., Relationship of diet to diverticulosis of the colon in rats, *Gastroenterology*, 12, 108, 1949.

22. Brodribb, A. J. M., Condon, R. E., Cowles, V., and DeCosse, J. J., Effect of dietary fiber on intraluminal pressure and myoelectrical activity of the left colon in monkeys, *Gastroenterology*, 77, 70, 1979.

23. Jaskiewicz, K., Rossouw, J. E., Kritchevsky, D., van Rensburg, S. J., Fincham, J. E., and Woodroof, C. W., The influence of diet and dimethylhydrazine on the small and large intestine of vervet monkeys, *Br. J. Exp. Pathol.*, 67, 361, 1986.

24. Wess, L., Eastwood, M. A., Edwards, C. A., Busuttil, A., and Miller, A., Collagen alteration in an animal model of colonic diverticulosis, *Gut*, 38, 701, 1996.

25. Wess, L., Eastwood, M., Busuttil, A., Edwards, C., and Miller, A., An association between maternal diet and colonic diverticulosis in an animal model, *Gut*, 39, 423, 1996.

26. Brodribb, A. J. M., Treatment of symptomatic diverticular disease with a high fiber diet, *Lancet*, 1, 664, 1977.

27. Eastwood, M. A., Smith, A. N., Brydon, W. G., and Pritchard, J., Comparison of bran, ispaghula, and lactulose on colon function in diverticular disease, *Gut*, 19, 1144, 1978.

28. Srivastava, G. S., Smith, A. N., and Painter, N. S., Sterculia bulk-forming agent with smooth muscle relaxant versus bran in diverticular disease, *Br. Med. J.*, 1, 315, 1976.

29. Ornstein, M. H., Littlewood, E. R., Baird, I. M., Fowler, J., North, W. R. S., and Cox, A. G., Are fibre supplements really necessary in diverticular disease of the colon? A controlled clinical trial, *Br. Med. J.*, 282, 1353, 1981.

30. Weinreich, J., Controlled studies with dietary fibre in the therapy of diverticular disease and irritable bowel syndrome, in *Colon and Nutrition*, Goebell, H. and Kasper, H., Eds., Falk Symposium 32, MTP Press, Lancaster, England, 1982, 239.

31. Ewerth, S., Ahlberg, J., Holmstrom, B., Persson, U., and Uden, R., Influence of symptoms and transit time of Vi-Siblin in diverticular disease, *Acta. Chir. Scand. Suppl.*, 500, 49, 1980.

32. Hodgson, W. J. B., The placebo effect, is it important in diverticular disease?, *Am. J. Gastroenterol.*, 67, 157, 1977.

33. Hyland, J. M. P. and Taylor, I., Does a high fibre diet prevent the complication of diverticular disease?, *Br. J. Surg.*, 67, 77, 1980.

34. Aldoori, W. H., Giovannucci, E. L., Rimm, E. B., Wing, A. L., Trichopoulos, D. V., and Willett, W. C., A prospective study of diet and risk of symptomatic diverticular disease in men, *Am. J. Clin. Nutr.*, 60, 753, 1994.

35. Aldoori, W. H., Giovannucci, E. L., Rockett, H. R., Sampson, L., Rimm, E. B., and and Willett, W. C., A prospective study of dietary fiber types and symptomatic diverticular disease in men, *J. Nutr.*, 128, 714, 1998.

Fiber and Inflammatory Bowel Diseases (Ulcerative Colitis And Crohn's Disease)

Hugh J. Freeman

Inflammatory bowel disease (IBD) refers to that group of conditions in which inflammation involves the small or large intestine or both. In common usage, IBD is restricted to those conditions whose etiology is unknown and generally includes Crohn's disease (CD) and ulcerative colitis (UC). As with many other intestinal conditions of undetermined or uncertain etiology, dietary factors, including fiber, have been proposed to play an important role in pathogenesis.

The low incidence of Crohn's disease in less-industrialized third-world countries and its apparently increasing incidence in more industrialized Western countries have led to speculation that dietary changes in the Western world that have developed in the past few decades may be partly responsible. For example, a consistent dietary difference between patients with CD and controls is the high refined-carbohydrate intake observed in CD, a finding which was first reported in 1976[1] and which has subsequently been confirmed.[2,3]

FIBER STUDIES IN CD

Fiber consumption in CD has also been examined in some studies (Table 5.7.1). Kasper and Sommer employed an experienced dietitian to perform dietary histories in CD patients and controls over 7 successive days.[4] They reported that patients with CD consumed slightly, but significantly, more fiber than control subjects (26.6 vs. 22.3 g). This increase was largely in the form of a significantly increased consumption of non-cellulose polysaccharide (17.3 vs. 14.5 g). In contrast, Thornton and co-workers reported that pre-illness dietary fiber intake of 30 patients with CD were significantly less than that of 30 controls.[5] While the median duration of symptoms in the CD patients was only 15 months, the range was wide, from 1 to 92 months; this confirmed the well-appreciated phenomenon that the validity of recall in some patients with longstanding symptoms may not be precise. Of interest was the finding that the CD patients consumed only about 25% of the raw fruit and vegetable fiber as the controls (0.6 vs. 2.3 g/d). A further study by Mayberry and co-workers found no difference between the dietary fiber intakes of patients with CD compared with normal controls.[2]

Table 5.7.1   Fiber Intake in Crohn's Disease

| No. Patients | Disease Duration | Fiber Intake (g/day) | | Ref. |
		Pre-Illness	Current	
35 Crohn's	1 year (av.)		26.6 (17.7[a])	4
70 Control			22.3 (14.5[a])	
30 Crohn's	5 mo	17.3 (0.2[b])		5
30 Control	(range: 1–92)	19.2 (2.3[b])		
16 Crohn's	Not stated		14	2
16 Control			20	

[a] Non-cellulose polysaccharides.
[b] Raw fruit and vegetable fiber.

The observations by Thornton et al.[5] that the pre-illness diet of Crohn's patients may have been low in fiber, especially raw fruit and vegetable fiber, led to several further studies (Table 5.7.2). Heaton et al.[6] reported the effects of treating 32 CD patients with a fiber-rich diet for a period of 4 years and 4 months. CD patients who were not provided with dietary instruction served as retrospective controls. While the study reports higher refined carbohydrate intake in controls compared to CD patients on the diet, no figures for dietary fiber intake in controls were given. The CD patients on the modified high-fiber, low-sugar diet had significantly fewer hospital admissions and total days in hospital compared to the control patients. While the number of operations in those patients on the special diet was fewer (1 vs. 5), the statistical significance of this was not defined.

Table 5.7.2   Fiber Trials in Crohn's Disease

No. Patients	Study Duration	Daily Fiber (g)	Daily Sugar (g)	Patient Admissions	Operations	Ref.
Retrospective controls						
32 Fiber	52 mo	33.4	39	11 (111 d)	1	6
32 Control			90	18 (533 d)	5	
Prospective, randomized						
30 Normalized	29 mo	13[a]			4	7
28 Low-residue		3			5	
190 High-fiber	2 yr	27.9[a]	9	18	7	8
162 Low-fiber		15.7	92	21	14	

[a] Low refined carbohydrate, high vegetable, and fruit fiber ("Bristol diet").

The apparent success of this "Bristol diet" led to a prospective study by Levenstein et al.[7] Thirty patients with CD placed on a "normalized" diet were compared to 28 patients given the "usual" low-residue diet prescribed in Italy. The number of portions of fiber consumed by those on the "normalized" diet was significantly higher than the number taken by those on the "usual" diet, but the significance of the difference in the total fiber intake (13 vs. 3 g) was not stated. Over a period of 29 months, there were no differences in outcome with respect to symptoms, hospitalizations, operations, complications, nutritional status, or postoperative recurrence. A second prospective randomized controlled study was reported by Ritchie et al.,[8] in which 190 patients with CD received the high fiber "Bristol diet" while 162 received the "low-fiber" diet. Patients in the "high-fiber" group also restricted their intake of refined carbohydrate, while those in the "low-fiber" group were encouraged to eat refined carbohydrate. No differences were found in clinical outcome over the two-year study period. Significantly more patients in the high-fiber group withdrew from the trial for reasons other than disease deterioration.

More recently, a population-based case-control study on dietary habits of patients with inflammatory bowel disease in Stockholm was reported.[9] Retrospective dietary habits over a five-year period were evaluated in 152 patients with Crohn's disease and compared to 145 ulcerative colitis patients and 305 controls. The relative risk of Crohn's disease was decreased in those consuming a high intake of fiber (15 g or more per day). Later, Geerling et al.[10] observed that the mean daily intake of fiber was significantly lower in Crohn's disease patients than in controls from the Netherlands.

FIBER STUDIES IN UC

Only limited studies have examined the effects of dietary fiber in UC (Table 5.7.3). Davies and Rhodes divided 39 patients with UC in remission on sulfasalazine into two groups.[11] Fifteen patients continued on sulfasalazine and their regular diet, while 20 of the 24 patients who tolerated a high-fiber diet were continued on that diet with sulfasalazine being stopped. The increased fiber was taken in the form of whole wheat bread, vegetables, and a supplement of 25 g bran supplied as Kellogg's All Bran or Allinson's Bran Plus. The cumulative relapse rates of the sulfasalazine group and the fiber group were 20 and 70%, respectively, over 6 months. The relapse rate on the high-fiber diet was similar to that expected in UC patients treated with placebo. A second study by Thornton et al.[12] examined the "pre-illness" diet of 30 patients with UC diagnosed within the previous 3 months. No differences were detected in refined carbohydrate or fiber intakes between these UC patients and 30 control subjects. Later, Hallert et al.[13] reported that ispaghula husk may relieve gastrointestinal symptoms in patients with UC.

Table 5.7.3   Fiber in Ulcerative Colitis

No. Patients	Disease Duration	Daily Fiber (g) Pre-Illness	Trial	Daily Sugar (g)	Relapse No. (rate, %)	Ref.
Retrospective controls						
30 UC	2 mo	19.9		97		12
30 Control		18.3		96		
Prospective, randomized						
15 Sulfasalazine	8.5 yr		13[a]		3 (15%)	11
20 High-fiber			3		15 (75%)	

[a] Fiber added as bran cereal, whole wheat bread, and vegetables.

In a recent randomized clinical trial of dietary fiber (administered in the form of Plantago ovata seeds), a Spanish group[14] described its effectiveness in maintaining remission in UC, being equivalent to mesalamine, a commonly prescribed anti-inflammatory pharmacologic agent. Finally, the effects of different forms of fiber have been evaluated in UC patients that have been surgically treated with an ileal pouch–anal anastomosis.[15] In a study from Seattle, no definite effects were documented on pouch function with either pectin or methyl cellulose.

SHORT-CHAIN FATTY ACIDS IN IBD

While only limited data are available to support a prominent role for fiber in the treatment of IBD, renewed interest has resulted from the recognition that important metabolic by-products of fiber, i.e., short-chain fatty acids (SCFAs), in the colon may be very relevant in disease pathogenesis and, possibly, therapy. Several studies in ileostomy subjects have shown that about 90 to 100% of orally admininstered fiber is recoverable in the ileostomy effluent.[16,17] When the fiber reaches the colon, anaerobic bacteria metabolize a varying amount to gases (CO_2, H_2, CH_4) and SCFAs (predominately butyrate, propionate, and acetate).[18] The SCFAs which are produced have been shown to be important sources of energy for colonocytes.[19] In addition, SCFAs stimulate colonic sodium and water absorption.[20,21] Diversion of the fecal stream as occurs, e.g., following colostomy, may result in an inflamed distal excluded segment, called "diversion colitis." Harig and co-workers[22] have reported improvement in diversion colitis using rectal SCFA irrigations.

In addition to a possible role for fiber in the generation of SCFAs in various colonic disorders, unabsorbed complex carbohydrates *per se* have been hypothesized to play a part in the diarrhea pathogenesis in IBD. Of course, totally undigested fiber probably has minimal effects, since fiber has very little osmotic activity. Metabolism of fiber entering the colon to SCFAs and lactic acid, however, would increase the osmotic load and provide a mechanism for diarrhea in IBD. However, as noted above, SCFA production may not lead to diarrhea due to their rapid absorption by the colon, their use as a colonic fuel, and their stimulation of sodium and water absorption.

Vernia et al.[23,24] have shown that fecal lactic acid concentrations are increased in both Crohn's colitis and UC, but that fecal weights correlate with lactic acid concentrations only in UC. Fecal SCFA concentrations were found to be much lower in patients with UC than in those with Crohn's colitis, in whom fecal concentrations were similar to those of normal controls. Holtug and co-workers have reported that some of the changes in SCFA pattern in UC may be due to bacterial fermentation of blood.[25] Indeed, other investigators have found higher SCFA levels in severe UC when compared with normal controls.[26] The reasons for the discrepancy in these studies are not clear but may relate to differences in methods or severity of disease.

The abnormalities in SCFAs in UC led Breuer et al.[27] to perform rectal irrigation of SCFAs in patients with distal UC. Twelve patients were treated with SCFA rectal irrigation over a period of 6 weeks in a non-blinded fashion. Nine were judged to be much improved. Clearly, a blinded, randomized, controlled trial will need to be conducted. If SCFAs are found to be better than placebos, the importance of these substances in UC will be confirmed.

REFERENCES

1. Martini, G. A. and Brandes, J. W., Increased consumption of refined carbohydrates in patients with Crohn's disease, *Klin. Wochenschr.*, 54, 367, 1976.
2. Mayberry, J. F., Rhodes, J., and Allan, R., Diet in Crohn's disease. Two studies of current and previous habits in newly diagnosed patients, *Dig. Dis. Sci.*, 26, 444, 1981.
3. Janerot, G., Jarnmark, I., and Nilsson, K., Consumption of refined sugar by patients with Crohn's disease, ulcerative colitis or irritable bowel syndrome, *Scand. J. Gastroenterol.*, 18, 999, 1983.
4. Kasper, H. and Sommer, H., Dietary fiber and nutrient intake in Crohn's disease, *Digestion*, 20, 323, 1979.
5. Thornton, J. R., Emmett, P. M., and Heaton, K. W., Diet and Crohn's disease: characteristics of the pre-illness diet, *Br. Med. J.*, 2, 762, 1979.
6. Heaton, K. W., Thornton, J. R., and Emmett, P. M., Treatment of Crohn's disease with an unrefined-carbohydrate, fibre-rich diet, *Br. Med. J.*, 2, 764, 1979.
7. Levenstein, S., Prantera, C., Luzi, C., and D'Ubaldi, A.., Low residue or normal diet in Crohn's disease: a prospective controlled study in Italian patients, *Gut*, 26, 989, 1985.
8. Ritchie, J. K., Wadsworth, J., Lennard-Jones, J. E., and Rogers, E., Controlled multicentre therapeutic trial of an unrefined carbohydrate, fibre-rich diet in Crohn's disease, *Br. Med. J.*, 295, 517, 1987.
9. Persson, P. G., Ahlbom, A., and Hellers, G., Diet and inflammatory bowel disease: a case-control study, *Epidemiology*, 3, 47, 1992.
10. Geerling, B. J., Badart-Smook, A., Stockbrugger, R. W., and Brummer, R. J., Comprehensive nutritional status in patients with long-standing Crohn disease in remission, *Am. J. Clin. Nutr.*, 67, 919, 1998.
11. Davies, P. S. and Rhodes, J., Maintenance of remission in ulcerative colitis with sulfasalazine or a high-fibre diet: a clinical trial, *Br. Med J.*, 1, 1524, 1978.
12. Thornton, J. R., Emmett, P. M., and Heaton, K. W., Diet and ulcerative colitis, *Br. Med. J.*, 280, 293, 1980.

13. Hallert, C., Kaldma, M., and Petersson, B. G., Ispaghula husk may relieve gastrointestinal symptoms in ulcerative colitis in remission, *Scand. J. Gastroenterol.*, 26, 747, 1991.

14. Fernandez-Banares, F., Hinojosa, J., Sanchez-Lombrana, J. L., Navarro, E., Martinez-Salmeron, J. F., Garcia-Puges, A., Gonzalez-Huix, F., Riera, J., Gonzalez-Lara, V., Dominguez-Abascal, F., Gine, J. J., Moles, J., Gomollon, F., and Gassull, M. A., Randomized clinical trial of Plantago ovata seeds (dietary fiber) as compared with mesalamine in maintaining remission in ulcerative colitis. Spanish Group for the Study of Crohn's disease and ulcerative colitis, *Am. J. Gastroenterol.*, 94, 427, 1999.

15. Thirlby, R. C. and Kelly, R., Pectin and methyl cellulose do not affect intestinal function in patients after ileal pouch-anal anastomosis, *Am. J. Gastroenterol.*, 92, 99, 1997.

16. Englyst, H. N. and Cummings, J. H., Digestion of the carbohydrates of banana (Musa paradisiacal sapientum) in the human small intestine, *Am. J. Clin. Nutr.*, 44, 42, 1986.

17. Englyst, H. N. and Cummings, J. H., Digestion of polysaccharides of potato in the small intestine of man, *Am. J. Clin. Nutr.*, 45, 423, 1987.

18. Cummings, J. H., Short chain fatty acids in the human colon, *Gut*, 22, 763, 1981.

19. Roediger, W. E. W., Utilization of nutrients by isolated epithelial cells of the rat colon, *Gastroenterology*, 83, 424, 1982.

20. Ruppin, H., Bar-Meir, S., Soergel, K. H., Wood, C. M., and Schmitt, M. G., Absorption of short-chain fatty acids by the colon, *Gastroenterology*, 78, 424, 1980.

21. Roediger, W. E. W. and Rae, D. A., Trophic effect of short chain fatty acids on mucosal handling of ions by the defunctioned colon, *Br. J. Surg.*, 69, 23, 1982.

22. Harig, J. M., Sorgel, K. H., Komorowski, R. A., and Woods, C.M., Treatment of diversion colitis with short chain fatty acid irrigation, *N. Engl. J. Med.*, 320, 23, 1989.

23. Vernia, P., Gnaedinger, A., Hauck, W., and Breuer, R. I., Organic anions and the diarrhea of inflammatory bowel disease, *Dig. Dis. Sci.*, 33, 1353, 1988.

24. Vernia, P., Caprilli, R., Latella, G., Barbetti, F., Magliocca, F. M., and Cittadini, M., Fecal lactate and ulcerative colitis, *Gastroenterology*, 95, 1564, 1988.

25. Holtug, K., Rasmussen, H. S., and Mortensen, P. B., Short chain fatty acids in inflammatory bowel disease. The effect of bacterial fermentation of blood, *Scand. J. Clin. Lab. Invest.*, 48, 667, 1988.

26. Roediger, W. E. W., Heyworth, M., Willoughby, P., Piris, J., Moore, A., and Truelove, S. C., Luminal ions and short chain fatty acids as markers of functional activity of the mucosa in ulcerative colitis, *J. Clin. Pathol.*, 35, 323, 1982.

27. Breuer, R. I., Buto, S. K., and Christ, M. L., Rectal irrigation with short chain fatty acids for distal ulcerative colitis, *Dig. Dis., Sci.*, 36, 185, 1991.

CHAPTER **5.8**

Disease Patterns in Japan and Changes in Dietary Fiber (1930–1980)

Keisuke Tsuji and Bunpei Mori

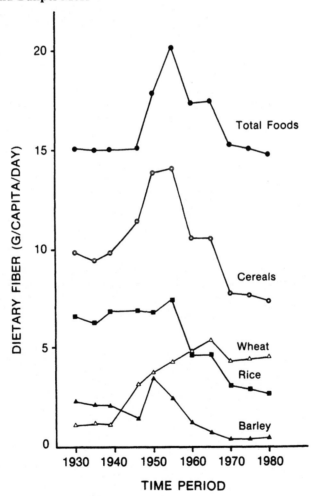

Figure 5.8.1 Dietary fiber (DF) intake by the Japanese people since 1930, where DF intake (grams per capita per day) = food intake × DF content. Food intake values are from Food Balance Tables of Japan.[1] DF content values are rice, 1.18 to 2.70%;[2] wheat, 1.02%;[3] and barley, 4.86%.[4]

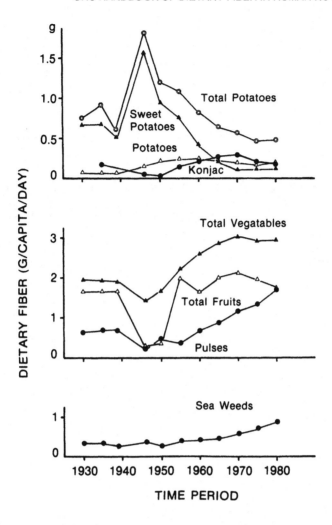

Figure 5.8.2 Dietary fiber (DF) intake by the Japanese people from potatoes, vegetables, fruit, pulses, and seaweeds since 1930 where DF intake (grams per capita per day) = food intake × DF content. Food intake values are from Food Balance Tables of Japan.[1] DF content values are sweet potatoes, 1.01%;[5] potatoes, 0.54%;[5] pulses as soybeans, 7.77%;[5] total vegetables, 0.96%;[2] total fruits, 1.14%;[2] seaweeds, 23.6%;[2] and konjac flour, 80%.[6]

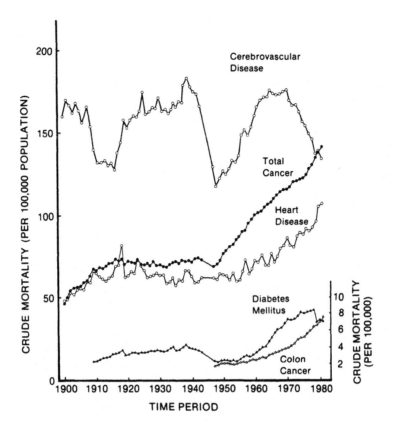

Figure 5.8.3 Changes of death rates from adult disease in Japan.[7]

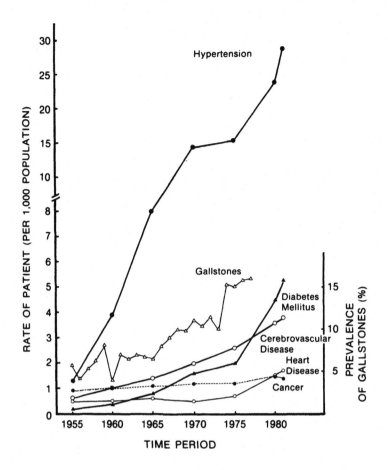

Figure 5.8.4 Number of patients in Japan suffering from adult diseases[8] and from gallstones.[9]

REFERENCES

1. Food Balance Tables of Japan, 1930–1980.
2. Mori, B., Contents of dietary fiber in some Japanese foods and the amount ingested through Japanese meals, *Nutr. Rep. Int.,* 26, 159, 1982.
3. Paul, A. A. and Southgate, D. A. T., McCance and Widdowson's *The Composition of Foods,* 4th ed., Her Majesty's Stationary Office, London, 1978.
4. Ayano, Y., *Chori Kagaku,* 15, 16, 1982.
5. Hoshi, S. and Takehitsa, F., Insoluble dietary fiber contents of foodstuffs, *Eiyo to Shokuryo,* 35, 133, 1982.
6. Tsuji, K. et al., unpublished data.
7. Japan Vital Statistics (1900–1980).
8. Japan Patient Survey (1955–1982).
9. Kameta, H. et al., *Jpn. Med. J.,* 2924, 24, 1980.

Dietary Fiber Modification of Toxin- or Carcinogen-Induced Effects on Intestinal and Mammary Tissues*

Hugh J. Freeman and Gene A. Spiller

The possible antitoxic effect of dietary fiber or fiber-rich foods and, more specifically, the possible protective role of dietary fiber in carcinogenesis has been the subject of many studies. After the hypothesis that colon cancer may be less common in populations consuming a high-fiber diet was proposed (see Chapter 5.5), the number of laboratory animal model studies on chemically induced carcinogenesis in the presence of various types of dietary fiber increased rapidly. Many of the early studies were done by Erschoff,[1,4,9,11] who demonstrated that otherwise-toxic levels of various substances in foods became either less toxic or non-toxic if the subject was fed with foods high in dietary fiber or some of the fiber polymers. This complex function of the fiber polymers, or high-fiber foods, is an important one. The long-term effects of low fiber compared to high fiber intakes on the toxic effects of food components, food contaminants, and, in general, environmental toxic substances, can have major implications on the etiology and/or pathogenesis of some diseases, specifically those that might be induced by carcinogens. It is interesting to note that some dietary fibers or dietary fiber-rich foods are protective for some toxic substances but not for others, and Erschoff showed that other beneficial effects such as the hypocholesterolemic effect of some fibers is often not connected to their antitoxic effects.[8] An example is locust bean gum, which is hypocholesterolemic but does not prevent cyclamate toxicity in rats when cyclamate is fed at the 5% level. Other examples of the specificity of the antitoxic effect of high-fiber substances are given in Tables 5.9.1 and 5.9.2. These studies emphasize that the effect of dietary fiber depends on the composition of its fiber components.

A problem instrinsic to these animal studies is that the same toxicity experiments cannot be done in humans. As a result, their limitation is the extrapolation to humans from animal studies. Table 5.9.1 summarizes some of the studies of protection against toxicity in general and some early carcinogenesis studies. Table 5.9.2 focuses on more recent studies on carcinogenesis and the possible protective effect of dietary fiber polymers or high-fiber foods. Caution is required in the interpretation of results with high-fiber foods, as other non-fiber components of food might be responsible for the antitoxic or cancer-preventing effect. Differences in research protocols, diet composition, and many other factors are certainly responsible for the differences in some results obtained. The interaction between dietary fiber polymers and other components of the diet means that the composition of the entire diet is a key factor in carcinogenesis and toxicity studies.

---

* This chapter is an updated version of Chapter 7.10, Modification by Dietary Fiber of Toxic or Carcinogenic Effects, by Bandaru S. Reddy and Gene A. Spiller, in the second edition of the Handbook.

Table 5.9.1   Studies on the Antitoxic Effect of Dietary Fiber or High-Fiber Foods and Early Carcinogenesis Studies in Experimental Animals

Toxic Substance	Dietary Fiber Source	Amount in Diet (%)	Animal	Effect[a]	Ref.
Tween 60	Soybean meal	15	Rats	+	3
Glucoascorbic acid (4%)	Alfalfa meal	20	Rats	+	4
Tween 20	Alfalfa meal	10	Rats	+	5
Tween 60	Rye grass	10		+	
	Wheat grass	10		+	
	Fescue grass	10		+	
	Orchard grass	10		+	
	Purified cellulose	10		+	
Span 20	Alfalfa meal	20		−	
2,5-Di-t-butyl-hydroquinone	Stock diet[b] vs. purified diet		Rats	+	6
Chlorazanil hydrochloride	Alfalfa		Rats	+	7
Sodium cyclamate	Locus bean gum	10	Rats	−	8
	Purified cellulose	10		−	
	Psyllium seed powder	10		+	
	Alfalfa meal	20		+	
	Carrot root powder	20		+	
	Gum karaya	10		+	
Tween 60	Sodium alginate	15	Rats	+	8
	Psyllium seed	2.5 or 5		+	
	Alfalfa meal	10		+	
	Rice straw	10		+	
	Carrot root powder	10		+	
	Purified cellulose	10		−	
FD & C Red #2	Alfalfa meal	10	Rats	+	9
	Watercress powder	10		+	
	Parsley powder	10		+	
Calcium (CdCl₂)	Increased fiber[c] but differing diets		Rats	+	10
Tween 60	Alfalfa meal	10	Mice	+	11
	Wheat grass meal	10		+	
	Rye grass meal	10		+	
	Sodium alginate	5		+	
	Agar	5		+	
	Alfalfa juice[b]			−	
	Locust bean gum	10		−	
	Apple powder	10		−	
2-Acetylaminofluorene	Stock diets[c] vs. purified diets		Rats	+	12

Note: This table summarizes only selected results of the cited studies. In many of these studies, many other high-fiber substances and polymers were tested.

[a] "+" indicates a general protective effect (such as weight maintenance or survival) when compared to controls on fiber-free or lower-fiber diets, without specific studies on tumorigenesis; "−" indicates no protective effect.
[b] Amount corresponding to the alfalfa meal fed.
[c] The term "stock diet" refers to diets based on natural foods (grains, alfalfa, etc.). These diets were usually compared to diets based on purified ingredients such as casein, starch, and glucose.

Table 5.9.2   Studies on the Protective Effect of Dietary Fiber or High-Fiber Foods in Chemical Carcinogenesis Studies

Carcinogen	Dietary Fiber Source (%)	Amount in Diet (%)	Animal	Effect[a]	Ref.
		Colon Studies			
1,2-DMH	Oat bran	20	SD rats	– –	26
1,2-DMH	Guar gum	10	SD rats	– –	26
1,2-DMH	Guar gum	5	SD rats	– –	27
AOM	Phytic acid	1	Fischer rats	+++	28
1,2-DMH	Wheat bran	20	SD rats	+++	13
AOM	Wheat bran	15	Fischer rats	+++	14
AOM	Wheat bran	15	Fischer rats	+++	15
3,2-DM-4-ABP	Wheat bran	15	Fischer rats	+++	16
AOM	Wheat bran	20	SD rats	+++	17
AOM	Wheat bran	30	SD rats	+++	17
1,2-DMH	Wheat bran	20	SD rats	+++	18
1,2-DMH	Wheat bran	20	Fischer rats	+++	19
1,2-DMH	Wheat bran	20	SD rats	– –	20[b]
1,2-DMH	Wheat bran	20	SD rats	– –	18[c]
1,2-DMH	Wheat bran	20	Balb/c mice	– –	21[d]
MNU	Wheat bran	15	Fischer rats	– –	14[e]
AOM	Wheat bran		Fischer rats	+++	40[f]
AOM	Citrus fiber	15	Fischer rats	+++	15
3,2-DM-4-ABP	Citrus fiber	15	Fischer rats	+++	16
3,2-DM-4-ABP	Corn bran	15	Fischer rats	–	22
1,2-DMH	Corn bran	20	Balb/c mice	–	21[d]
1,2-DMH	Corn bran	20	Fischer rats	–	19
1,2-DMH	Rice bran	20	Fischer rats	–	19
1,2-DMH	Soybean bran	20	Fischer rats	–	19
1,2-DMH	Soybean bran	20	Balb/c mice	–	21[d]
AOM	Alfalfa	20	SD rats	+++	17
AOM	Alfalfa	30	SD rats	+++	17
AOM	Alfalfa	15	Fischer rats	–	14
MNU	Alfalfa	15	Fischer rats	–	14[c]
1,2-DMH	Barley fiber		SD rats	+++	33
AOM	Coffee fiber	10	Fischer rats	+++	34[a]
1,2-DMH	Carrot fiber	20	SD rats	–	20[b]
AOM	Pectin	15	Fischer rats	+++	14
1,2-DMH	Pectin	4.5	Wistar rats	–	23
1,2-DMH	Pectin	9	Wistar rats	–	23
1,2-DMH	Pectin	6.5	SD rats	–	20[b]
1,2-DMH	Pectin	4.5	Wistar rats	–	35
1,2-DMH	Pectin	9	Wistar rats	–	35
1,2-DMH	Hemicellulose	4.5	Wistar rats	+++	36
1,2-DMH	Cellulose	4.5	Wistar rats	+++	24
1,2-DMH	Cellulose	4.5	Wistar rats	+++	23
1,2-DMH	Cellulose	9	Wistar rats	+++	23
1,2-DMH	Cellulose	4.5	Wistar rats	+++	35
1,2-DMH	Cellulose	9	Wistar rats	+++	35
AOM	Cellulose	40	Fischer rats	+++	25
AOM	Cellulose	20	SD rats	+++	17
AOM	Cellulose	30	SD rats	+++	17

Table 5.9.2 (Continued) Studies on the Protective Effect of Dietary Fiber or High-Fiber Foods in Chemical Carcinogenesis Studies

Carcinogen	Dietary Fiber Source (%)	Amount in Diet (%)	Animal	Effect[a]	Ref.
AOM	Cellulose	20	Fischer rats	–	25
3,2-DM-4-ABP	Lignin	7.5	Fischer rats	+++	22
1,2-DMH	Cellulose		SD rats	+++	37
1,2-DMH	Lignin		SD rats	–	37
1,2-DMH	Cellulose	5	SD rats	+++	38
1,2-DMH	Cellulose	15	SD rats	+++	38
1,2-DMH	Cellulose	10	SD rats	+++	39

Mammary Studies

MNU	Wheat bran	10	Fischer rats	+++	26

Note: Listed studies refer to chemically induced carcinogenesis, but genetic model of intestinal polyposis (Apc knockout mice) shows protective role of high-fiber-containing diet for small and large intestinal neoplasia.[41]

[a] "+++" indicates a protective effect against tumorigenesis in the cited study (compared to fiber-free or lower-fiber diets); "–" indicates no protective effect in the cited study; "– –" indicates enhancing effect in the cited study.

[b] Experimental fiber diets were fed to animals 3 days before, during, and 14 days after carcinogen treatment. The animals were then transferred to standard rat pellets and fed this diet until termination of the experiment.

[c] Effect of wheat bran on stage of initiation was studied. Wheat bran was fed to rats during carcinogen treatment only. They were transferred to fiber-free diet until termination of the experiment.

[d] Animals fed the control diet or fiber-free diet had very low colon tumor incidence.

[e] MNU, methylnitrosourea is a direct-acting carcinogen. Other abbreviations used for indirect-acting carcinogens include 1,2-DMH, 1,2-dimethylhydrazine; AOM, azoxymethane; 3,2-DM-4-ABP, 3,2-dimethyl-4-amino-biphenyl.

[f] Study showed lipid portion of wheat bran critical for protective effect, with associated reduction in nitric oxide synthase and total cyclooxygenase activities (COX-1, COX-2).

REFERENCES

1. Ershoff, B. H., Antitoxic effects of plant fibers, *Am. J. Clin. Nutr.*, 27, 1395, 1974.
2. Kritchevsky, D., Modification by fiber of toxic dietary effects, *Fed. Proc. Fed. Am. Soc. Exp. Biol.*, 36, 1692, 1977.
3. Chow, B. F., Burnett, J. M., Ling, C. T., and Barrows, L., Effect of basal diet on the response of rats to certain dietary non-ionic surface-active agents, *J. Nutr.*, 49, 563, 1953.
4. Ershoff, B. H., Beneficial effect of alfalfa and other succulent plants on glucoascorbic acid toxicity in the rat, *Proc. Soc. Exp. Biol. Med.*, 95, 656, 1957.
5. Ershoff, B. H., Beneficial effect of alfalfa meal and other bulk-containing or bulk-forming materials on the toxicity of nonionic surface-active agents in the rat, *J. Nutr.*, 70, 484, 1960.
6. Ershoff, B. H., Comparative effects of a purified and stock diet on DBH (2,5-di-*t*-butylhydroquinone), toxicity in the rat, *Proc. Soc. Exp. Biol. Med.*, 141, 857, 1972.
7. Ershoff, B. H., Beneficial effect of alfalfa meal on chlorazanil hydrochloride toxicity in the rat, *Exp. Med. Surg.*, 17, 204, 1959.
8. Ershoff, B. H. and Marshall, W. E., Protective effect of dietary fiber in rats fed toxic doses of sodium cyclamate and polyoxyethelene sorbitan monostearate (Tween 60), *J. Food Sci.*, 40, 357, 1975.
9. Ershoff, B. H. and Thurstun, E. W., Effects of diet on amaranth (FD & C Red No.2) toxicity in the rat, *J. Nutr.*, 104, 937, 1974.
10. Wilson, R. H. and De Eds, F., Importance of diet in studies of chronic toxicity, *Arch. Ind. Hyg. Occup. Med.*, 1, 73, 1950.

11. Ershoff, B. H. and Hernandez H. J., Beneficial effects of alfalfa meal and other bulk-containing or bulk-forming materials on symptoms of Tween 60 toxicity in the immature mouse, *J. Nutr.*, 69, 172, 1959.
12. Engel, B. W. and Copeland, D. H., Protective action of stock diets against the cancer-inducing action of 2-acetylaminofluorene in rats, *Cancer Res.*, 12, 211, 1952.
13. Wilson, R. B., Hutcheson, D. P., and Wideman, L., Dimethylhydrazine-induced colon tumors in rats fed diets containing beef fat or corn oil with and without wheat bran, *Am. J. Clin. Nutr.*, 30, 176, 1977.
14. Watanabe, K., Reddy, B. S., Weisburger, J. H., and Kritchevsky, D., Effect of dietary alfalfa, pectin, and wheat bran on azoxymethane- or methynitrosourea-induced colon carcinogenesis in F344 rats, *J. Natl. Cancer Inst.*, 63, 141, 1979.
15. Reddy, B. S., Mori, H., and Nicolais, M., Effect of dietary wheat bran and dehydrated citrus fiber on azoxymethane-induced intestinal carcinogenesis in Fischer F344 rats, *J. Natl. Cancer Inst.*, 66, 553, 1981.
16. Reddy, B. S. and Mori, H., Effect of dietary wheat bran and dehydrated citrus fiber on 3,2-dimethyl-4-aminobiphenyl-induced intestinal carcinogenesis in F344 rats, *Carcinogenesis*, 2, 21, 1981.
17. Nigro, N. D., Bull, A. W., Klopfer, B. A., Pak, M. S., and Campbell, R. L., Effect of dietary fiber on azoxymethane-induced intestinal carcinogenesis in rats, *J. Natl. Cancr Inst.*, 62, 1097, 1979.
18. Jacobs, L. R., Enhancement of rat colon carcinogenesis by wheat bran consumption during the stage of 1,2-dimethylhydrazine administration, *Cancer Res.*, 43, 4057, 1983.
19. Barnes, D. S., Clapp, N. K., Scott, D. A., and Berry, S. G., Effects of wheat, rice, corn, and soybean bran on 1,2-dimethylhydrazine-induced large bowel tumorigenesis, *Nutr. Cancer*, 5, 1, 1983.
20. Bauer, H. G., Asp, N., Oste, R., Dahlquist, A., and Fredlund, P. E., Effect of dietary fiber on induction of colorectal tumors and fecal B-glucuronidase activity in the rat, *Cancer Res.*, 39, 3752, 1979.
21. Clapp, N. K., Henke, M. A., London, J. F., and Shock T. L., Enhancement of 1,2-dimethylhydrazine-induced large bowel tumorigenesis in Balb/c mice by corn, soybean and wheat bran, *Nutr. Cancer*, 6, 77, 1984.
22. Reddy, B. S., Maeura, Y., and Wayman, M., Effect of dietary corn bran and autohydrolyzed lignin on 3,2-dimethyl-4-aminobiphenyl-induced intestinal carcinogenesis in male F344 rats, *J. Natl. Cancer Inst.*, 71, 419, 1983.
23. Freeman, H. J., Spiller, G. A., and Kim, Y. S., A double-blind study on the effects of differing purified cellulose and pectin fiber diets on 1,2-dimethylhydrazine-induced rat colonic neoplasia, *Cancer Res.*, 40, 2661, 1980.
24. Freeman, H. J., Spiller, G. A., and Kim, Y. S., A double-blind study on the effects of purified cellulose dietary fiber on 1,2-dimethylhydrazine-induced rat colonic neoplasia, *Cancer Res.*, 38, 2912, 1978.
25. Ward, J. M., Yamamoto, R. S., and Weisburger, J. H., Cellulose dietary bulk and azoxymethane-induced intestinal cancer, *J. Natl. Cancer Inst.*, 51, 713, 1973.
26. Jacobs, L. R. and Lupton, J. R., Relationship between colonic luminal pH, cell proliferation, and colon carcinogenesis in 1,2-dimethylhydrazine treated rats fed high fiber diets, *Cancer Res.*, 46, 1727, 1986.
27. Bauer, H. G., Asp, N. G., Dahlquist, A., Fredlund, P. E., Nyman, M., and Oste, R., Effect of two kinds of pectin and guar gum on 1,2-dimethylhydrazine initiation of colon tumors and on fecal B-glucuronidase activity in the rat, *Cancer Res.*, 41, 2518, 1981.
28. Ullah, A. and Shamuddin, A. M., Dose-dependent inhibition of large intestinal cancer by inositol hexaphospate in F344 rats, *Carcinogenesis*, 11, 2219, 1990.
29. Cohen, L. A., Kendall, M. E., Zang, E., Meschter, C., and Rose, D. P., Modulation of N-nitrosomethylurea-induced mammary tumor promotion by dietary fiber and fat, *J. Natl. Cancer Inst.*, 83, 496, 1991.
30. Reddy, B. S., Dietary fiber and colon carcinogenesis: a critical review, in *Dietary Fiber in Health and Disease*, Vahouny, G.V. and Kritchevsky, D., Eds., Plenum Press, New York, 1982, 265.
31. Freeman, H. J., Experimental animal studies in colon carcinogenesis and dietary fiber, in *Medical Aspects of Dietary Fiber*, Spiller, G. A. and McPherson-Kay, R., Eds., Plenum Press, New York, 1980, 83.
32. Pilch, S. M., Physiological Effects and Health Consequences of Dietary Fiber, Life Sciences Research Office, Federation of American Societies for Experimental Biology, Bethesda, MD, 1987.
33. McIntosh, G. H., Jorensen, L., and Royle, P., The potential of an insoluble dietary fiber-rich source from barley to protect from DMH-induced intestinal tumors in rats, *Nutr. Cancer*, 19, 213, 1993.

34. Rao, C. V., Chou, D., Simi, B., Ku, H., and Reddy, B. S., Prevention of colonic aberrant crypt foci and modulation of large bowel microbial activity by dietary coffee fiber, inulin and pectin, *Carcinogenesis*, 19, 1815, 1998.

35. Freeman, H. J., Effects of differing purified cellulose, pectin and hemicellulose fiber diets on fecal enzymes in 1,2-dimethylhydrazine-iduced rat colon carcinogenesis, *Cancer Res.*, 46, 5529, 1986.

36. Freeman, H. J., Spiller, G. A., and Kim, Y. S., Effect of high hemicellulose corn bran on 1,2-dimethylhydrazine-induced rat intestinal neoplasia, *Carcinogenesis*, 5, 261, 1984.

37. Sloan, D. A., Fleiszer, D. M., Richards, G. K., Murray, D., and Brown, R. A., The effect of the fiber components cellulose and lignin on experimental colon neoplasia, *J. Surg. Oncol.*, 52, 77, 1993.

38. Hertman, D. W., Ord, V. A., Hunter, K. E., and Cameron, I. L., Effect of dietary cellulose on cell proliferation and progression of 1,2-dimethylhydrazine-induced colon carcinogenesis in rats, *Cancer Res.*, 49, 5581, 1989.

39. Sakamoto, J., Nakaji, S., Sugawara, K., Iwane, S., and Munakata, A., Comparison of resistant starch with cellulose diet on 1,2-dimethylhydrazine-induced colonic carcinogenesis in rats, *Gastroenterology*, 110, 116, 1996.

40. Reddy, B. S., Hirose, Y., Cohen, L. A., Simi, B., Cooma, I., and Rao, C. V., Preventive potential of wheat bran fractions against experimental colon carcinogenesis: implications for human colon cancer prevention, *Cancer Res.*, 60, 4792, 2000.

41. Hioki, K., Shivapurkar, N., Oshima, H., Alabaster, O., Oshima, M., and Taketo, M. M., Suppression of intestinal polyp development by low-fat and high-fiber diet in Apc (delta716) knockout mice, *Carcinogenesis*, 18, 1863, 1997.

Effect of Whole Grains, Cereal Fiber, and Phytic Acid on Health

CHAPTER **6.1**

Whole Grain, Fiber, and Antioxidants

Gene Miller

INTRODUCTION

Considerable scientific data suggest that the risk of cancer, heart disease, and other chronic diseases of aging is reduced by diets high in fruits, whole grain products, and vegetables.[1-6] Several decades of research have focused on identification of food components and mechanisms to explain the positive health effect. Lignans have been the subject of considerable study,[7-9] but for grain products, most research centered on fiber as the efficacious agent. Such studies demonstrate the benefits of grain fiber, and sound mechanisms have been proposed to explain biological function.[10-13] Still, it has been suggested that fiber alone does not explain the full effect of whole grain products.[11,14,15] Epidemiological studies regarding fruits and vegetables clearly indicate their positive impact on health regarding chronic, degenerative disease.[16-18] Natural antioxidants such as vitamin C, vitamin E, and β-carotene were identified as potential active components. Experimental studies with individual compounds validate their importance but do not explain completely the efficacy of fruits and vegetables. The French paradox observation, where heart disease is relatively low for a wine-drinking population with high saturated fat intake,[19] draws attention to the wide variety of phenolic antioxidants that may act to prevent disease. In fact, flavonoids were recognized by Szent-Györgyi[20] in 1937 to have vitamin-like activity. In spite of sometimes-ambiguous results from experiments to test ability of pure compounds to inhibit cancer or coronary heart disease, it is generally accepted that natural antioxidants are important to good health.

WHOLE GRAIN ANTIOXIDANTS

Whole grains contain numerous antioxidants of different structural types.[21] Many are common among plants, but some are unique. Examples of a few grain antioxidant structures are shown in Figure 6.1.1. Cinnamic acids, benzoates, flavonoids, and tocopherols are basic antioxidant compounds common to grains, fruits, and vegetables in diverse structural combinations. Avenanthramides are unique to oats. Tocotrienols, long-chain mono- and diol-esters of ferulic and caffeic acids and alkyl resorcinols, are abundant in most grains. In addition, there are many other antioxidant compounds that occur in lesser amounts in grains. These compounds vary in solubility from freely soluble in water to fat soluble. Insoluble antioxidants include phenolic acids covalently bound by ester linkages to the arabinose side chains of arabinoxylan fiber polymers of cell walls.[22,23] These esters are about 90% ferulate and 10% coumarate, which together constitute about 1% of the grain

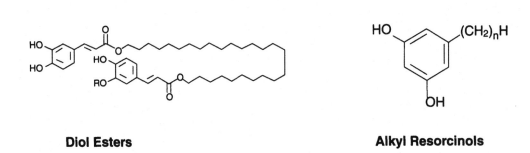

Cinnamic Acids

Tocopherols

Flavonoids

Avenanthramides

Diol Esters

Alkyl Resorcinols

Figure 6.1.1 Plant antioxidants.

seed coat. A substantial part of ferulate esters dimerizes to form diferulate bridges between fiber strands and give structural strength to the cell walls. Seven different diferulates have been identified that could be formed by a radical mechanism.[24]

Fiber-bound phenolic esters are common to grains and grasses but are found in only a few of the dicots, spinach and beets being familiar examples.[25] Antioxidants esterified to grain fiber are not available for absorption unless freed by enzymatic hydrolysis in the colon. The majority of grain antioxidants are found in outer layers of grain seeds, as are most other phytonutrients. Components of grain contained in thick-walled bran cells are hindered from absorption. Even soluble materials may be carried to the colon with bran, where they may or may not be released for absorption, dependent on microflora activity. In this respect, results from studies on physiological effects of diets that contain raw grain and bran or intact cooked grain could differ from studies using the same grains but that have been processed in ways that disrupt cellular structure.

ANTIOXIDANT CONTENT OF FOOD PRODUCTS

Since grains contain many different antioxidants with potential for health benefit, it was of interest to estimate total activity in grain products, fruits, and vegetables. The relative amount of antioxidant activity in these foods is an indication of potential contribution to disease reduction by antioxidant mechanisms. Analysis of antioxidant activity was done using a stable free radical, 1,1-diphenyl-2-picrylhydrazyl (DPPH), in 50% aqueous methanol.[26] DPPH has been thoroughly studied as an analytical reagent for antioxidants.[27,28] A significant part of the antioxidants in grains is not readily soluble in 50% aqueous methanol, is trapped in coarse cells of the bran, or is covalently bound to cell walls. Because of this, DPPH was reacted directly with finely ground sample in warm aqueous methanol for 4 hours.[29] This procedure measures soluble antioxidants and also allows the DPPH to react with insoluble antioxidants distributed throughout the food matrix. In addition to solubility issues, antioxidants have a wide range of activity, from highly reactive to very weak activity. The significance to human health of different antioxidant compounds that have diverse chemical properties is unknown, but a variety of compounds and activities offer potential protection for a range of human disease mechanisms.

Fruits, grains, vegetables, processed products, and ingredients were analyzed for antioxidant activity using the DPPH method. Results shown in Table 6.1.1 are expressed as Trolox equivalents per 100 g (TE) of sample. It is apparent that whole grain products average higher in antioxidant activity than fruits or vegetables on an *as is* basis. Similar results were reported for aqueous extracts of foods using ORAC (oxygen radical absorption capacity) technology.[30] The same kinds of fruits and vegetables were analyzed in both studies, but average activity for vegetables was similar to fruits by the ORAC method. This may be due to differences in products analyzed, solvent systems, or methodology. The ORAC method utilizes a high-energy free radical (2,2′-azobis(2-amidinopropane) dihydrochloride), which can react with weak antioxidants. DPPH is a bulky, stable free radical that reacts slowly with some antioxidants, and not at all with very weak proton radical donors. For example, DPPH reacts very slightly with β-carotene and only slowly with vanillic acid. This may partially explain why ORAC values on aqueous extracts of cereal products were similar to DPPH results of the whole product. Regardless, whole grain products are substantially higher in antioxidant activity than commonly consumed fruits and vegetables.

Table 6.1.1   Average Antioxidant Activity for Food Products

Food Material	Average TE/100 g
Common vegetables	400
Common fruits	1200
Whole wheat bread	2000
Whole grain breakfast cereals	2800

Antioxidant activity of different fruits, grains, and vegetables varies considerably, as previously reported.[26] Vegetables range from 1400 TE for red cabbage to 50 TE for celery; fruits vary from 2200 TE for red plums to 100 TE for melons. Antioxidant activity was 3000 TE for a whole wheat cereal and 1300 TE for a cereal made from refined rice. Consumption of a variety of foods is important to ensure a balanced intake of phytonutrients including antioxidants.

Antioxidant activity for common grains is shown in Table 6.1.2. As for fruits and vegetables, there are significant differences in activity between different grains. White rice with no bran has significant antioxidant activity but is considerably lower than brown rice with bran. Red wheat is higher in antioxidant activity than white wheat or oat groats. Pearled barley with partially removed bran is higher in antioxidant activity than red wheat. Rye is exceptionally high in antioxidant activity but, unfortunately, is a minor grain in most Western diets. Annual consumption of rye is

Table 6.1.2 Antioxidant Activity of Grains

Grain	TE/100 grams
White rice	700
Whole white wheat	1400
Brown rice	1500
Oat groats	1800
Whole red wheat	2500
Pearled barley	3100
Rye	4700

high in Finland, and it is believed to have important health benefits due to lignans and other phytonutrients.[7,31] All whole grains contain substantial antioxidant activity when compared to an average value for common fruits or vegetables. There is not a convenient way to evaluate the relative health significance of antioxidant mixtures in different foods, but it is reasonable to assume that very low activity foods have less potential for benefit than the medium or high activity foods.

Antioxidant activities calculated for an average serving of fruit, vegetable, whole wheat bread, or whole grain breakfast cereal are compared in Table 6.1.3. The amount of antioxidants from a serving of whole grain product is similar to that from an average serving of fruit and greater than an average serving of vegetables. Since Western diets typically contain relatively little whole grain products and are low in fruits and vegetables, antioxidant intake could be increased significantly by modest diet changes such as eating whole grain breakfast cereals and whole grain breads in place of refined grain products.

Table 6.1.3 Antioxidant Content For Average Servings of Whole Grain Products, Fruits, and Vegetables

Product	Serving (g)	TE Activity
Whole grain breakfast cereals	50	1400
Whole wheat bread	50	1000
Average fruit	100	1200
Average vegetable	100	630

Antioxidant activity is compared for grain fractions and grain products in Table 6.1.4. Antioxidants are concentrated in bran fractions, although the endosperm has significant activity. It is not possible from these results to determine how much of total bound or insoluble antioxidants is measured by DPPH, but DPPH analysis indicates that there is significant antioxidant activity associated with fiber of cereal grains. Even oat hulls that were extracted with aqueous alkali retained high antioxidant activity. Whole grain cereal that was extracted with 50% aqueous methanol had about 65% of starting activity. Insoluble antioxidants have not been completely identified, but it is reasonable to assume a significant part is from phenolic acids esterified to fiber. Tannins, which have very high antioxidant activity,[32] and lignins may explain some of the activity.

Table 6.1.4 Antioxidant Activity of Grain Fractions and Products

Ingredient	TE/100 grams
Red wheat flour	900
Red wheat bran	11000
Whole red wheat	2500
Alkali extracted oat hulls	6000
Aq. MeOH ext'd wheat cereal	1700
White bread (dry)	1600
Bread, crust (dry)	2050
Bread, white (dry)	1100

PROCESSING AND ANTIOXIDANTS

Another aspect of grain antioxidant activity is that it does not appear to decrease during bread making or processing for breakfast cereals. For example, antioxidant activity in baked bread is higher than the starting flour (Table 6.1.4). It appears that there is essentially no loss of natural antioxidants while there is formation of new antioxidant activity, most likely Maillard reaction products. This is demonstrated by comparison of crust antioxidant activity to that of crust-free white bread. The crust is about double in antioxidant activity compared to the crust-free part. The crust-free part is about the same as flour on an equal moisture basis. This suggests that there is little change in antioxidants in the interior of the bread loaf during baking. High temperature conditions at the loaf surface promote crust browning. Reductone products are characteristic of the Maillard reaction and may explain the increase in crust antioxidant activity. A similar effect is seen for breakfast cereals. Antioxidant activity increases gradually during cooking steps of breakfast cereal processing, but the biggest increase is from toasting.

ANTIOXIDANT ABSORPTION AND METABOLISM

It has been shown that natural antioxidants are bioavailable and that the level of antioxidant activity in blood increases on a diet high in fruits and vegetables or after consumption of foods high in antioxidants such as tea, wine, or fruits.[33-35] And it is known that antioxidants released in the colon by microbial action can be absorbed.[36] However, bioavailability of grain antioxidants in food products has not been determined specifically. Potential health benefit of unique antioxidants, including Maillard reaction products, is not known. It is reasonable to assume that many of the grain and grain product antioxidants are bioavailable and can function as free radical scavengers in the body. In addition, these compounds may also participate in other mechanisms suggested for specific antioxidants, such as reducing platelet adhesion, vasorelaxation, cell apoptosis, and induction of detoxification enzymes.[37-42] Further, antioxidants in the digestive tract have potential to react with nitrites and free radicals existing in food when consumed or generated by biological processes.

Bran fiber is of interest because of how it may effect the distribution and absorption of phytonutrients. If the bran of whole grains is essentially intact when it is consumed, the contents of cells will be much less available for absorption. Small molecules, readily soluble in water, may diffuse out of the bran cells, but other constituents would not be available at all except after fiber degradation by bacteria in the colon. Covalently bound phenolics are resistant to digestion in the stomach and small intestine, but enzymatic hydrolysis is possible in the colon.[43-45] Arabino-ferulates and free phenolic acids are released by microorganism fermentation. Diferulate release is possible but is more difficult because of attachment to two fiber chains.

From experiments with rats fed ^{14}C-labeled bound phenolics in spinach, it was determined that 19% of the label was excreted in the feces, 20% was excreted in urine, and over 34% of the label was retained in body tissues after 18 hours.[45] These results demonstrate that bound phenolics, after release in the colon by enzymatic hydrolysis, are bioavailable. High-protein and fatty diets reduce the abundance of colon microorganisms as compared to a high-fiber diet. In addition, antibiotics can inhibit growth of colon microflora that ferment fiber for over 30 days.[46] This suggests that availability of phytonutrients in whole grain will be reduced unless the grain is processed to open bran cells and colon microflora are healthy. It is essential that the everyday diet is relatively high in fiber to help sustain a microflora that is optimum for obtaining maximum health benefit from grain phytonutrients.

Fiber-bound phenolics were identified many years ago and have been the subject of considerable study in recent years.[22,44,47,48] Grain fiber material has significant antioxidant activity. This activity is consistent with reports for phenolic content in bran fractions, with consideration for natural variability and activity from insoluble polyphenolics such as lignin or tannins.[32,44,49] Antioxidant activity for a very pure sample of corn bran was 20,000 TE by DPPH analysis. This calculates for 3.9% ferulic acid if all activity is due to ferulates. It may be that corn bran contains high levels of ferulate, and it may contain small amounts of highly active compounds such as tannins.[32] The sample of very pure red wheat bran (Table 6.1.4) was 11,000 TE, equivalent to 2.1% ferulate. Although high, this is in the range of ferulate concentrations reported for wheat bran.[44,49,50] It is of interest that carob hulls, which are known to be high in tannin compounds, analyzed for 160,000 TE. Based on the activity measured for tannic acid (1,400,000 TE), carob could contain roughly 11% tannic acid that is reactive with DPPH in 50% aqueous methanol.

Processed whole grain products contain considerable antioxidant activity in the form of phenolic acids covalently bound to cell wall fiber. Grain products provide many phytonutrients, including antioxidants that are concentrated in the bran. It is possible that there is a synergistic relationship with fiber that goes beyond a simple combination of chemical compounds. In the case of antioxidants, there are several ways they can be utilized by the body. Fat-soluble antioxidants can be absorbed through the lymphatic system, and water-soluble antioxidants can be absorbed in the small intestine. Antioxidants covalently bound to cell wall fiber and compounds contained within cellular structures are transported to the large intestine, to be released by fermentation in the presence of appropriate microorganisms. Antioxidants released in this manner are available to scavenge free radicals present in the colon. Epithelial cells of the colon absorb free phenolics and can benefit from their antioxidant activity. In this manner, whole grain antioxidants can act as free radical scavengers through the entire digestive tract and in colon tissues. When fiber carries bound antioxidants to the colon, there is time-delayed activity present in the digestive tract. This activity, along with the protective effect of fiber and fiber fermentation products, may provide unique protection that is not possible by any single component. Transport of antioxidants to the colon is characteristic to whole grain materials because of covalently bound phenolics but is possible for only a few vegetables and fruits.

CONCLUSION

It is well established that grain fiber is important to human health. In addition, there are many other potential health-supporting phytonutrients in whole grains, including antioxidants, lignans, phytates, sterols, sphingolipids, tocotrienols, vitamins, and minerals. The health contribution of antioxidants in grain products has received little attention. Whole grain products provide equal or greater antioxidant activity compared to fruits or vegetables on a per-serving basis. Whole grain antioxidants represent a variety of structural types, including significant amounts of phenolic acids esterified to cell wall fiber. Covalently bound antioxidants are transported to the colon along with fiber and remain functional agents for an extended time period. Enzymatic hydrolysis in the colon can free phenolics for absorption into the epithelium. It is hypothesized that bound antioxidants, in synergy with fiber, deliver a unique functionality to the colon and are an important part of the overall health benefit provided by whole grain products. These hypothetical mechanisms offer additional possibilities to explain the efficacy of whole grain products to reduce chronic disease.

REFERENCES

1. National Academy of Sciences, *Diet and Health, Implications for Reducing Chronic Disease*, National Academy Press, Washington, DC, 1989.
2. World Cancer Research Fund and American Institute for Cancer Research, *Food, Nutrition and Prevention of Cancer: A Global Perspective*, AICR, Washington, DC, 1997.

3. Rimm, E. B., Ascherio, A., Giovannucci, E., Spiegleman, D., Stampfer, M. S., and Willet, W.C., Vegetable, fruit and cereal fiber intake and risk of coronary heart disease among men, *JAMA*, 275, 447, 1996.

4. Jacobs, D. R., Meyer, K. A., Kushi, L. H., and Folsom, A. R., Is whole grain intake associated with reduced total and cause-specific death rates in older women, the Iowa Women's Health Study, *Am. J. Public Health*, 89, 322, 1999.

5. Greenberg, E. R. and Sporn, M. B., Antioxidant vitamins, cancer and cardiovascular disease, *N. Eng. J. Med.*, 334, 1189, 1996.

6. Bruce, B., Spiller, G. A., Klevay, L. M., and Gallagher, S. K., A diet high in whole and unrefined foods favorably alters lipids, antioxidant defenses and colon function, *J. Am. College Nutr.*, 19(1), 61, 2000.

7. Adlercreutz, H. and Mazur, W., Phyto-oestrogens and western diseases, *Ann. Med.*, 29, 95, 1997.

8. Ford, J. D., Davin, L. B., and Lewis, N. G., Plant lignans and health: chemoprevention and biotechnoloical opportunities, in *Plant Polyphenols 2: Chemistry, Biology, Pharmacology, Ecology*, Gross et al., Eds., Kluwer Academic/Plenum Publishers, New York, 1999, 675–694.

9. COST 916, Phyto-estrogens: exposure, bioavailability, health benefits and safety concerns, Bausch-Goldbohm, S., Kardinal, A., and Serra, F., Eds., Office for Official Publications of the European Communities, Luxembourg, 1999.

10. Spiller, G. A., Ed., *CRC Handbook of Dietary Fiber in Human Nutrition*, 2nd ed., CRC Press, Boca Raton, FL, 1993.

11. Wolk, A., Manson, J. E., Stampfer, M., Colditz, G. A., Hu, F. B., Speizer, F. E., Hennekens, C. H., and Willet, W. C., Long-term intake of dietary fiber and decreased risk of coronary heart disease among women, *JAMA*, 281(21), 1998, 1999.

12. Andlauer, W. and Fürst, P., Does cereal reduce the risk of cancer?, *Cereal Foods World*, 44(2), 76, 1999.

13. Anderson, J. W. and Hanna, T. J., Whole grains and protection against coronary heart disease: what are the active components and mechanisms, *Am. J. Clin. Nutr.*, 70, 307, 1999.

14. Folino, M., McIntyr, A., and Young, G. P., Dietary fibers differ in their effects on large bowel epithelial proliferation and fecal fermentation-dependent events in rats, *J. Nutr.*, 125(6), 1521, 1995.

15. Jacobs, D. R., Marquart, L., Slavin, J., and Kushi, L. H., Whole grain intake and cancer: an expanded review and meta-analysis, *Nutr. Cancer*, 30(2), 85, 1998.

16. Steinberg, D., Antioxidants and atherosclerosis: a current assessment, *Circulation*, 84, 1420, 1991.

17. Gey, K. F., The antioxidant hypothesis of cardiovascular disease, epidemiology and mechanisms, *Biochem. Soc. Trans.*, 18, 1041, 1990.

18. Ames, B. M., Shigena, M. K., and Hagen, T. M., Oxidants, antioxidants and the degenerative diseases of aging, *Proc. Natl. Acad. Sci. USA*, 90, 7915, 1993.

19. Renaud, S. and de Lorgeril, M., Wine, alcohol, platelets and the French paradox for coronary heart disease, *Lancet*, 339, 1523, 1992.

20. Bentsath, A., Rusznyak, S., and Szent-Györgi, A., Vitamin P, *Nature*, 139, 326, 1937.

21. Collins, F. W., Oat phenolics: structure, occurrence and function, in *Oat Chemistry and Technology*, Webster, F. H., Ed., American Association of Cereal Chemists, St. Paul, 1986, chap. 9.

22. Fulcher, R. G., Morphological and chemical organization of the oat kernel, in *Oat Chemistry and Technology*, Webster, F. H., Ed., American Association of Cereal Chemists, St. Paul, 1986, chap. 3.

23. Andreasen, M. F., Christensen, L. P., Meyer, A. S., and Hanson, A., Content of phenolic acids and ferulic dehydrodimers in 17 rye (*secale cereale* L.) varieties, *J. Agric. Fd. Chem.*, 48, 2837, 2000.

24. Ralph, J., Quideau, S., Grabber, J. H., and Hatfield, R., Identification and synthesis of new ferulic acid dehydrodimers present in grass cell walls, *J. Chem. Soc. Perkin Trans. I*, 3485, 1994.

25. Saulnier, L. and Thibault, J. F., Ferulic acid and diferulic acid as components of sugar beet pectins and maize bran heteroxylans, *J. Sci. Fd. Agric.*, 79, 396, 1999.

26. Miller, H. E., Rigelhof, F., Marquart, L., Prakash, A., and Kanter, M., Antioxidant content of whole grain breakfast cereals, fruit and vegetables, *J. Am. Coll. of Nutr.*, 19(S), 3125, 2000.

27. Brand-Williams, W., Cuvelier, M. E., and Berset, C., Use of a free radical method to evaluate antioxidant activity, *Lebensm-Wiss U-Technol*, 28, 25, 1995.

28. Fukumoto, L. R. and Mazza, G., Assessing antioxidant and prooxidant activities of phenolic compounds, *J. Agric. Food Chem.*, 48, 3597, 2000.

29. Miller, H. E., Rigelhof, F., Marquart, L., Prakash, A., and Kanter, M., Whole grain products and antioxidants, *Cereal Foods World*, 45(2), 59, 2000.
30. Prior, R. L., Cao, G., and Inglett, G., Antioxidant content of cereal grain ingredients and commercial breakfast cereals, *Abstr. Papers Am. Chem. Soc.*, 216, 119, 1998.
31. Poutanen, K. and Liukkonan, K., Rye: a Nordic focus, *Func. Fd. Neutraceut.*, 3, 30, 2000.
32. Hagerman, H. E., Riedl, K. M., Jones, A., Sovik, K. N., Ritchard, N. T., and Hartzfeld, B. W., High molecular weight polyphenolics (tannins) as biological antioxidants, *J. Agric. Fd. Chem.*, 46, 1887, 1998.
33. Cao, G., Russel, R. M., Lischner, N., and Rrior, R. L., Serum antioxidant capacity is increased by consumption of strawberries, spinach, red wine or vitamin C in elderly women, *J. Nutr.*, 128, 2383, 1998.
34. Bourne, L. C. and Rice-Evans, C., Bioavailability of ferulic acid, *Biochem. Biophys. Res. Commun.*, 253, 222, 1998.
35. Hollman, C. H., Tijburg, L. B. M., and Yang, C. S., Bioavailability of flavanoids from tea, *Crit. Rev. Fd. Sci. Nutr.*, 37, 719, 1997.
36. Ohta, T., Semboku, N., Kuchi, A., Egashira, Y., and Sanada, H., Antioxidant activity of corn bran cell wall fragments in the LDL oxidation system, *J. Agric. Fd. Chem.*, 45, 1664, 1997.
37. Ursini, F., Tubaro, F., Rong, J., and Sevanian, A., Optimization of nutrition: polyphenols and vasculer protection, *Nutr. Rev.*, 57(8), 241, 1999.
38. Bravo, L., Polyphenols: chemistry, dietary source, metabolism and nutritional significance, *Nutr. Rev.*, 56(11), 317, 1998.
39. Slavin, J. L., Martini, M. C., Jacobs, J. R., and Marquart, L., Plausible mechanisms for the protectiveness of whole grains, *Am. J. Clin. Nutr.*, 70(5), 4595, 1999.
40. Ferguson, L. R. and Harris, P. J., Protection against cancer by wheat bran: role of dietary fibre and phytochemicals, *Eur. J. Cancer Prev.*, 8, 17, 1999.
41. Zhu, M., Phillipson, J. D., Greengrass, P. M., Bowery, N. E., and Cai, Y., Plant polyphenols: biologically active compounds or nonselective binders to protein?, *Phytochemistry*, 44, 441-447, 1997.
42. Kamal-Eldin, A., Frank, J., Razdan, A., Teugblad, S., Basu, S., and Vessby, B., Effects of dietary phenolic compounds on tocopherol, cholesterol, and fatty acids in rats, *Lipids*, 35(4), 427-435, 2000.
43. Chesson, A., Provan, G. J., Russell, W. R., Scobbie, L., Richardson, A. J., and Stewart, C., Hydroxycinnamic acids in the digestive tract of livestock and humans, *J. Sci. Fd. Agric.*, 79, 373, 1999.
44. Kroon, P. A., Faulds, C. B., Ryden, P., Robertson, J. A., and Williamson, G., Release of covalently bound ferulic acid from fiber in the human colon, *J. Agric. Fd. Chem.*, 45(3), 661, 1997.
45. Buchanan, C. J., Wallace, G., Fry, S. C., and Eastwood, M. C., In vivo release of ^{14}C-labeled penolics groups from intact dietary spinach cell walls during passage through rat intestine, *J. Sci. Fd. Agric.*, 71, 459, 1996.
46. Adlercreutz, H., personal communication, 2000.
47. Kroon, P. A. and Williamson, G., Hydroycinnamates in plants and food: current and future perspectives, *J. Sci. Fd. Agric.*, 79, 355, 1999.
48. Shiyi, O., Yan, L., and Kongron, G., A study on OH radical scavenging activity of dietary fibre from wheat bran, *Acta Nutrimenta Sinica*, 21(2), 191, 1999.
49. Andreasen, M. F., Christensen, L. P., Meyer, A. S., and Hansen, A., Release of hydroxycinnamic and hydroxybenzoic acids in rye by commercial plant cell wall degrading enzyme preparations, *J. Sci. Fd. Agric.*, 79, 411–413, 1999.
50. Smith, M. M. and Hartley, R. D., Occurrence and nature of ferulic acid substition of cell-wall polysaccharides in graminaceous plants, *Carb. Res.*, 118, 65, 1983.

Whole Grains, Cereal Fiber, and Chronic Diseases: Epidemiologic Evidence

Mark A. Pereira, Joel J. Pins, David R. Jacobs, Jr.,
Leonard Marquart, and Joseph Keenan

INTRODUCTION

The finding on cereal fibre illustrates one of the uses of epidemiology — in exploration.

J. N. Morris et al., *British Medical Journal*, 1977

The hypothesis that dietary fiber may reduce the risk for chronic diseases was extrapolated from the ecological observations of Burkitt et al.,[1] who compared and contrasted the diets and disease patterns of Westernized and non-Westernized cultures. This hypothesis came from whole plant foods, with fruits and vegetables historically and contemporaneously receiving much public health attention, and less attention being given to whole grain foods. Over the past few decades, important epidemiologic observations have been made on the topic of dietary fiber and chronic disease risk, thus fueling a reductionist approach rather than a "whole food" one. Recent epidemiologic findings on whole grain foods allow us to evaluate the food source of fiber, with its nutrient-rich complex still somewhat intact, in association with chronic disease risk. As such, we have developed a nontraditional hypothesis that fiber alone is only one potentially efficacious component of whole grains and other appropriately processed plant foods.

As indicated by the quote above by Morris and colleagues,[2] exploratory findings for cereal fiber intake and CHD risk were in need of support by candidate mechanisms, which we describe in Chapter 6.3, and confirmation from other studies in similar and different populations, which we describe herein. The goal of this chapter is to review the observational epidemiologic evidence for the potential role of cereal fiber and its primary food source — whole grains — in reducing risk for chronic diseases.

GRAIN INTAKE AND DEFINITIONS FOR EPIDEMIOLOGIC STUDIES

At the base of the Food Guide Pyramid, grains compose approximately 25% of the food supply in the U.S.[3] However, very little grain is available in whole or minimally refined form, with at least 95% being stripped of its bran and germ.[4,5] It has been estimated that average intake of whole grain products in the U.S. is ~0.5 eating occasions per day, with total grain products (whole + refined) being less than 3 per day in comparison to the recommended intake of 6 to 11 servings per day.[6]

In observational epidemiologic studies based on self-reported dietary intake, we are limited to rather crude differentiation between whole and refined grain intake. Foods coded as whole grain are those that we know or suspect to include bran and/or germ and therefore are a potentially nutrient-rich fiber complex. These include commercially available "dark" or "mixed grain" breads, brown rice, or brand-name breakfast cereals with a whole grain (or whole grain flour) as the first ingredient or elsewhere on the ingredient list with at least 2 g of fiber per serving.[7,8] In contrast, refined grains are defined for epidemiologic purposes as those foods that are known or strongly suspected to have no bran or germ due to the refining process and only the fiber-poor, nutrient-poor endosperm present. These include white bread, white rice, and brand-name breakfast cereals with a refined grain as the first ingredient and less than 2 g of fiber per serving. Table 6.2.1 summarizes the foods contributing to whole and refined grain intake for epidemiologic studies utilizing databases of self-reported intake.

The loss of critical nutrients in the bran and germ during the refining process is acknowledged by the enrichment of refined grains with many vitamins and minerals by the food industry in an attempt to replace natural nutrients. However, enrichment is insufficient when one considers that fiber, unsaturated fatty acids, and many micronutrients and phytochemicals, including some unidentified, are not able to be replaced. We have hypothesized that these nutrients present in grains in their natural form may act together, perhaps synergistically, in the body to modify risk for chronic diseases such as cardiovascular disease, diabetes, and cancer (see Chapter 6.3).[9] Epidemiologic evidence reviewed in this chapter, and experimental evidence of the accompanying chapter, may help to provide further impetus for modification of the current dietary guidelines in Westernized countries.

BRIEF METHODOLOGIC OVERVIEW OF NUTRITIONAL EPIDEMIOLOGY

The methodologic nuances of nutritional epidemiology should be reviewed prior to embarking on a critical evaluation of the published studies. We have arranged tables in this chapter to guide the reader through the salient features of many studies of dietary fiber, whole grain foods, and chronic disease risk. A quick review on the interpretation of the studies described in these tables and the accompanying text may help in judging strengths and weaknesses of the literature. For a thorough review of nutritional epidemiologic methods, the reader is referred to Willett.[10]

Study Design

Prospective studies are stronger than cross-sectional, because with cross-sectional studies it is not possible to establish temporality — that is, that the exposure (diet) precedes disease onset. Furthermore, the presence of frank disease in cross-sectional studies may result in reverse causality — real changes in diet due to secondary prevention efforts or consequences of illness or medication use — or self-report bias in dietary recall due to knowledge of diet and health. Prospective studies have the capability to exclude those with the disease of interest at baseline, or time 0, and follow them through time to track the number of cases (e.g., incidence of myocardial infarction), thereafter conducting analyses to determine if self-reported diet at baseline is associated with incidence of disease. Given the wealth of longitudinal studies on fiber, whole grains, and CVD and type 2 diabetes, we will not thoroughly review the cross-sectional studies.

Case-control studies have commonly been done for cancer, as this study design is more efficient for less common diseases. Case-control studies are particularly prone to bias, however, especially recall bias and other biases related to the selection of controls and interviews that probe for exposure status. Cases, because of their disease status, may recall dietary and other exposures differently

Table 6.2.1 Description and Relative Consumption of Common Whole and Refined Grain Foods in Epidemiologic Studies

Food Group	Whole Grain		Refined Grain	
	Foods	Estimated Relative Contribution to Food Group	Foods	Estimated Relative Contribution to Food Group
Bread and bread products	Dark, brown, mixed grain bread	60%	White bread	30%
Breakfast cereal	Whole grain or bran as first ingredient; Whole grain or bran elsewhere in ingredient list AND at least 2 g fiber per serving; Oatmeal and other hot whole grain cereals	25%	Refined grain or sugar as first ingredient; Whole grain or bran elsewhere in ingredient list AND less than 2 g of fiber per serving; Cream of wheat and other hot refined grain cereals	4%
Other breakfast items	Whole wheat, rye, and bran muffins; Whole wheat pancakes and waffles	1%	Regular white flour muffins, rolls, donuts, and croissants; Regular pancakes and waffles	10%
Pizza, pasta, tortillas, etc.	Made from whole wheat or other whole grain	—	Made from white or semolina flour or other refined grain flour	8%
Rice	Brown and wild rice	1%	White rice	3%
Snacks and desserts	Popcorn, corn chips, whole wheat or rye crackers, and pretzels	13%	White wheat flour crackers and pretzels, cakes, cookies and brownies	45%

Source: Adapted from Jacobs et al.[5,30] and Pereira et al.[8]

(overestimating or underestimating exposure) than controls. However, some comprehensive meta-analyses of whole grain and cancer have considered these biases in their methods, and the discrepancies between these case-control studies and the few prospective studies of fiber and cancer will be discussed.

Measurement of Diet

There is a large degree of error in self-reported diet in epidemiologic studies. This error is generally agreed by nutritional epidemiologists to be random in nature, thus biasing associations toward the null hypothesis of no association between diet and disease, and increasing the probability of missing a true association (type II error). Therefore, when one finds a statistically significant and biologically meaningful association in support of some *a priori* hypothesis, especially after control for potentially confounding factors (see below), the association is likely to be real. In fact, there is evidence that adjustment for this measurement error may sometimes strengthen associations,[10] depending on the nature and quality of the measurement error adjustment and, of course, whether there is a true association as hypothesized.

Adjustment for Other Potential Confounders

Adjustment for confounders is especially critical with such self-reported behaviors as intake of fiber-rich foods, which correlates strongly with important lifestyle behaviors such as cigarette smoking, physical activity, vitamin supplement use, and other dietary factors. Not only must epidemiologists control for these potential confounders in their statistical modeling, but they must have measured these potential confounders accurately to minimize susceptibility to residual confounding. For example, if a certain study of fiber and risk for coronary heart disease has a crude measure of physical activity, such as classifying participants, into two categories — sedentary vs. active — physical activity level could still confound associations between fiber and incidence of coronary disease. Within the physically active group of participants there may be a broad distribution of physical activity and dietary fiber intake, leaving open the possibility of confounding within subgroups of physical activity. This potential problem would be minimized if a study had a very detailed measure of physical activity, such as a continuous metabolic index derived from a series of questions about type, frequency, and intensity of activity. Many studies discussed in some detail in this chapter have rigorously controlled for potential confounders. In addition, if one also finds support for physiologic effects from animal experiments and human trials, as reviewed in Chapter 6.3, residual confounding is less likely to be operating to explain the observational findings.

Sample Size and Characteristics

The larger the sample size and the more representative the sample is of the overall population, the more likely the sample is to have a broad distribution of dietary intake and the greater the number of disease endpoints that will be accumulated over time. These factors will increase the likelihood of detecting an association between exposure (fiber or food intake) and endpoint (risk factor or incidence rate of disease). However, depending on the sampling strategy and age, gender, and racial composition of the sample, a larger sample size may not always result in an unbiased and representative sample of the population in terms of dietary intake and characteristics. The overall population from which the participants are recruited may be an entire country (e.g., National Health Interview Survey) or a population subgroup (e.g., the Nurses Health Study). Although female nurses may be a relatively homogenous group, such a sample has internal validity due to the comprehensive and careful methods. The high response rate and very large sample size in the Nurses Health Study also contribute to the enhanced likelihood of detecting important associations between diet and health and generalizing these findings to middle-aged and older women who have similar characteristics. Indeed, as will be discussed below, some nutritional findings from the Nurses Health Study and another study of postmenopausal women from the state of Iowa (the Iowa Women's Health Study) are consistent.

Magnitude and Nature of Association

Generally, with such common diseases as cardiovascular disease, a 20% reduction in risk may have public health relevance, especially if this risk reduction is observed between groups within the study population consuming realistic, generalizable amounts of a nutrient or food. For example, one might ask: What is the relative risk reduction for coronary heart disease for each increase in cereal fiber of five grams per day — or the equivalent of one or two servings of whole grain breakfast cereal? If a dose-response curve is also observed across increments of increasing nutrient intake (whereby risk for the disease is decreased with increasing intake), then the findings are more likely to be real rather than spurious or confounded.

DIETARY FIBER AND CHRONIC DISEASE RISK FACTORS

In this section we will provide a brief overview of observational studies of dietary fiber or whole grain intake and risk factors for chronic disease, while a more thorough review of associations between fiber (and its food sources) and actual incidence of frank disease will follow. The cross-sectional studies of dietary fiber reviewed herein do not include frank cases of disease. Instead, these studies have examined associations between dietary fiber and risk factors or biomarkers for chronic disease. Risk factors for cardiovascular disease and type 2 diabetes will not be differentiated, because these diseases have many risk factors in common. Indeed, these diseases are thought to have a common etiology in the insulin resistance syndrome, including hyperinsulinemia, impaired glucose metabolism, dyslipidemia, hypertension, hypofibrinolysis, obesity, and central fat patterning.[11] Risk factors for cancer are less clear, in part because cancer is a much more heterogenous set of diseases than CVD and type 2 diabetes. There are a few biomarkers reflecting risk for CVD and type 2 diabetes that also may be important in the etiology of certain cancers. These may include blood insulin concentration, systemic inflammation, and antioxidant capacity. Insulin may promote the growth of tumors, markers of inflammation may reflect an immune response, and reduced antioxidative capacity may indicate susceptibility to free-radical damage of tissue or DNA. Fiber-rich foods, for reasons discussed in the accompanying chapter along with a review of the experimental evidence, have the potential to affect all of these risk factors for the three main chronic diseases — cardiovascular disease, type 2 diabetes, and certain cancers.

Although the cholesterol-lowering effect of dietary fiber appears to be modest and dependent on its solubility (as discussed in the accompanying chapter), there are many other potential mechanisms whereby dietary fiber–rich foods may reduce risk for chronic diseases. One of the most promising fiber–risk factor associations is that of glucose control and insulin sensitivity. Such effects of dietary fiber may operate systemically, resulting in benefits on blood pressure and hemostatic factors through the clustering of related abnormalities as mentioned above. However, because of the difficulty in measuring diet by self-report and the expense of collecting good risk factor data in large samples of individuals for epidemiologic purposes, few studies have provided good detail of fiber–risk factor associations. The few cross-sectional and longitudinal studies of dietary fiber and fasting insulin and other markers of insulin sensitivity have revealed that fiber appears to be favorably associated with insulin sensitivity.[12–15] This association appears to be independent of other dietary and lifestyle factors.

Humble et al.[16] have identified possible mechanisms to explain their associations between intake of crude fiber and coronary heart disease incidence (included in the next section) in hypercholesterolemic middle-aged men. Across quintiles of increasing fiber intake at baseline of the study, a strong inverse linear trend was observed for post-challenge glucose concentration ($p = .001$), with a weaker inverse ($p = .06$) and positive ($p = .11$) trend for body mass index and HDL cholesterol. No association was found for systolic blood pressure, and insulin was not measured. It should also be noted that these associations were not adjusted for potential confounding factors, such as physical activity habits.

A prospective study was recently undertaken to assess the relative capacity of the major macronutrients to predict changes in cardiovascular disease risk factors over a 10-year period (1985/6 to 1995/6).[17] Total dietary fiber from all sources was used, as source of fiber was not available for analyses. Study participants were 2909 young black and white adults enrolled in the Coronary Artery Risk Development in Young Adults (CARDIA) Study. In addition to comparing fiber to saturated fat, unsaturated fat, protein, and carbohydrate in this regard, these authors hypothesized that dietary fiber may exert its beneficial effects on attenuating atherogenesis through its effects on circulating insulin concentrations. As such, the findings may also apply to type 2 diabetes and certain hormonally mediated cancers in which insulin levels may be important. Dietary fiber intake was consistently associated in a protective dose response manner with 10-year body weight gain.[17] Those in the highest 20% of dietary fiber intake (>21 g/2000 kcal) gained approximately 8 fewer pounds of weight over the 10-year period than those in the lowest 20% of dietary fiber intake (<12 g/2000 kcal). Similar results were found for the waist–hip ratio. Fasting and 2-hour post-glucose insulin concentrations demonstrated graded inverse associations with dietary fiber intake in both black and white women and men, even after adjustment for all known potential cofounders as well as body mass index. Furthermore, 10-year changes in blood pressure, LDL cholesterol, HDL cholesterol, and triglycerides, as well as cross-sectional associations with fibrinogen (a marker of hemostasis as well as inflammation), were all associated with dietary fiber intake in a dose–response manner in whites. (Weaker but consistent associations were observed in blacks.) Most of these associations could be explained by adjustment for fasting insulin concentration, supporting a mechanistic role of insulin sensitivity in the effect of fiber intake on CVD risk factors. In comparison, while a recent cross-sectional study found no association between dietary fiber intake and fibrinogen, a graded inverse association between fiber intake and PAI-1 concentration was reported.[18] These findings from the Family Heart Study[18] are consistent with the PAI-1 and fibrinogen findings for our human experiments discussed in the accompanying chapter.

In the study described above,[17] not only were these associations for dietary fiber and risk factors stronger than those for saturated fat, unsaturated fat, carbohydrate, and protein, but the few associations that were observed between total or saturated fat and body weight or insulin were considerably attenuated and no longer statistically significant after adjustment for dietary fiber intake. This is a classic example of confounding that has often been overlooked with respect to the classic diet–heart hypothesis. Previous studies have demonstrated that fiber may have stronger associations with risk for coronary disease than saturated fat or cholesterol,[19,20] and that the association between saturated fat intake and coronary disease risk may in fact be confounded by intake of dietary fiber.[19,21] Dietary fat and fiber intake are inversely and moderately correlated — high-saturated-fat diets almost invariably include little dietary fiber. Therefore, it may not be the saturated fat itself that is the most pernicious factor in the Westernized diet, but rather the lack of fiber and associated nutrients, such as minerals, antioxidants, and phytoestrogens, or other factors (e.g., red meat and its processing) related to a high-saturated-fat dietary pattern.

While the above study did not examine intake of whole foods, the dietary fiber consumed by this population came predominantly from whole grains, fruits, and vegetables, and some contributions from nuts and legumes.[22] In fact, a previous report from the CARDIA Study described inverse dose–response associations between whole grain intake and fasting plasma insulin concentration.[8] These associations were independent of many other lifestyle factors associated with whole grain intake and fasting insulin. Factors potentially on the causal pathway between whole grain intake and fasting insulin—body mass index (through satiety or insulin itself), magnesium (abundant in whole grains and potentially an important nutrient for type 2 diabetes evolution), and dietary fiber — were each shown to explain some of the observed association between whole grain intake and fasting insulin.[8] Only when all three of these variables were added to the model simultaneously was all of the association explained.

DIETARY FIBER AND INCIDENCE OF CHRONIC DISEASE

Cardiovascular Disease

Table 6.2.2 describes the salient features of epidemiologic studies of dietary fiber and coronary heart disease. The studies are heterogenous in that they span a time period of 23 years and include small and large numbers of men and women, differing in characteristics from male British men[2] to U.S. nurses.[23] The studies are relatively homogenous in their dietary and analytic methods, having followed healthy individuals over time to accumulate cases and deaths of coronary heart disease, and regress these events on categories fiber intake derived from self-reports at baseline. All studies have adjusted for potential confounders, such as age, cigarette smoking, alcohol intake, energy intake, body mass index, and physical activity. Some studies have adjusted for additional dietary factors — a particular strength of those studies — such as fruit and vegetable intake when regressing heart disease incidence on whole grain intake or cereal fiber, or intake of fatty acids and cholesterol.

The early study by Morris et al.[2] is particularly intriguing, for several reasons. This is a very small study sample of English men ($n = 337$) whom the authors had to follow for 20 years in order to have the minimal number of events (45) for which to conduct their analyses. They reported a graded inverse association between intake of cereal fiber and incidence of CHD events over the 20-year period such that men in the middle tertile of cereal fiber intake had a relative risk of 0.57, or a 43% reduction in risk of CHD in comparison to the reference group — men in the lowest tertile of cereal fiber intake. Those men in the highest tertile of cereal fiber intake had an 82% lower risk than those in the lowest tertile. Although these estimates of relative risk have wide confidence intervals (not shown) due to the small sample size of this study, the p-value for this observation was very low, suggesting that the chances of this finding being spurious were 5 out of 1000. Still, Morris and colleagues admitted that they didn't have an *a priori* hypothesis for this finding. They proceeded to investigate this finding further by stratification for potential confounders as one alternative to multivariate adjustment. The findings were startling. For every stratum of smoking status and occupation and for duration of follow-up (years since baseline in intervals of 5 and 10 years), the same inverse association persisted for cereal fiber and incidence of coronary heart disease. Upon examination of the foods that contribute to dietary cereal fiber, brown breads were found to be the most influential, while white (refined) bread was found to have no correlation with CHD incidence.

Studies by Kushi et al.[24] and Khaw and Barrett-Connor[25] in the mid-1980s examined CHD deaths over 23 and 13 years, respectively, regressed on total dietary fiber intake in their respective populations. Kushi et al.[24] observed a 43% reduction in CHD risk for the highest tertile of fiber intake, whereas Khaw and Barrett-Connor[25] observed a 15% (not significant) reduction in men and a 33% reduction in women. Humble et al.[16] reported weaker findings for quintiles of fiber intake, with a nonsignificant 8% reduction for the highest vs. lowest quintile of intake. However, a limitation of these studies was that they did not examine the type of dietary fiber. If the observations of Morris et al.[2] were real, then total dietary fiber should have a weaker association with coronary disease incidence than cereal fiber.

From 1996 to the present, there have been a series of studies with very consistent findings for risk of CHD according to intake of cereal fiber and whole grain foods. The one exception is the study by Mann et al.,[26] which did not include type of fiber in the analyses. Although Mann et al.[26] observed a nonsignificant increased risk of CHD with increasing total fiber consumption, this finding may have been spurious due to the small number of events. In support of this possibility of a spurious finding, these authors reported no association between dietary fiber intake and all-cause mortality.

Table 6.2.2 Prospective Epidemiologic Studies of Dietary Fiber and Risk of Coronary Heart Disease

Study	Sample	Outcome	Exposure	Relative Risks per Increasing Category of Intake					p Value
				1	2	3	4	5	
Morris et al.[2]	337 English men	45 cases over 20 years	Cereal	1.0	0.57	0.18			<.005
			Fruit, veg., pulses, and nuts	1.0	1.29	0.93			NS
Kushi et al.[24]	1001 Irish/American men	110 deaths over 23 years	Tertiles of fiber intake	1.0	0.88	0.57			<.05
Khaw et al.[25]	356 U.S. men	65 deaths over 13 years	Difference in fiber intake of 6 g	1.0	0.85				.15
	503 U.S. women			1.0	0.67				.05
Humble et al.[16]	1801 U.S. men	249 cases over 10 years	Highest and lowest quintiles of fiber intake	1.0				0.92	<.10
Pietinen et al.[27]	21,930 Finish smoking men	635 deaths over 6 years	Quintiles of fiber intake from cereal, vegetable, and fruit — Cereal	1.0	0.91	0.90	0.83	0.78	.01
			Vegetable	1.0	0.86	0.89	0.66	0.88	.08
			Fruit	1.0	1.09	1.39	1.26	1.16	.77
Rimm et al.[20]	43,757 U.S. male health professionals	734 cases over 6 years	Quintiles of fiber intake from cereal, vegetable, and fruit — Cereal	1.0	0.96	0.88	0.86	0.71	.007
			Vegetable	1.0	1.08	0.99	1.00	0.83	.05
			Fruit	1.0	0.93	0.83	0.84	0.81	.10
Mann et al.[26]	10,802 U.K. men and women	64 deaths over 13 years	Tertiles of fiber intake	1.0	1.92	2.25			NS
Todd et al.[28]	5754 Scottish men	296 cases	Quartiles of dietary fiber intake	1.0	0.68	0.70	0.64		Not given
	5875 Scottish women	97 cases over 9 years		1.0	0.94	0.60	0.56		
Wolk et al.[23]	68,782 U.S. female nurses	591 cases over 10 years	Quintiles of fiber intake from cereal, vegetable, and fruit — Cereal	1.0	1.06	0.71	0.76	0.66	<.001
			Vegetable	1.0	1.05	1.11	1.10	1.13	.63
			Fruit	1.0	0.92	0.82	1.00	0.94	.51

Note: All studies adjusted for potentially confounding variables, including demographics, other dietary factors, body mass, and lifestyle factors. Cases = fatal + nonfatal events. *p*-values are for tests of linear trend for relative risks across categories of intake for studies with three or more categories.

Pietinen et al.[27] compared the rate of CHD deaths across quintiles of cereal fiber, vegetable fiber, and fruit fiber intake among 21,930 male Finnish smokers enrolled in the ATBC Study. These authors found a reduced rate of death with increasing quintile of cereal fiber intake that reached a 26% reduction in risk for men in the highest quintile (consuming an average of 26 g of cereal fiber per day) relative to those in the lowest quintile of intake (consuming an average of 9 g per day). Findings for vegetable fiber appeared to be somewhat weaker, with some of the association being explained by intake of antioxidant vitamins. Although fruit fiber also appeared to be protective for coronary death, the protective associations were entirely explained by antioxidant intake, suggesting that it may not be the fiber in fruit that is responsible for reducing risk. Alternatively, because fruits and vegetables contain a great deal of water and relatively little fiber per unit volume, the amount of fiber obtained from fruit may be insufficient in most diets to observe an association with disease risk. Following this line of thought, in this population intake of cereal fiber was much greater than for fiber from vegetables and fruits, and this may partly explain why findings were more robust for cereal fiber. Also, findings were weaker and not statistically significant when the endpoint used was all major coronary events (fatal and nonfatal). A possible explanation for this discrepancy is that dietary fiber intake reduces the case-fatality rate in men with coronary disease and has less impact on the incidence of coronary disease in a population at high risk, such as male smokers in Finland.

Rimm et al.[20] reported findings from the Health Professionals Follow-up Study in the U.S. very similar to those just described from the ATBC Study. The distribution of dietary fiber intake, unlike the ATBC Study, was relatively similar across food groups (vegetable, fruit, and cereal), although total intake appeared to be lower than in the ATBC Study. The authors did note that age-adjusted findings were stronger for fatal than for non-fatal myocardial infarction but that fatal and nonfatal categories were grouped together due to a limited number of cases. Shown in Table 6.2.2 are the relative risk estimates from this study from a regression model which simultaneously included cereal, fruit, and vegetable fiber and a long list of potential confounding variables. Although all three types of fiber appeared to reduce risk for myocardial infarction, the findings were strongest and statistically significant for cereal fiber, with a reduced risk of 29% (95% confidence interval = 46% to 8%) in the highest quintile of intake relative to the lowest quintile. Interestingly, the average intake in this quintile was only 9.7 g per day — similar to the lowest quintile from the ATBC Study. Although cross-cultural comparisons are of interest in evaluating consistency among studies, caution should be used in such endeavors for cultural and methodologic reasons. For example, Finnish smoking men generally eat few fruits and vegetables and a lot of whole grain rye bread; and the method of quantifying dietary intake in the ATBC Study is much more comprehensive than the food frequency questionnaire used in the HPFS Study.

From the Scottish Heart Health Study, Todd et al.[28] reported the relative risk of CHD incidence for men and women. Although the sample size (n = 3,833 women and 4,036 men available for analysis) and number of events (n = 97 women) were small in comparison to the other studies in Table 6.2.1, these authors observed a consistent decrease in CHD risk with increasing quartile of dietary fiber intake that reached a magnitude of 44% reduced risk for the highest quartile of women. Although the confidence interval around this estimate was wide and not statistically significant, the reduced risk across quintiles was graded and appeared to be stronger than the association in men. This possible gender difference is consistent with the findings of Khaw and Barrett-Connor.[25] The findings for men, with more statistical power due to a larger number of cases, were statistically significant for each of the second through fourth quartiles of fiber intake when compared to the lowest quartile.

Wolk et al.[23] reported particularly robust associations between intake of cereal fiber and CHD risk in a large cohort (n = 68,782) of women from the Nurses Health Study. In comparison to women in the lowest quintile of intake, women in the highest quintile were observed to have a relative risk of CHD of 0.66, indicating a 34% reduction in risk of coronary heart disease. Furthermore, for every increase of 5 g of cereal fiber intake, it was estimated that risk of heart disease was reduced by 37% (95% confidence interval = 51% to 19%). In comparison, 10 g of cereal fiber per day appeared to be necessary to reduce the risk of CHD by a similar amount in the men of the Health Professionals Follow-up Study, for which the same dietary questionnaire and analytical methods were used.[20] Consistent with the findings of Rimm et al.[20] and Pietinen et al.,[27] the corresponding relative risks for fruit and vegetable fiber were weaker and not statistically significant in the Nurses Health Study.[23]

Table 6.2.3 describes findings from prospective epidemiologic studies of whole and refined grain intake and risk for coronary heart disease as well as total cardiovascular disease. Morris and colleagues described the relative contribution of various grain products to dietary cereal fiber intake and their qualitative association with CHD risk. Brown bread and some whole meal breads and breakfast cereals were found to be strongly associated with cereal fiber intake and were therefore presumed to explain the robust association between intake of cereal fiber and CHD risk. However, no association was found between intake of other grains and white bread and CHD incidence.

From the Seventh-Day Adventists Study, Fraser et al.[29] supported the earlier findings by Morris et al.,[2] demonstrating a 43% reduction in risk of CHD for men and women who endorsed whole grain bread intake relative to those endorsing white bread consumption. Those endorsing mixed grain breads also appeared to have a reduction in risk of 41% compared to white bread eaters, although this finding was not statistically significant.

In their study of fiber and coronary disease incidence in the ATBC Study, Pietinen et al.[27] examined dietary intake of various food groups and food sources which contribute fiber as well as many other nutrients. The only food group that appeared to offer protection from CHD incidence was vegetables, whereas vegetables, fruits and berries, and rye products in particular were all associated with reduced risk for coronary death in a dose–response manner. The contrast between rye products, primarily consumed in whole grain form in Finland, and other cereal products, which probably included a lot of refined grain foods, is displayed in Table 6.2.3 for this study. While rye products were associated with a reduced risk for CHD death of 25% in the highest (172 g per day) in comparison to the lowest (16 g per day) quintile, no such apparent protection was observed for other cereal products (215 vs. 47 g per day).

Using data on postmenopausal women from the Iowa Women's Health Study, Jacobs et al.[5,30] published studies of whole grain intake and mortality from cardiovascular disease and other causes. Whereas the previous studies[2,27,29] had made simple observations regarding specific whole grain breads, Jacobs et al.[5,30] developed an algorithm for breakfast cereals according to whole grain content described earlier and incorporated these cereals along with breads and many other types of whole grain foods into food groups of whole and refined grains. Reductions in risk for CHD mortality were observed within increasing whole grain intake, whereas no such protection was observed for refined grain intake. Women who reported consuming more than one serving of whole grains per day had a 30% lower risk (95% confidence interval = 50% to 2%) of ischemic heart disease death than those women who reported one-half or fewer servings per day. This association was attenuated but could not be entirely explained by adjustment for selected constituents of whole grain (dietary fiber, vitamin E, folic acid, phytic acid, iron, magnesium, and manganese). Recently, Jacobs et al.[5] expanded these analyses to include all CVD deaths (as well as deaths from cancers and all causes). These findings were confirmed by Liu et al.,[31,32] using the same food groups for whole and refined grain, in 75,521 women in the Nurses Health Study for endpoints of coronary disease[31] and incident ischemic stroke.[32] Most of the protective association of whole grain intake with CHD risk in the study by Liu et al.[31] was observed for whole grain breakfast cereals, brown rice, and bran, whereas in the study by Jacobs et al.,[30] considerable CHD risk reduction was also observed specifically for intake of "dark bread." These findings are summarized in Table 6.2.3. The consistent reduction in risk for cardiovascular disease incidence or mortality, as well as the lack of any association between refined grain intake and these endpoints, is apparent.

In summary, observations from epidemiologic cohort studies reported over the past few years are novel and important in two respects: (1) whole grain foods appear to offer protection from

Table 6.2.3 Prospective Epidemiologic Studies of Whole and Refined Grain Intake and Risk of Cardiovascular Disease

Study	Sample	Outcome	Exposure		Relative Risks per Increasing Category of Intake					p-Value
					1	2	3	4	5	
Morris et al.[2]	337 English men	45 CHD cases over 20 years	Intake of brown and whole meal breads, breakfast cereals, cakes, biscuits, and white bread		Analyses were described qualitatively. Largest differences across tertiles of cereal fiber intake were observed for brown and whole meal breads and breakfast cereals. No association was observed between white bread and other refined carbohydrates and CHD incidence.					
Fraser et al.[29]	31,208 U.S. Seventh-Day Adventists	134 CHD cases	Whole wheat and mixed grain bread relative to white bread	Whole	1.0	0.56				<.01
				Mixed	1.0	0.59				NS
Pietinen et al.[27]	21,930 Finnish smoking men	635 CHD deaths over 6 years	Rye products		1.0	0.87	0.86	0.79	0.75	.02
			Other cereal products		1.0	0.94	0.93	1.03	1.05	.83
Jacobs et al.[30]	34,492 U.S. women	438 CHD deaths over 9 years	Quintiles of whole and refined grain intake	Whole	1.0	0.96	0.71	0.64	0.70	.02
				Refined	1.0	0.99	1.14	1.04	1.12	.57
Jacobs et al.[5]	38,740 U.S. women	1,097 CVD deaths over 9 years	Quintiles of whole and refined grain fiber intake	Whole	1.0	1.01	0.85	0.78	0.82	.02
				Refined	1.0	1.08	1.03	0.96	1.09	.70
Liu et al.[31]	75,521 U.S. female nurses	761 CHD cases over 10 years	Quintiles of whole grain intake	Whole	1.0	0.92	0.93	0.83	0.75	.01
Liu et al.[32]	75,521 U.S. female nurses	352 ischemic stroke cases over 12 years	Quintiles of whole and refined grain intake	Whole	1.0	0.72	0.78	0.60	0.69	.08
				Refined	1.0	1.11	1.18	0.94	0.97	.58

Note: All studies adjusted for potentially confounding variables, including demographics, other dietary factors, body mass, and lifestyle factors. CHD = coronary heart disease. CVD = cardiovascular disease (heart disease + stroke and other events). Cases = fatal + nonfatal events. p-values are for tests of linear trend for relative risks across categories of intake for studies with three or more categories.

cardiovascular disease above and beyond the effects that may be explained by fiber or dietary fat, and (2) the benefits of dietary fiber and whole grain foods have been observed in women with magnitudes of association that may be stronger than those in men. Previous studies in the U.S. and Finland had suggested that cereal fiber, coming primarily from whole grain foods, may be associated with coronary heart disease more consistently and strongly than fiber from fruits and vegetables. The stronger associations of cereal fiber, if real, could possibly be due to a synergy of nutrients in the bran and germ that cannot be explained by quantifying the fiber itself or a few common nutrients in the diet.[33] As discussed in the chapter on mechanisms and experimental evidence, there may be many yet-to-be identified biologically active constituents in these parts of the plant that tend to be retained in whole grain foods.

Type 2 Diabetes

As discussed above, cardiovascular disease and type 2 diabetes share common etiologies in which diet appears to play an important role. Therefore, given the evidence described above for cereal fiber, whole grains, and heart disease risk, it is not surprising that recent epidemiological evidence from prospective studies suggests that intake of dietary fiber, and especially cereal fiber and whole grain foods, is inversely associated with risk for developing type 2 diabetes. These recent observations may have great public health importance because of the rising incidence of type 2 diabetes in the Westernized world.[34,35]

An early study reported no differences in dietary fiber intake or foods providing dietary fiber between women who did and did not develop type 2 diabetes in the future.[36] However, this study used a single 24-hour recall of diet, which is known to be a poor measure of habitual dietary intake and would have considerably biased any real association toward the null hypothesis.

Findings from the Nurses Health Study,[37] the Health Professionals Follow-up Study,[38] and the Iowa Women's Health Study[39] have revealed that cereal fiber, but not fruit and vegetable fiber, is inversely associated with risk of type 2 diabetes in a dose–response manner in both women and men (Table 6.2.4). The magnitude of the risk reduction observed for the highest quintile of cereal fiber intake (median intake of ~7–10 g/day) was 30–35% relative to the lowest quintile (median intake ~2–4 g/day). An interesting aspect of these studies was that the association between cereal fiber and type 2 diabetes incidence was independent of the dietary glycemic index or glycemic load, which is an estimate of potential for the diet to increase blood glucose acutely, primarily through amount and type of carbohydrate reported. However, the nature of the joint associations of cereal fiber and glycemic load on risk for type 2 diabetes is not clear from these three studies. The results from the Nurses Health Study[37] suggested that cereal fiber and the dietary glycemic load were additive in their association with type 2 diabetes; women in the lowest tertile of cereal fiber intake and the highest tertile of glycemic load were 2.5 times more likely to develop diabetes over the 6-year period in comparison to women in the highest tertile of cereal fiber and lowest tertile of glycemic load. Although the Health Professionals Follow-Up Study confirmed this additive finding for cereal fiber and glycemic load on risk of type 2 diabetes, it also appeared that cereal fiber had no association with risk for type 2 diabetes in those men in the lowest tertile of glycemic load, whereas glycemic load had no association with diabetes in those men in the top two tertiles of cereal fiber intake. Meyer et al.[39] observed no association between glycemic load or glycemic index and incidence of type 2 diabetes in the Iowa Women's Health Study, with fiber intake appearing to protect women from type 2 diabetes at all levels of the glycemic load.

Finally, the study by Meyer et al.[39] and an additional report from the Nurses Health Study[40] have confirmed that whole grain intake is inversely associated with risk of type 2 diabetes, while refined grain intake is not associated with risk of type 2 diabetes. This risk reduction was approximately 20%[39] and 25%[40] for women in the highest quintile of whole grain intake in comparison to those in the lowest quintile in these two studies. In the Nurses Health Study, the apparent protection conferred by whole grain foods was observed for virtually every whole grain food item

Table 6.2.4 Prospective Epidemiologic Studies of Dietary Fiber, Whole Grain Foods, and Risk of Type 2 Diabetes

Study	Sample	Outcome	Exposure		Relative Risks per Increasing Category of Intake					
					1	2	3	4	5	p-Value
Salmeron et al.[38]	42,759 U.S. men	523 cases over 6 years	Quintiles of fiber intake	Cereal	1.0	1.14	0.95	0.91	0.70	.01
				Fruit	1.0	1.01	0.89	1.14	1.01	.68
				Vegetable	1.0	1.12	1.22	1.10	1.12	.65
Salmeron et al.[37]	65,173 U.S. female nurses	915 cases over 6 years	Quintiles of cereal fiber intake	Cereal	1.0	1.01	0.85	0.82	0.72	<.01
				Fruit	1.0	0.87	0.95	0.94	0.87	.39
				Vegetable	1.0	1.40	1.23	1.29	1.27	.54
Meyer et al.[39]	35,988 U.S. women	1,141 cases over 11 years	Quintiles of fiber and whole and refined grain intake	Cereal	1.0	0.93	0.88	0.77	0.64	<.01
				Fruit	1.0	0.98	1.14	1.06	1.17	.08
				Vegetable	1.0	1.07	1.12	1.12	0.97	.77
				Whole	1.0	0.99	0.98	0.92	0.79	.01
				Refined	1.0	0.96	0.81	0.98	0.87	.36
Liu et al.[40]	75,521 U.S. female nurses	1,879 cases over 10 years	Quintiles of whole and refined grain intake	Whole	1.0	0.91	0.94	0.75	0.74	<.01
				Refined	1.0	1.10	1.02	1.10	1.11	.26

Note: All studies adjusted for potentially confounding variables, including demographics, other dietary factors, body mass, and lifestyle factors. *p*-values are for tests of linear trend for relative risks across categories of intake.

(dark bread, whole grain breakfast cereal, popcorn, cooked oatmeal, brown rice, wheat germ, bran, and other whole grains).[40] In the Iowa Women's Health Study, cereal fiber and dietary magnesium intake appeared to explain most of the protective associations between whole grain intake and risk of type 2 diabetes.[39] This is not to say that there aren't other possible mechanisms or constituents of whole grains for which cereal fiber and magnesium serve as markers in epidemiologic data. As described earlier in this chapter, Pereira et al.[8] observed an inverse association between whole grain intake and fasting insulin concentration in young adult men and women that was explained by fiber intake, magnesium intake, and body mass index. Each of these factors may be on the causal pathway between whole grain intake and glucose control, which is important to remember when interpreting studies because most of the studies on fiber and chronic diseases have adjusted the associations for body mass index. The reader is referred to Chapter 6.3, which provides insight into the experimental evidence on this important topic.

Cancer

Studies of dietary fiber and cancer have revealed mixed findings. Therefore, this area of nutrition research remains very controversial. Case-control and prospective studies of dietary fiber and colorectal cancer have been inconsistent.[41-49] Few studies have explored other types of cancer, because dietary fiber has been thought to reduce risk for colorectal cancer through actions in the colon that are described in the accompanying chapter. Until recently there has been little development of biological plausibility for fiber and other cancers.

The most rigorous prospective epidemiologic analysis on this topic to date, from the Nurses Health Study, found no association between dietary fiber intake and the incidence of colorectal cancer in 88,757 women followed for 16 years, in which 787 cases of colorectal cancer were documented and 1,012 adenomas of the distal colon and rectum were identified by endoscopy.[49] These authors attempted to uncover many methodologic barriers that may have masked a real association. They examined types of fiber (fruit, vegetable, and cereal) and many subgroups of women, but no association emerged between intake of fiber and risk for colorectal cancer. This finding is probably not explained by inaccuracies in dietary reporting because, as discussed above, there have been strong associations between cereal fiber and whole grains with risk of heart disease and type 2 diabetes in this same study.

Jacobs and colleagues have conducted a meta-analysis of 40 case-control studies of cancer in order to estimate the odds of having various cancers contingent upon dietary whole grain intake.[50] Although case-control studies of diet and cancer may be particularly susceptible to recall bias, most of the case-control studies included in this meta-analysis did not have a hypothesis about whole grain intake or a specific hypothesis about diet in general. Therefore, Jacobs et al.[50] took advantage of existing dietary data in the published reports where whole grain was not a main focus of any of the studies. It is the main exposure of interest that would be most susceptible to recall or interviewer bias in these studies. A further strength is the inclusion of many types of cancers in this meta-analysis.

The findings from the meta-analysis of Jacobs et al.[50] revealed that individuals who reported habitual diets including whole grain foods were at significantly reduced odds of having 18 types of cancer. Whole grain intake was observed to reduce the odds of having colorectal cancer by 21% (95% confidence interval = 31% to 11%). The pooled odds ratio for all cancers was 0.66, or a 34% reduction in odds (95% confidence interval = 40% to 28%) for whole grain eaters compared to non-eaters. These results were similar after excluding six instances of design/reporting flaws or low intake and were also similar when examined in studies that adjusted for the most covariates.

A meta-analysis by Chatenoud et al.[51] revealed findings very similar to those reported by Jacobs et al.[50] Using data from an integrated series of case-control studies in northern Italy from 1983 to 1996, these authors observed odds ratios less than 1.0 for whole grain eaters in comparison to non-eaters for 17 of 18 cancers (the one exception being thyroid cancer). It is important to note that the authors selected 7990 controls who were admitted to the hospitals for acute, non-neoplastic conditions, unlikely to have been caused by diet, tobacco use, or alcohol. These observations were strengthened by the documentation of a dose–response association in comparing odds of cancers across low, intermediate, and high consumption of whole grain intake.

Slattery et al.[52,53] used data from a population-based study conducted in Northern California, Utah, and Minnesota to examine associations between dietary eating patterns and risk of developing colon cancer among 1993 cases and 2410 controls. Total fruit intake was not associated with colon cancer risk.[52] Among men, higher levels of whole grain intake were associated with a 40% reduction in the odds of having colon cancer (95% confidence interval, 60%–10%).[52] Dietary fiber intake was associated with a 50% reduction in the odds of having colon cancer for older men, 30% reduction in older women, 40% reduction for men with proximal tumors, and 50% reduction for women with proximal tumors.[52] A "prudent" dietary pattern, identified by factor analysis, was associated with higher levels of vigorous leisure-time physical activity, smaller body size, and higher intakes of dietary fiber and folate.[53] This dietary pattern appeared to confer protection from colon cancer, with the strongest associations being observed among people diagnosed prior to age 67 years (men, 47% reduction in odds of colon cancer, 95% confidence interval = 57%–8%; women, 42% reduction in odds, 95% confidence interval = 62%–13%) and among people with proximal tumors (men, 45% reduction in odds, 95% confidence interval = 62%–20%; women, 36% reduction in odds, 95% confidence interval = 55%–8%).[53]

In summary, findings of cereal fiber, whole grains, and risk of colorectal cancer have been inconsistent, with the clearest evidence for a potentially protective association coming from case-control studies of whole grains, dietary fiber, and cancer. If cereal fiber really does protect against colorectal cancers, why hasn't this been borne out in prospective studies as it has for heart disease and type 2 diabetes? There may be etiological as well as methodologic reasons for this discrepancy. Colorectal cancer may depart from heart disease and type 2 diabetes in its long latency period. Risk factors for cardiovascular disease and type 2 diabetes may be modified over relatively short periods of time, such as weeks, whereas slow-growing colon polyps may be less mutable and may require longer periods of dietary stimulus to affect their growth and malignant potential. Perhaps case-control studies, although susceptible to recall bias and interviewer bias (important issues discussed in some detail above), have more accurate reports of long-term diet, potentially including early adulthood, than prospective studies which may span only a decade or two at most. Certainly there have been secular trends toward improving diet in the U.S. over the past few decades, such that diet as reported for the past month or year may not reflect the habitual diet of 5 years or 10 years or longer. Perhaps most importantly, there is a need to examine the association between whole grain intake and risk for colorectal cancer prospectively. Only fiber and colorectal cancer have been examined in prospective studies. Beyond fiber, there are many constituents, nutrients, and phytochemicals present in whole grain foods that may offer protection from colorectal cancer.[9] That the case-control meta-analyses by Jacobs et al.[50] and Chatenoud et al.[51] both demonstrate decreased risk for many types of cancer in addition to colorectal provides evidence that whole grains are offering much more than just cereal fiber. Chapter 6.3 discusses in greater detail these possible mechanisms, as well as the animal experiments and a few randomized trials in humans on this topic.

Total Mortality

Given the epidemiologic studies reviewed in the previous sections, one would expect that studies which have included all-cause mortality as an endpoint would reveal that dietary fiber, and therefore foods providing fiber, would appear to extend life. This would, of course, be true even if there is no benefit from these foods for cancer risk, because the inverse associations with cardiovascular disease and type 2 diabetes are quite consistent across various populations with different study methods. Some of the studies described above have, in fact, examined the association between types of dietary fiber and whole grain foods in association with the risk of all-cause mortality. The findings have been generally consistent, although not as strong as for cardiovascular disease and type 2 diabetes.

Recently, fiber and fiber-rich foods have been more closely examined in studies examining cardiovascular disease incidence in older women. In the Iowa Women's Health Study, we asked: "Does the association between cereal fiber and risk for disease depend on its source?" While this issue has been partly addressed in studies evaluating associations of fruit, vegetable, and cereal fiber with risk for coronary disease, this trial used a unique approach: partitioning cereal fiber eaters into those consuming cereal fiber from refined grains vs. those consuming cereal fiber from whole grains. A subset of 11,040 women was selected on their similar consumption of cereal fiber (total = 5.8 g/day), with one group consuming predominantly whole grain cereal fiber (71% of cereal fiber, $n = 7481$) and the other consuming predominantly refined grain cereal fiber (77% of cereal fiber, $n = 3559$).[33] From 1986 to the end of 1997, 1341 deaths were observed among these women. Those reporting consumption of mostly whole grain fiber had an average death rate that was 17% lower (95% confidence interval = 27% to 6%) than those consuming mostly refined grain fiber, after adjustment for potentially confounding factors including demographics, other dietary factors, body habitus measures, physical activity, smoking, alcohol use, and hormone replacement therapy.[33] Although this subset analysis had limited statistical precision to evaluate cause-specific mortality, death rates from coronary disease and other cardiovascular diseases as well as cancer also appeared to be lower for the whole grain fiber consumers compared to their refined-grain-consuming counterparts.

The results of this study were very enlightening and, in fact, confirmed the findings of Jacobs et al.[5,30] and Liu et al.[31] in that fiber itself does not explain all of the association between whole grains and risk for CVD. One might ask that, if the previous studies were able to explain all of the associations between whole grain intake and coronary disease by fiber intake, then why would it matter if the fiber came from the starchy nutrient-poor endosperm exclusively (refined grain) or also from the nutrient-packed bran and germ (whole grain)? As discussed earlier, we submit that, while fiber itself may have many important physiologic effects that may modulate risk for coronary disease, the fiber- and nutrient-dense structures of certain plants, such as the germ and bran of grains, may be particularly efficacious for controlling cardiovascular disease risk factor evolution.

Taken together, the epidemiologic findings for disease incidence and for death suggest that a diet rich in minimally or appropriately processed plant foods, and perhaps whole grains, may improve the quality (delaying disease incidence) and the quantity (delaying death, especially due to cardiovascular diseases) of life.

CONCLUSIONS, POTENTIAL APPLICATIONS, AND FUTURE RESEARCH NEEDS

What have we learned by reviewing the epidemiology of dietary fiber, fiber-rich foods, and chronic disease risk? Do we now know, with this wealth of data from studies around the world, what Morris and his colleagues[2] felt that they knew 23 years ago?

> The finding on cereal fibre illustrates one of the uses of epidemiology — in exploration.... The physical and chemical properties of cereal and fruit and vegetable fibre differ substantially, so different physiological effects are to be expected.... The linoleate is only one possibility that cereal fibre may be the vehicle for other effectual nutrients. So, meanwhile, no mechanisms can be postulated of the present observation (which could be tested fairly quickly); and since we ourselves are only now and painfully learning about "fibre", we shall not speculate. Historically, the observation makes sense: *if* dietary fibre is related to the "modern epidemic" of CHD, the link should be with the fibre in cereals. It is the intake of that which has fallen; potatoes apart, consumption of fruit and vegetables has if anything increased. To those who wilt at the possibility of yet another behavioural risk factor for CHD it may be said that what is presently known by no means accounts for the occurrence of heart attack

and immunity from it; that this one would be easier to put right than some; and, as in so much of today's health and prevention, makes good sense in itself.[2]

So what is new in 2001? We have confirmed Morris's findings[2] for coronary disease and extended them to the newer epidemic of type 2 diabetes — a disease with much in common, etiologically, with heart disease. We have also, as described in Chapter 6.3, heeded the call of Morris et al.[2] in conducting experiments in animals and humans to identify many promising and possible biological mechanisms through which dietary fiber, and cereal fiber and whole grain foods in particular, may reduce risk for these diseases. Finally, we are making progress toward changing dietary patterns in the population by specifying whole grain intake rather than simply total grain intake. And we are setting population goals to strive toward increased whole grain consumption (Healthy People 2010, U.S. Department of Health and Human Services, Office of Disease Prevention and Health Promotion), which has lagged far behind the promotion of fruit and vegetable intake.

One area of continued controversy is the role of dietary fiber in the etiology of colorectal cancer. Results have been inconsistent, without sufficient support for either increased or decreased risk for cancer according to intake of dietary fiber. The potential mechanisms are many, but it is difficult to make recommendations specific to cancer when benefit has not been consistently observed in observational studies of free-living humans. Cancer may be more etiologically heterogenous than cardiovascular disease and type 2 diabetes, and the progression of cancer may be less mutable in response to behavioral modification. Risk for type 2 diabetes and coronary disease, on the other hand, may be effected in weeks or less in response to diet or exercise.

While the jury is still out on cancer, findings for cardiovascular disease and diabetes and total mortality are sufficiently strong to warrant continued public health efforts, primarily on the part of government and industry, to promote the consumption of foods rich in dietary fiber — especially whole grains. As such, in 1999 the U.S. Food and Drug Admistration allowed the following health claim: "Diets rich in whole-grain foods and other plant foods and low in total fat, saturated fat and cholesterol may reduce the risk for heart disease and certain cancers." (FDA Docket #99P-2209).

REFERENCES

1. Burkitt, D. P., Walker A. R., and Painter N. S., Dietary fiber and disease, *JAMA*, 229, 1068, 1974.
2. Morris, J. N., Marr, J. W., and Clayton, D. G., Diet and heart: a postscript, *BMJ*, 2, 1307, 1977.
3. Putnam, J. J. and Allshouse, J. E., Food consumption, prices, and expenditures, 1996. Annual data, 1970-94. USDA Economic Services Report, Statistical Bulletin #928.
4. Gerrior., S., Personal communication, January 29, 1997, based on Census of Manufacturers, Grain Mill Products, Industry Series, MC92-1-20D, USDA.
5. Jacobs D. R., Jr. et al., Is whole grain intake associated with reduced total and cause-specific death rates in older women? The Iowa Women's Health Study, *Am. J. Pub. Health*, 89, 322, 1999.
6. Albertson, A. M. and Tobelmann, R. C., Consumption of grain and whole-grain foods by an American population during the years 1990 to 1992, *J. Am. Diet. Assoc.*, 95, 703, 1995.
7. Jacobs, D. J., Jr. et al., Whole-grain intake and cancer: an expanded review and meta-analysis, *Nutr. Cancer*, 30, 85, 1998.
8. Pereira, M. A. et al., The association of whole grain intake and fasting insulin in a biracial cohort of young adults: the CARDIA Study, *CVD Prevention*, 1, 231, 1998.
9. Slavin, J. L. et al., Plausible mechanisms for the protectiveness of whole grains, *Am. J. Clin. Nutr.*, 70, 459S, 1999.
10. Willett, W. C., *Nutritional Epidemiology*, 2nd ed., Oxford University Press, New York, 1998.
11. Reaven, G., Role of insulin resistance in human disease, *Diabetes*, 37, 1595, 1988.
12. Lovejoy, J. and DiGiroloama, M., Habitual dietary intake and insulin sensitivity in lean and obese adults, *Am. J. Clin. Nutr.*, 55, 1174, 1992.
13. Feskens, E. J. M., Loeber, J., and Kromhout, D., Diet and physical activity as determinants of hyperinsulinemia: the Zutphen Elderly Study, *Am. J. Epidemiol.*, 140, 350, 1994.

14. Vitelli, L. L. et al., Association of dietary composition with fasting serum insulin level: the ARIC Study, *Nutr. Metab. Cardiovasc. Dis.*, 6, 194, 1996.

15. Marshall, J. A., Bessesen, D. H., and Hamman, R. F., High saturated fat and low starch and fibre are associated with hyperinsulinemia in a non-diabetic population: the San Luis Valley Diabetes Study, *Diabetologia*, 40, 430, 1997.

16. Humble, C. G., Malarcher, A. M., and Tyroler, H. A., Dietary fiber and coronary heart disease in middle-aged hypercholesterolemic men, *Am. J. Prev. Med.*, 9, 197, 1993.

17. Ludwig, D. S. et al., Dietary fiber, weight gain, and cardiovascular disease risk factors in young adults, *JAMA*, 282, 1539, 1999.

18. Djousse, L. et al., Relationship between dietary fiber consumption and fibrinogen and plasminogen activator inhibitor type 1: the National Heart, Lung, and Blood Institute Family Heart Study, *Am. J. Clin. Nutr.*, 68, 568, 1998.

19. Ascherio, A. et al., Dietary fat and risk of coronary heart disease in men, *BMJ*, 313, 84, 1996.

20. Rimm, E. B. et al., Vegetable, fruit, and cereal fiber intake and risk of coronary heart disease among men, *JAMA*, 275, 447, 1996.

21. Pietinen, P. et al., Intake of fatty acids and risk of coronary heart disease in a cohort of Finnish men. The Alpha-Tocopherol, Beta-Carotene Cancer Prevention Study, *Am. J. Epidemiol.*, 145, 876, 1997.

22. Ludwig, D. S., Pereira, M. A., and Jacobs, D. R., Dietary fiber and weight gain [letter to the editor], *JAMA*, 283, 1821, 2000.

23. Wolk, A. et al., Long-term intake of dietary fiber and decreased risk of coronary heart disease among women, *JAMA*, 281, 1998, 1999.

24. Kushi, L. H. et al., Diet and 20-year mortality from coronary heart disease. The Ireland-Boston Diet-Heart Study, *N. Engl. J. Med.*, 31, 811, 1985.

25. Khaw, K. T. and Barrett-Connor, E., Dietary fiber and reduced ischemic heart disease mortality rates in men and women: a 12-year prospective study, *Am. J. Epidemiol.*, 126, 1093, 1987.

26. Mann, J. I. et al., Dietary determinants of ischaemic heart disease in health conscious individuals, *Heart*, 78, 450, 1997.

27. Pietinen, P. et al., Intake of dietary fiber and risk of coronary heart disease in a cohort of Finnish Men. The Alpha-Tocopherol, Beta-Carotene Cancer Prevention Study, *Circulation*, 94, 2720, 1996.

28. Todd, S. et al., Dietary antioxidant vitamins and fiber in the etiology of cardiovascular disease and all-cause mortality: results from the Scottish Heart Health Study, *Am. J. Epidemiol.*, 150, 1073, 1999.

29. Fraser, G. E. et al., A possible protective effect of nut consumption on risk of coronary heart disease, *Arch. Intern. Med.*, 152, 1416, 1998.

30. Jacobs D. R., Jr. et al., Whole grain intake may reduce risk of coronary heart disease death in postmenopausal women: the Iowa Women's Health Study, *Am. J. Clin. Nutr.*, 68, 248, 1998.

31. Liu, S. et al., Whole-grain consumption and risk of coronary heart disease: results from the Nurses' Health Study, *Am. J. Clin. Nutr.*, 70, 412, 1999.

32. Liu, S. et al., Whole grain consumption and risk of ischemic stroke in women, *JAMA*, 284, 1534, 2000.

33. Jacobs, D. J., Jr. et al. Fiber from whole grains, but not refined grains, is inversely associated with all-cause mortality in older women: the Iowa Women's Health Study, *J. Am. Coll. Nutr.*, 19, 326S, 2000.

34. Centers for Disease Control and Prevention, Trends in the prevalence and incidence of self-reported diabetes mellitus–US 1980–84, *MMWR*, 46, 1014, 1997.

35. Burke, J. P. et al., Rapid rise in the incidence of type II diabetes from 1987 to 1996, *Arch. Intern. Med.*, 159, 1450, 1999.

36. Lundgren, H. et al., Dietary habits and incidence of noninsulin-dependent diabetes mellitus in a population of women in Gothenburg, Sweden, *Am. J. Clin. Nutr.*, 49, 708, 1989.

37. Salmerón, J. et al., Dietary fiber, glycemic load, and risk of noninsulin-dependent diabetes mellitus in women, *JAMA*, 277, 472, 1997.

38. Salmerón, J. et al., Dietary fiber, glycemic load, and risk of noninsulin-dependent diabetes mellitus in men, *Diabetes Care*, 20, 545, 1997.

39. Meyer, K. A. et al., Carbohydrates, dietary fiber, and incident type II diabetes mellitus in older women, *Am. J. Clin. Nutr.*, 71, 921, 2000.

40. Liu, S. et al., A prospective study of whole-grain intake and risk of type II diabetes mellitus in U.S. women, *Am. J. Pub. Health*, 90, 1409, 2000.

41. Howe, G. R. et al., Dietary intake of fiber and decreased risk of cancers of the colon and rectum: evidence from the combined analysis of 13 case-control studies, *J. Natl. Cancer Inst.*, 84, 1887, 1992.

42. Friedenreich, C. M., Brant, R. F., and Riboli, E., Influence of methodologic factors in a pooled analysis of 13 case-control studies of colorectal cancer and dietary fiber, *Epidemiology*, 5, 66, 1994. [Erratum, *Epidemiology*, 5, 385, 1994.]

43. Giovannucci, E. et al., Intake of fat, meat, and fiber in relation to risk of colon cancer in men, *Cancer Res.*, 54, 2390, 1994.

44. Goldbohm, R. A. et al., Prospective study on alcohol consumption and the risk of cancer of the colon and rectum in the Netherlands, *Cancer Causes Control*, 5, 95, 1994.

45. Heilbrun, L. K. et al., Diet and colorectal cancer with special reference to fiber intake, *Int. J. Cancer*, 44, 1, 1989.

46. Kato, I., et al., Prospective study of diet and female colorectal cancer: the New York University Women's Health Study, *Nutr. Cancer*, 28, 276, 1997.

47. Steinmetz, K. A. et al., Vegetables, fruit, and colon cancer in the Iowa Women's Health Study, *Am. J. Epidemiol.*, 139, 1, 1994.

48. Thun, M. J. et al., Risk factors for fatal colon cancer in a large prospective study, *J. Natl. Cancer Inst.*, 84, 1491, 1992.

49. Fuchs et al., Dietary fiber and the risk of colorectal cancer and adenoma in women, *New Engl. J. Med.*, 340, 169, 1999.

50. Jacobs, D. J., Jr. et al., Whole grains intake and cancer: an expanded review and meta-analysis, *Nutr. Cancer*, 30, 85, 1998.

51. Chatenoud, L. et al., Whole grain food intake and cancer risk, *Int. J. Cancer*, 77, 24, 1998.

52. Slattery, M. L. et al., Plant foods and colon cancer: an assessment of specific foods and their related nutrients (United States), *Cancer Causes Control*, 8, 575, 1997.

53. Slattery, M. L. et al., Eating patterns and risk of colon cancer, *Am. J. Epidemiol.*, 148, 4, 1998.

Whole Grains, Cereal Fiber, and Chronic Diseases: Experimental Evidence and Possible Biologic Mechanisms

**Joel J. Pins, Mark A. Pereira, David R. Jacobs, Jr.,
Len Marquart, and Joseph M. Keenan**

INTRODUCTION

Despite the efforts of early health advocates, grain consumption in the U.S. fell throughout the 1900s until 1972, with some recovery since then. Recent data indicate that grain intake currently composes about 25% of total energy consumption, with whole grain intake providing only 1% of our total energy.[1-3] Nevertheless, evidence continues to amass supporting the health benefits of increased whole grain intake. The evidence was sufficiently strong that in 1999 the U.S. Food and Drug Administration (FDA) allowed the following health claim: "Diets rich in whole-grain foods and other plant foods and low in total fat, saturated fat and cholesterol may reduce the risk for heart disease and certain cancers" (FDA Docket #99P-2209). Based on the same evidence, the USDA Dietary Guidelines for Americans were amended to include specific mention of whole grains: "Eat a variety of grains daily, especially whole grains" (pp. 29–30, Dietary Guideline Advisory Committee Rationale, *http://www.ars.usda.gov/dgac/dgac_ration.pdf*).

The current research on whole grain intake and health tends to be nonspecific as to mechanisms. More research is warranted to understand how whole grain foods might produce health benefits. Historically, most of the research in this field has focused on the "magic bullet" approach — testing a single grain component rather than foods rich in whole grains. Such methodology is built on many assumptions and fails to recognize the possible interactive and/or additive effects of all whole grain components.[4] The "whole food" approach does make studying biological mechanisms challenging, but it likely is a more realistic model for testing outcomes. Few clinical trials have been done investigating the causal relationships and the potential biological pathways by which whole grains might modify chronic disease and possibly mortality. This chapter will provide a working definition of whole grains as well as explore several possible biological mechanisms linking whole grain intake with coronary heart disease (CHD), type II diabetes, and cancer.

WHOLE GRAINS: WHAT ARE THEY?

In terms of production, the major cereal grains are wheat, rice, and corn, with minor grains including oats, rye, barley, triticale, sorghum, and millet.[5] Though minor in terms of pounds of production, oats are generally eaten whole and contribute disproportionately to whole grain consumption. Moreover, wheat and rice account for over 50% of total grain production.[5] In developed countries, to increase shelf life and palatability, most grains undergo considerable refinement. Such processing includes, but is not limited to, milling, heat extraction, cooking, parboiling, extruding, puffing, flaking, and other techniques.[5] Prior to processing, all grains are similar in structure — composed of an endosperm, germ, and bran layer. The percentage of bran and germ varies between grains, but the endosperm consistently represents a little more than 80% of the kernel. In milling, the most common of the refinement processes listed above, the bran and germ are stripped from the endosperm and the latter is ground into flour.

Refined flour products contribute a significant percentage of total carbohydrate intake in the U.S. Unfortunately, most nutrients, dietary fiber, and phytochemicals are disproportionately concentrated in the bran and germ and are therefore lost in milling.[5] For example, one of the more recently researched whole grain phytochemicals is a family of compounds named *phenolic acids*. Recent data indicate that refinement of whole grains results in significant reduction of the content of phenolic acids.[6] Based on this information, grain foods that are unrefined (retain the bran and germ) can be classified as "whole." Whether the bran and the germ are removed, modification of the harvested kernel occurs in almost all cases prior to human consumption. Whole grains must then, by definition, be minimally processed grains. More specifically, the American Association of Cereal Chemists has created the following working definition: "Whole grains shall consist of the intact, ground, cracked, or flaked caryopsis, whose principal anatomical components, the starchy endosperm, germ, and bran, are present in substantially the same relative proportions as they exist in the intact caryopsis."[7] Furthermore, the FDA has adopted a definition in the health claim mentioned above that whole grain foods must consist of at least 51% whole grain flour (containing bran, germ, and endosperm) by weight. Examples of foods made with whole grain flours include some breakfast cereals, whole grain pasta, and a few commercial breads.

CORONARY HEART DISEASE

As described in our accompanying chapter, numerous epidemiologic studies have demonstrated that increased whole grain consumption is associated with reduced CHD.[8–10] Many of the protective effects of whole grains have been attributed to their dietary fiber content; in fact, most of the research focuses on the lipid-modifying effects of soluble fibers. Additionally, dietary fibers have been shown to directly and indirectly affect other CVD-related factors such as hyperinsulinemia, hyperglycemia, hypertension, obesity, and hemostatic factors. These fiber effects may be related to the nondigestible constituents themselves, such as hemicellulose, but they are equally likely related to the many phytochemicals that are found intermixed with the nondigestible constituents. For example, whole grains are also rich in antioxidants such as tocotrienols, phytoestrogens, and phenolic acids. Antioxidant intake has been shown to decrease the incidence of CHD by slowing the rate of low-density lipoprotein (LDL) oxidation and exhibiting other vaso-protective properties. This section of the chapter will focus on the CHD-altering effects of the fiber and antioxidant components of whole grains.

Lipid-Modifying Effects

Since the publication of the first oat-feeding trial in the early 1960s, the beneficial cholesterol-lowering effects of soluble fiber have been well documented: especially among hyperlipidemics, they reduce total and LDL cholesterol in serum, without lowering high-density lipoprotein (HDL) cholesterol or significantly altering serum triglyceride (Tg) concentrations.[11] Whole grains are also rich in fructans, oligosaccharides classified as dietary soluble fibers, because they resist digestion in the upper gastrointestinal tract and are fermented in the large intestine by indigenous bacteria. Results from a recent trial suggest that inulin and oligofructose (the most common fructans) might independently improve serum lipid concentration.[12] Additionally, very few human and animal trials have suggested that wheat and other cereal brans significantly reduce serum triglyceride concentrations.[13] Isoflavones from soy foods have also been shown to beneficially affect serum lipids.[14] Analogous phytoestrogens in whole grains might then also produce beneficial effects on serum triglyceride and HDL cholesterol concentrations.

Unfortunately, very few clinical trials have been conducted directly testing the lipid-altering effects of whole vs. refined grains. In a recent crossover clinical trial, Leinonen et al.[15] examined the lipid-lowering effects of unrefined rye bread — a rich source of dietary fiber including arabinoxylan, a viscous soluble fiber, which accounts for approximately 60% of the total fiber content. During each trial phase, the healthy young participants were asked to consume either refined wheat or whole rye bread in addition to their normal diet. Whereas no lipid changes occurred during the wheat phase, LDL and total cholesterol reductions of 12% and 10%, respectively, were observed in the rye phase. This effect was observed only in men, which the authors suggest may be due to the difference in total rye bread consumed by men vs. women.

The hypocholesterolemic effects of whole grains rich in dietary fibers and oligosaccharides appear to work via one or more of four primary pathways. Though not all fibers affect each of these pathways equally, all mechanisms generally rely on the viscous nature of these fibers. Consider, for example, that hydrolyzed guar gum, which does not possess the viscous properties of unmodified guar gum, and non-viscous soluble fibers such as gum arabic are ineffective in reducing serum cholesterol.[16,17]

The primary mechanism (see Figure 6.3.1) by which some viscous fibers reduce serum cholesterol is by binding bile acids in the small intestine and thereby altering enterohepatic bile acid recycling. This decreases the bile acid pool and requires more endogenous hepatic bile acid synthesis. To do so, the liver must either up-regulate endogenous sterol synthesis or increase LDL particle uptake from circulation.[18] A second mechanism of action is stimulated by the fermentation of fibers, oligosaccharides, and undigested starches in the large intestine by indigenous bacteria. One of the by-products of this process is short-chain fatty acids (SCFAs), including acetate, butyrate, and propionate. Some of these SCFAs (primarily propionate) enter the system via portal circulation and are delivered to the liver, where they inhibit hepatic cholesterol synthesis by limiting the action of HMG-CoA reductase.[19] A recent animal trial demonstrated increased bacterial propionate production after feeding of poorly digestible resistant starches. Elevated levels of propionic acid resulted in reduced serum total cholesterol, serum LDL cholesterol, hepatic cholesterol, and hepatic triglyceride in rats.[20] Viscous soluble fibers have also been suggested to slow gastric emptying and the digestion/absorption of carbohydrates in the small intestine. Such action results in the reduction of postprandial insulin and a decrease in the activity of HMG-CoA reductase.[21] A final hypothesis is that decreased absorption of dietary fats and cholesterol due to increased intestinal viscosity by soluble fibers might result in serum cholesterol reduction.[22]

As mentioned above, the total lipid-modifying effects of whole grains might be due to the combined effect of the fiber, oligosaccharides, and resistant starches as well as the bran fraction and the phytoestrogens. Whether cereal bran and phytoestrogens improve lipid profile, as well as the mechanism by which they might do so, has not yet been fully established.

Hypotensive Effects

The blood pressure–modifying effects of whole grains and their associated components have not been studied as extensively as their hypocholesterolemic effects. Some epidemiologic studies

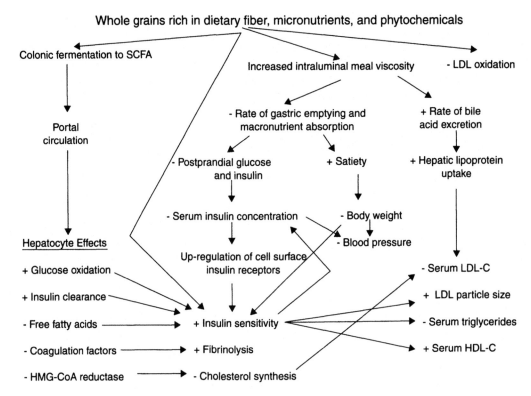

Figure 6.3.1   Whole grains and CHD/diabetes; theoretical model of mechanisms of action. Legend: + signifies an increase in the variable after the pathway has been initiated; - signifies a decrease in the variable after the pathway has been initiated.

have suggested that increased dietary fiber intake is associated with a decreased incidence of hypertension as well as lower blood pressure, while other studies have failed to show an effect. Limited clinical trials have been conducted with blood pressure as the primary outcome variable, using whole grains rich in fiber or fiber supplements as the sole intervention. In a recent study among diabetics, Vuksan et al.[23] added a viscous soluble fiber (glucomannan) to the AHA Step 2 diet of type 2 diabetics. Participants were crossed to a wheat fiber control after 3 weeks of intervention. Compared to the control period, the soluble fiber–rich intervention reduced systolic blood pressure (sBP) 9.4 mmHg (6.9%). Keenan et al.[24] reported that oat-based cereals — oats that are rich in the soluble fiber beta-glucan — reduced both sBP and diastolic blood pressure (dBP) by 7.5 mmHg and 5.5 mmHg, respectively, when compared to refined wheat-based cereals. In a follow-up trial, our group demonstrated that whole grain oat-based cereals significantly reduced the need for antihypertensive medication compared to a refined grain cereal control.[25]

The mechanism (see Figure 6.3.1) by which soluble fibers exert their hypotensive effect is poorly understood. It has been proposed that the increase in insulin sensitivity induced by soluble fiber results in lower circulating insulin levels. In animal models, reduced insulin levels have been shown to result in improved endothelial cell function and reduced blood pressure.[26]

Additionally, Scherrer et al.[27] have reported that hyperinsulinemia causes increased renal tissue sodium reabsorption, which subsequently increases plasma volume, enhances stimulation of the sympathetic nervous system, and induces hypercatecholaminemia. Both conditions result in increased vasoconstriction and further sodium retention, leading to increased blood pressure.

Antithrombotic Effects

Various studies have noted a strong association between rates of coagulation and fibrinolysis and CHD. Specifically, research suggests that increased concentrations of plasma fibrinogen, plasminogen activator inhibitor type 1 (PAI-1), and factor VIIc increase CHD risk; however, the effect of whole grains and dietary fiber on these risk factors is less clear. Animal trials have indicated that increased dietary fiber intake might reduce both PAI-1 and fibrinogen. Our recently completed crossover feeding experiment compared whole vs. refined grain diets in 11 overweight insulin-resistant adults. The washout period was 6 to 9 weeks, and the non-grain part of the diets was matched between treatments. Grain intake included 6 to 10 servings per day of breakfast cereal, bread, rice, pasta, and various snacks.[28] PAI-1 concentration was significantly reduced at weeks 2, 4, and 6 during treatment with whole grains (mean difference = 28.1 ng/ml, $p < .001$). This effect appeared to be due, at least in part, to an improvement in insulin sensitivity during the whole grain diet. Additionally, fibrinogen levels were consistently lower during all weeks of the feeding of whole vs. refined grains, though these differences did not reach statistical significance.

The mechanism (see Figure 6.3.1) by which whole grains and dietary fibers increase fibrinolytic activity is not well elucidated. Some have suggested that increased insulin sensitivity is pivotal in the relationship. It has been proposed that regardless of the pathway to increased insulin sensitivity (i.e., up-regulation of cell surface insulin receptors or suppression of hepatic free fatty acid release), the condition may inhibit hepatic synthesis of certain coagulation factors.[29]

Body Weight Effect

Excessive body fatness is a primary predictor of CHD as well as type 2 diabetes. Numerous trials to date have investigated the effects of dietary fibers or whole grains on satiety and/or body weight. Rigaud et al.[30] recently investigated the satiating effects of a psyllium supplement (7.4 g/day) in addition to the normal diet of healthy volunteers. Compared to a placebo, the psyllium treatment reduced feelings of hunger by 13% and decreased energy intake by 17%. Pins et al.[31] recently investigated the satiety effects of a whole grain barley product vs. a refined grain wheat product. After 1 week on the whole grain supplement treatment, participants in the whole grain group reported a much greater feeling of fullness and being less hungry. At the end of the 4-week study, there was a nonsignificant weight loss of 2 pounds in the whole grain group. In a controlled feeding study of whole vs. refined grains, Pereira et al.[32] reported that participants had a tendency to be less hungry between meals on the whole grain diet. Additionally, there was a nonsignificant trend toward weight loss on the whole grain diet when compared to the refined grain diet, even though both diet phases were designed to maintain constant body weight. Here again, the biological effects of whole grains rich in soluble fibers might largely be attributed to their viscous nature and their slowing of gastric emptying; a recent trial investigating the satiating effects of a hydrolyzed guar gum (non-viscous fiber) found no effect on various measures of satiety.

The mechanism (see Figure 6.3.1) relating whole grain and dietary fiber consumption to greater feelings of fullness is likely related to the rate of gastric emptying as well as the rate of total carbohydrate digestion and absorption. Bourdon et al.[33] recently demonstrated that carbohydrate digestion and absorption were significantly slowed in response to a high-soluble-fiber meal. Additionally, cholecystokinin (CCK), which reduces the rate of gastric emptying, was elevated for a longer time after the high-soluble-fiber meal compared to the low-fiber meal. This finding might help explain the mechanism by which dietary fibers increase satiety and ultimately facilitate weight loss.

Antioxidant Effects and Other Vasoprotective Effects

Various experimental and clinical data support the hypothesis that modification (oxidation or glycation) of the LDL particle increases the atherogenicity of the particle and is a major step in CHD.[34] Whole-grain foods are a rich source of antioxidants,[35-37] including vitamins, trace minerals, and various nonnutrients such as phenolic acids, phytoestrogens, and phytic acid.[38] Whole grains are especially rich sources of vitamin E, specifically tocotrienols and (depending on the soil content) selenium, as well. Vitamin E is incorporated into the LDL particle and can reduce oxidative modification of LDL via its activity as a reducing agent.[39] Vitamin E also keeps selenium in the reduced state, allowing it to function as a co-factor for glutathione peroxidase. This enzyme complex is responsible for the clearance of lipid hydroperoxides (i.e., malondialdehyde), which are known to be atherogenic. Various phytic acids have also been shown to exhibit antioxidant properties *in vivo*.

The mechanism (see Figure 6.3.1) by which antioxidants protect against CHD is fairly well understood. Antioxidants are known to delay the onset of lipoprotein oxidative modification or at least slow the rate at which it occurs. In comparison to unmodified particles, oxidatively modified particles are known to be major contributors to plaque formation in the subendothelial space and subsequent CHD.[34] Vitamin E, via its functions as an antioxidant or in other capacities, has also been shown to modify other risk factors for CHD such as smooth muscle cell proliferation, decreased activation of protein kinase C, decreased platelet aggregation, as well as provide beneficial effects on eicosanoid metabolism.[40] Homocysteine is another known risk factor for CHD and might be reduced by increased consumption of whole grains.[41,42] Whole grains are rich in folate, which is the primary agent responsible for lowering homocysteine levels. Some whole grain foods and all refined grain flours are now fortified with folate in the U.S.

Another important contributor to CHD is abnormal vascular reactivity. Moreover, exogenous estrogen has been shown to improve vascular response after an injury as well as vasodilatation.[43] Recent data indicate that some plant estrogens share various chemical properties with estradiol. Certain plant estrogens called lignans are found in whole grains, yet limited information is available on food concentrations. However, data indicate that urinary excretion is associated with fiber intake, suggesting that they are located in the outer layer of the grain.[44] It is known that once ingested, plant lignans (secoisolariciresinol and matairesinol) are converted to mammalian lignans (enterolactone and enterodiol) via the action of endogenous gut bacteria. The lignans of whole grains share chemical properties with soy isoflavones, which have been more extensively studied. In a recent animal trial, rhesus monkeys with known atherosclerotic disease were treated for 6 months with soy isoflavones. Arterial response to acetylcholine was enhanced, as well as endothelium-modulated dilatation.[45] In a more recent animal trial, soy isoflavones were shown to significantly reduce the development of atherosclerosis in disease-free rabbits.[46] Rabbits in the treatment group experienced a significant reduction in various measures of lipid oxidation, as well as 37% less cholesterol deposition in the aortic arch when compared to controls.

Based on these data, it is apparent that whole grains and their many constituents may reduce the risk of CHD via their effects on multiple variables. The exact mechanisms, and the extent to which they are operative, need much further exploration. Nevertheless, it is well accepted that whole grains improve serum lipids, decrease blood pressure, improve fibrinolysis, improve antioxidant status, as well as improve vascular reactivity. Whole grain may help in weight loss, at least to the extent that isovolumic replacement of refined grain flour with whole grain flour leads to a 15–20% reduction in energy intake from the grain food. Whole grains also improve insulin sensitivity, which reduces risk for CHD. This aspect will be discussed in the next section on type 2 diabetes.

TYPE 2 DIABETES

As is the case with CHD, epidemiologic cohort studies have shown that whole grains reduce the risk of type 2 diabetes (see Chapter 6.2). Whole grains and/or their components have been shown to exert a significant effect on glucose and insulin metabolism. The majority of this effect might be due to fiber content or, more specifically, the fermentable fiber content of whole grains. Of interest, a recent epidemiologic study[47] (described in detail in the accompanying chapter) found that insoluble fiber was as predictive of reduced diabetes incidence as soluble fiber. Recent studies have shown that certain foods possess a low glycemic index, that is, they have less postprandial effects toward glycemia and insulinemia. Thus, the lower glycemic index of foods that contain whole grain particles might partially explain the beneficial effects of these foods in terms of type 2 diabetes. Additionally, it is just as likely that an unknown component of whole grains or an unexpected interaction between grain components might be responsible for the reduced risk of diabetes observed in the epidemiologic studies. For example, numerous plant lignans were just discovered in whole grain rye at many times the concentration of those traditionally thought to be the most prevalent of these phytoestrogens.[48] Moreover, in our recent feeding trial, we noted a significant improvement in insulin sensitivity in response to a whole grain diet rich in foods with a moderate to high glycemic index. Such findings suggest that many "unknowns" might at least in part help to explain the beneficial effects of whole grains in terms of diabetes. The following section will focus on the glycemic and insulinemic effects of whole grains as well as their fermentable components.

Glycemic and Insulinemic Effects

Due to their viscous nature and gastrointestinal effects, soluble fibers have been shown to exert significant glycemic and insulinemic effects. Dietary fiber-rich interventions lower serum insulin and glucose concentrations as well as improve insulin sensitivity.[49,50] More recent trials have studied the long-term glycemic effects of purified fibers.

The acute effects of soluble fibers on glucose and insulin have been fairly well established, as illustrated by recent trials. Braaten et al. were one of the first to demonstrate a significant reduction in serum glucose and insulin when oat gum was added to a glucose load. This same group showed that both oat gum and oat bran, when added to wheat farina, significantly reduced both glucose and insulin responses.[51] More recently, other fibers have been investigated for their glucose- and insulin-modifying properties. Lu et al.[52] investigated the postprandial effects of arabinoxylan in a normoglycemic population. Fourteen healthy individuals were asked to consume three isoenergetic breakfast meals — containing either 0, 6, or 12 g of soluble fiber — on nonconsecutive days after an overnight fast. The arabinoxylan-rich meals reduced peak postprandial glucose from 7.2 mmol/l to 6.3 and 5.9 mmol/l for participants on the 6 g and 12 g fiber plans, respectively. Similarly, in each case, the area under the curve for glucose (20.2% and 41.4%) and insulin (17.0% and 32.7%) was significantly reduced by the arabinoxlyan soluble fiber. In another study, psyllium supplementation produced analogous reductions in all-day and postprandial glucose levels when added to the traditional diabetic diet in men with type 2 diabetes ($n = 34$).[53] In a third study, glucomannan, a less frequently studied soluble fiber, was reported to improve long-term glycemic control, reducing serum fructosamine levels by 5.7% after a 3-week intervention at 0.7 g per 100 kcal.[23]

Whole grains rich in total and soluble fiber can also improve glucose and insulin metabolism. Granfeldt et al.[54] tested the effects of raw rolled oats, boiled rolled oats, and boiled intact oat kernels vs. white bread in older men. Only the intact oats resulted in a significant reduction in postprandial glucose and insulin compared to white bread. Chandalia et al.[55] demonstrated significant glucose and insulin effects in a diabetic population after increasing dietary fiber intake to 25 g of soluble and 25 g of insoluble fiber daily, some of which was provided by whole grains. Reductions were observed in mean daily glucose (13 mg/dl) and urinary glucose (1.3 g), as well as 24-hour glucose (10%) and insulin (12%) areas under the curve.

Our research group conducted a trial comparing whole grain oat cereal intake with refined grain cereals. In addition to the blood pressure reductions noted above, after 6 weeks of whole grain cereal supplementation, the treatment group experienced a significant reduction in the amount of insulin needed to clear a glucose load, suggesting improved insulin sensitivity.[24] As described above, Pereira et al.[32] also tested the insulin-modifying effects of a whole grain vs. a refined grain diet. The study diets included six to ten daily servings of grains. By 2 weeks into the whole grain diet, fasting insulin was lower, although most of the whole grain foods consumed were made from whole grain flour, with a moderate to high glycemic index. Insulin levels remained suppressed and significantly lower than the refined grain diet through 6 weeks ($p < .05$). Results of euglycemic hyperinsulinemic clamp tests in 9 of the 11 subjects confirmed that the average insulin sensitivity of these subjects was improved by the whole grain diet.

Two primary mechanisms (see Figure 6.3.1) have been proposed for the glucose- and insulin-improving actions of whole grains rich in fiber. The first pathway has to do with the glycemic index of whole grain foods. The glycemic index is the elevation in plasma glucose after the consumption of a specific carbohydrate-rich food as compared to white bread or a glucose solution.[56,57] One of the primary predictors of the glycemic index of a whole grain is the structure of food components and soluble fiber content.[58] Any processing, such as refinement, that disrupts the food structure and/or decreases the soluble fiber content results in increased glucose and insulin responses. Therefore, whole grains (not whole meal) tend to reduce the glycemic response.[59]

In fact, Jarvi et al. recently published a study showing that simply altering the structure of starch-rich foods (decreasing glycemic index) resulted in a 30% reduction in area-under-the-curve for glucose and insulin, as well as a significant decrease in fructosamine and PAI-1.[60] Intact whole grains have lower glycemic indexes than refined grains, with grains richest in soluble fiber having the lowest indexes.[61] Independent of their delivery medium, soluble fibers decrease the rate of gastric emptying and slow the digestion of macronutrients. These phenomena result in a significant reduction in postprandial glycemia. Reduced serum glucose levels decrease the amount of insulin needed to clear the glucose load; over time, the reduced ambient insulin levels may result in an up-regulation of cell surface insulin receptors, thereby increasing insulin sensitivity.[62]

A recent animal trial suggested that soluble fibers may also directly increase the translocation of GLUT 4 receptors to the cell surface, resulting in improved insulin sensitivity without affecting PI3 kinase activation.[62] The second pathway involves the fermentation of soluble fibers, oligosaccharides, and resistant starches by bacteria in the large intestine, producing SCFAs which then enter the portal circulation. There is some evidence that hepatocytes, when exposed to an increase in SCFAs, may increase glucose oxidation, decrease free fatty acid release, and increase insulin clearance — all of which might improve insulin sensitivity.[63,64] In closing, again, it is likely that other whole grain constituents or interactions between known and unknown constituents beneficially modify risk for diabetes via the mechanisms highlighted above or via other currently unexplored pathways.

CANCER

It has long been thought that dietary fiber is very protective against the incidence of colon cancer. However, findings from both a recent prospective epidemiologic study and two clinical trials of polyp recurrence prevention have raised serious questions about this relationship.[65–67] Yet various animal experiments and epidemiologic studies suggest that whole grains provide significant protection against gastrointestinal cancers and possibly other systemic cancers as well. Such findings suggest that other whole grain components or a synergy between components provide protection against carcinogenesis. The following section will look at the anticarcinogenic effects of various components in whole grains, including the fermentable fraction, antioxidants, and phytoestrogens. Additionally, the cumulative effect of whole grains on insulin metabolism will be explored.

Gastrointestinal Effects

Most of the research to date has investigated the effects of dietary fiber on colorectal cancer. More recently other whole grain components, such as the lipid fraction or oligosaccharides, have been shown to decrease risk of this cancer. The lipid fraction of whole grains is known to contain omega-3 fatty acids, and the feeding of a diet containing 5% energy from n-3 fatty acids has been shown to decrease the incidence of aberrant crypt foci in rats.[68] Moreover, a recent interesting animal trial demonstrated that feeding male F344 rats a 10% wheat bran diet fortified with 2% bran oil and dephytinized resulted in a significant decrease in colon tumor incidence, multiplicity, and volume.[69]

Total fiber and oligosaccharides (which are known to be more concentrated in whole vs. refined grain) are known to exert various gastrointestinal effects, most of which appear to be protective against colorectal cancer. Much of the action has to do with the fermentability of these agents. For example, insoluble lignified fiber found in the outer bran of whole grains is only slightly degraded but greatly increases fecal bulk due to its physicochemical properties and water-holding capacity.[70] Highly fermentable carbohydrates such as soluble fibers and oligosaccharides also affect fecal weight by affecting bacterial metabolism and increasing the formation of bacterial biomass.[71] Importantly, increased fecal bulk has also been shown to greatly reduce intestinal transit time.[72] Additionally, increased intake of fermentable carbohydrate results in corresponding increases in the concentration of bifidobacteria and decreases in E. coli and clostridia. Certain bacteria exhibit differential enzyme activity (i.e., beta-glucuronidase) whose by-products might be carcinogenic, suggesting that dietary fibers might affect the cancer process by encouraging the colonization of certain types of bacteria. Moreover, intestinal bacteria convert primary bile acids into secondary bile acids, which have been suggested to promote the tumorigenesis process related to colon cancer.[73] Moreover, gut bacteria increase intestinal diacylglycerol content via the catabolism of dietary fatty acids and phospholipids.[74] Diacylglycerol content is further increased in the presence of secondary bile acids. As indicated above, one of the end products of bacterial fermentation is increased formation of SCFAs. It has been suggested that butyrate, the preferred fuel of colonocytes, may be a protective factor in colon carcinogenesis.[75]

To date, only one human trial has been conducted to investigate the effects of whole grains on risk for colon cancer. Grasten et al.[76] compared the effects of whole-meal rye vs. white wheat bread on some putative colon cancer risk markers in 17 healthy Finnish study participants. Test breads provided a minimum of 20% of daily energy intake and were consumed for two 4-week feeding periods separated by a 4-week washout. Compared to the white bread control, whole-meal rye bread significantly increased fecal output and frequency as well as reduced mean intestinal transit time in both men and women. Total and secondary bile acid concentrations were significantly lower during the rye bread period. The findings from this human trial are congruent with many animal and in vitro trials, suggesting that whole grains improve gastrointestinal function and reduce colon cancer risk.

Several mechanisms (see Figure 6.3.2) help explain the protective nature of whole grain components against colon cancer. Dietary fibers and, to a lesser extent, oligosaccharides dilute colonic contents by increasing fecal weight, accelerate intestinal transit time, and increase fecal frequency. Such actions decrease the opportunity for fecal mutagens to interact with intestinal epithelial cells, thereby reducing the likelihood of cellular mutation. Colonocyte proliferation is promoted by secondary bile acids. Hyperproliferation increases the opportunity for DNA mutations and subsequent replication of abnormal cells. Dietary fibers protect colonocytes by binding or diluting secondary bile acids. Additionally, the fermentable fraction of whole grains increases SCFA

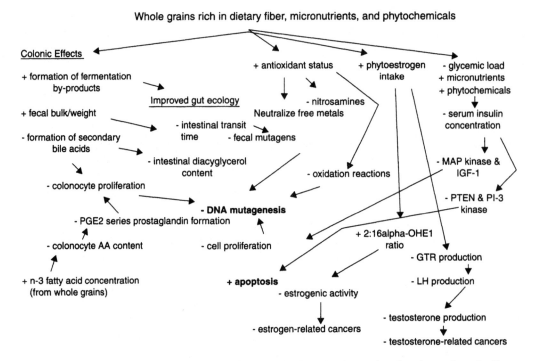

Figure 6.3.2　Whole grains and cancer; theoretical model of mechanisms of action. Legend: + signifies an increase in the variable after the pathway has been initiated; - signifies a decrease in the variable after the pathway has been initiated.

concentrations, which lowers colonic pH and results in a decreased conversion of primary to secondary bile acids.

Fermentable agents also alter gut ecology. In doing so, concentrations of certain bacteria, such as bifidobacteria, increase while others decrease. Bifidobacteria possess a low beta-glucuronidase activity, and end products of this enzyme have been suggested to be carcinogenic.[77] Other bacterial enzymes including urease (produces ammonia from urea) have been implicated in colon cancer due to the tumor-promoting actions of their end products. However, the effect of whole grains on these enzymes is unknown. The type of bacteria in the colon also affects intestinal concentrations of diacylglycerols. Diacylglycerols have been shown to activate protein kinase C isozymes,[78] and different isozymes stimulate cell proliferation, increasing subsequent cancer risk.[79] Wheat bran compared to a low-fiber diet has been shown to decrease the total intestinal diacylglycerol concentration, possibly via its effects on bacterial metabolism.[80]

The lipid fraction of whole grain includes n-3 fatty acids. These fatty acids may exert their anticarcinogenic effects via their influence of arachidonic acid metabolism. This 20-carbon fatty acid is the precursor of the dienoic prostaglandins. The PGE2 series of prostaglandins have been shown to increase colon cancer cell proliferation and inhibit apoptosis.[81,82] n-3 fatty acids decrease arachidonic acid concentration by competitive substitution and thereby decrease the production of the PGE2 series prostaglandins. This is one of the anticarcinogenic effects of n-3 fatty acids. These fatty acids have also been shown to alter oncogene expression, apoptosis, and intracellular signal transduction pathways.

Antioxidant Effects

Antioxidants from a variety of food sources have been shown to decrease the incidence of various types of cancer. Whole grains which contain a variety of antioxidants such as vitamin E, some trace minerals, phenolic acids, and phytoestrogens, and antinutrients such as phytic acid, have also been shown to effect the carcinogenesis process (see Chapters 6.1 and 6.5). Antioxidants function to reduce or delay the rate of oxidation reactions. In doing so, less oxidative damage occurs in the cell and the likelihood of forming cancer cells is reduced.

Whole grains are thought to be particularly rich sources of phenolic acids, especially ferulic acid.[35-37] Phenolic acids are concentrated in the bran fraction of the grain. Wheat bran and ready-to-eat cereals containing bran have been shown to exhibit significant antioxidant activity. Phytic acid is another antioxidant, which is concentrated in whole grains. Phytic acid is often classified as an antinutrient due to its ability to bind various minerals in the intestinal tract, thereby making then unabsorbable. However, such activity might explain the anticancer properties of phytic acid. Metals such as iron and copper have been shown to initiate oxidation reactions via the formation of reactive oxygen or nitrogen species such as the hydroxyl radical. Iron has been shown to be in its unbound form in the intestinal tract and thereby capable of initiating such reactions. Phytic acid, with its known chelating properties, might decrease the availability of metals and subsequent oxidation reactions.

Grains are also potentially rich sources of vitamin E and selenium. However, the concentration of both compounds is significantly reduced by the refining process. Under numerous experimental conditions, vitamin E has been shown to protect electron-dense cellular components (i.e., polyunsaturated fatty acids and genetic material) from oxidation reactions. This vitamin has also been shown to inhibit nitrosation reactions in the gut, thereby decreasing the availability of nitrosamines for absorption. The antioxidant enzyme glutathione peroxidase requires selenium as a cofactor, and compromised selenium status has been shown to decrease the activity of this enzyme.

The mechanisms (see Figure 6.3.2) by which the antioxidants in whole grains provide protection against cancer are many. In general, antioxidants protect genetic material from oxidative damage and subsequent mutation. If such mutations become part of the permanent genetic code, the initiation stage of cancer is said to have begun. In addition to their general antioxidant properties, phenolic acids protect against carcinogenesis via the induction of detoxification systems, specifically the Phase II conjugation reactions. Moreover, certain phenolic acids (caffeic and ferulic acids) have been defined as inhibitors of cancer cell initiation. They appear to act by preventing the formation of carcinogens from precursor compounds and by blocking the interaction of carcinogens with critical subcellular components.[83] By chelating metals, phytic acid greatly reduces the oxidant load in the gastrointestinal tract. Colonic bacteria also produce a significant amount of reactive nitrogen species, which might be reduced by phytic acid. Such activities reduce the oxidant exposure of intestinal epithelial cells and possible genetic mutation. Vitamin E, in addition to its general antioxidant capacities, has been classified as a cancer inhibitor due to its ability to inhibit the formation of carcinogens from precursor compounds such as nitrosamines.[83] As mentioned above, the action of glutathione peroxidase is a function of the availability of selenium. This enzyme has been shown to inhibit cell proliferation and, in general, selenium is considered a suppressing agent when it comes to its anticarcinogenic activity. Suppressing agents prevent the expression of neoplasia in cells that have previously been exposed to a carcinogen.[83]

Phytoestrogen Effects

Lignans, isoflavones, and coumestans (phytoestrogens) are compounds found in plants that exhibit estrogenic activity due to their structural similarity with endogenous estrogens. Certain whole grains such as wheat, oats, and rye are known to be concentrated sources of lignans.[84] Lignans are known to be associated with the fiber components of grains and therefore are thought to be lost in the refining process. This suggests that only whole grains, and not refined grains, are a significant dietary source. Phytoestrogens have been shown to exhibit certain cancer-protecting properties. At least some of these effects are due to their effect on endogenous sex hormone production, metabolism, and biological activity.[84]

Modification of estrogen metabolism has been suggested to alter the etiology of breast and other hormone-related cancers. For example, in women, significant lengthening of the overall cycle duration has been shown to reduce the risk of hormone-related cancers. Due to the concentration of lignans in flaxseed, that has been the delivery agent studied most often. Flaxseed powder supplementation has been shown to increase the average luteal phase length of the menstrual cycle in premenopausal women.[85] Additionally, changes in endogenous estrogen metabolism products might explain the chemoprotective effects of lignans. Estradiol and estrone are metabolized along two irreversible and competing pathways. The end products of these hydroxylation pathways are 2-hydroxylated and the 16-alpha-hydroxylated metabolites. Due to the different biological activities of these products, it has been proposed that an elevated ratio of 2-hydroxyestrogen to 16-alpha-hydroxyestrone (2:16alpha-OHE1) would reduce the risk of hormone-related cancers in women. In two recent human trials, daily consumption of 10 g of flaxseed significantly increased the urinary 2:16alpha-OHE1 ratio in premenopausal and postmenopausal women.[86,87] Flaxseed has also been shown to delay the progression of mammary tumorigenesis in a recent animal trial as well as reduce early markers of risk for mammary and colon carcinogenesis.[88] Similarly, changes in testosterone metabolism have been suggested to protect men against hormone-related cancers, such as prostate cancer. The phytoestrogen family of isoflavones has been studied to this end. In a recent animal trial, the spontaneous development of prostate cancer was significantly reduced in male Lobund-Wistar rats after the feeding of isoflavones for 22 months.[89]

The mechanisms (see Figure 6.3.2) by which phytoestrogens might protect against the occurrence of hormone-related cancers are poorly understood. Preliminary reports indicate that lignans directly inhibit the growth of human mammary tumor cells as well as reduce mammary and prostate tumor initiation. Additionally, 2-OHE metabolites are thought to exhibit very little estrogenic activity and might even possess antiestrogenic properties. Conversely, the 16-alpha-OHE1 demonstrates significant estrogenic activity and subsequently increases risk of breast cancer.[90] The ratio of these metabolites is a fair measure of total estrogenic activity and is decreased in women with breast cancer.[91] In men, phytoestrogens act as agonists for the action of testosterone in the prostate and related tissues and thereby possibly reduce carcinogenesis. It has been proposed that phytoestrogens result in decreased hypothalmic production of gonadotrophin-releasing hormone, which in turn inhibits the production of luteinizing hormone in the anterior pituitary with a subsequent decrease in the production of circulating testosterone by the Leydig's cells of the testes.[89,92] Additionally, genistein, a specific phytoestrogen, has been shown to reduce the activity of 5-alpha reductase, thereby decreasing the production of the powerful androgen dehydrotestosterone from testosterone.[93] Phytoestrogens, and specifically lignans, probably exhibit many other anticarcinogenic properties, thereby explaining their powerful cancer-reducing effects, but currently these are unknown.

Insulinemic Effects

Epidemiologic studies have reported that higher serum insulin levels are associated with increased risk of colon, breast, and possibly other cancers.[94-97] As mentioned above, refined grains on average exhibit a higher glycemic response than whole grains. Over time, a higher glycemic index diet has been shown to decrease insulin sensitivity and results in increased serum insulin levels.[98] Therefore, whole grains might reduce the risk of certain types of cancer by preventing acute and chronic states of hyperinsulinemia. It is also known that increased deep visceral adiposity decreases insulin sensitivity. This may explain in part why obesity is a risk factor for cancer. Modification of the glycemic index has been shown to affect satiety, which ultimately might affect weight gain and subsequent insulin resistance. Either directly or indirectly, emerging evidence suggests that increased whole grain consumption might protect against future cancers.

As might be expected, very little empirical data exist to explain the mechanism (see Figure 6.3.2) by which insulin is related to the carcinogenesis process. Most of the evidence comes from animal studies investigating the effect of insulin on colon carcinogenesis. Hyperinsulinemia has been shown to induce cell proliferation, possibly through the mitogen-activated protein (MAP) kinase pathway.[99] Decreased apoptosis has also been associated with elevated insulin levels, and modification of the phophatidylinositol 3-kinase and PTEN pathways might explain this effect.[100] Additionally, serum insulin growth factor-I (IGF-I) levels are elevated in response to insulin. IGF-I has also been shown to increase cell proliferation and reduce apoptosis. Other metabolic effects (elevated triglycerides and free fatty acids) may explain the carcinogenic effects associated with states of hyperinsulinemia; however, most of these pathways are currently poorly understood.

Chronic hyperinsulinemia and related metabolic consequences might increase risk of future breast, prostate, and colon cancer, but future elucidation of this relationship is necessary. More prospective epidemiologic data are needed as well as human trials investigating the relationship between insulin and risk markers for these cancers. Finally, more animal work is needed to determine the possible mechanisms by which insulin and related variables might induce carcinogenesis.

CONCLUSIONS

Based on this review, two things are apparent: (1) the possible mechanisms by which whole grains and their components modify risk for CHD and type 2 diabetes are better elucidated than are mechanisms which might relate to cancer; and (2) more studies testing whole grains as the primary intervention rather than a whole grain component are greatly needed. In terms of the latter issue, it has become clear in recent years that the "magic bullet" approach for investigating the disease-modifying effects of diet is not the best model. It is very possible that gastrointestinal and/or systemic interactions occur between dietary components to, at least in part, explain their physiological effects. More mechanistic work is certainly needed, but it is imperative that more studies are conducted using whole grains as the primary intervention. In the future, this will allow a clearer discussion of the relationship between whole grain intake and CHD, type 2 diabetes, and cancer, as well as other diseases. Finally, it is clear from this review that the "whole" is greater than the sum of its parts, and the recent health claims and public health recommendations to increase whole grain intake appear justified.

REFERENCES

1. Putnam, J. J. and Allshouse, J. E., *Food Consumption, Prices and Expenditures, 1996*, Statistical Bulletin 928, U.S. Department of Agriculture, Washington D.C., 1996.
2. Gerrior, S., Written communication, January, 1997.
3. Jacobs, D. R. Jr. et al., Is whole grain intake associated with reduced total and cause-specific death rates in older women? The Iowa Women's Health Study, *Am. J. Public Health*, 89, 322, 1999.
4. Potter, J. D., Food and phytochemicals, magic bullets and measurement error: a commentary, *Am. J. Epidemiol.*, 144, 1026, 1997.
5. Pedersen, B., Knudsen, K. E. B., and Eggum, B. O., Nutritive value of cereal products with emphasis on the effect of milling, *World Rev. Nutr. Diet*, 60, 1, 1989.
6. Hatcher, D. W. and Kruger, J. E., Simple phenolic acids in flours prepared from Canadian wheat: relationship to ash content, color, and polyphenol oxidase activity, *Cereal Chem.*, 74, 337, 1997.
7. American Association of Cereal Chemists, AACC whole grain ingredient definition, *Cereal Foods World*, 45, 79, 2000.
8. Jacobs, D. R. Jr. et al., Whole grain intake may reduce risk of coronary heart disease death in postmenopausal women: the Iowa Women's Health Study, *Am. J. Clin. Nutr.*, 68, 248, 1998.
9. Liu, S. et al., Whole-grain consumption and risk of coronary hear disease: results from the Nurses' Health Study, *Am. J. Clin. Nutr.*, 70, 412, 1999.

10. Rimm, E. B. et al., Vegetable, fruit, and cereal fiber intake and risk of coronary heart disease among men, *JAMA*, 275, 447, 1996.

11. Glore, S. R. et al., Soluble fiber and serum lipids: a literature review, *J. Am. Diet Assoc.*, 94, 425, 1994.

12. Davidson, M. H. and Maki, K. C., Effects of dietary inulin on serum lipids, *J. Nutr.*, 129, 1474S, 1999.

13. Heaton, K. W. and Pomare, E. W., Effect of bran on blood lipids and calcium, *Lancet*, 1, 49, 1979.

14. Anderson, J. W., Johnstone, B. M., and Cook-Newell, M. E., Meta-analysis of effects of soy protein intake on serum lipids in humans, *N. Engl. J. Med.*, 333, 276, 1995.

15. Leinonen, K. S., Poutanen, K. S., and Mykkanen, H. M., Rye bread decreases serum total and LDL cholesterol in men with moderately elevated serum cholesterol, *J. Nutr.*, 130, 164, 2000.

16. Anderson, S. A., Fisher, K. D., and Talbott, J. M., Evaluation of the health aspects of using partially hydrolyzed guar gum as a food ingredient, Life Sciences Research Office, Federation of American Societies for Experimental Biology, Bethesda, MD, 1990.

17. Davidson, M. H. et al., A low-viscosity soluble-fiber fruit juice supplement fails to lower cholesterol in hypercholesterolemic men and women, *J. Nutr.*, 128, 1927, 1998.

18. Marlett, J. A. et al., Mechanism of serum cholesterol reduction by oat bran, *Hepatology*, 20, 1450, 1994.

19. Cummings, J. H. and Macfarlane, G. T., Colonic microflora: nutrition and health, *Nutrition*, 13, 476, 1997.

20. Cheng, H. and Lai, M., Fermentation of resistant rice starch produces propionate reducing serum and hepatic cholesterol in rats, *J. Nutr.*, 130, 1991, 2000.

21. Wurch, P. and Pi-Sunyer, F. X., The role of viscous soluble fiber in the metabolic control of diabetes, *Diabetes Care*, 20, 1774, 1997.

22. Spiller, R. C., Pharmacology of dietary fibre, *Pharmacol Ther.*, 62, 407, 1994.

23. Vuksan, V. et al., Konjac-mannan (Glucomannan) improves glycemia and other associated risk factors for coronary heart disease in type 2 diabetes, *Diabetes Care*, 22, 913, 1999.

24. Keenan, J. M. et al., Oat ingestion reduces systolic and diastolic blood pressure among moderate hypertensives: a pilot trial, *J. Fam. Prac.*, 2001, in press.

25. Pins, J. J. et al., Whole grain cereals reduce antihypertensive medication need, blood lipids and plasma glucose levels (Abstract #39), *J. Am Coll. Nutr.*, 18, 529, 1999.

26. Katakam, P. et al., Endothelial dysfunction preceeds hypertension in diet induced insulin resistance, *Am. J. Physiol.*, 275, R788, 1998.

27. Scherrer, U. and Sartori, C., Defective nitric oxide synthesis: a link between metabolic insulin resistance, sympathetic overactivity and cardiovascular morbidity, *Eur. J. Endocrinol.*, 142, 315, 2000.

28. Pereira, M. A. et al., The effect of whole grains on inflammation and fibrinolysis (Abstract #3), *CVD Epi. Prev. Prog.*, 40, 8, 2000.

29. Yudkin, J. S., Abnormalities of coagulation and fibrinolysis in insulin resistance. Evidence for a common antecedent?, *Diabetes Care*, 22, C25, 1999.

30. Rigaud, D. et al., Effect of psyllium on gastric emptying, hunger feeling and food intake in normal volunteers: a double blind study, *Eur. J. Clin. Nutr.*, 52, 239, 1998.

31. Pins, J. J. et al., A comparison of barley and wheat products on blood lipids, satiety, and markers of oxidation (Abstract #49), *J. Am. Coll. Nutr.*, 19, 686, 2000.

32. Pereira, M. A. et al., The effect of whole grains on insulin sensitivity in overweight adults (Abstract #150.2), *FASEB J.*, 14, A203, 2000.

33. Bourdon, I. et al., Postprandial lipid, glucose, insulin, and cholecystokinin responses in men fed barley pasta enriched with β-glucan, *Am. J. Clin. Nutr.*, 69, 55, 1999.

34. Navab, M. et al., The yin and yang of oxidation in the development of the fatty streak, *Arterioscler. Thromb. Vasc. Biol.*, 16, 831, 1996.

35. Baublis, A., Decker, E. A., and Clydesdale, F. M., Antioxidant effect of aqueous extracts from wheat based ready-to-eat breakfast cereals, *Food Chem.*, 10, 1, 1999.

36. Miller H. E. et al., Antioxidant content of whole grain breakfast cereals, fruits and vegetables, *J. Am. Coll. Nutr.*, 19, 312S, 2000.

37. Miller, H. E. et al., Whole-grain products and antioxidants, *Cereal Foods World*, 45, 59, 2000.

38. Thompson, L. U., Antioxidants and hormone-mediated health benefits of whole grains, *Crit. Rev. Food Sci. Nutr.*, 34, 473, 1994.

39. Dieber-Rotheneder, M. et al., Effect of oral supplementation with d-alpha-tocopherol on the vitamin E content of human low density lipoproteins and resistance to oxidation, *J. Lipid Res.*, 32, 1325, 1992.

40. Chan, A. C., Vitamin E and atherosclerosis, *J. Nutr.*, 128, 1593, 1998.
41. Eikelboom, J. W. et al., Homocyst(e)ine and cardiovascular disease: a critical review of the epidemiologic evidence, *Ann. Intern. Med.*, 131, 363, 1999.
42. Malinow, M. R. et al., Reduction of plasma homcyst(e)ine levels by breakfast cereals fortified with folic acid in patients with coronary heart disease, *N. Engl. J. Med.*, 338, 1009, 1998.
43. Mendelsohn, M. E. and Karas, R. H., The protective effects of estrogen on the cardiovascular system, *N. Engl. J. Med.*, 340, 1801, 1999.
44. Adlercreutz, H. et al., Determination of urinary lignans and phytoestrogen metabolites, potential antiestrogens and anticarcinogens in urine of women on various habitual diets, *J. Steroid Biochem.*, 25, 971, 1986.
45. Williams, J. K. and Clarkson, T. B., Dietary soy isoflavones inhibit in-vivo constrictor responses of coronary arteries to collagen-induced platelet activation, *Coron. Artery Dis.*, 9, 759, 1998.
46. Yamakoshi, J. et al., Isoflavone aglycone-rich extract without soy protein attenuates atherosclerosis development in cholesterol-fed rabbits, *J. Nutr.*, 130, 1887, 2000.
47. Liukkonen, K. et al., Formation of enterolactone during *in vitro* fermentation of rye, Data presented at American Association of Cereal Chemists annual meeting, Kansas City, MO, Nov. 2000.
48. Meyer, K. A. et al., Carbohydrates, dietary fiber, and incident type 2 diabetes in older women, *Am. J. Clin. Nutr.*, 71, 921, 2000.
49. Anderson, J. W. et al., Metabolic effects of high-carbohydrate, high-fiber diets for insulin-dependent diabetic individuals, *Am. J. Clin. Nutr.*, 54, 936, 1991.
50. Fukagawa, N. K. et al., High-carbohydrate, high-fiber diets increase peripheral insulin sensitivity in healthy young and old adults, *Am. J. Clin. Nutr.*, 52, 524, 1990.
51. Braaten, J. T. et al., High beta-glucan oat bran and oat gum reduce postprandial blood glucose and insulin in subjects with and without type 2 diabetes, *Diabet. Med.*, 11, 312, 1994.
52. Lu, Z. X. et al., Arabinoxylan fiber, a byproduct of wheat flour processing, reduces the postprandial glucose response in normoglycemic subjects, *Am. J. Clin. Nutr.*, 71, 1123, 2000.
53. Anderson, J. W. et al., Effects of psyllium on glucose and serum lipid responses in men with type 2 diabetes and hypercholesterolemia, *Am. J. Clin. Nutr.*, 70, 466, 1999.
54. Granfeldt, Y., Drews, A., and Bjorck, I., Arepas made from high amylose corn flour produce favorably low glucose and insulin responses in healthy humans, *J. Nutr.*, 125, 459, 1995.
55. Chandalia, M. et al., Beneficial effects of high dietary fiber intake in patients with type 2 diabetes mellitus, *N. Engl. J. Med.*, 342, 1392, 2000.
56. Reaven, G. and Miller, R., Study of the relationship between glucose and insulin responses to an oral glucose load in man, *Diabetes*, 17, 560, 1968.
57. Wolever, T. M. S. et al., The glycemic index: methodology and clinical implications, *Am. J. Clin. Nutr.*, 54, 846, 1991.
58. Bjorck, I. et al., Food properties affecting the digestion and absorption of carbohydrates, *Am. J. Clin. Nutr.*, 59S, 688S, 1994.
59. Jenkins, D. J. A. et al., Low glycemic response to traditionally processed wheat and rye products: bulgur and pumpernickel bread, *Am. J. Clin. Nutr.*, 43, 516, 1986.
60. Jarvi, A. E. et al., Improved glycemic control and lipid profile and normalized fibrinolytic activity on a low-glycemic index diet in type 2 diabetic patients, *Diabetes Care*, 22, 10, 1999.
61. Jenkins, D. J. A. et al., Wholemeal versus wholegrain breads: proportion of whole or cracked grain and the glycaemic response, *Brit. Med. J.*, 297, 958, 1988.
62. Song, Y. J. et al., Soluble dietary fibre improves insulin sensitivity by increasing muscle GLUT-4 content in stroke-prone spontaneously hypertensive rats, *Clin. Exp. Pharmacol. Physiol.*, 27, 41, 2000.
63. Thorburn, A., Muir, J., and Proietto, J., Carbohydrate fermentation decreases hepatic glucose output in healthy subjects, *Metabolism*, 42, 780, 1993.
64. Venter, C. S., Vorster, H. H., and Cummings, J. H., Effects of dietary propionate on carbohydrate and lipid metabolism in healthy volunteers, *Am. J. Gastroenterol.*, 85, 549, 1990.
65. Fuchs, C. S. et al., Dietary fiber and the risk of colorectal cancer and adenoma in women, *N. Engl. J. Med.*, 340, 169, 1999.
66. Bonithon-Kopp, C. et al., Calcium and fibre supplementation in prevention of colorectal adenoma recurrence: a randomised intervention trial, *Lancet*, 356, 1300, 2000.

67. Alberts, D. S. et al., Lack of effect of a high-fiber cereal supplement on the recurrence of colorectal adenomas, *N. Engl. J. Med.*, 342, 1156, 2000.
68. Bartoli, R. et al., Effect of olive oil on early and late events of colon carcinogenesis in rats: modulation of arachidonic acid metabolism and local prostaglandin E2 synthesis, *Gut*, 46, 191, 2000.
69. Reddy, B. S. et al., Preventive potential of wheat bran fractions against experimental colon carcinogenesis: implications for human colon cancer prevention, *Cancer Res.*, 60, 4792, 2000.
70. Bach, K. K. E., Johansen, H. N., and Glitso, V., Rye dietary fiber and fermentation in the colon, *Cereal Foods World*, 72, 690, 1997.
71. Stephen, A. M. and Cummings, J. H., The microbial contribution to human fecal mass, *J. Med. Microbiol.*, 13, 45, 1980.
72. Cummings, J. H. et al., Fecal weight, colon cancer risk and dietary intake of non-starch polysaccharides (dietary fiber), *Gastroenterology*, 103, 1783, 1992.
73. Reddy, B. S. and Watanabe, K., Effect of cholesterol metabolites and promoting effect of lithocholic acid in colon carcinogenesis in germ-free and conventional F344 rats, *Cancer Res.*, 39, 1521, 1979.
74. Morotomi, M. et al., Production of diacylglycerol, an activator of protein kinase C, by human intestinal flora, *Cancer Res.*, 50, 3539, 1990.
75. Scheppach, W., Butyrate and the epithelium of the large intestine, in *Functional Properties of Non-Digestible Carbohydrates*, Guillon, F. et al., Eds., Nantes, France, 1998, 215.
76. Grasten, S. M. et al., Rye bread improves bowel function and decreases the concentrations of some compounds that are putative colon cancer risk markers in middle-aged women and men, *J. Nutr.*, 130, 2215, 2000.
77. Hawksworth, G., Drasar, B. S., and Hill, M. J., Intestinal bacteria and the hydrolysis of glycoside bonds, *J. Med. Microbiol.*, 4, 451, 1971.
78. Nishizuka, Y., Intracellular signaling by hydrolysis of phospholipids and activation of protein kinase C, *Science*, 258, 608, 1992.
79. Chapkin, R. S. et al., Dietary fibers and fats alter rat colon protein kinase C activity: correlation to cell proliferation, *J. Nutr.*, 123, 649, 1993.
80. Reddy, B. S., Simi, B., and Engle, A., Biochemical epidemiology of colon cancer: effects of types of dietary fiber on colonic diacylglycerols in women, *Gastroenterology*, 106, 883, 1994.
81. Qiao, L. et al., Selected eicosanoids increase the proliferation rate of human colon carcinoma lines and mouse colonocytes in vivo, *Biochem. Biophys. Acta*, 1258, 215, 1995.
82. Sheng, H. et al., Modulation of apoptosis and Bcl-2 expression by prostaglandin E_2 in human colon cancer cells, *Cancer Res.*, 58, 362, 1998.
83. Wattenberg, L. W., Chemoprevention of cancer, *Cancer Res.*, 45, 1, 1985.
84. Adlercreutz, H. and Mazur, W., Phyto-oestrogens and Western diseases, *Ann. Med.*, 29, 95, 1997.
85. Fishman, J., Bradlow, H. L., and Gallagher, T. F., Oxidative metabolism of estradiol, *J. Biol. Chem.*, 235, 3104, 1960.
86. Haggans, C. J. et al., Effect of flaxseed consumption on urinary estrogen metabolites in postmenopausal women, *Nutr. Cancer*, 33, 188, 1999.
87. Haggans, C. J. et al., The effect of flaxseed and wheat bran consumption on urinary estrogen metabolites in premenopausal women, *Cancer Epidemiol. Biomarkers Prev.*, 9, 719, 2000.
88. Rickard, S. E. et al., Dose effects of flaxseed and its lignan on N-methyl-N-nitrosourea-induced mammary tumorigenesis in rats, *Nutr. Cancer*, 35, 50, 1999.
89. Pollard, M. and Wolter, W., Prevention of spontaneous prostate-related cancer in Lobund-Wistar rats by a soy protein isolate/isoflavone diet, *Prostate*, 45, 101, 2000.
90. Schneider, J. et al., Abnormal oxidative metabolism of estradiol in women with breast cancer, *Proc. Natl. Acad. Sci. USA*, 79, 3047, 1982.
91. Ho, G. H. et al., Urinary 2/16-hydroxyestrone ratio: correlation with serum insulin-like growth factor binding protein-3 and a potential biomarker of breast cancer risk, *Ann. Acad. Med. Singapore*, 27, 294, 1998.
92. Norman, A. W. and Litwack, G., *Hormones*, Academic Press, New York, 1997, 513.
93. Evans, B. A. J., Griffith, K., and Morton, M. S., Inhibition of 5α reductase and 17β hydroxysteroid dehydrogenase in genital skin fibroblasts by dietary lignans and isoflavinoids, *Endocrinology*, 147, 295, 1995.

94. Schoen, R. E. et al., Increased blood glucose and insulin, body size and incident colorectal cancer, *JNCI*, 91, 1147, 1999.

95. Krazer, R. R., Insulin resistance, insulin like growth factor I and breast cancer: a hypothesis, *Int. J. Cancer*, 62, 403, 1995.

96. McKeown-Eyssen, G., Epidemiology of colorectal cancer revisited: are serum triglycerides and/or plasma glucose associated with risk?, *Cancer Epi. Bio. Prev.*, 3, 687, 1994.

97. Giovannucci, E., Insulin and colon cancer, *Cancer Causes Control*, 6, 164, 1995.

98. Frost, G. et al., Insulin sensitivity in women at risk of coronary heart disease and the effect of a low glycemic diet, *Metabolism*, 47, 1245, 1998.

99. Kahn, C. R., Banting Lecture, Insulin action, diabetogenes, and the cause of type II diabetes, *Diabetes*, 43, 1066, 1994.

100. Maehama, T. and Dixon, J. E., PTEN: a tumor suppressor that functions as a phospholipid phosphatase, *Trends Cell Biol.*, 9, 125, 1999.

Bioavailability of Minerals from Cereals

Wenche Frølich

INTRODUCTION

Whole grain cereals and cereal products are some of the best sources not only for dietary fiber, but also for minerals and trace elements in our diet. An increased consumption of flours with high extraction rates of these compounds is therefore a nutritional aim in many countries. Most minerals and trace elements in the cereals are closely related to the outer layers, especially the aleurone cells, where dietary fiber and phytic acid are also recovered. All these components have therefore, to a certain extent, been defined as a part of the dietary fiber complex.

The complexity of interactions that may take place between minerals and different components in the dietary fiber complex makes it very difficult to predict the bioavailability of minerals in whole grain cereals by chemical determinations of minerals and trace elements present in the cereal products. Due to the chelating properties of the dietary fiber components and the phytic acid, there has been a lot of concern about the effect of an unrefined high-fiber diet with respect to mineral bioavailability. An increasing knowledge of the complexity of nutrient interactions and the number of dietary components that can influence bioavailability makes this field very complicated. This includes both the difficulties in the analysis of dietary fiber and the various physical and chemical conditions which may alter the interactions between the nutrients.

MINERALS STUDIED

Bioavailability problems of practical significance are known for some minerals of long established nutritional importance such as calcium, zinc, and iron, but there seem to be similar problems for other minerals and trace elements such as selenium, chromium, copper, and nickel. New knowledge of bioavailability is constantly being discovered, and it seems that currently only a small fraction of these problems are recognized and corrected for.

MINERALS AND UNREFINED CEREAL PRODUCTS

It has been claimed that the bioavailability of minerals and trace elements in diets rich in whole grain products can be reduced in comparison with diets rich in refined cereal products. Great

0-8493-2387-8/01/$0.00+$1.50

controversies, in terms of mineral interactions, have been connected with the chelating properties of dietary fiber vs. phytic acid. In earlier studies it was claimed that the phytic acid present in the whole grain cereal products was the component chiefly responsible for the chelating of divalent minerals. More recently it has been suggested that phytic acid is not the component which is solely responsible for the decreased mineral availability. Fiber itself or other polysaccharides seem to a great extent to complex with minerals. However, the results in the literature are conflicting, and it is still debatable whether it is the fiber components, the phytic acid, or both that are responsible for the decreased absorption of minerals from whole grain cereal products.

Dietary fiber is often divided into a soluble and an insoluble fraction due to relative solubilities and other chemical properties. The solubilities of the minerals may be decreased as a result of chelation to fiber components. Dietary fibers could increase the viscosity and reduce the rate of migration of minerals, which, in addition to reduced transit time, could result in changes in the bioavailability of minerals.

The binding behavior of different minerals to cereal fibers seems to be extremely variable, probably due to the various chelating properties of the different fiber components. The various cereals also have quite different dietary fiber compositions with different chemical structure and binding capacities, making the chelating properties of the same mineral special for each cereal. As dietary fiber and phytic acid most often occur together in the cereal foods, it is difficult to distinguish between the effect of the different dietary fiber components and the phytic acid.

In many studies isolated fiber components and phytic acid have been added to the diet to study the effects of the individual components on the mineral bioavailability. It is important to realize that addition of isolated components to the diet only indicates the effect of the same amount of native dietary fiber or phytate present in the original food item.

Generalization about the bioavailability of minerals can be misleading, because the chelating properties are not the same in different cereals due to different amounts of fiber, different fiber composition, and different amounts of phytate present in the different cereals.

It is also important to stress that the refining of cereals leads to a marked fall in the mineral content. Therefore, an inhibition of the percent uptake of minerals and trace elements from the whole grain cereal products does not necessarily mean a decreased absolute intake, due to the considerably higher amount of minerals present in the whole grain.

BINDING BEHAVIOR OF MINERALS

The binding behavior of different minerals to cereal fibers seems to be quite variable, probably due to various chelating properties of the minerals. Little information on minerals other than Ca, Zn, Fe, Cu, and P is available, and no agreement exists for the different minerals studied. Much of the older work is still relevant today and has been taken into consideration when conclusions have been drawn.

ENRICHMENT STUDIES

When a single mineral is added to the food, as has been done in various enrichment studies, the balance between this mineral and the rest of the minerals and trace elements present is changed. This type of enrichment study has given quite different results from studies with the corresponding amount of the mineral naturally occurring in the food, even if the same amounts of dietary fiber and phytic acid were present in the studies.

In many studies, both human and animal studies, dosages of dietary fiber and phytic acid which are not physiological have been used. The interpretation of these studies is difficult and extrapolation to normal diets is often impossible.

HUMAN STUDIES/ANIMAL STUDIES

Much less is known about the mineral requirement and bioavailability in humans than in animals. Only limited studies on minerals connected with deficiency states can be carried out in humans. It is also difficult to carry out long-term studies, and studies which might cause risks to humans cannot be performed from an ethical point of view, e.g., studies on children and pregnant women. Evidence suggests, however, that many observations carried out in animals do have relevance to man. On the other hand, direct extrapolations from animals to humans do not give correct answers in all cases, and before any definite conclusions can be drawn, human studies are needed.

IN VITRO/IN VIVO STUDIES

The mechanisms by which dietary fiber chelates to the minerals are largely unknown. Several *in vitro* studies have been published concerning dietary fiber components that are responsible for the mineral association. The different isolated fiber components have been shown to have different cation exchange potentials, and several factors must be taken into consideration when interpreting the results: (1) presence of different chelators such as phytic acid, oxalic acid, tannins, citrate, and amino acids, (2) pH in the solution, (3) concentration of minerals, (4) heat treatment that may affect the binding, (5) presence of type and amount of various dietary fiber components, and (6) concentration of minerals. It is important to realize that great care is needed when extrapolating results from *in vitro* studies to *in vivo* conditions. The ability of minerals to bind or chelate to the different cereal components or isolated fiber fractions seems to be different in an *in vitro* system than when ingested alone or together with a composite diet.

INFLUENCE OF PROCESSING

The heat treatment during processing of cereal foods, both during the milling procedure and baking of bread, also influences the bioavailability of the minerals present in the final product. This is mainly due to the breakdown of phytic acid, but reorganization of dietary fiber components is also a factor, changing the chelating properties of these components. This is important to bear in mind when conclusions concerning the final cereal products (e.g., bread) are to be drawn on the basis of the cereal ingredients like flour and bran. Fermentation and leavening seem to improve the utilization of the minerals.

OTHER FACTORS INFLUENCING BIOAVAILABILITY

The bioavailability, which is a measure of the degree of both absorption and utilization, is shown to be affected by both intrinsic and extrinsic factors. The individual needs for the mineral due to nutritional and health status, sex, and age are intrinsic factors. Components in the diet are the extrinsic factors and could have both promoting and inhibitory effects. It is of importance to bear in mind that when studying mineral bioavailability, the composite diet should be taken into consideration and not only a single food component or fraction of the food. Studies on a single food item, on the other hand, can be used to identify the dietary components that are responsible for the changes in the mineral absorption.

The studies made with respect to the influence of other food items on mineral absorption from cereals are mainly done with respect to iron, with only a few studies on zinc. Ascorbic acid seems to be the most potent enhancer of iron absorption, while animal protein improves both zinc and iron absorption. Tea, on the other hand, seems to depress iron absorption.

LONG-TERM STUDIES NEEDED

Adaptation to a diminished availability of minerals is probably of importance after continuous addition of fiber from unrefined cereals. In experiments with a duration longer than 3 to 4 weeks, no change in mineral availability from whole grain cereals is observed. Most of the studies published are, however, short-term experiments, and it is therefore difficult to draw any definite conclusions about the inhibitory/promoting factors until more long-term studies have been performed.

CONCLUSIONS

There seems to be an inhibitory effect on the bioavailability of some minerals due to some of the components in the dietary fiber complex in cereals. Different cereals have different chelating properties due to different fiber components present in the various cereals. In the numerous human, animal, and *in vitro* studies on the effect of dietary fiber on mineral bioavailability, more controversy than consensus is found. There is a general agreement in the literature that further research is needed to clarify a number of questions still not solved.

In countries where the intake of minerals is limited and whole grain cereals account for the main part of energy, the somewhat decreased absorption could be of importance. In diets with extremely high dietary fiber and phytic acid content, deficiencies in both zinc and iron are likely to occur. There is, however, no evidence that the dietary fiber intake from a fiber-rich Western diet will interfere sufficiently with mineral absorption to cause deficiency in a healthy population. Such a diet is usually well balanced with a good quality standard, and animal products are a natural part of the diet. It is important to stress that a natural high-fiber diet contains more minerals and trace elements than a low-fiber diet, as fiber and minerals are located together in the cereals. On the other hand, if the increase in the dietary fiber content is due to increased intake of isolated fiber components, there is no additional intake of minerals. The chelating properties of these isolated dietary fiber components could have an influence on the utilization of minerals and trace elements. However, much work is still needed in this field. The studies completed so far only give us an idea of the complexity of the mineral bioavailability from cereals.

Table 6.4.1 References to Minerals Studied with Respect to Bioavailability from Cereals

Mineral	Increased Absorption, Ref. No.	Decreased or Low Absorption, Ref. No.	No Change in Availability, Ref. No.
Ca	16, 106, 130	6, 13, 16, 17, 18, 19, 33, 48, 58, 59, 61, 66, 74, 83, 87, 88, 89, 106, 108, 114, 121, 159, 163, 177, 184	4, 5, 11, 43, 44, 64, 75, 82, 84, 91, 94, 96, 99, 106, 109, 113, 115, 152, 153, 158, 169, 175, 176, 182, 183, 186
P	151	87, 157, 167, 168	4, 82, 96, 106, 114, 115, 158, 175, 182
Zn	52, 72, 97, 98, 111, 276	12, 20, 34, 42, 47, 48, 65, 69, 70, 71, 73, 84, 85, 87, 88, 89, 90, 96, 114, 115, 121, 125, 136, 138, 140, 149, 154, 158, 159, 173, 178	4, 5, 11, 14, 31, 38, 45, 81, 82, 89, 97, 99, 103, 113, 123, 152, 156, 177, 182, 183, 184
Mn			64, 158, 159,160
Cu		21, 65, 115	69, 97, 152, 159, 177, 182
Mg	16, 77, 106, 113	12, 16, 48, 66, 93, 106, 115, 159	5, 19, 64, 79, 82, 96, 99, 110, 115, 152, 160, 175, 177, 184, 186
Se			182
Fe	83, 87, 88, 89, 3, 15, 39, 40, 53, 63, 95, 101, 116, 120, 130, 158, 178, 186, 187	1, 2, 7, 8, 10, 12, 13, 22, 23, 24, 28, 32, 37, 46, 47, 49, 51, 54, 55, 56, 75, 78, 80, 81, 86, 88, 100, 104, 105, 107, 117, 119, 131, 132, 133, 137, 171, 172, 179	4, 9, 16, 27, 30, 35, 36, 43, 57, 68, 82, 89, 96, 97, 99, 101, 106, 112, 113, 115, 122, 123, 124, 134, 135, 145, 156, 159, 160, 177, 182, 183, 184

Table 6.4.2   Description of Mineral Bioavailability Studies from Cereals

Mineral	Subject	Exp. Design	Time	Diet	Fiber Source	Result	Ref.
Fe	Human, 8 people	Balance	49–91 days	Controlled, 40–50% of energy from white flour	Whole wheat meal (extraction rate 92%) replaces white bread	Decreased iron absorption by brown bread, but mean balance positive	107
Fe	Rat	Hgb-relation			Whole wheat bread	Lowered availability; iron from bread less available than inorganic iron	80
Fe	Human, 154 people	Radioisotope technique	2-week period		Rice	Increased absorption with fortification with FeSO$_4$	39
Fe	Human	Hgb, serum iron, IBC radioassay, ^{59}Fe, ^{56}Fe	15 days	Controlled, meal	Corn	Decreased Fe absorption	55
Fe, Ca, Mg	Human, 3 people	Balance	7-day period, 3–5 weeks		Brown bread (1 lb)	Fe, P not affected; Mg, Ca, absorption negative after 4 weeks; Mg, Ca absorption positive after 8 weeks	106
Fe	Human, 66 people	Radioassay, food intrinsically labeled with ^{55}Fe		Controlled, 1 meal	Rice	Low availability	100
Fe	Human, 116 people	Radio-Fe erythrocyte utilization method	14 days	Controlled, 1 meal	Maize meal porridge	Very low absorption (3.8%)	22
Fe	Human, 66 people	Radio-Fe, erythrocyte utilization method		Controlled, 1 meal	Maize, wheat	Low absorption	101
Fe	Human, 42 children	^{59}Fe-labeled maize, whole body counter		Controlled, 1 meal	Maize	Low absorption (4.3%)	2
Fe, Mg, Ca	Human, 12 people	Balance	3 weeks		Unpolished rice (27 oz)	Ca, Mg absorption lowered on unpolished rice for 3 weeks; long term (18 weeks): Ca, Mg retention improved, Fe not affected	16
Fe, Zn, Cu	Human, 5 people	Balance	28–30 days		26 g corn bran, 26 g wheat bran	No significant effect of bran; Cu absorption better because of higher intake	97
Fe	Human	Hgb-measurements			Wheat bread	Not affected	43
Fe	Human	Balance			Different cereals	Affected by phytic acid	1
Fe	Human	Serum iron measurements			Whole wheat bread	Affected, possible binder phytic acid	24

Mineral	Subject	Method	Duration	Diet	Material	Result	Ref
Fe	Human, 21 people	Radioisotope technique; blood samples	17 days		Chapathi from whole meal wheat flour or white flour	Affected, but not significantly absorption higher from white flour than whole grain (3.2% contra 1.7%), possible binder phytate	27
Fe	Human, 6 people, 28 people	Radioisotope	10 days	Self-selected	1. Rolls containing 10 or 40% bran 2. Rolls containing 0.3 to 10% bran	Decreased Fe absorption	7
Fe	Human, 6 people	Metabolic balance, serum Fe measurement	3 weeks	Metabolically controlled	36 g bran of wheat	Serum Fe level fell, hemoglobin decreased	49
Fe	Rat	Hgb-repletion test	3 weeks repletion		Whole grain wheat bread	Fe utilization negatively affected, unrelated to phytic acid or fiber	78
Fe, Ca	Human, 14 people	Serum measurements	6 weeks	Self-controlled	20 g wheat bran	Serum iron fell, Ca unaltered	75
Fe, Zn, Ca, Mg	Human, 10 people	Blood samples, serum mineral levels	6–12 weeks	Self-controlled	20 g wheat bran 1. Low phytate 2. Normal phytate level	Not affected by wheat bran, phytic acid no influence	99
Fe	Human, 9 people	Radioassay			Bread, enriched with ferrum reductum or ferric ammonium citrate	Decreased absorption with bread	10
Fe	Rat	1. Chemical balance measurement 2. Radioassay	14 days	Semisynthetic, 310 g bread/kg diet	Bread/white, 60.5 g fiber/kg; brown, 130.2 g fiber/kg; whole meal, 221.2 g fiber/kg	No differences in Fe absorption	30
Fe	Human, 2 people	Balance experiment, serum iron		Bread 60% of energy	Wheat bread; white bread, 2 g fiber; brown bread, 15 g fiber; whole grain, 22 g fiber	Serum Fe decreased, decreased Fe balance	32
Fe					Oatmeal	Low availability, no correlation with phytate, possible binder phosphor	104

Table 6.4.2 (Continued) Description of Mineral Bioavailability Studies from Cereals

Mineral	Subject	Exp. Design	Time	Diet	Fiber Source	Result	Ref.
Fe	Human, 4 people	Radioactivity measurements	10–15 days	Self-selected, 28 g bread	White bread, exchanged for whole meal bread	Lowered Fe absorption in wheat Fe from bran	28
Fe	Rat	Repletion experiment	24 days		Bread, wheat	Fe better absorption from $FeSO_4$ than bread	63
Fe	Human, 11 people	Radioiron absorption		200 g rice (2 mg iron)	Rice	Low Fe absorption	54
Fe	Human, 42 people	Radioiron absorption		Controlled, pancakes	Whole meal from wheat	Geometric mean wheat Fe absorption 5.1%; $1/4$ of that of $FeSO_4$	46
Fe	Human, 4 people			Self-selected, meal + bread	Bran	Fe absorption 6.4; in one iron deficient 19%	9
Fe	Rat	Hemoglobin regeneration technique			Monoferric phytate from bran	Relative biological value of Fe the same from bran and ferrous ammonium sulfate	68
Fe	Human, 60 people	Double isotope technique		Controlled	Whole wheat bran, 12 g bran	Decreased Fe absorption 51 to 74%; not phytic acid, but the soluble fraction more than insoluble	105
Fe	Human	Isotope technique			Unmilled rice	Fe four times better absorption from milled than unmilled rice	8
Fe	Dog	Double radioisotope method, total body counting			Monoferric phytate	Absorption not influenced by phytic acid	57
Fe	Human	Radioisotope technique		Controlled, meal; 100 g bread	Whole meal bread	Significantly lower Fe absorption from whole meal bread	51
Fe	Rat	Hemoglobin repletion			Corn, NFD up to 15%	Fe 50% less available than ferrous sulfate	37
Fe, Zn	Rat	Isotope dilution technique, fecal and urinary Zn		Semisynthetic diet; 180 g bran/kg diet	Bran	No differences in Fe absorption due to particle size; small effect on Zn retention due to particle size	14
Fe	Pig	Hemoglobin repletion	7–9 weeks	Controlled, Fe intake constant	Wheat bran 20% of diet	No differences in Fe absorption	35

		Phytate			Bread		
Mg					Bread	May be affected, caused by phytate	93
Zn, Ca, Mg, P	Rat	Balance experiment	41 days, 2-week adaptation period	Controlled	Wheat bran, 10% and 15%	No adverse effect on mineral absorption; favored P retention, adaptation	5
Zn, Cu	Human, 7 people	Balance	32 days	Controlled	Rice, corn, wheat	Cu absorption not affected; Zn negatively affected by fiber and phytate	69
Zn	Rat	Growth response, absorption in femur and serum	4 weeks	Controlled	Wheat bread	Not affected, probably due to completely hydrolyzed phytate during breadmaking	81
Zn, Ca, P	Human, 3 people	Balance	28–32 days	Bread, 350 g	Whole meal bread	Negative effect on Zn	90
Zn, Ca, P	Human	Balance, urine, feces	6 days	Controlled, bread, 40% of energy; phytate content 680 and 1040 mg/day	Whole meal bread, unleavened	Negative effect on Ca, Zn, P	87
Zn	Swine	Growth measurements				Depressed growth due to phytic acid	70
Zn, Ca	Human	Balance, feces, plasma	20 days	Controlled, 500 g bread (60% of energy)	Whole meal bread (25 g fiber)	Negative Zn balance, negative Ca balance but not significant, binder is cellulose	84
Zn	Human, 4 people	Balance	4 weeks	Self-selected + bran	Wheat bran, 14 g	Not significantly affected by bran	38
Zn, Mg	Human, 7 people	Balance	7 days	Controlled	Wheat bran (10–20 g), cellulose, hemicellulose	Tendency to increase fecal Zn loss	72
Zn	Human, 28 people	Balance, plasma	15 weeks	Controlled, Zn intake constant	Wheatflakes, wheat bran	Negatively affected	42
Ca, Zn	Human, 2 people	Balance	20 days	Controlled, metabolic ward, 50% of energy from bread	Whole wheat bread	Negative balance of Ca, Mg, Zn, P	85

Table 6.4.2 (Continued) Description of Mineral Bioavailability Studies from Cereals

Mineral	Subject	Exp. Design	Time	Diet	Fiber Source	Result	Ref.
Zn	Human, 66 people	Radioisotope technique; whole-body counter		Controlled	Whole grain bread	Decreased percent absorption but increased total absorption; possible binder phytic acid	98
Zn	Chicken	Growth response	4 weeks	Controlled	Corn	Decreased absorption; only 60% Zn utilized; possible binder phytic acid	71
Zn	Rat	Femur Zn measurement		Controlled	Rice, barley	Barley poorer source than mixed infant cereal (wheat, corn, oat); rice poorer than standard; no correlation between Zn availability and fiber/phytate	103
Zn	Rat	Repletion experiment and growth response	28 days		Wheat bran 50 g fiber/kg	Reduced growth; decreased zinc absorption (phytate possible binder)	20
Zn	Rat	Weight gain, femur Zn content			Iranian flat bread, bread and dough	Bread better Zn source than unfermented dough; no differences on dough with different fermenting time; no correlation between Zn and fiber/phytate	31
Zn	Rat	Growth response			Selected cereals	Phytic acid inversely related to Zn availability; ratio of Zn to phytate important; Zn availability; more inhibition of phytic acid in cereals than legumes	34
Zn	Rat				Grain	Availability of Zn in grain better than in legumes; phytic acid not the only factor responsible for decreased availability	52

Mineral	Species	Study	Control	Duration	Cereal	Effect	Ref.
Zn	Rat	Balance experiment and ^{65}Zn kinetic			Cereal	Phytic acid naturally occurring in food; affects Zn metabolism to the same extent as Na phytate	45
Zn	Rat	Balance; growth response	Controlled		Breakfast cereals: rice, corn	If molar ratio > 15, depressed growth; biological response not directly correlated to dietary fiber in cereals; phytate-to-Zn ratio major factor affecting Zn availability	67
Zn, Ca	Rat	Metabolic balance			Wheat bran 0.5%, 10%, 15%	No significant changes	4
Zn	Rat	Balance studies			Rye	Apparent Zn absorption and retention in absolute values, higher from flour with high extraction rate	73
Ca, Mg, Na, Cl, K	Human, 6 people	Balance experiment	Controlled	3 weeks	Different cereals, fiber intake increased from 17 to 45 g/day (bran, whole meal)	Decreased Ca absorption; K, Na, Cl small changes, fecal Mg increased, but probably due to higher Mg intake	19
Ca	Human	Balance studies		4–9 weeks	Whole meal bread	No change or adaptation	106
Zn, Ca, Mg	Human, 2 people	Balance		5–6 weeks	Whole meal bread	Negatively affected Ca absorption, Ca, Zn adaptation	11
Ca	Human, 19 people	Serum measurements	Controlled, 230 g bread	19 weeks	Whole meal bread	Not affected	43
Ca	Human, 27 people	Balance		6 weeks	Bran (10–20 g)	Lowered Ca in serum	74
Ca	Human	Balance			Wheat whole meal bread, unleavened	Decreased Ca absorption, possible binder phytic acid	6
Ca	Human	Balance			Whole meal bread chapathi	Decreased Ca absorption	83
Ca	Human	Balance		7 weeks	Whole meal bread	Decreased Ca absorption	33
Ca	Human	Balance		3 weeks	Whole meal bread, bran (22 g → 53 g fiber)	Negative Ca balance even if increased Ca intake	18
Ca	Human				Whole grain	Decreased Ca absorption	108

Table 6.4.2 (Continued) Description of Mineral Bioavailability Studies from Cereals

Mineral	Subject	Exp. Design	Time	Diet	Fiber Source	Result	Ref.
Ca	Human, 9 people	Balance	9 month periods: 2–3 weeks	Flour, 40–50% of energy	Whole grain flour (extraction rate 92%)	Negative Ca balance; possible binder phytate; dephytinization gives better absorption	59
Zn, Ca, P	Human, 3 people	Balance	28 + 32 days	Controlled	Whole grain bread, unleavened or leavened	Unleavened bread: negative Ca and Zn balance; high phytate intake can cause negative disturbance in Zn and Ca adaptation for serum Fe and serum Zn	89
Ca	Human, 4 people	Balance	3 weeks		Wheat fiber, 31 g fiber	Negative Ca balance	17
Ca	Human, 6 people	Balance	11 days	Controlled	Whole meal wheat bread fiber, 123 g (standard 106 g)	Negative Ca balance	58
Ca	Human, 14 people	Balance (serum)	4–9 weeks	Controlled	Wheat bran, 38 g bran per day	No changes in plasma Ca	44
Ca	Human, 25 people	Balance (serum)	5 weeks	Controlled	Wheat bran, 24 g bran per day	No changes in serum Ca	109

Minerals	Subjects	Method	Duration	Diet	Food	Result	Ref
Ca	Survey, children	Balance		Self-selected	Whole meal bread	Ca adaptation	94
Ca, Mg, Zn, P	Human, 2 people	Balance	1940–1948	Controlled, 60% of energy from bread	Whole meal bread; fiber, 12.6 g/day	Negative Zn balance, negative Ca balance, negative Mg balance	48
Zn, Cu, Fe, Mg	Rat	Balance			Phytic acid	Decreased absorption	21
Mg	Rat	Balance		Wheat flour, 55% Mg; the rest of Mg from magnesium carbonate	Whole grain wheat bread	Mg available	110
Mg	Rat	Balance	3 weeks		Whole grain wheat bread	Mg available	79
Mg	Rat	Balance	4 weeks		Whole grain wheat flour	Mg available; higher absorption from flour than from the same amount of added salt	77
Ca, P, Zn, Mg	Human, 68 people	13 months		Self-selected	3 tsp bran per day	No influence on mineral balance; bran does not cause deficiency	82
P, Ca, Zn, Mg, Fe	Human, 8 people (ileostomy)	Metabolic balance technique	2–3 weeks	Controlled	Wheat bran, 16 g/day	No effect on mineral absorption except Zn	96

Table 6.4.2a   Description of Mineral Bioavailability Studies from Cereals (References After 1984)

Mineral	Subject	Exp. Design	Time	Diet	Fiber source	Result	Ref.
Fe	Rat	Hgb regeneration assay in weanling anemic rats		Controlled, ± juice	Baked/unbaked wheat bran muffins	Baking + organic acids increased bioavailability	116
Fe	Rat	Whole body counter			Extruded maize	Extrusion no effect on Fe absorption	124
Fe	Rat	Hgb regeneration			Bran cereal, corn meal	Cereals significant contribution to available Fe in diet	187
Fe	Rat	Hgb repletion		Corn tortillas and cooked beans	Maize, beans	Fe availability reduced with 15% NDF; correlation between soluble Fe and repletion; Fe from corn tortillas, 50% less available than $FeSO_4$	132
Fe, Mn, Cu, Zn, Mg, Ca	Human	Balance study	45 days	Controlled	Three levels of phytate	No effect on absorption of Fe, Mn, Cu; decreased absorption for Zn, Mg, Ca	159
Fe	Human	Isotope study, absorption test			Muffins baked with wheat bran	Fiber not the major determinant of food Fe availability, but Fe absorption lowered in bran muffins; fruit enhanced	119
Fe, Zn, Ca	Human	Metabolic balance	26 days	Controlled	Wheat bran, corn bran, soybean husk	Increased Fe excretion	120
Fe, Zn, Ca	Chicks	Metabolic balance and tissue conc	18 days	Controlled	Wheat bran	Minerals not affected	183
Fe	Rats	Balance	10 days	Controlled	Whole wheat, wheat bran	Digestibility lowest with wheat bran; no significant relation between Fe and phytate absorption	112
Fe	Rat	Hgb regeneration		Controlled	Wheat bran	No change	134
Fe	Rat	Balance technique		Controlled	White bread 6% DF, brown bread 13% DF, whole meal bread 22% DF	Fe absorption higher in control, but no difference within the breads; fiber itself no effect	122
Fe, Zn	Human	Balance study	12 weeks	Controlled	Cereals, fruits, vegetables increased from 20–30 g	No change in Fe or Zn absorption	156
Fe	Rat	Whole body radioassay procedure			Different wheat varieties	Selection of wheat for high protein content, no effect on Fe bioavailability	145

Mineral	Species	Method	Duration	Diet	Material	Results	Ref.
Fe	Rat	Retention study on rat intestine			Maize and wheat fiber	Retention lowered by presence of fiber, polymerization	171
Fe	Human	Erythrocytes utilization of radioactive Fe			Sorghum	Polyphenol and phytate decreased Fe absorption; hemicellulose and lignin possible inhibitors of Fe absorption	133
Zn, Fe	Human	Isotopic retention from fecal extraction	4–7 Days	40 g extruded/not extruded cereal + milk	Wheat bran and flour	Extrusion cooking, no effect on absorption	123
Zn	Rat	Balance	4 weeks	Dosa + milk	Dosa (rice and dal)	Zn absorption higher in plain dosa diet than in raw dosa mixture	111
Zn, Fe, Ca, Mg, P	Human	Whole body counter			Extruded high-fiber cereals	The total effects of extrusion on bioavailability are small but observable; negative effect on Zn, Ca, Mg; no effect on Fe	150
Zn	Human, 33 people	Whole body counter		Controlled	20 or 30% wheat bran	Zn absorption improved when extrusion was performed after phytate reduction	149
Zn	Rat	Growth response, Zn retention, Zn concentration in serum and bone	25 weeks	ad lib	Endosperm, whole grain, bran-enriched crisp bread	DF and phytate from bran; limit availability of Zn to minor degree when Zn is needed	138
Zn	Rat	Growth response, bone-Zn deposition	3 weeks	Controlled	Whole meal, wheat bread, and crisp bread	Lowered Zn absorption when high phytic acid/Zn ratio; improvement by enrichment of Zn	140
Zn	Human	Whole body counter		Meals based on 60 g cereals + milk	Rye, barley, oatmeal, triticale, whole wheat	Food preparation that decreases the phytic acid improves Zn absorption	173
Zn, P	Rat	Balance study, femur consistency of Zn, Ca, P	9–12 days		Wheat bran, barley husk	Both sources had more negative effect on Zn than Ca absorption; phytate did not appear as a major factor affecting mineral absorption in barley husk	121
Zn	Human	Radioisotope technique			Browned and unbrowned corn products	Reduced Zn absorption in browned products, probably due to Maillard products	154
Zn, Se	Rat	Whole body isotope study		Controlled	Wheat grain	Se and Zn have antagonistic effects on each other	146

Table 6.4.2a (Continued)   Description of Mineral Bioavailability Studies from Cereals (References After 1984)

Mineral	Subject	Exp. Design	Time	Diet	Fiber source	Result	Ref.
Zn	Human	Rise in plasma zinc	6 hours		Wheat bran, phytate-reduced bran rice (low-phytate, low-fiber)	Decreased Zn, rise mainly due to phytate	136
Zn, Cu, Ca, Mg	Human	Metabolic balance	4 weeks	Controlled	Wheat bran (0.4 g/kg/day)	No change in mineral balance	152
Zn	Human	Zinc tolerance test, whole body monitor		Controlled	Wheat bran	Wheat bran leads to significant reduction in Zn absorption	125
Zn, Fe	Rat	Whole body retention using radioisotopes	19 days	Controlled	Sorghum products	Fe highly available; Zn more available from fermented products with lower phytic acid	178
Ca	Rat	Balance study; bioavailability measured by TIBIA, Ca content reflecting retention	27 days	Controlled, ad lib	Whole wheat bread (enriched with Ca)	Ca bioavailability 95% from bread, same as milk diet	169
Ca, P, Mg	Rat	Balance study, urine, feces, tissue	7 months	ad lib	Cellulose, wheat bran, oat bran, corn bran at 4 of 14% TDF	Diets did not appreciably affect mineral levels	175
Ca	Human	Balance		Controlled	Oat bran	No impact on Ca intake	176
Ca, Fe, Zn, Na, Mg	Human	Metabolic balance	72 days	Controlled	Wheat bran	Fecal excretion for minerals not changed, except Mg which increased	113
Ca, P, Mg, Fe, Zn, Cu, Se	Human	Balance serum, urine	3 months	Controlled	Wheat bran bread, guar gum bread	No change in serum or urinary concentration of any of the minerals	182
Ca, P, Mg, Na, K, Zn, Fe	Pig	Balance study	26 days	Controlled, + 15% fiber	Oat husk, soybean husk	No effect on mineral utilization; Zn balance lower with oat husk: Fe balance higher with soya husk	158
Ca	Rat	Balance	6 weeks	Controlled	5, 10, 15% processed oat husk	No effect on Ca absorption	153
Ca, Zn, Cu, Fe, Mg	Human	Balance study		Controlled	Hard red wheat bran baked in yeast leavened bread, 20–45 g DF/day	Increased loss of Ca, but not of Zn, Cu, Fe, or Mg for the increased DF	177

Mineral	Species	Method	Duration	Treatment	Source	Comments	Ref.
Ca	Human	Urinary Ca excretion	1–36 months		Rice bran	Phytic acid in rice bran decreased Ca absorption	163
Ca, Mg, Zn, Fe	Human	Balance	21 days	Controlled	Fiber 50 g/day; bread w/barley fiber; bread w/whole wheat bran; fruits, vegetables	No effects on mineral balance; improved absorption of Fe, Zn	186
Ca, Mg, Fe, Cu, Zn, Mn, Se	Pig	Balance study, urine, feces	2 weeks	Controlled cereals/milk	Wheat, oat, barley	In comparison with mixed cereal diet: *barley* — decreased loss due to lower content of minerals; *wheat* — increased loss of minerals, no change of intake; *oat* — higher absorption, especially Fe, Ca	130
P, Ca, Zn	Pig	Balance study		Marginal Ca and P (0.5 and 0.35%), addition of Zn (20 vs. 100 mg/kg)	Barley, wheat, corn	Absorption of P high in wheat; Zn supplement affected phytase activity in small intestine; Ca absorption influence negative by Zn supplement; mineral absorption different in different cereals	151
P	Pig	Balance study	6 weeks	Controlled wheat diets	Corn triticale wheat	The higher the phytase activity of the diet, the greater the phytate P availability and the lower the bone mineral disorder; triticale and wheat higher in phytase than corn	167
P, Ca, Mg, Zn	Pig	Balance study	3 weeks	Controlled	Wheat bran, 20% DF	Wheat bran, a source of available P and Mg, but might have an unfavorable effect on the utilization of Ca and Zn; Low-methoxylated pectin has deleterious effect on mineral balances	114
P	Pig	Balance	6 weeks	Controlled	Wheat or corn + 0.3% P	P utilization 1.7 times higher in wheat than corn due to phytase activity	168

Table 6.4.2a (Continued) Description of Mineral Bioavailability Studies from Cereals (References After 1984)

Mineral	Subject	Exp. Design	Time	Diet	Fiber source	Result	Ref.
P, Ca, Mg, Zn, Cu	Rat	Balance		Controlled corn, soybean meal + fiber	Wheat bran, rice, rice bran cellulose	Phytate more reduced in wheat bran diet than rice; cellulose no effect on serum or tissue mineral concentration; rice bran no effect on serum levels of Ca, P, Mg; lower concentration of Zn, Mg, Cu	115
Mg, Cu, Ca, Fe, Zn	Human	Metabolic balance	22 days	Controlled	Coarse bran bread (35 g NDF, 22 g NDF)	Balance value for Mg, Fe, Zn, and Cu did not differ by type of bread; Ca balance was negative; excretion significance greater when consuming coarse than fine bran bread	184
Na, K, P	Human	Balance	14 days	Controlled	Brown rice	P balance lower in brown rice, other minerals not affected	157
Various minerals	Human (10 men)	Balance study	15 days		Whole or dephytinized wheat bran	No effect on mineral bioavailability	160

Note: OH = oat husk; NDF = neutral detergent fiber.

Table 6.4.3 *In Vitro* Binding Studies

Mineral	Fiber Source	Result	Ref.
Ca, Mg. Zn, Fe	Wheat bran and fractions of dietary fiber	Lignin, pectin; high metal-binding capacity; metal binding; pH dependent	13
Fe, Cu, Zn	Rice bran	All three metals bound, probably to hemicellulose sequence of binding; Cu > Zn > Fe. Metals released with enzyme incubation; Zn affected dietary Cu binding	65
Zn, Fe	Whole meal wheat bread	Bran high binding capacity for Zn and Fe. Zn binding pH dependent; lignin and two fractions of hemicellulose high capacity for Zn; complexes with wheat fiber; can to some extent explain decreased availability of Fe and Zn	47
Fe	Wheat, rice	Ionizable iron nearly twice as high when compared with that from chapathi (wheat); percentage ionizable iron was lower in the parboiled rice than in raw rice, but actual amount the same; cereal, twofold increase of ionizable iron when germinating; cooking of rice/wheat did not influence ionizable iron	76
Fe	Wheat, maize	Neutral detergent fiber accounts for all binding capacity of iron. Binding pH dependent; iron binding by fiber is strongly inhibited by ascorbic acid, citric acid, phytic acid, EDTA, cysteine, phosphate, and calcium; iron in wheat and maize strongly inhibited	86
Fe	Wheat bran	Ascorbic acid inhibits complete binding of ferrous iron; boiling for 1 h no effect on phytic acid; toasting for 1 h: 19% destruction of phytic acid; boiling 1 h in 1 N HCL: 36% destruction of phytic acid	12
Zn	Rye bread and whole wheat bread	Higher availability with increased rising time	41
Zn	Whole wheat bread	Dephytinized fiber did bind Zn; adding of phytic acid lowered the ability to bind Zn	84
Zn	Bran, and components of bran	Soluble components responsible for 39% of total binding power of wheat bran; possible binder: phytate. Hemicellulose, cellulose, starch, pectin contribute only 10% of total binding capacity	32
Zn, Fe, Ca, Mg	Wheat bran	Zn, Fe, the only soluble metals of wheat bran associated with phytic acid; at least 70% of phytate does not exist as Ca_5Mg-phytate	26
Ca	Wheat bran	Only weakly binding; no important contribution to Ca binding; increased binding with lowered pH (pH under 5)	91
Ca, Mg	Cell wall fraction	Cellulose, hemicellulose: low availability	66
Mg, Mn, Ca	Rice bran	Minerals available for absorption; minerals released with incubation for 16 h	64
Fe	Phytate, oatmeal	No correlation with phytate and Fe absorption; oatmeal low availability, phosphate?	104

Table 6.4.3 (Continued) *In Vitro* **Binding Studies**

Mineral	Fiber Source	Result	Ref.
Ca, Zn, Fe	Bread	Cellulose important binder; fiber responsible more than phytic acid	88
Ca, Mg, Zn, Fe	Wheat bran	Binding to cellulose and lignin not affected by cooking; pH-dependent Ca binding diminished by boiling, not affected by toasting; Zn affected significantly by pH and type of cooking (toasting had no effect), boiling no effect at pH 6, decreasing binding by boiling pH 7	13
Zn, Cu, Fe	Corn	Cornflakes bound more Cu and less Fe than corn grits at pH 5, 6, 7	50
Na, K, Ca, Mg, P	Wheat bran	Ash associated with soluble fiber, coprecipitation due to isolation procedure of fiber partly responsible; dependent on ionic strength and different buffers	102
Ash	Different cereals	Ash associated with soluble fiber components	36
Zn	Wheat bran	Soluble components responsible for 37% of total binding power of wheat bran; possible binder phytate; hemicellulose, cellulose, starch, pectin contribute only 10% of total binding capacity	92
Fe	Wheat bread	Insoluble iron generated due to baking process; the differences found between iron sources prior to baking vanished in final baked product	56

Table 6.4.3a *In Vitro* Binding Studies (References After 1984)

Mineral	Fiber Source	Method	Result	Ref.
Fe	Breakfast cereals w/wheat bran and germ	*In vitro* procedure simulating gastro intestinal digestion	Wheat bran, germ reduced availability; processing affects availability	117
Fe	Sorghum	Solubility study	Germination, soak, fermentation increased soluble Fe	179
Fe	Maize	Solubility boiling	Availability of Fe same as for soluble Fe	135
Fe	Maize	Diffusing across a semipermeable membrane	Increased availability after extrusion-cooking procedure, mainly due to refining of maize	142
Fe	Wheat roll	Digestion under similar physical conditions	Degradation of inositol hexa- and penta-phosphates significantly reduced inhibitory effect on Fe availability	172
Fe	Wheat flake cereal	Solubility during sequential pH treatment	Acid incubation to form an organic acid chelate with iron improved bioavailability with Fe fortification of cereals	161
Fe	Cereals with 0–973 mg tannins	Measurements of ionizable iron	Tannins as well as phytates may be responsible for low absorption of iron in Indian diets	131
Fe, Zn, Mg, Ca, P	Wheat bran and whole wheat flour	Isolation procedure	The different minerals chelated to different DF components; only 10% Fe associated with phytic acid; 60% Fe associated with insoluble fractions; 24% Zn, 60% Ca, 9% Mg associated with phytic acid	126
Zn	Polished rice	*In vitro* digestion; separation of gel; filtration of soluble Zn components	More than 30% of rice zinc-solubilized; proteinaceous components increases soluble Zn	147
Zn, Cd, Cu	Wheat, barley, rye, oat	^{31}P-NMR spectroscopy; potentiometric methods; isolation procedures	Minerals associated with soluble fiber fractions; phytate potent inhibitor in wheat, but not in the other cereals studied	131
Ca, Mg, Zn, Cu	Different cereal products	Extraction precipitation	Organic ligand, EDTA, and citric acid prevented precipitation; naturally occurring soluble ligands important controlling factors for bioavailabilities	155
Ca, Cu, Fe, K, Mg, Mn, P, Zn	Whole oat grain	Isolation procedures	70% of minerals present in kernel associated with soluble fiber fractions, most probably phytic acid/glucans; Fe and Cu the only minerals that are associated with insoluble fraction	127
Ca, Zn	Ca-fortified wheat flake	Solubility during sequential pH treatment (pH 2–7)	Citric acid increased solubility of Zn and Ca; his, cyst, alone and in combination, enhanced Zn solubility, but not Ca; malate, citrate + malate, lactate + malate, citrate + lactate, glucan did not affect Zn and Ca solubility	118

Table 6.4.3a (Continued) *In Vitro* Binding Studies (References After 1984)

Mineral	Fiber Source	Method	Result	Ref.
Cu, Cd, Zn	Soluble fiber of wheat bran, whole wheat grain, inolaxol, cellulose	Potentiometric method	Phytic acid in wheat interacted strongly with minerals	165
Cu, Cd, Zn	Barley, rye, oat	Potentiometric method	Considerable association found between minerals and soluble fractions of all three cereals; the ability to bind was in order Cu (II) > Zn (II) > Cd (II) for cereals barley > oats = rye; between pH 3.5–5, phytic acid important chelator for oats; pure β-glucan from barley no complexing agent	166
	Wheat bran, oat	^{31}P-NMR	Phytase present in oats; breakdown of phytic acid in oats same as for wheat	129

Table 6.4.4 Effect of Addition of Other Foods on Bioavailability of Minerals

Mineral	Fiber Source	Subject	Food Addition	Result	Ref.
Fe	Rice	Human	Fish	Increased absorption	39
Fe	Corn maize, bread	Human	Vitamin C	Increased absorption	15
Fe	Rice	Human	Fruit, meat	Absorption increased 5 times	40
Fe	Maize	Human	50 g meat; 100 g fish; 150 g papaya (66 mg vitamin C)	Absorption increased 2 times with meat and fish, 5 times with papaya	53
Fe	Corn	Human	Fish or food of animal origin	Increased availability	55
Fe	Bread	Human	Tea	Decreased availability	23
Fe	Rice	Human	Ascorbic acid	Improved availability	100
Fe	Maize	Human	Tea, ascorbic acid	Tea reduced absorption from 3.8 to 2.1%; ascorbic acid increased absorption 10 times; inhibitory effect of tea overcome if ascorbic acid given	22
Fe	Maize, wheat	Human	Ascorbic acid	Enhanced absorption from maize, not from wheat	101
Fe	Cereals	Human	Ascorbic acid	Improved nonheme iron absorption	29
Zn	Whole grain bread	Human	Animal protein, milk (Ca)	Both improved absorption	71
Fe	Whole grain bread	Human	Tea, orange juice, egg yolk	Tea reduced to half; orange juice increased 2 times; egg yolk inhibitor	95
Fe	Whole meal bread	Human	Fruit juice, egg	Fruit juice enhanced absorption, egg no effect	28
Fe	Rice	Human	Fish	Absorption improved with fish	3
Fe	Wheat bread	Human	Orange juice	Improved absorption	10
Fe	Whole meal bread	Human	Ascorbic acid	Enhanced absorption	51
Zn	Flat bread	Rat	Protein (animal)	Could prevent complexation of Zn with phytic acid	31
Fe	Breakfast cereal foods	In vitro	Milk	Enhanced bioavailability	174
Fe	Whole wheat flour	In vitro (diffusion across a semipermeable membrane)	Various beverages and condiments	Choice of beverage and condiments influence Fe availability in either reducing or enhancing	144
Fe	Processed foods of white and whole meal bread, wheat bran, maize meal, corn flakes	In vitro (diffusion across a semipermeable membrane)	Fruit juices	Processing increased bioavailability compared to raw materials; Fe diffusibility was enhanced by fruit juices	143
Fe	Rice	Rats fed ad libitum	Various carbohydrates	Bioavailability higher in diets containing starch and lactose	150

Table 6.4.4 (Continued) Effect of Addition of Other Foods on Bioavailability of Minerals

Mineral	Fiber Source	Subject	Food Addition	Result	Ref.
Fe	Breakfast cereals	In vitro	Sugar, orange juice, citric acid	Sugar slight increase; orange juice dramatically enhanced; citric acid more potent enhancer than ascorbic acid	117
Fe	Cereal-based	1. In vitro solubilization 2. Isotope experiments on humans	Milk	1. Soluble Fe increased with milk 2. No change in Fe absorption	181
Fe	Wheat bran	Isotope experiments on humans	Ascorbic acid or meat	Iron absorption inhibited 50% by phytate; ascorbic acid/meat counteract the inhibition	137
Zn	Corn germ	Rat depletion experiments; growth development	Citric acid	Citric acid improved Zn availability	164
Zn	Corn germ (0.5% phytate)	Depletion experiment with rats	1% citric acid	Improved absorption with citric acid	164

REFERENCES

1. Apte, S. V. and Venkatachalam, P. S., Iron absorption in human volunteers using high phytate cereal diet, *Ind. J. Med. Res.*, 50, 516, 1962.
2. Ashworth, A., Milner, P. F., Waterlow, J. C., and Walker, R. B., Absorption of iron from maize *(Zea mays L.)* and soya beans *(Glycine hispida Mx)* in Jamaican infants, *Br. J. Nutr.*, 29, 269, 1973.
3. Aung-Than-Batu, Thein-Than, and Thave-Toe, Iron absorption from South East Asia rice based meals, *Am. J. Clin. Nutr.*, 29, 219, 1976.
4. Bagheri, S. M. and Gueguen, L., Effects of wheat bran on the metabolism of ^{46}Ca and ^{65}Zn in rats, *J. Nutr.*, 112, 2047, 1982.
5. Bagheri, S. M. and Gueguen, L., Influence of wheat bran diets containing unequal amounts of calcium, magnesium, phosphorus and zinc upon the absorption of these minerals in rats, *Nutr. Rep. Int.*, 24, 47, 1981.
6. Berlyne, G. M. , Ari, J. B., Nord, E., and Shainkin, R., Bedouin osteomalacia due to calcium deprivation caused by high phytic acid content of unleavened bread, *Am. J. Clin. Nutr.*, 26, 910, 1973.
7. Björn-Rasmussen, E., Iron absorption from wheat bread. Influence of various amount of bran, *Nutr. Metab.*, 16, 101, 1974.
8. Björn-Rasmussen, E., Hallberg, L., and Walker, R., Isotopic exchange of iron between labelled foods and between a food and iron salt, *Am. J. Clin. Nutr.*, 26, 1311, 1973.
9. Callender, S. T. and Warner, G. T., Iron absorption from brown bread, *Lancet*, 1, 546, 1970.
10. Callender, S. T. and Warner, G. T., Iron absorption from bread, *Am. J. Clin. Nutr.*, 21, 1170, 1968.
11. Campell, G. J., Reinhold, J. G., Cannell, J. S., and Nourmana, I., The effect of prolonged consumption of whole meal bread upon metabolism of calcium, magnesium, zinc and phosphorus of two young American adults, *Pahlavi Med. J.*, 7, 1, 1976.
12. Camire, A. L. and Clydesdale, F. M., Interactions of soluble iron with wheat bran, *J. Food Sci.*, 47, 1296, 1982.
13. Camire, A. L. and Clydesdale, F. M., Effect of pH and heat treatment on the binding of calcium, magnesium zinc and iron to wheat bran and fraction of dietary fiber, *J. Food Sci.*, 46, 548, 1981.
14. Caprez, A. and Fairweather-Tait, S. J., The effect of heat treatment and particle size of bran on mineral absorption in rats, *Br. J. Nutr.*, 48, 467, 1982.
15. Cook, J. D. and Monsen, E. R., Vitamin C, the common cold and iron absorption, *Am. J. Clin. Nutr.*, 35, 235, 1977.
16. Cullumbine, M., Basnayake, V., Le Motte, J., and Wickramanayaka, T. W., Mineral metabolism on rice diets, *Br. J. Nutr.*, 4, 101, 1950.
17. Cummings, J. M., Hill, M. J., Jivraj, T., Houston, H., Branch, W. J., and Jenkins, D. J. A., The effect of meat protein and dietary fiber on colonic function and metabolism. I. Changes in bowel habit, bile acid excretion and calcium absorption, *Am. J. Clin. Nutr.*, 32, 2086, 1979.
18. Cummings, J. M., Nutritional implications of dietary fiber, *Am. J. Clin. Nutr.*, 31, S21, 1978.
19. Cummings, J. M., Hill, M. J., Jenkins, D. J. A., Pearson, J. R., and Wiggins, H. S., Changes in fecal composition and colonic function due to cereal fiber, *Am. J. Clin. Nutr.*, 29, 1468, 1976.
20. Davis, N. T., Hristic, V., and Flett, A. A., Phytate rather than fibre in bran as the major determinant of zinc availability to rats, *Nutr. Rep. Inc.*, 15, 207, 1977.
21. Davis, N. T. and Nightingale, R., The effects of phytate on intestinal absorption and secretion of zinc and whole body retention of zinc, copper, iron, manganese in rats, *Br. J. Nutr.*, 34, 243, 1975.
22. Derman, D., Sayers, M., Lynch, S. R., Charlton, R. W., Bothwell, T. M., and Mayet, F., Iron absorption from cereal based meal containing cane sugar fortified with ascorbic acid, *Br. J. Nutr.*, 38, 261, 1977.
23. Disler, P. B., Lynch, S. R., Charlton, R. W., Torrance, J. D., Bothwell, T. M., Walker, R. B., and Mayet, F., The effect of tea on iron absorption, *Gut*, 16, 193, 1975.
24. Dobbs, R . J. and Baird, I. M., Effect of wholemeal and white bread on iron absorption, *Br. Med. J.*, 2, 1641, 1977.
25. Drews, L. M., Kies, C., and Fox, H. M., Effect of dietary fiber on copper, zinc, magnesium utilization by adolescent boys, *Am. J. Clin. Nutr.*, 32, 1893, 1979.
26. Ellis, R. and Morris, E. R., Relation between phytic acid and trace metals in wheat bran and soy bean, *Cereal Chem.*, 58, 367, 1981.

27. Elwood, P. C., Benjamin, I. T., Fry, F.-A., Eakins, J. D., Brown, D. A., De Kock, P. C., and Shah, J. V., Absorption of iron from chapathi made from wheat flour, *Am. J. Clin. Nutr.*, 23, 1267, 1970.

28. Elwood, P. C., Newton, D., Eakins, J. D., and Brown, D. A., Absorption of iron from bread, *Am. J. Clin. Nutr.*, 21, 1162, 1968.

29. Erdman, J. W., Jr., Bioavailability of nutrients from food, *Contemp. Nutr.*, 3, 1, 1978.

30. Fairweather-Tait, S. J., The effect of different levels of wheat bran on iron absorption in rats from bread containing similar amounts of phytate, *Br. J. Nutr.*, 47, 243, 1982.

31. Faridi, H. A., Finney, P. L., and Rubenthaler, G. L., Iranian flat breads: relative bioavailability of zinc, *J. Food Sci.*, 48, 107, 1983.

32. Faradji, B., Reinhold, J. G., and Abadi, P., Human studies of iron absorption from fiber-rich Iranian flatbreads, *Nutr. Rep. Int.*, 23, 267, 1981.

33. Ford, J. A., Colhoun, E. M., McIntosh, W. B., and Dunningan, M. G., Biochemical response of late rickets and osteomalacia to a chapathi-free diet, *Br. Med. J.*, 3, 446, 1972.

34. Franz, K. B., Kennedy, B. M., and Feller, F. A., Relative bioavailability of zinc from selected cereals and legumes using rat growth, *J. Nutr.*, 110, 2272, 1980.

35. Frølich, W. and Lysø, A., Bioavailability of iron from wheat bran in pigs, *Am. J. Clin. Nutr.*, 37, 31, 1983.

36. Frølich, W. and Asp, N. G., Dietary fiber content in cereals in Norway, *Cereals Chem.*, 58, 524, 1981.

37. Garcia-Lopez, S. and Wyatt, C. J., Effect of fiber in corn tortillas and cooked beans on iron availability, *J. Agric. Food Chem.*, 30, 724, 1982.

38. Guthrie, B. E. and Robinson, M. F., Zinc balance studies during wheat bran supplementation, *Fed. Proc. Fed. Am. Soc. Exp. Biol.*, 37, 254, 1978.

39. Hallberg, L., Bjorn-Rasmussen, E., and Garby, L., Iron absorption from South-East Asian diets and the effect of iron fortification, *Am. J. Clin. Nutr.*, 31, 1403, 1978.

40. Hallberg, L., Garby, L., Suwanik, R., and Bjorn-Rasmussen, E., Iron absorption from South-East Asian diets, *Am. J. Clin. Nutr.*, 27, 826, 1974.

41. Harland, B. F. and Harland, J., Fermentative reduction of phytate in rye, white and whole wheat breads, *Cereal Chem.*, 57, 226, 1980.

42. Harland, B. F., Stringfellow, D. E., Connor, D. H., Foster, W. D., and Heggie, C. M., Lower plasma zinc in humans ingesting wheat bran products, *Fed. Proc. Fed. Am. Soc. Exp. Biol.*, 38, 548, 1979.

43. Heaton, K. W., Manning, A. P., and Hartog, M., Lack of effect on blood lipids and calcium concentrations of young mean on changing from white to wholemeal bread, *Br. J. Nutr.*, 35, 55, 1976.

44. Heaton, K. W. and Pomare, E. W., Effect of bran of blood lipids and calcium, *Lancet*, 1, 49, 1974.

45. House, W. E., Welch, R. M., and Van Campen, D. R., Effect of phytic acid on the absorption, distribution and endogenous excretion of zinc in rats, *J. Nutr.*, 112, 941, 1982.

46. Hussain, R., Walker, R. B., Layrisse, M., Clark, P., and Finch, C. A., Nutritive value of food iron, *Am. J. Clin. Nutr.*, 16, 464, 1965.

47. Ismail-Beigi, F., Faradji, B., and Reinhold, J. G., Binding of zinc and iron to wheat bread, wheat bran and their components, *Am. J. Clin. Nutr.*, 30, 1721, 1977.

48. Ismail-Beigi, F., Reinhold, J. G., Faradji, B., and Abadi, P., Effect of cellulose added to diets of low and high fiber content upon the metabolism of calcium, magnesium, zinc and phosphorus by man, *J. Nutr.*, 107, 510, 1977.

49. Jenkins, D. J. A., Hill, M. S., and Cummings, J. H., Effect of wheat fiber on blood lipids, fecal steroid excretion arid serum iron, *Am. J. Clin. Nutr.*, 28, 1408, 1975.

50. Johnson, P. E., Lykken, G., Mahalko, J., Milne, D., Inman, L., Sanstead, H. H., Garcia, W. J., and Inglett, G. E., The effect of browned and unbrowned corn products on absorption of zinc, iron and copper in humans, presented at ACS Meeting, Las Vegas, NV, 1982.

51. Kobza, K. and Steenblock, V., Effect of wholemeal and white bread on iron absorption in normal people, *Br. Med. J.*, 1, 1641, 1977.

52. Lantzsch, M. J., Schenkel, H., and Nickel, I., Zn availability in grains and legumes, in *Trace Element Metabolism in Man and Animals*, Vol. 3, Kirchgessner, M., Ed., Arbeitskries Teir ernährungsforgschung Weihen stephan (ATW) Freising-Weihenstephan, West Germany, 1978, 460.

53. Layrisse, M., Martinez-Torres, C., and Gonzales, M., Measurement of the total daily dietary iron absorption by intrinsic tag model, *Am. J. Natur.*, 27, 152, 1974.

54. Layrisse, M. and Martinez-Torres, C., Food iron absorption: iron supplementation of food, *Preg. Hematol.*, 7, 137, 1971.

55. Layrisse, M., Martinez-Torres, C., and Roche, M., Effect of interaction of various foods on iron absorption, *Am. J. Clin. Nutr.*, 21, 1175, 1968.

56. Lee, K. and Clydesdale, F. M., The effect of baking on the iron in iron enriched flour, *J. Food Sci.*, 45, 1500, 1980.

57. Lipschitz, D. A., Simpson, K. M., Cook, J. D., and Morris, E. R., Absorption of monoferric phytate by dogs, *J. Nutr.*, 109, 1154, 1979.

58. McCance, R. A. and Walsham, C. M., The digestibility and absorption of calories, proteins, purines, fat and calcium in wholemeal wheaten bread, *Br. J. Nutr.*, 2, 26, 1948.

59. McCance, R. A. and Widdowson, E. M., Mineral metabolism of healthy adults on white and brown bread dietaries, *J. Physiol.*, 101, 44, 1942.

60. McHale, A., Kies, C., and Fox, H. M., Calcium and magnesium nutritional status of adolescent humans fed cellulose and hemicellulose supplement, *J. Food Sci.*. 44, 1412, 1979.

61. Mellanby, E., Anti-calcifying action of phytate, *J. Physiol.*, 109, 488, 1949.

62. Miller, J., Effect of heat processing diet mixtures on bioavailability of iron, *Nutr. Res.*, 3, 351, 1983.

63. Miller, J., Study of experimental conditions for most reliable estimates of relative biological value of iron in bread, *J. Agric. Food Chem.*, 25, 154, 1977,

64. Mod, R. R., Ory, R. L., Morris, N. M., and Normand, F. L., In vitro interaction of rice hemicellulose with trace minerals and their release by digestive enzymes, *Cereal Chem.*, 59, 538, 1982.

65. Mod, R. R., Ory, R. L., Morris, N. M., and Normand, F. L., Chemical properties and interactions of rice hemicellulose with trace minerals in vitro, *J. Agric. Food Chem.*, 29, 449, 1981.

66. Molloy, L. F. and Richards, E. L., Complexing of calcium and magnesium by organic constituents of Yorkshire Fog (*Holcus lanatus*). II. Complexing of Cal^{2+} and Mg^{2+} by cell wall fraction and organic acid, *J. Food. Agric.*, 22, 397, 1971.

67. Morris, E. R. and Ellis, R., Phytate-zinc molar ratio of breakfast cereals and bioavailability of zinc to rats, *Cereal Chem.*, 58, 363, 1981.

68. Morris, E. R. and Ellis, R., Isolation of monoferric phytate from wheat bran and its biological value as an iron source to the rat, *J. Nutr.*, 106, 753, 1976.

69. Obizoba, I. C., Zinc and copper metabolism of human adults fed combinations of corn, wheat, beans, rice and milk containing various levels of phytate, *Nutr. Rep. Int.*, 42, 203, 1981.

70. Oberleas, D., Muhrer, M. E., and O'Dell, B. L., Some effects of phytic acid on zinc availability and physiology of swine, *J. Anim. Sci.*, 21, 57, 1962.

71. O'Dell, B. L., Effect of dietary components upon zinc availability, *Am. J. Clin. Nutr.*, 22, 1315, 1969.

72. Papakyrikos, H., Kies, C., and Fox, H. M., Zinc and magnesium utilization as affected by graded levels of hemicellulose, cellulose and wheat bran, *Fed. Proc. Fed. Am. Soc. Exp. Biol.*, 38, 549, 1979.

73. Pedersen, B. and Eggum, B. O., The influence of milling on the nutritive value of flour cereal grains. I. Rye, *Qual. Plant Foods Hum. Nutr.*, 32, 185, 1983.

74. Persson, I. K., Raby, P., Fønt-Beck, P., and Jensen, E., Effect of prolonged bran administration on serum levels of cholesterol, ionized calcium and iron in the elderly, *J. Am. Gerontol. Soc.*, 24, 334, 1976.

75. Persson, I., Raby, K., Fonns-Beck, P., and Jensen, E., Bran and blood-lipids, *Lancet*, 2, 1208, 1975.

76. Prabhavathi, T., and Narasinga Rao, B. S., Effect of domestic preparation of cereals and legumes on ionizable iron, *J. Sci. Food Agric.*, 30, 597, 1979.

77. Ranhotra, G. S., Loewe, R. J., and Puyat, L. V., Bioavailability of magnesium from wheat flour and various organic and inorganic salts, *Cereal Chem.*, 53, 770, 1976.

78. Ranhotra, G. S., Lee, C., and Gelroth, J. A., Bioavailability of iron in some commercial variety breads, *Nutr. Rep. Int.*, 19, 851, 1979.

79. Ranhotra, G. S., Lee, C., and Gelroth, J. A., Expanded cereal fortification: bioavailability and functionality (flavor) of magnesium in bread, *J. Food Sci.*, 45, 915, 1980.

80. Ranhotra, G. S., Lee, C., and Gelroth, J. A., Bioavailability of iron in high-cellulose bread, *Cereal Chem.*, 56, 156, 1979.

81. Ranhotra, G. S., Lee, C., and Gelroth, J. A., Bioavailability of zinc in soy-fortified wheat bread, *Nutr. Rep. Int.*, 18, 487, 1978.

82. Rattan, J., Levin, N., Graff, E., Weizer, N., and Gilat, T., A high fiber diet does not cause mineral and nutrient deficiencies, *J. Clin. Gastroenterol.*, 3, 339, 1981.

83. Reinhold, J. G., Rickets in Asian immigrants, *Lancet*, 2, 1132, 1976.
84. Reinhold, J. G., Faradji, B., Abadi, P., and Ismail-Beigi, F., Binding of zinc to fiber and other solids of whole-meal bread, in *Trace Elements in Human Health and Disease*, Vol. 1., Prasad, A.-S. and Oberleas, D., Eds., Academic Press, New York, 1976, 163.
85. Reinhold, J. G., Faradji, B., Abadi, P., and Ismail-Beigi, F., Decreased absorption of calcium, magnesium, zinc and phosphorus by humans due to increased fiber and phosphorus consumption as wheat bread, *J. Nutr.*, 106, 493, 1976.
86. Reinhold, J. G., Garcia, J. S., and Garzon, P., Binding of iron by fiber of wheat and maize, *Am. J. Clin. Nutr.*, 34, 1384, 1981.
87. Reinhold, J. G., Hedayati, H., Lahimgarzadeh, A., and Nasr, K., Zinc, calcium, phosphorus and nitrogen balances of Iranian villagers following a change from phytate-rich to phytate-poor diets, *Ecol. Food Nutr.*, 2, 157, 1973.
88. Reinhold, J. G., Ismail-Beigi, F., and Faradji, B., Fiber vs phytate as determinant of the bioavailability of calcium, zinc and iron of bread stuff, *Nutr. Rep. Int.*, 12, 75, 1975.
89. Reinhold, J. G., Lahimgarzadeh, A., Nasr, K., and Hedayati, M., Effects of purified phytate and phytate rich bread upon metabolism of zinc, calcium, phosphorus and nitrogen in man, *Lancet*, 1, 283, 1973.
90. Reinhold, J. G., Nasr, K., Lahimgarzadeh, A., and Hedayati, M., Effect of purified phytate and phytate rich bread upon metabolism of zinc, calcium, phosphorus and nitrogen in man, *Lancet*, 1, 283, 1973.
91. Rendelman, J. A., Cereal complexes: binding of calcium by bran and components of bran, *Cereal Chem.*, 59, 302, 1982.
92. Rendelman, J. A. and Grobe, C. A., Cereal complexes: binding of zinc by bran and components of bran, *Cereal Chem.*, 59, 310, 1982.
93. Roberts, A. H. and Yudkin, J., Dietary phytate as a possible cause of magnesium deficiency, *Nature* (London), 185, 823, 1960.
94. Robertson, I., Ford, J. A., McIntosh, W. B., and Dunnigan, M. G., The role of cereals in the aetiology of nutritional rickets, the lesson of the Irish National Nutrition Survey 1943–1948, *Br. J. Nutr.*, 45, 17, 1981.
95. Rossander, L., Hallberg, L., and Björn-Rasmussen, E., Absorption of iron from breakfast meals, *Am. J. Clin. Nutr.*, 32, 2484, 1979.
96. Sandberg, A. S., Hasselblad, C., Hasselblad, K., and Hultén, L., The effect of wheat bran on the absorption of minerals in the small intestine, *Br. J. Nutr.*, 48, 185, 1982.
97. Sandstead, M. M., Munoz, J. M., Jacob, R. A., Klevay, L. M.. Reck, S. J., Logan, G. M., Dintzis, F. R., Inglett, G. E., and Shuey, W. C., Influence of dietary fiber on trace elements balance, *Am. J. Clin. Nutr.*, 31, S180, 1978.
98. Sandström, B. M., Arvidsson, B., Cederblad, Å., and Björn-Rasmussen, E., Zinc absorption from composite meals. I. The significance of wheat extraction rate, zinc, calcium and protein content in meals based on bread, *Am. J. Clin. Nutr.*, 33, 739, 1980.
99. Sandström, B. M., Andersson, H., Bosaeus, I., Falkheden, B. T., Göransson, H., and Melkersson, M., The effect of wheat bran on the intake of energy and nutrients and on serum mineral levels in constipated geriatric patients, *Hum. Nutr. Clin. Nutr.*, 37, 295, 1983.
100. Sayers, M. H., Lynch, S. R., Chariton, R. W., Bothwell, T. M., and Mayet, F., Iron absorption from rice meals cooked with fortified salt containing ferrous sulfate and ascorbic acid, *Br. J. Nutr.*, 31, 367, 1974.
101. Sayers, M. H., Lynch, S. R., Jacob, P., Charlton, R. W., Bothwell, T. M., Walker, R. B., and Mayet, F., The effects of ascorbic acid supplementation on the absorption of iron in maize, wheat, soya, *Br. J. Haematol.*, 24, 209, 1973.
102. Schweizer, T. F., Frølich, W., Del Vedovo, S., and Besson, R., Minerals and phytic acid in the analysis of dietary fiber from cereals, *Cereal Chem.*, 61(2), 116, 1983.
103. Shah, B. G., Giroux, A., and Belonje, B., Bioavailability of zinc in infant cereals, *Nutr. Metab.*, 23, 286, 1979.
104. Sharpe, M.. Peacock, W. C., Cooke, R., and Harris, R. S., The effect of phytate and other foods on iron absorption, *J. Nutr.*, 41, 435, 1950.
105. Simpson, K. S., Morris, E. R., and Cook, J. D., The inhibitory effect of bran on iron absorption in man, *Am. J. Clin. Nutr.*, 34, 1469, 1981.

106. Walker, A. R. P., Fox, F. W., and Irving, J. T., Studies in human mineral metabolism. I. The effect of bread rich in phytate phosphorus on the metabolism of certain mineral salts with special reference to calcium, *Biochem. J.*, 42, 452, 1948.

107. Widdowson, E. M. and McCance, R. A., Iron exchanges of adults on white and brown bread diet, *Lancet*, 1, 588, 1942.

108. Widdowson, E. M., Interactions of dietary calcium with phytates, phosphates and fats, *Nutr. Dieta*, 15, 38, 1970.

109. Weinreich, J., Pedersen, O., and Dinesen, K., Role of bran in normals, *Acta Med. Scand.*, 202, 125, 1977.

110. Winterringer, G. L. and Ranhotra, G. S., Relative bioavailability of magnesium from mineral and soy-fortified breads, *Cereal Chem.*, 60, 14, 1983.

111. Ajit Kaur Labana and Kawatra, B. L., Studies on protein quality and availability of zinc from Dosa, *J. Food Sci. Technol.*, 23, 224, 1986.

112. Akhtar, D., Begum, N., and Sattar, A., Effect of dietary phytate on bioavailability of iron, *Nutr. Res.*, 7, 833, 1987.

113. Andersson, H., Navert, B., Bingham, S. A., Englyst, H. N., and Cummings, J. H., The effects of breads containing similar amounts of phytate, but different amounts of wheat bran on calcium, zinc and iron balance in man, *Br. J. Nutr.*, 50, 503, 1983.

114. Bagheri, S. and Gueguen, L., Effect of wheat bran and pectin on the absorption and retention of phosphorus. calcium, magnesium and zinc by the growing pig, *Reprod. Nutr. Rev.*, 25, 705, 1985.

115. Ballam, G. C., Nelson, T. S., and Kirby, L. K., The effect of phytate and fiber source on phytate hydrolysis and mineral availability in rats, *Nutr. Rep. Int.*, 30, 1089, 1984.

116. Buchowski, M., Vanderstoep, J., and Kitts, D. D., Effects of heat treatment and organic acids on bioavailability of endogenous iron from wheat bran in rats, *Can. Inst. Food Sci. Technol. J.*, 21, 161, 1988.

117. Carlson, B. L. and Miller, D. D., Effects of product formulation, processing and meal composition on *in vitro* estimated iron availability from cereal-containing breakfast cereals, *J. Food Sci.*, 48, 1211, 1983.

118. Clydesdale, F. M., Effectiveness of organic chelators in solubilizing calcium and zinc in the fortified cereals under simulated gastrointestinal pH conditions, *J. Food Proc. Preserv.*, 13, 307, 1989.

119. Cook, J. D., Noble, N. L., Morck, T. A., Lynch, S. R., and Petersburg, S. J., Effect of fiber on nonheme iron absorption, *Gastroenterology*, 85, 1354, 1983.

120. Dintzis, F. R., Watson, P. R., and Sandstead, H. H., Mineral content of brans passed through the human G.I. tract, *Am. J. Clin. Nutr.*, 113, 653, 1983.

121. Donangelo, C. M. and Eggum, B. O., Comparative effects of wheat bran and barley husk on nutrient utilization in rats. II. Zinc, calcium and phosphorus, *Br. J. Nutr.*, 56, 269, 1986.

122. Fairweather-Tait, S. J., The effect of different levels of wheat bran on iron absorption in rats from bread containing similar amounts of phytate, *Brit. J. Nutr.*, 47, 243, 1982.

123. Fairweather-Tait, S. J., Portwood, D. E., Symss, L. L., Eagles, J., and Minski, M. J., Iron and zinc absorption in human subjects from a mixed meal of extruded and non-extruded wheat bran and flour, *Am. J. Clin. Nutr.*, 49, 151, 1989.

124. Fairweather-Tait, S. J., Symss, L. L., Smith, A. C., and Johnson, I. T., The effect of extrusion cooking on iron absorption from maize and potato, *J. Sci. Food Agric.*, 38, 73, 1987.

125. Farah, D. A., Hall, M. J., Mills, P. R., and Russel, R. I., Effect of wheat bran on zinc absorption, *Hum. Nutr. Clin. Nutr.*, 38, 433, 1984.

126. Frølich, W. and Asp, N.-G., Minerals and phytate in the analysis of dietary fiber from Cereals. III, *Cereal Chem.*, 62, 238, 1985.

127. Frølich, W. and Nyman, M., Minerals, phytate and dietary fiber in different fractions of oat grain, *J. Cereal Sci.*, 7, 73, 1988.

128. Frølich, W., Drakenberg, T., and Asp, N.-G., Enzymic degradation of phytate (myo-inositol hexaphosphate) in whole grain flour suspension and dough. A comparison between ^{31}P-NMR spectroscopy and a ferric ion method, *J. Cereal Sci.*, 4, 325, 1986.

129. Frølich, W., Wahlgren, M., and Drakenberg, T., Studies on phytate in oats and wheat using ^{31}P-NMR spectroscopy, *J. Cereal Sci.*, 8, 47, 1988.

130. Frølich, W. et al., Phytic acid, dietary fiber and minerals in wheat, oats and barley, Proc. 23rd Nordic Cereal Conf. 1987, 327, 1988.

131. Frølich, W., Chelating properties of dietary fiber and phytate. The role for mineral availability, *Adv. Exp. Med. Biol.*, 270, 83, 1990.

132. Garcia-Lopez, S. and Wyatt, C. J., Effect of fiber in corn-tortillas and cooked beans on iron availability, *J. Agric. Food Chem.*, 30, 724, 1982.

133. Gillooly, M., Bothwell, T. H., Charlton, R. W., Torrance, J. D., Bezwoda, W. R., MacPhail, A. P., Derman, D. P., Novelli, L., Morrall, P., and Mayet, F., Factors affecting the absorption of iron from cereals, *Br. J. Nutr.*, 51, 37, 1984.

134. Gordon, D. T. and Chao, L. S., Relationship of components in wheat bran and spinach to iron availability in the anemic rat, *J. Nutr.*, 114, 526, 1984.

135. Gupta, H. O., Iron and its availability in maize (*Zea mays L.*), *J. Food Sci. Technol.*, 25, 179, 1988.

136. Hall, M. J., Downs, L., Ene, M. D., and Farah, D., Effect of reduced phytate wheat bran on zinc absorption, *Eur. J. Clin. Nutr.*, 43, 4431, 1989.

137. Hallberg, L., Wheat fiber, phytase and iron absorption, *Scand. J. Gastroenterol. Suppl.*, 129, 73, 1987.

138. Hallmans, G., Sjöström, R., Wetter, L., and Wing, K. R., The availability of zinc in endosperm, whole grain and bran-enriched wheat crispbreads fed to rats on a zinc-deficient diet, *Br. J. Nutr.*, 62, 165, 1989.

139. Harland, B. F. and Morris, E. R., Fiber and mineral absorption, in *Dietary Fibre Perspectives. Reviews and Bibliography*, Leeds, A. R., Ed., John Libbey, London, 1985, 72.

140. Harmuth-Hoene, A. E. and Meuser, F., Improvement of the bioavailability of zinc in wholemeal bread and crispbread, *Z. Ernaehrungswiss.*, 27, 244, 1988.

141. Harmuth-Hoene, A. E., Dietary fiber and bioavailability of essential trace elements, a controversial topic, in *Trace Element—Analytical Chemistry in Medicine and Biology*, Vol. 4, Walter de Gruyter, Berlin, 1987, 108.

142. Hazell, T. and Johnson, I. T., Influence of food processing on iron availability *in vitro* from extruded maize-based snack foods, *J. Sci. Food Agric.*, 46, 365, 1989.

143. Hazell, T. and Johnson, I. T., Effects of food processing and fruit juices on *in vitro* estimated iron availability from cereals, vegetables and fruit, *J. Sci. Food Agric.*, 38, 73, 1987.

144. Hazell, T. and Johnson, I. T., The influence of beverages and condiments on *in vitro* estimate of iron availability from wheat flour and potato, *Food Chem.*, 27, 151, 1988.

145. House, W. A. and Welch, R. M., Bioavailability to rats of iron in six varieties of wheat grain intrinsically labeled with radio iron, *J. Nutr.*, 117, 476, 1987.

146. House, W. A. and Welch, R. M., Bioavailability of and interactions between zinc and selenium in rats fed wheat grain intrinsically labelled with ^{65}Zn and ^{75}Se, *J. Nutr.*, 119, 916, 1989.

147. Ikeda, S., Characterization of zinc components on *in vitro* enzymatic digestion of foods, *J. Food Sci.*, 49, 1297, 1984.

148. Ink, S., Fiber. Mineral and fiber-vitamin interaction, in *Nutrient Interactions*, Bodwell, C. E. and Erdman, J. W., Eds., Marcel Dekker, New York. 1988, 253.

149. Kivistö, B., Cederblad, A., Davidsson, L., Sandberg, A.-S., and Sandström, B. M., Effect of meal composition and phytate content on zinc absorption in humans from an extruded bran product, *J. Cereal Sci.*, 10, 189, 1989.

150. Kivistö, B., Anderson, H., Cederblad, G., Sandberg, A. S., and Sandström, B. M., Extrusion cooking of a high-fiber cereal product. II. Effects on apparent absorption of zinc, iron, calcium, magnesium and phosphorus in humans, *Br. J. Nutr.*, 55, 255, 1986.

151. Lantzsch, H.-J., Scheuermann, S. E., and Menke, K.-H., Influence of various sources on the phosphorus, calcium and zinc metabolism of young pigs at different dietary levels, *J. Anim. Physiol. Anim. Nutr.*, 60, 146, 1988.

152. Liu, Z. Q., Chao, C. S., and Wu, H. W., Investigation of the effect of a diet with wheat bran on the metabolic balances of Zn, Cu, Ca and Mg in diabetics, *Chung Hua Nei Ko Tsa Chih*, 28, 741, 1989.

153. Lopez-Guisa, J. M., Harrned, M. C., Dubielzig, R., Rao, S. C., and Marlett, J. A., Processed oat hulls as potential dietary fiber sources in rats, *J. Nutr.*, 118, 953, 1988.

154. Lykken, G. I., Mahalko, J., Johnson, P. E., Milne, D., Sandstead, H. H., Garcia, W. J., Dintzis, F. R., and Inglett, G. E., Effect of browned and unbrowned corn products intrinsically labeled with zinc-65 on absorption of zinc-65 in humans, *J. Nutr.*, 116, 7955, 1986.

155. Lyon, D. B., Studies on the solubility of Ca, Mg, Zn and Cu in cereal products, *Am. J. Clin. Nutr.*, 39, 190, 1984.
156. Mason, P. M., Judd, P. A., Fairweather-Tait, S. J., Eagles, J., and Miniski, M. J., The effect of moderately increased intakes of complex carbohydrates (cereals, vegetables and fruit) for 12 weeks on iron and zinc metabolism, *Br. J. Nutr.*, 63, 597, 1990.
157. Miyoshi, H., Okuda, T., Okuda, K., and Koishi, H., Effects of brown rice apparent digestibility and balance of nutrients in young men on low protein diets, *J. Nutr. Sci. Vitaminol.* (Tokyo), 33, 207, 1987.
158. Moore, R. J. and Kornegay, E. T., Effect of dietary fiber level and duration of feeding on fiber digestibility and mineral utilization by growing pigs fed high-fiber diets, *Animal Sci.*, Virginia Agric. Exp. Station, Virginia Polytech. Inst. and State Univ., 6, 96, 1986/1987.
159. Morris, E. R., Ellis, R., Hill, A. D., Cottrell, S., Steele, P., Moy, T., and Moser, P. B., Trace elements nutriture of adult men consuming three levels of phytate, *Fed. Proc.*, 43, 846, 1984.
160. Morris, E. R., Ellis, R., Steele, P., and Moser, P. B., Mineral balance of adult men consuming whole or dephytinized wheat bran, *Nutr. Res.*, 8, 445, 1988.
161. Nadeau, D. B. and Clydesdale, F. M., Effect of acid pretreatment on the stability of citric and malic acid complexes with various iron sources in a wheat flake cereal, *J. Food Biochem.*, 10, 241, 1986,
162. Narasinga Rao, B. S. and Prabhavathi, T., Tannin content of foods commonly consumed in India and its influence on ionizable iron, *J. Sci. Food Agric.*, 33, 889, 1982.
163. Ohkawa, T., Ebisuno, S., Kitagawa, M., Morimoto, S., Miyazaki, Y., and Yasukawa, S., Rice bran treatment for patients with hypercalciuric stones: experimental and clinical studies, *J. Urol.*, 132, 1140, 1984.
164. Pallauf, J., Kraemer, K., Markwitan, A., and Ebel, D., Effect of citric acid supplementation on the bioavailability of zinc from corn germs, *Z. Ernaehrungswiss.*, 29, 27, 1990.
165. Persson, H., Nair, B. M., Frølich, W., Nyman, M., and Asp, N.-G., Binding of mineral elements by some dietary fibre components *in vitro*. II, *Food Chem.*, 26, 139, 1987.
166. Persson, H., Nyman, M., Liljeberg, H., Önning, G., and Frølich, W., Binding of mineral elements by dietary fibre components in cereals—*in vitro*. III, *Food Chem.*, 40, 169, 1991.
167. Pointillaert, A., Fourdin, A., and Fountaine, N., Importance of cereal phytase activity for phytate phosphorus utilization by growing pigs fed diets containing triticale or corn, *J. Nutr.*, 117, 907, 1987.
168. Pointillart, A., Fontaine, N., and Thomasset, M., Phytate phosphorus utilization and intestinal phosphatases in pigs fed low phosphorus: wheat or corn diets, *Nutr. Rep. Inter.*, 29, 473, 1984.
169. Poneros-Schneier, A. G. and Erdman, J. L., Bioavailability of calcium from sesame seeds, almond powder, whole wheat bread, spinach and non-fat dry milk in rats, *J. Food Sci.*, 54, 150, 1989.
170. Reddy, N. S. and Reddy, P. R., Effect of different carbohydrates on the availability of iron from rice, *Nutr. Rep. Int.*, 31, 1117, 1985.
171. Reinhold, J. G., Garcia Estrada, J., Garcia, P. M., and Garzon, P., Retention of iron by rat intestine *in vivo* as affected by dietary fiber, ascorbate and citrate, *J. Nutr.*, 116, 1007, 1986.
172. Sandberg, A. S., Carlsson, N. G., and Svanberg, U., Effects of inositol tri-, tetra-, penta- and hexaphosphates on *in vitro* estimation of iron availability, *J. Food Sci.*, 54, 159, 1989.
173. Sandström, B. M., Almgren, A., Kivistö, B., and Cederblad, A., Zinc absorption in humans from meals based on rye, barley, oatmeal, triticale and whole wheat, *J. Nutr.*, 117, 1898, 1987.
174. Saxena, A. and Seshadri, S., The effect of whole milk, milk protein and some constituent amino acids on the *in vitro* availability of iron from cereal meals, *Nutr. Res.*, 8, 717, 1988.
175. Shah, B. G., Malcolm, S., Belonje, B., Trick, K. D., Brassard, R., and Monge, A. R., Effect of dietary cereal brans on the metabolism of calcium, phosphorus and magnesium in a long term rat study, *Nutr. Res.*, 10, 1015, 1990.
176. Spencer, H., Derler, J., and Osis, D., Calcium requirement, bioavailability and loss, *Fed. Proc.*, 46, 631, 1987.
177. Spiller, G. A., Story, J. A., Wong, L. G., Nunes, J. D., Alton, M., Petro, M. S., Furumoto, E. J., Whittam, J. H., and Scala, J., Effect of increasing levels of hard wheat fiber on fecal weight, minerals and steroids and gastrointestinal transit time in healthy young women, *J. Nutr.*, 116, 778, 1986.
178. Stuart, S. M. A., Johnson, P. E., Hamaker, B., and Kirleis, A., Absorption of zinc and iron by rats fed meals containing sorghum food products, *J. Cereal Sci.*, 6, 81, 1987.

179. Svanberg, U. and Sandberg, A. S., Improved iron availability in weaning foods through the use of germination and fermentation, Household level food tech. Proceedings of a workshop held in Narirobi, Kenya, FSTA 22, 10G9, 1987.
180. Toma, R. B. and Curtis, D. J., Effect on mineral bioavailability, *Food Technol.*, 111, 1986.
181. Turnlund, J. R., Smith, R. G., Kretsch, M. J., Keyes, W. R., and Shah, A. G., Milk's effect on the bioavailability of iron from cereal-based diets in young women by use of *in vitro* and *in vivo* methods, *Am. J. Clin. Nutr.*, 652, 373, 1990.
182. Vaaler, S., Aaseth, J., Hanssen, K. F., Dahl-Jørgensen, K., Frølich, W., Ødegaard, B., and Agenaes, Ø., Trace elements in serum and urine of diabetes patients given bread enriched with wheat bran or guar gum, in Int. Symp. Trace Element Metabolism in Man and Animals, TEMA-5, 1985, 142.
183. Van der Aar, P. J., Fahey, G. C., Bricke, S. C., Allen, S. E., and Berger, L. L., Effects of dietary fibers on mineral status of chicks, *J. Nutr.*, 113, 653, 1983.
184. van Dokkum, W., Wesstra, A., and Schippers, F. A., Physiological effects of fibre-rich types of breads. I. The effect of dietary fibre from bread on mineral balance of young men, *Br. J. Nutr.*, 47, 451, 1982.
185. Walker, A. R. P., Dietary fibre and mineral metabolism, *Molec. Aspects Med.*, 6, 69, 1987.
186. Wisker, E., Schweizer, T. F., and Feldheim, W., Effects of dietary fiber on mineral balance in humans, in *Dietary Fibre, Chemical and Biological Aspects*, Southgate, D. A. T., Waldron, K., Johnson, I. T., and Fenwick, G. R., Eds., Royal Society of Chemistry, Norwich, Special Publication No. 83, 1990, 23.
187. Zhang, D., Henricks, D. G., Mahoney, A. W., and Cornforth, D. P., Bioavailability of iron in green peas, spinach, bran cereal and corn meal fed to anemic rats, *J. Food Sci.*, 50, 426, 1985.

Phytic Acid and Cancer

Mazda Jenab and Lilian U. Thompson

INTRODUCTION

Many epidemiological studies,[1-3] meta-analyses,[4-6] and reviews[7-15] suggest that diets high in fiber and low in fat may be associated with a decreased risk of many cancers. However, not all epidemiological findings are able to establish a clear, definitive role for all dietary fibers in cancer prevention.[16-20] Differences in environmental factors, experimental design, and models used may account for some, but not all, of the inconsistencies, suggesting that some dietary fiber–associated components rather than dietary fiber *per se* may, in part, be responsible for the suggested cancer protective effects of high-fiber diets.

Phytic acid (PA) is one fiber-associated component, found in high concentrations in cereals, legumes, and oilseeds, that has been suggested to have cancer-protective effects. It is myoinositol with six phosphate moieties attached and is a ubiquitous plant component often complexed with calcium, potassium, or magnesium in cereals or a crystalline globule inside protein bodies in legumes, nuts, and oilseeds.[21] In many cereals and oilseeds, PA constitutes up to 1 to 5% of the weight and serves as the chief storage form of phosphorus.[22-24]

Because of its highly negatively charged phosphorylated structure, PA is able to bind with many divalent cations, proteins, and starch and consequently reduce their bioavailability.[24,25-27] For this reason, PA has traditionally been considered an antinutrient,[28] and many ways of removing it from foods have been suggested.[29-32] However, in the last two decades, several studies suggest that this same reactivity may confer on PA some health-beneficial effects, particularly the reduction of cancer risk.[33-37]

In this chapter, *in vitro* and *in vivo* studies on the effect of PA on cancer risk, along with its potential mechanisms of action, will be reviewed. A majority of the *in vivo* studies were conducted in animal models using purified PA added to either the diet or drinking water. Only a few studies have been conducted comparing the effect of purified PA (exogenous) to that of the naturally occurring PA (endogenous) in foods. The limitations of these different experimental approaches to prove the effects of PA are also discussed.

IN VITRO STUDIES

Table 6.5.1 summarizes the *in vitro* cell culture studies showing the antineoplastic action of purified PA on various cell types. PA inhibited cell growth and increased cell differentiation and maturation of HT-29 human colon carcinoma cells,[38,39] K-562 human erythroleukemia cell lines,[40] human PC-3 prostate adenocarcinoma,[41] human rhabdosarcoma,[42] human HepG2 liver cancer,[43] and estrogen receptor positive MCF-7 and estrogen receptor negative MDA-MB-231 human breast cancer cells.[44] In the latter experiment, significant inhibition was achieved with 1mM PA after 6 h of treatment, while other studies[39,41] have shown a dose-dependent decrease.

Eggleton[45] has shown that PA does not directly activate neutrophil inflammatory events but does enhance immune cell response to inflammatory stimuli. In a number of the above studies,[38–41] PA caused a reversion of malignant phenotype, i.e., decrease in expression of tumor markers within the cells (HT-29 cells) or change to a "normal" cellular appearance (K-562 erythroleukemia cells). In addition, pure PA added to HT-29 cells has been shown to upregulate the expression of p53, a tumor suppressor gene, and p21[wafl/cip1], a growth inhibitor,[46] suggesting that the antineoplastic action of PA may involve the direct modulation of genes controlling the growth and maturation of the cell.

ANIMAL STUDIES

A strong cancer-protective effect of purified PA has been shown in a large number of animal studies done under various experimental conditions, models, time periods, and endpoints ranging from preneoplastic markers such as cell proliferation and aberrant crypt foci (ACF) parameters to tumorigenesis (summarized in Table 6.5.2).

Colon Cancer

In colon cancer studies, pure PA has been shown to reduce the rate of colonic cell proliferation at early (2–14 weeks)[33,35,37,47] and late (36–40 weeks)[48,49] time points and to reduce various ACF parameters when provided in the diet[37,50] or in the drinking water.[51]

When provided in the drinking water, 1% PA has been shown to significantly decrease both the number of tumors and the tumor volume of azoxymethane-treated (AOM-treated) rats when treatment was commenced in the pre-initiation phase.[34,52] When administered to AOM-treated rats up to 5 months post-initiation, PA (2%, supplied in the drinking water) again significantly reduced the number of colon tumors, tumor size, and mitotic rate when compared to the control group,[49] suggesting that PA can have protective effects at both the initiation and promotion stages of colon carcinogenesis. Pretlow et al.[51] also found that post-initiation administration (1 week) of PA (2%, supplied in the drinking water) reduced the number of colon tumors (by 58%) and the tumor volume (by 76%). Similar colon cancer protective effects were observed when PA was provided in the diet.[53,54]

Mammary Cancer

Cell proliferation in the mammary gland was reduced by dietary PA supplementation (1.2%), with the reductions being more dramatic when the PA was added to diets supplemented with high levels of iron and calcium[35] (Table 6.5.2). Although an initial study showed only a non-statistically significant decrease in mammary tumors,[55] subsequent experiments[36,56] have shown that pure PA, supplemented in the drinking water, can effectively decrease mammary tumor incidence in dimethylbenzanthracene (DMBA)-treated rats. Similar effects have been observed with pure PA provided in the diet.[53,57]

Table 6.5.1 *In Vitro* Studies on the Effects of Phytic Acid on Various Cell Lines

Reference	Study Details	Amount of PA Used	PA Effect
Colon			
Saied and Shamsuddin[46]	HT-29 human colon carcinoma cell line	3.3, 5.0, 8.0 mM	Increase in expression of p53 and p21[waf1/cip1] with 3.3 and 5 mM PA at 3 and 6 days
Sakamoto et al[38]	HT-29 human colon carcinoma cell line	0.66–10.0 mM	Decrease in cell proliferation and markers of cell differentiation
Yang and Shamsuddin[39]	HT-29 human colon carcinoma cell line	0.33–20.0 mM	Decrease in cell growth and proliferation at 1 and 5 mM; increased differentiation and reversion to normal phenotype; inhibition of PA breakdown within the cell did not alter growth inhibition
Breast, Mammary			
Shamsuddin et al.[44]	MCF-7, MDA-MB-231 human breast cancer cells	1–5.0 mM	Dose-dependent decrease in growth; decrease in DNA synthesis; increase in differentiation
Liver			
Vucenik et al.[43]	HepG2 human liver cancer cells	0.25–5.0 mM	Dose-dependent decrease in growth; increase in differentiation; decrease in expression of mutant p53 protein and increase in p21[waf1/cip1]
Soft Tissue			
Vucenik et al.[42]	Rhabdomyosarcoma (soft tissue sarcoma) cells	0.1–10.0 mM	Dose-dependent decrease in growth with resumption after removal of PA from media
Blood			
Eggleton[45]	Neutrophils adherent to plastic or laminin	100.0, 250.0 µM	In presence of PA, stimulated cells increased interleukin-8 production and sustained assembly of F-actin; no effect of PA on non-stimulated cells
Shamsuddin et al.[40]	K-562 erythroleukemia cell line	0.05% and 0.1%	PA decreased growth and increased differentiation, intracellular Ca and lower IP concentrations
Prostate			
Shamsuddin and Yang[41]	PC-3 human prostate cancer cells	0.1–1.0 mM	Dose-dependent decrease in growth; increase in cell differentiation

Table 6.5.2 *In Vivo* Studies on the Effects of Phytic Acid on Various Cancers

Reference	Study Details	Disease Parameter Studied	Amount of PA Given	Mode of PA Administration	PA Effect
Colon — Early Risk Markers					
Nielsen et al.[33]	Male Wistar rats; no carcinogen; 2 wk	Cell proliferation	0.6, 1.2, 2.0%	Diet	Decrease in colonic cell proliferation
Thompson and Zhang[35]	Female C57BL/6J mice; DMBA; 3 wk	Cell proliferation	1.2%	Diet	Decrease in colon cell proliferation
Pretlow et al.[51]	Male F344 rats, AOM, 4,12, and 36 wk	ACF; tumor	2.0%	Drinking water	Decrease in number of ACF with multiplicity ≥ 4 at 12 wk
Owen et al.[70]	Adenoma patients	Cell proliferation	Variable amounts of dietary PA	N/A	No association between fecal PA levels and colon cell proliferation, mineral levels, or lipid content
Shivapurkar et al.[53]	Female SD rats; AOM; MNU; 9 and 30 wk	ACF	2.0%	Diet	Decrease in total number of ACF and ACF with multiplicities ≥ 4
Challa et al.[50]	Male F344 rats; AOM; 13 wk	ACF	1.0 and 2.0%	Diet	Decrease in incidence of ACF
Corpet et al.[47]	Female SD rats; AOM; 4 wk	ACF; cell proliferation	2.0%	Drinking water	Decrease in proliferation of normal crypts but not of ACF
Jenab and Thompson[37]	Male F344 rats; AOM; 14.3 wk	ACF; SIM ACF; cell proliferation	1.0%	Diet	Decrease in number of ACF and SIM ACF; decrease in cell proliferation and crypt height
Colon — Tumorigenesis					
Shamsuddin et al.[34]	Male F344 rats; AOM; 36 months	Tumor	2.0%	Drinking water; treatment commenced after 12 wk of carcinogen	Decrease in tumor number
Shamsuddin et al.[34]	Male F344 rats; AOM; 24 wk	Tumor	1.0%	Drinking water; treatment commenced prior to carcinogen	Decrease in tumor frequency (34.7%), volume (min. 63%), and colonic mitotic rate; decrease in hydroxyl radical formation by PA
Nelson et al.[54]	Male SD rats; DMH; 24 wk	Tumor	0.25%	Diet	Inhibit the colon cancer–promoting effect of iron
Shamsuddin and Ullah[49]	Male F344 rats; AOM; 40 wk (20 wk of PA treatment)	Tumor; mitotic rate	2.0%	Drinking water; treatment commenced 20 wk after carcinogen induction	Decrease in tumor number, size, and volume; decreased colonic mitotic rate
Shamsuddin et al.[48]	Male CD-1 mice; DMH; 19 and 36 wk	Tumor; mitotic rate	1.0%	Drinking water	Decrease in tumor number; decrease in mitotic rate

Reference	Model	Endpoint	Dose	Route	Results
Ullah and Shamsuddin[52]	Male F344 rats; AOM; PA provided prior to carcinogen administration; 38 wk	Tumor	0.1% and 1.0%	Drinking water	Decrease in tumor prevalence and size with 0.1% PA; 1.0% PA reduced tumor frequency and size
Prettlow et al.[51]	Male F344 rats; AOM; 4,12, and 36 wk	ACF; tumor	2.0%	Drinking water	Decrease in tumor number and volume at 36 wk
Mammary — Early Risk Markers					
Thompson and Zhang[35]	Female C57BL/6J mice; DMBA; 3 wk	Cell proliferation; nuclear aberration	1.2%	Diet	Decrease in mammary cell proliferation and nuclear aberrations; decrease in promotional effect of Ca and Fe
Mammary — Tumorigenesis					
Vucenik et al.[55]	Female SD rats; DMBA; PA provided prior to carcinogen administration; 18 wk	Tumor	15 mM	Drinking water	Non-statistically-significant reductions in tumor frequency, multiplicity, and size
Hirose et al.[57]	Female SD rats; DMBA; 35 wk	Tumor	2.0%	Diet	Decrease in size of palpable tumors; increase in number of surviving animals
Vucenik et al.[56]	Female SD rats; DMBA; 45 wk	Tumor	15 mM	Drinking water	Decrease in tumor incidence; decrease in tumor multiplicity and burden when PA combined with 15 mM inositol
Shivapurkar et al.[53]	Female SD rats; AOM; MNU; 9 and 30 wk	Tumor	2.0%	Diet	Decrease in number of tumors
Vucenik et al.[36]	Female SD rats; DMBA; 29 wk	Tumor	0.4%	Drinking water	Decrease in tumor incidence and number
Liver					
Vucenik et al.[58]	Male BALB/c nude mice inoculated with HepG2 human liver cancer cells; 1.7 wk	Tumor	40 mg/kg of body weight	Intra-tumoral injection	Decrease in tumor weight
Vucenik et al.[58]	Male BALB/c nude mice inoculated with HepG2 human liver cancer cells pretreated with PA; 8.9 wk	Tumor	NA	N/A	No tumors in mice receiving cells pretreated with PA vs. 71% tumor incidence in mice receiving untreated cells

Table 6.5.2 (Continued) *In Vivo* Studies on the Effects of Phytic Acid on Various Cancers

Reference	Study Details	Disease Parameter Studied	Amount of PA Given	Mode of PA Administration	PA Effect
Soft Tissue					
Jariwalla et al.[59]	Female F344 rats injected with fibrosarcoma cells	Tumor	12.0% pentapotassium dimagnesium phytate (equiv. to 8.9% PA)	Diet	Decrease in incidence and growth rate of cell transplant–induced fibrosarcomas
Vucenik et al.[60]	Male C3H/Jsed mice with transplanted tumor from FSA-1 fibrosarcoma cells; up to 6.9 wk	Tumor	0.25%	i.p. injection	Decrease in tumor growth; prolonged survival
Vucenik et al.[60]	Male C3H/Jsed mice injected i.p. with FSA-1 fibrosarcoma cells; 4 wk	Metastatic tumor	0.25%	i.p. injection	Decrease in number of pulmonary metastases
Vucenik et al.[42]	Male NIH athymic nude mice inoculated with rhabdomyosarcoma cells; 2 and 5 wk	Tumor	40 mg/kg of body weight	Peritumoral injection	Decrease in time of tumor appearance, tumor incidence, and growth
Skin					
Ishikawa et al.[61]	Female ICR mice; DMBA; 3 and 22 wk	Papillomas; cell proliferation	2.0%	Drinking water	Decrease in number of papillomas and number of tumor-bearing mice at 3 wk; decreased cell proliferation after 1 wk

Multi-Organ, Wide Spectrum, Bladder, and Adverse

Reference	Animal model		Dose	Route	Results
Hirose et al.[62]	Male F344 rats TTAD, DHPN, EHEN, DMAB, 32 wk	Tumor	2.0%	Diet	Increase in urinary bladder papillomas, weak decrease in neoplastic lesions in liver and pancreas; no effect in lung, colon, esophagus, forestomach, small intestine, kidney, and thyroid gland
Hiasa et al.[120]	Male and female F344, 100–108 wk	Tumor	1.25, 2.5%	Drinking water	Necrosis and calcification of renal papillae with papillomas in some of the high-dose rats
Takaba et al.[73]	Male F344 rats; BBN; 32 wk	Tumor	2.0%	Diet	Sodium-PA increased development of pre- and neoplastic urinary bladder lesions; Mg-PA and pure PA had no effect
Takaba et al.[76]	Male F344 rats; DHPN, EHEN, DMAB; 36 wk	Tumor	1.0%	Diet	No modifying effects when dietary treatment commenced during initiation stage of multi-organ carcinogenesis
Hirose et al.[72]	Male F344 rats; DHPN, EHEN, DMAB, BBN	Tumor	2.0%	Drinking water	Decrease in hepatic tumors; no difference in incidence or multiplicity but decrease in diameter of mammary tumors; increase in bladder carcinogenesis with sodium salt of PA

Note: Abbreviations: AOM – azoxymethane; ACF – aberrant crypt foci; BBN – *N*-butyl-*N*-(4-hydroxybutyl)nitrosamine; DHPN – 2,2′-dihydroxy-di-*n*-propylnitrosamine; DMAB – 3,2′-dimethyl-4-aminobiphenyl; DMBA – dimethylbenzanthracene; EHEN – *N*-ethyl-*N*-hydroxy-ethylnitrosamine; F344 – Fisher344; MNU – methylnitrosourea; N/A – not applicable; PA – phytic acid; SD – Sprague-Dawley; SIM – sialomucin producing; TTAD – *n*-tritriacontane-16,18 dione.

Other Cancers

Injection of pure PA directly into HepG2 liver cancer tumors inhibited their growth in immunodeficient mice.[58] Also, HepG2 cells treated with PA prior to inoculation into the mice developed substantially fewer tumors than untreated cells, even though PA was not provided to the mice.[58] PA reduced the growth of rat fibrosarcoma[59] as well as subcutaneously transplanted mice fibrosarcoma cells and the number of pulmonary metastases established after their injection.[60] Furthermore, PA delivered by injection directly into the tumor inhibited growth of human rhabdomyosarcoma, an aggressive soft tissue tumor cell line, in immunodeficient mice.[42] Supplementation of PA (2%) in the drinking water has protective effects in skin 2-step papillomas,[61] while dietary supplementation of the same amount has inhibited hepatocellular carcinomas in the liver as well as eosinophilic foci, which are putative preneoplastic lesions, in the pancreas.[62]

Mode of PA Administration

Diet vs. Distilled Water

A majority of the studies on PA and cancer used pure PA at the level of 1–2% given either in a low-fiber diet or in the drinking water (Table 6.5.3). Since most of these studies show positive effects of PA on cancer prevention (Table 6.5.4), it can be argued that either mode of PA administration is effective. However, animals fed 1% PA in the diet may be receiving different amounts of PA than animals receiving 1% PA in the drinking water, as the intake depends on how much they eat or drink. Very few of the studies listed in Table 6.5.2 provide an assessment of overall amount of PA consumed or information about amount of food or drinking water intake. Thus, it is difficult to compare effective PA levels in studies that provide PA in the diet vs. in the drinking water.

Pure (Exogenous) vs. Food (Endogenous) PA

When administered as part of the diet, pure PA may form complexes with the mineral, protein, or starch components in the diet. When given in the drinking water, the ability of PA to bind with other dietary components depends on whether it is consumed concurrently with diet or at different time periods than the diet. On the other hand, endogenous PA in a high-fiber food source, such as wheat bran, may already be tightly bound to the fiber, proteins or minerals, making it less available for absorption or interaction with other dietary components or the colonic mucosa. Hence, the cancer-protective effect of PA may theoretically differ depending on whether it is provided in the pure form (exogenous) or as a natural component (endogenous) of a high-fiber food such as wheat bran. However, to date only a few studies[36,37,63] have attempted to make a comparison between endogenous and exogenous PA.

Vucenik et al.[36] showed that levels of wheat bran up to 20% were ineffective in reducing rat mammary tumorigenesis, while an amount of PA equivalent to that in 20% wheat bran (0.4%) added in pure form to the drinking water caused a significant reduction in tumor incidence. Nevertheless, although the authors matched the level of pure PA in the drinking water of one group to the level of PA present in the 20% wheat bran diet of the other group, they provided no data on the total amount of PA consumed by each group nor gave any assurance that the total amounts consumed were equal. Thus, as discussed earlier, in such cases it is very difficult to effectively compare the effects of the endogenous PA in wheat bran to exogenous pure PA given in the drinking water.

Suggestions have been made that to reduce cancer risk, supplementing a diet with pure PA may be better than eating fiber-rich foods.[36,64] However, high-fiber diets provide many more phytochemicals than PA and are also associated with reduction in risk of diseases other than cancer. Therefore,

Table 6.5.3 Number of *In Vivo* Studies Using Different Levels and Modes of Phytic Acid (PA) Administration

Amount of PA Used in Study	Number of Studies Using Each Mode of PA Administration		
	Diet	Drinking Water	Intratumoral or I.P. Injection
< 1 %	1	2	0
1 to <2 %	6	4	0
2 %	6	6	0
> 2 %	1	1	0
15 mM	0	2	0
40 mg/kg body weight	0	0	2
Total	14	15	2

Note: Values represent number of studies using a certain level of PA with each mode of PA administration. Some studies with more than one level of PA intake were repeated in the count.

Table 6.5.4 Summary of All *In Vivo* Studies on Phytic Acid and Cancer

Organ and Endpoint	Number of Studies			
	Total	Protective Effects	No Effects/Equivocal	Promotive/Adverse Effects
Colon				
Early risk markers	8	7	1	0
Tumor	7	7	0	0
Mammary				
Early risk markers	1	1	0	0
Tumor	4	3[a]	1	0
Liver				
Tumor	2	2	0	0
Soft tissue				
Tumor	4	4	0	0
Bladder				
Necrosis/calcification	1	0	0	1
Tumor	4	0	0	4
Skin				
Tumor	1	1	0	0
Multi-organ (except bladder)	2	0	2	1

Note: Values represent number of studies. Some studies with more than one timepoint or endpoint were repeated in the count.

[a] One study was effective only when phytic acid was combined with inositol.

it is still more practical to eat diets containing high-fiber foods than a refined diet supplemented with just one phytochemical.

Jenab and Thompson[37] tried to differentiate the role of endogenous versus vs. PA by determining the effect of diets supplemented with either 25% wheat bran, 1.0% pure PA (equivalent to the amount of PA in the 25% wheat bran diet), 25% dephytinized wheat bran (wheat bran with the endogenous PA removed), or dephytinized wheat bran with 1.0% pure PA. The effect of endogenous PA was indicated by a comparison of wheat bran and dephytinized wheat bran, while the effect of exogenous PA in a high- or low-fiber diet was indicated by a comparison of the 1% PA and the 25% dephytinized wheat bran plus 1% PA diets. In this study, the actual intake of pure PA (exogenous) was the same as the intake of endogenous PA. Results showed a significant reduction in the number of sialomucin-producing (SIM-producing) ACF, an important early biomarker of colon cancer risk, by all the treatment diets (Table 6.5.5). In addition, exogenous

PA added to the low-fiber diet significantly reduced the number of ACF and size of ACF vs. the control diet. All the treatment diets also significantly reduced the labeling index of cell proliferation in the top 40% of the crypt vs. the control diet, but wheat bran, with its endogenous PA, was significantly more effective than the other diets (Table 6.5.5). The removal of PA from the wheat bran caused an increase in the rate of cell proliferation (Table 6.5.5), suggesting that the colon cancer–protective effects of wheat bran may be due, in part, to its PA. The rate of cell proliferation with the 1% PA diet was significantly lower relative to the control group but significantly higher than the wheat bran group and not different from the other diets. This differential effect of endogenous and exogenous PA suggests that, although both are effective, they may be acting through different mechanisms.

Table 6.5.5 Number of Aberrant Crypt Foci and Labeling Index of Cell Proliferation in the Distal Colon of Rats on Wheat Bran or Phytic Acid Diets

Groups	Number of ACF	Number of Sialomucin ACF	Labeling Index in the Top 40%
BD	64.67 ± 4.59[a]	34.33 ± 3.58[a]	18.45 ± 1.38[a]
WB	51.09 ± 2.37[ab]	15.64 ± 1.83[b]	7.97 ± 0.99[d]
DWB	54.55 ± 3.28[ab]	18.64 ± 2.16[b]	13.71 ± 1.48[bc]
DWBPA	54.82 ± 3.46[ab]	18.55 ± 3.64[b]	9.69 ± 0.91[cd]
PA	44.93 ± 4.01[b]	12.57 ± 3.13[b]	12.69 ± 1.19[bc]

Note: Values are means ± SEM on a sample size of 15 rats per group for aberrant crypt foci data and 24 crypts per rat with 6 rats per group for labeling index of cell proliferation data; values with different superscripts are significantly different, $p < 0.05$. BD = basal diet, control group; WB = 25% wheat bran diet; DWB = 25% dephytinized wheat bran diet; DWBPA = 25% dephytinized wheat bran plus 1.0% added PA diet; PA = 1.0% added PA diet.

Source: Adapted from Jenab, M. and Thompson, L. U., *Carcinogenesis*, 19, 1087, 1998.

Reddy et al.[63] found that a diet supplemented with 10% defatted and dephytinized wheat bran had an effect on colon tumorigenesis which did not differ from that of a diet supplemented with a similar amount (10%) of wheat bran with its endogenous PA and oil intact. Likewise, addition of 0.4% exogenous PA to a dephytinized and defatted wheat bran (10%) diet did not cause any significant changes in colon tumorigenesis compared to a 10% wheat bran diet. Although this study was not designed to compare the role of endogenous and exogenous PA, the results do suggest that PA may not be a strong factor in the protective effects of wheat bran, since removal of endogenous PA and addition of exogenous PA did not significantly affect colon tumorigenesis. However, the amount of PA tested in this study (0.4%) is much less than the amount (1–2%) in most of the other studies listed in Table 6.5.2, as well as in the Jenab and Thompson[37] study cited above. Since most of the colon cancer–protective effects of wheat bran have been found at levels of intake much higher than 10%,[65–69] levels of PA greater than 0.4%, which is the amount in a 10% wheat bran diet, may be required for reduction in risk of colon cancer. Perhaps the most important finding of this study is that removal of both the oil and PA components of wheat bran caused a significant increase in the number of adenocarcinomas, suggesting that the colon cancer–protective effects of wheat bran may be associated with many of its components and not just its endogenous PA. In the same study, addition of 2% wheat bran oil (an amount in excess of that found in 10% wheat bran) alone or with 0.4% exogenous PA to a 10% dephytinized and defatted wheat bran diet significantly reduced the number of adenocarcinomas vs. the 10% wheat bran diet, suggesting that wheat bran oil may also be an important colon cancer–protective component of wheat bran. However, because the amount of oil added in this study was largely in excess of the amount found in 10% wheat bran, making direct comparisons with the wheat bran is difficult.

The results of the above studies suggest that endogenous PA derived from wheat bran, as well as exogenous PA added back to wheat bran or to a low-fiber diet, may be cancer protective, depending on the concentration of PA. They also highlight the point that the cancer-protective effects of high-fiber diets may stem from more than just one important component.

HUMAN STUDIES

Limited clinical studies have been conducted on the role of PA in cancer prevention. Owen et al.[70] observed a strong correlation between fecal PA and fecal minerals, particularly iron, but no relationship between the rate of cell proliferation and fecal PA content in adenoma patients. They attributed the lack of an effect possibly to the presence of adenomas affecting colorectal cell kinetics.[71] However, it is unclear from this study whether the colonic sampling for the rate of cell proliferation was performed at the same time as fecal collection or whether the patients were maintained on the same diets as they were at the time of fecal collection, factors which may influence the relationships. Any effects of dietary PA on cell proliferation probably require long-term exposure to constant levels of dietary PA and, therefore, clinical experiments in this area will require long-term consumption of controlled diets with known levels of PA and minerals. Owen et al.[70] did not relate fecal PA levels to dietary PA intake. It is possible that it is the PA that is broken down within the colon to lower inositol phosphates or the PA that is absorbed by the colonocytes that may be having protective effects and not the essentially unreactive PA that is complexed with other dietary components that is excreted in the feces.

ADVERSE EFFECTS

While most of the studies on PA show a protective effect (Table 6.5.2, Table 6.5.4), an exception is an adverse effect of PA on bladder cancer.[62,72,73] Since most of these studies use the sodium salt of PA, it may be possible that the sodium-PA alters urinary sodium ion concentration or pH, with negative consequences for the bladder,[62,74] or it may directly affect transitional cell epithelial growth in the bladder.[75] Furthermore, Hirose et al.[72] and Takaba et al.[76] (Table 6.5.2) have found that these bladder cancer–promotive effects are observed only with sodium-PA and not with unchelated PA or other PA chelates. Thus, there may be little risk from consuming food sources rich in PA, such as wheat bran. Nonetheless, the potential negative effects of PA, particularly diets supplemented with sodium-PA, need to be further studied prior to any recommendations on its intake.

POTENTIAL MECHANISMS OF ACTION

Evidently, PA has a cancer-protective effect on different tissues, as seen in various cancer models under different experimental conditions. However, the mechanisms behind the action of PA are not clear, although several have been suggested.

Interactions with Protein and Starch — Enzyme Inhibition and Malabsorption

PA may potentially bind important proteins and enzymes within the cell and thus alter its growth characteristics. PA has been shown *in vitro* to inhibit the activity of several enzymes such as serine/threonine protein phosphatases[77] as well as a number of intracellular proteins.[78–80] However, the effects of PA may be different *in vivo*.

Within the digestive tract, PA can potentially bind dietary proteins and digestive enzymes such as trypsin, thus inhibiting protein digestion and absorption.[81,82] PA may also reduce the rate of digestion and absorption of starches,[83,84] either by hydrogen binding to starch, indirectly by binding to proteins that starch is bound to,[82,84] or by binding amylase or enzyme cofactors such as Ca^{2+}.[24] A negative correlation has been observed between PA intake level from cereal and legume foods and the glycemic index,[85] suggesting reduced absorption of dietary starch with increasing levels of PA. Furthermore, re-addition of PA to dephytinized navy bean flour caused a reversion of the increased rate of digestion and blood glucose response seen upon dephytinization.[86] The undigested and unabsorbed starch reaches the colon and contributes to increased fecal bulk or is fermented to short-chain fatty acids (SCFAs) and decreases pH. These, in turn, may have protective effects on the colon.[24] The SCFA butyrate has been shown in several studies to reversibly prolong the doubling time and to slow down the growth rates of human colorectal cancer cell lines;[87,88] to reduce DNA synthesis;[89] to induce apoptosis in human colon cancer cell lines[90] and in rats fed butyrate pellets;[91] and to suppress colon tumor formation.[92] Any starch that is not digested and absorbed in the small intestine would also lessen the glucose absorption and potentially decrease the insulin response. This is of consequence not only to diabetes but also to colon cancer in light of the insulin hypothesis of colon carcinogenesis, whereby lesser insulin response is related to decreased tumor growth promotion.[93–95]

The extent of the protein–starch–PA interactions depends on the ability of PA to also interact with other dietary compounds. For example, the inhibitory effects of PA on starch digestibility and absorption have been reversed by the addition of calcium, which is preferentially chelated by the PA.[96] The PA is then unable to bind to or interact with starches in the ingested food. Thus, the effects of reactive pure PA, i.e., exogenous PA, added to a diet or drinking water may be different from the same amount of PA present within the matrix of a foodstuff, i.e., endogenous PA, which may already be bound to other food components.

Interactions with Minerals and Antioxidative Effects

PA can chelate polyvalent cations, such as iron, calcium, and zinc,[97] which are required for vital cellular functions such as cofactors for enzymes and metalloproteins involved in gene regulation and expression.[98] For example, zinc supplementation has been shown to reverse inhibition of colonic epithelial cell proliferation,[33] suggesting that chelation of zinc by PA was inhibiting DNA synthesis, for which zinc is required. This may also be a mechanism in the recently observed protective effects of PA on human rhabdomyosarcoma[42] and HepG2 liver cancer cells in athymic mice, whereby PA was injected directly into the tumor daily.

Individuals consuming less dietary fiber have been shown to produce significantly more hydroxyl radicals.[99] Such oxygen-derived free radicals, generated in fecal material close to colonic epithelium, may play a role in the etiology of colon carcinogenesis by causing either direct cellular and genetic damage or by promoting the conversion and oxidation of procarcinogens to carcinogens or mitogenic tumor promoters.

Iron has been associated with both the initiation and promotion stages of carcinogenesis by enhancing oxidative damage,[100] since the formation of hydroxyl radicals within the colon depends on iron for catalysis.[101] The amount of iron necessary for such reactions can be diet-derived.[102] Thus, removal of iron, perhaps via chelation with PA, may inhibit the production of hydroxyl radicals and may be protective. PA is a particularly effective chelator of iron since it does not allow the iron to be soluble, making it completely bio-unavailable[22] and incapable of participating in free-radical-generating pathways. PA also catalyzes the oxidation of ferrous to ferric iron, thus removing the substrate for the Fenton reaction.[23] A correlation has been observed between fecal PA and iron content, indicating that PA is capable of binding iron within the digestive tract.[70,103]

In vitro addition of PA to a superoxide radical-generating system inhibits the hydroxyl radical formation, although at different ratios of PA to iron.[22,104] PA has also been shown to completely inhibit iron-catalyzed lipid peroxidation[23] and the production of reactive oxygen species[103] *in vitro*. However, the latter has only been shown to be true for EDTA-depleted systems, suggesting that

EDTA may be a stronger chelator of iron than PA. This is important, since it shows that the inhibitory effects of PA may be strong only in the absence of other chelating agents. Thus, in the *in vivo* situation, if dietary iron is already chelated or bound, and with the mostly anaerobic environment of the colon, the antioxidant effects of PA seen *in vitro* may not be strongly reproducible *in vivo*. For example, Rimbach and Pallauf [104] observed no effect of PA on liver oxidant or antioxidant status even in a high-iron situation, although Porres et al.[105] have shown that breakdown of endogenous PA in a corn–soy diet by addition of phytase enzyme can cause an increase in colonic lipid peroxidation.

It is evident that PA may act as a preventive antioxidant by chelating and insolubilizing iron to prevent its participation in free-radical-generating pathways *in vitro*, but more study is necessary to determine whether this is applicable *in vivo*.

Participation in the Inositol Phosphate Pool

PA has been shown to be rapidly absorbed and to be converted to lower inositol phosphates in various murine and human cells *in vitro*[106] and *in vivo*.[38] If PA can enter the cell, it can participate in the inositol phosphate pool and be converted to lower inositol phosphates (IP_{1-5}). PA added to the media of K-562 erythroleukemia cells *in vitro* results in a 41% increase and 26% decrease in intracellular IP_3 and IP_2, respectively, indicating both absorption and conversion of PA.[40] Similarly, PA has been shown *in vitro* to be absorbed and converted to IP_3 by WRK-1 rat mammary epithelial cells.[107]

The colon cancer–protective effects observed with PA supplementation are strengthened in the presence of myoinositol, the parent compound of PA.[48] Similar observations have been made in metastatic and mammary models of cancer,[55,56,62] with the PA + myoinositol group showing significantly greater reduction of tumor burden, number, and multiplicity than PA or inositol alone. Inositol produced from PA breakdown may also participate in the IP pool, contribute to lower IP production, and modulate signal transduction mechanisms. This possibility is strengthened by the observation that myoinositol protects against mammary cancer[56] and lung cancer.[108] In light of these observations, and since PA can be converted to lower inositol phosphates within mammalian cells,[106] it is also possible that the cancer-protective effects of PA are being mediated through the lower inositol phosphates or myoinositol itself.[109]

The full functions, secondary messenger roles, and intracellular importance of inositol phosphates still need much further clarification. Thus, with so many roles within the cell, it is conceivable that the dietary modulation of inositol phosphates by PA may play an as-yet undiscovered role in colon cancer prevention or inhibition.

Other Mechanisms

A number of *in vitro* (Table 6.5.1) and *in vivo* studies (Table 6.5.2) have shown that PA can reduce the rate of colonic cell proliferation,[33–35,37,47,52] suggesting that PA affects tumor growth through changes in the rate of cell division. Interestingly, Jenab and Thompson[110] have recently shown that both the endogenous PA in 25% wheat bran and exogenous PA (1%) added either to dephytinized wheat bran or to a low-fiber diet can increase the colonic rate of cell apoptosis and the degree of differentiation. These measures are important prognostic indicators of colon cancer risk and tumor development[111] and thus provide a mechanism whereby endogenous and exogenous PA may be protective of early biomarkers of colon cancer risk. Since there was no significant difference between any of the treatment groups, endogenous and exogenous PA as well as wheat bran fiber can all be considered to equally affect apoptosis and cell differentiation. These studies suggest that part of the beneficial effects of PA can be modulated through alterations in cell proliferation, apoptosis, and differentiation.

PA may also affect the process of tumor promotion by inhibiting 12-O-tetradecanoylphorbol-13-acetate-induced (TPA-induced) ornithine decarboxylase activity in HEL-30 keratinocytes and CD-1 mouse skin.[112] PA has also been shown to block TPA or epidermal growth factor–induced cell transformation in JB6 mouse epidermal cells by inhibiting phosphatidylinositol-3 (PI-3) kinase, an enzyme involved in the phosphorylation and hydrolysis of lipids involved in cellular signaling.[113]

Enhanced natural killer cell activity has been shown in carcinogen-treated mice fed with PA and *in vitro* when splenocytes from normal mice were treated with PA.[114] Such immune system effects may be another means by which PA can exert its actions.

PA may modulate cellular response at the receptor level. For example, PA has been shown to compete for binding sites on the IGF-II receptor,[115] which is over-expressed in certain tumors and cell lines.[116,117] Increased IGF-II levels have been linked to an increased risk for colorectal cancer.[118] Manousos et al.[118] suggest that IGF receptor activation plays a role in later stages of carcinogenesis, indicating that IGF receptor inhibition, possibly by PA, may be a favorable event. PA has also been shown to bind the basic fibroblast growth factor receptor (bFGF), sterically blocking its binding domain and thus disrupting its signals.[119]

CONCLUSIONS

It is evident from *in vitro* and animal studies that purified exogenous PA provided either in the drinking water or the diet has cancer-protective effects on a variety of tissues. From the limited number of studies conducted on the role of endogenous vs. exogenous PA, it appears that endogenous PA may be in part responsible for the cancer-protective effects of high-fiber foods, particularly wheat bran, a rich source of PA. Well-designed, prospective clinical studies still need to be conducted to validate the effects of PA observed in animal studies. Several mechanisms have been suggested for the cancer-protective effects of PA, including its ability to bind starch, proteins, enzymes, and minerals such as the pro-oxidant iron; potential participation in cellular inositol phosphate pools; and involvement in signal transduction, cell-signaling cascades, and gene expression. PA may have an important role in the reduction of cancer risk by high-fiber diets advocated by major health and government agencies. However, more research is needed to further distinguish the role of endogenous PA present within the matrix of a foodstuff and exogenous PA added in pure form either to the diet or drinking water and to relate experimental studies to data to be obtained from various human populations.

REFERENCES

1. Steinmetz, K. A., Kushi, L. H., Bostick, R. M., Folsom, A. R., and Potter, J. D., Vegetables, fruit, and colon cancer in the Iowa women's health study, *Am. J. Epidemiol.*, 139, 1, 1994.
2. Chatenoud, L., Tavani, A., La Vecchia, C., Jacobs, D. R., Jr., Negri, E., and Levi, F., Whole grain food intake and cancer risk, *Int. J. Cancer*, 77, 24, 1998.
3. Negri, E., Franceschi, S., Parpinel, M., and La Vecchia, C., Fiber intake and risk of colorectal cancer, *Cancer Epidemiol. Biomarkers Prev.*, 7, 667, 1998.
4. Howe, G. R., Benito, E., Castelleto, R., Cornee, J., Esteve, J., and Gallagher, R. P., Dietary intake of fiber and decreased risk of cancers of the colon and rectum: evidence from the combined analysis of 13 case control studies, *J. Natl. Cancer Inst.*, 84, 1887, 1992.
5. Trock, B., Lanza, E., and Greenwald, P., Dietary fiber, vegetables, and colon cancer: critical review and meta-analyses of the epidemiologic evidence, *J. Natl. Cancer Inst.*, 18, 650, 1990.
6. Gandini, S., Merzenich, H., Robertson, C., and Boyle, P., Meta-analysis of studies on breast cancer risk and diet: the role of fruit and vegetable consumption and the intake of associated micronutrients, *Eur. J. Cancer*, 36, 636, 2000.

7. McKeown-Eyssen, G. E. and Bright-See, E., Dietary factors in colon cancer: international relationships, *Nutr. Cancer*, 6, 160, 1984.

8. Greenwald, P., Lanza, E., and Eddy, G. A., Dietary fiber in the reduction of colon cancer risk, *J. Am. Diet. Assoc.*, 87, 1178, 1987.

9. Jacobs, L. R., Fiber and colon cancer, *Gastroenterol. Clin. North Am.*, 17, 747, 1988.

10. Higginson, J. and Sheridan, M. J., Nutrition and human cancer, in *Human Nutrition: A Comprehensive Treatise*, vol. 7, Alfin-Slater, R. B. and Kritchevsky, D., Eds., Plenum Press, New York, 1991, 1.

11. Wynder, E. L., Reddy, B. S., and Weisburger, J. H., Environmental factors in colorectal cancer: some unresolved issues, *Cancer*, 70, 1222, 1992.

12. Helzlsouer, K. J., Block, G., Blumberg, J., Diplock, A. T., Levine, M., Marnett, L. J., Schulplein, R. J., Spence, J. T., and Simic, M. G., Summary of the round table discussion on strategies for cancer prevention: diet, food, additives, supplements and drugs, *Cancer Res.*, 54(suppl.), 2044s, 1994.

13. Lipworth, L., Epidemiology of breast cancer, *Eur. J. Cancer Prev.*, 4, 7, 1995.

14. Potter, J. D., Nutrition and colorectal cancer, *Cancer Causes Control*, 7, 127, 1996.

15. Potter, J. D., Cancer prevention, epidemiology and experiment, *Cancer Lett.*, 114, 7, 1997.

16. Hill, M. J., MacLennan, R., and Newcombe, K., Diet and large bowel cancer in three socioeconomic groups in Hong Kong, *Lancet*, 1, 436, 1979.

17. Verhoeven, D. T., Assen, N., Goldbohm, R. A., Dorant, E., van't Veer, P., Sturmans, F., Hermus, R. J., and van den Brandt, P. A., Vitamins C and E, retinol, beta-carotene and dietary fibre in relation to breast cancer risk: a prospective cohort study, *Br. J. Cancer*, 75, 149, 1997.

18. Fuchs, C. S., Giovannucci, E. L., Colditz, G. A., Hunter, D. J., Stampfer, M. J., Rosner, B., Speizer, F. E., and Willett, W. C., Dietary fiber and the risk of colorectal cancer and adenoma in women, *N. Engl. J. Med.*, 340, 169, 1999.

19. Alberts, D. S., Martinez, M. E., Roe, D. J., Guillen-Rodriquez, J. M., Marshall, J. R., van Leeuwen, J. B., Reid, M. E., Ritenbaugh, C., Vargas, P. A., Bhattacharyya, A. B., Earnest, D. L., and Sampliner, R. E., Lack of effect of a high-fiber cereal supplement on the recurrence of colorectal adenomas, *N. Engl. J. Med.*, 342, 1156, 2000.

20. Schatzkin, A., Lanza, E., Corle, D., Lance, P., Iber, F., Caan, B., Shike, M., Weissfeld, J., Burt, R., Cooper, M. R., Kikendall, J. W., and Cahill, J., Lack of effect of a low-fat, high-fiber diet on the recurrence of colorectal adenomas. Polyp Prevention Trial Study Group, *N. Engl. J. Med.*, 342, 1149, 2000.

21. Reddy, N. R., Sathe, S., and Salunkhe, D. K., Phytates in legumes and cereals, *Adv. Food Res.*, 28, 1, 1982.

22. Graf, E. and Eaton, J. W., Effects of phytate on mineral bioavailability in mice, *J. Nutr.*, 114, 1192, 1984.

23. Graf, E., Empson, K. L., and Eaton, J. W., Phytic acid: a natural antioxidant, *J. Biol. Chem.*, 262, 11647, 1987.

24. Rickard, S. E. and Thompson, L. U., Interactions and biological effects of phytic acid, in *Antinutrients and Phytochemicals in Food*, Shahidi, F., Ed., American Chemical Society, Washington, D.C., 1997, 294.

25. Brune, M., Rossander, L., and Hallberg, L., Iron absorption: no intestinal adaptation to a high-phytate diet, *Am. J. Clin. Nutr.*, 49, 542, 1989.

26. Torre, M., Rodriguez, A. R., and Saura-Calixto, F., Effects of dietary fiber and phytic acid on mineral bioavailability, *Crit. Rev. Food. Sci. Nutr.*, 1, 1, 1991.

27. Zhou, J. R. and Erdman, J. W., Phytic acid in health and disease, *Crit. Rev. Food Sci. Nutr.*, 35, 495, 1995.

28. Cheryan, M., Phytic acid interactions in food systems, *Crit. Rev. Food Sci. Nutr.*, 13, 297, 1980.

29. Reinhold, J., Nasr, K., Lahimgarzadeh, A., and Hedayati, H., Effects of purified phytate and phytate rich bread upon metabolism of zinc, calcium, phosphorus and nitrogen, *Lancet*, 1, 283, 1973.

30. Morris, E. R. and Ellis, R., Bioavailability to rats of iron and zinc in wheat bran: response to low-phytate bran and effect of the phytate/zinc molar ratio, *J. Nutr.*, 110, 2000, 1980.

31. Sathe, S. K. and Salunkhe, D. K., Technology of removal of unwanted components of dry beans, *Crit. Rev. Food Sci. Nutr.*, 21, 263, 1984.

32. Thompson, L. U. and Cho, Y. S., Effect of acylation upon extraction of nitrogen, minerals and phytic acid in rapeseed flour and protein concentrate, *J. Food Sci.*, 49, 771, 1984.

33. Nielsen, B. K., Thompson, L. U., and Bird, R. P., Effect of phytic acid on colonic epithelial cell proliferation, *Cancer Lett.*, 37, 317, 1987.

34. Shamsuddin, A. M., Elsayed, A. M., and Ullah, A., Suppression of large intestinal cancer in F-344 rats by inositol hexaphosphate, *Carcinogenesis*, 9, 577, 1988.

35. Thompson, L. U. and Zhang, L., Phytic acid and minerals: effect on early markers of risk for mammary and colon carcinogenesis, *Carcinogenesis*, 12, 2041, 1991.

36. Vucenik, I., Yang, G. Y., and Shamsuddin, A. M., Comparison of pure inositol hexaphosphate and high-bran diet in the prevention of DMBA-induced rat mammary carcinogenesis, *Nutr. Cancer*, 28, 7, 1997.

37. Jenab, M. and Thompson, L. U., The influence of phytic acid in wheat bran on early biomarkers of colon carcinogenesis, *Carcinogenesis*, 19, 1087, 1998.

38. Sakamoto, K., Venkatraman, G., and Shamsuddin, A. M., Growth inhibition and differentiation of HT-29 cells in vitro by inositol hexaphosphate (phytic acid), *Carcinogenesis*, 14, 1815, 1993.

39. Yang, G. Y. and Shamsuddin, A. M., IP6-induced growth inhibition and differentiation of HT-29 human colon cancer cells: involvement of intracellular inositol phosphates, *Anticancer Res.*, 15, 2479, 1995.

40. Shamsuddin, A. M., Baten, A., and Lalwani, N. D., Effects of inositol hexaphosphate on growth and differentiation in K-562 erythroleukemia cell line, *Cancer Lett.*, 64, 195, 1992.

41. Shamsuddin, A. M., and Yang, G. Y., Inositol hexaphosphate inhibits growth and induces differentiation of PC-3 human prostate cancer cells, *Carcinogenesis*, 16, 1975, 1995.

42. Vucenik, I., Kalebic, T., Tantivejkul, K., and Shamsuddin, A. M., Novel anticancer function of inositol hexaphosphate: inhibition of human rhabdomyosarcoma in vitro and in vivo, *Anticancer Res.*, 18, 1377, 1998.

43. Vucenik, I., Tantivejkul, K., Zhang, Z. S., Cole, K. E., Saied, I., and Shamsuddin, A. M., IP6 in treatment of liver cancer. I. IP6 inhibits growth and reverses transformed phenotype in HepG2 human liver cancer cell line, *Anticancer Res.*, 18, 4083, 1998.

44. Shamsuddin, A. M., Yang, G. Y., and Vucenik, I., Novel anticancer function of IP6: growth inhibition and differentiation of human mammary cancer cell lines in vitro, *Anticancer Res.*, 16, 3287, 1996.

45. Eggleton, P., Effect of IP6 on human neutrophil cytokine production and cell morphology, *Anticancer Res.*, 19, 3711, 1999.

46. Saied, I. T. and Shamsuddin, A. M., Up-regulation of the tumor suppressor gene p53 and WAF1 gene expression by IP6 in HT-29 human colon carcinoma cell line, *Anticancer Res.*, 18, 1479, 1998.

47. Corpet, D. E., Tache, S., and Peiffer, G., Colon tumor promotion: is it a selection process? Effects of cholate, phytate and food restriction in rats on proliferation and apoptosis in normal and aberrant crypts, *Cancer Lett.*, 114, 135, 1997.

48. Shamsuddin, A. M., Ullah, A., and Chakravarthy, A., Inositol and inositol hexaphosphate suppress cell proliferation and tumor formation in CD-1 mice, *Carcinogenesis*, 10, 1461, 1989.

49. Shamsuddin, A. M. and Ullah, A., Inositol hexaphosphate inhibits large intestinal cancer in F344 rats 5 months after induction by azoxymethane, *Carcinogenesis*, 10, 625, 1989.

50. Challa, A., Rao, D. R., and Reddy, B. S., Interactive suppression of aberrant crypt foci induced by azoxymethane in rat colon by phytic acid and green tea, *Carcinogenesis*, 18, 2023, 1997.

51. Pretlow, T. P., O'Riordan, M. A., Somich, G. A., Amini, S. B., and Pretlow, T. G., Aberrant crypts correlate with tumor incidence in F344 rats treated with azoxymethane and phytate, *Carcinogenesis*, 13, 1509, 1992.

52. Ullah, A. and Shamsuddin, A. M., Dose-dependent inhibition of large intestinal cancer by inositol hexaphosphate in F344 rats, *Carcinogenesis*, 11, 2219, 1990.

53. Shivapurkar, N., Tang, Z. C., Frost, A., and Alabaster, O., A rapid dual organ rat carcinogenesis bioassay for evaluating the chemoprevention of breast and colon cancer, *Cancer Lett.*, 100, 169, 1996.

54. Nelson, R. L., Yoo, S. J., Tanure, G., Andrianopoulos, G., and Misumi, A., The effect of iron on experimental colorectal carcinogenesis, *Anticancer Res.*, 9, 1477, 1989.

55. Vucenik, I., Sakamoto, K., Bansal, M., and Shamsuddin, A. M., Inhibition of rat mammary carcinogenesis by inositol hexaphosphate (phytic acid). A pilot study, *Cancer Lett.*, 75, 95, 1993.

56. Vucenik, I., Yang, G. Y., and Shamsuddin, A. M., Inositol hexaphosphate and inositol inhibit DMBA-induced rat mammary cancer, *Carcinogenesis*, 16, 1055, 1995.

57. Hirose, M., Hoshiya, T., Akagi, K., Futakuchi, M., and Ito, N., Inhibition of mammary gland carcinogenesis by green tea catechins and other naturally occurring antioxidants in female Sprague-Dawley rats pretreated with 7,12-dimethylbenz[alpha]anthracene, *Cancer Lett.*, 83, 149, 1994.

58. Vucenik, I., Zhang, Z. S., and Shamsuddin, A. M., IP6 in treatment of liver cancer. II. Intra-tumoral injection of IP6 regresses pre-existing human liver cancer xenotransplanted in nude mice, *Anticancer Res.*, 18, 4091, 1998.

59. Jariwalla, R. J., Sabin, R., Lawson, S., Bloch, D. A., Prender, M., Andrews, V., and Herman, Z. S., Effect of dietary phytic acid (phytate) on the incidence and growth rate of tumors promoted in Fisher rats by magnesium supplement, *Nutr. Res.*, 8, 813, 1988.

60. Vucenik, I., Tomazic, V. J., Fabian, D., and Shamsuddin, A. M., Antitumor activity of phytic acid (inositol hexaphosphate) in murine transplanted and metastatic fibrosarcoma. A pilot study, *Cancer Lett.*, 65, 9, 1992.

61. Ishikawa, T., Nakatsuru, Y., Zarkovic, M., and Shamsuddin, A. M., Inhibition of skin cancer by IP6 in vivo: initiation-promotion model, *Anticancer Res.*, 19, 3749, 1999.

62. Hirose, M., Ozaki, K., Takaba, K., Fukushima, S., Shirai, T., and Ito, N., Modifying effects of the naturally occurring antioxidants gamma oryzanol, phytic acid, tannic acid and n-tritriacontane-16, 18-dione in a rat wide-spectrum organ carcinogenesis model, *Carcinogenesis*, 12, 1917, 1991.

63. Reddy, B. S., Hirose, Y., Cohen, L. A., Simi, B., Cooma, I., and Rao, C. V., Preventive potential of wheat bran fractions against experimental colon carcinogenesis: implications for human colon cancer prevention, *Cancer Res.*, 60, 4792, 2000

64. Shamsuddin, A. M. and Vucenik, I., Mammary tumor inhibition by IP6: a review, *Anticancer Res.*, 19, 3671, 1999.

65. Wilson, R. B., Hutcheson, D. P., and Wideman, L., Dimethylhydrazine induced colon tumors in rats fed diets containing beef fat or corn oil with or without wheat bran, *Am. J. Clin. Nutr.*, 30, 176, 1977.

66. Chen, W. F., Patchevsky, A. S., and Goldsmith, H. S., Colonic protection from dimethylhydrazine by a high fiber diet, *Surg. Gyn. Obs.*, 147, 503, 1978.

67. Reddy, B. S. and Mori, H., Effect of dietary wheat bran and dehydrated citrus fiber on 3,2-dimethyl-4-aminobiphenyl induced intestinal carcinogenesis in F344 rats, *Carcinogenesis*, 2, 21, 1981.

68. Barnes, D. S., Clapp, N. K., Scott, D. A., Oberst, D. L., and Berry, S. G., Effects of wheat, rice, corn and soybean bran on 1,2-dimethylhydrazine-induced large bowel tumorigenesis in F344 rats, *Nutr. Cancer*, 5, 1, 1983.

69. Maziya-Dixon, B. B., Klopfenstein, C. F., and Leipold, H. W., Protective effects of hard red wheat versus hard white wheats in chemically induced colon cancer in CF1 mice, *Cereal Chem.*, 71, 359, 1994.

70. Owen, R. W., Weisgerber, U. M., Spiegelhalder, B., and Bartsch, H., Faecal phytic acid and its relation to other putative markers of risk for colorectal cancer, *Gut*, 38, 591, 1996.

71. Risio, M., Lipkin, M., Candelaresi, G., Bertone, A., Coverlizza, S., and Rossini, F. P., Correlations between rectal mucosa cell proliferation and the clinical and pathological features of non-familial neoplasia of the large intestine, *Cancer Res.*, 51, 1917, 1991.

72. Hirose, M., Fukushima, S., Imaida, K., Ito, N., and Shirai, T., Modifying effects of phytic acid and gamma-oryzanol on the promotion stage of rat carcinogenesis, *Anticancer Res.*, 19, 3665, 1999.

73. Takaba, K., Hirose, M., Ogawa, K., Hakoi, K., and Fukushima, S., Modification of n-butyl-n(4-hydroxybutyl)nitrosamine-initiated urinary bladder carcinogenesis in rats by phytic acid and its salts, *Food Chem. Toxic.*, 32, 499, 1994.

74. Fukushima, S., Tamano, S., Shibata, M. A., Kurata, Y., Hirose, M., and Ito, N., The role of urinary pH and sodium ion concentration in the promotion stage of two-stage carcinogenesis of the rat urinary bladder, *Carcinogenesis*, 9, 1203, 1988.

75. Shibata, M. A., Yamada, M., Tanaka, H., Kagawa, M., and Fukushima, S., Changes in urine composition, bladder epithelial morphology, and DNA synthesis in male F344 rats in response to ingestion of bladder tumor promoters, *Toxicol. Appl. Pharmacol.*, 99, 37, 1989.

76. Takaba, K., Hirose, M., Yoshida, Y., Kimura, J., Ito, N., and Shirai, T., Effects of n-tritriacontane-16,18-dione, curcumin, chlorphyllin, dihydroguaiaretic acid, tannic acid and phytic acid on the initiation stage in a rat multi-organ carcinogenesis model, *Cancer Lett.*, 113, 39, 1997.

77. Larsson, O., Barker, C. J., Sjoholm, A., Carlqvist, H., Michell, R. H., Bertorello, A., Nilsson, T., Honkanen, R. E., Mayr, G. W., Zwiler, J., and Berggren, P. O., Inhibition of phosphatases and increased Ca²⁺ channel activity by inositol hexakisphosphate, *Science*, 278, 471, 1997.

78. Ali, N., Duden, R., Bembenek, M. E., and Shears, S. B., The interaction of coatomer with inositol polyphosphates is conserved in *Saccharomyces cerevisiae*, *Biochem. J.*, 310 (pt. 1), 279, 1995.

79. O'Rourke, F., Matthews, E., and Feistein, M. B., Isolation of InsP⁴ and InsP⁶ binding proteins from human platelets: InsP⁴ promotes Ca²⁺ efflux from inside-out plasma membrane vesicles containing 104 kDa GAP¹IP⁴BP protein, *Biochem. J.*, 315 (pt. 3), 1027, 1996.

80. Yamaguchi, Y., Ikenaka, K., Niinobe, M., Yamada, H., and Mikoshiba, K., Myelin proteolipid protein (PLP), but not DM-20, is an inositol hexakisphosphate-binding protein, *J. Biol. Chem.*, 271, 27838, 1996.

81. Singh, M. and Krikorian, A. D., Inhibition of trypsin activity in-vitro by phytate, *J. Ag. Food Chem.*, 30, 799, 1982.

82. Thompson, L. U., Phytic acid: a factor influencing starch digestibility and blood glucose response, in *Phytic Acid: Chemistry and Applications*, Graf, E., Ed., Pilatus Press, Minneapolis, MN, 1986, 173.

83. Gupta, M., Khetarpaul, N., and Chauhan, B. M., Rabadi fermentation of wheat: changes in phytic acid content and in vitro digestibility, *Plant Foods Hum. Nutr.*, 42, 109, 1992.

84. Thompson, L. U., Phytic acid and other nutrients: are they partly responsible for health benefits of high fiber foods, in *Dietary Fiber in Health and Disease*, Kritchevsky, D., and Bonfield, C., Eds., Egan Press, New York, 1995, 305.

85. Yoon, J. H., Thompson, L. U., and Jenkins, D. J. A., The effect of phytic acid on in vitro rate of starch digestibility and blood glucose response, *Am. J. Clin. Nutr.*, 38, 835, 1983.

86. Thompson, L. U., Button, C. L., and Jenkins, D. J., Phytic acid and calcium affect the in vitro rate of navy bean starch digestion and blood glucose response in humans, *Am. J. Clin. Nutr.*, 46, 467, 1987.

87. Coradini, D., Pellizzaro, C., Marimpietri, D., Abolafio, G., and Daidone, M. G., Sodium butyrate modulates cell cycle-related proteins in HT29 human colonic adenocarcinoma cells, *Cell Prolif.*, 33, 139, 2000.

88. Sakata, T., Stimulatory effect of short chain fatty acids on epithelial cell proliferation in rat intestine: a possible explanation for trophic effects of fermentable fiber, gut microbes and luminal trophic factors, *Br. J. Nutr.*, 58, 95, 1987.

89. Borenfreund, E., Schmid, E., Bendich, A., and Franke, W. S., Constitutive aggregates of intermediate sized filaments of the vimentin and cytokeratin type in cultured hepatoma cells and their dispersal by butyrate, *Exp. Cell Res.*, 127, 215, 1980.

90. Hague, A., Manning, A. M., Hanlon, K. A., Huschtscha, L. I., Hart, D., and Paraskeva, C., Sodium butyrate induces apoptosis in human colonic tumor cell lines in a p53-independent pathway: implications for the possible role of dietary fiber in the prevention of large bowel cancer, *Int. J. Cancer*, 55, 498, 1993.

91. Caderni, G., Luceri, C., Lancioni, L., Tessitore, L., and Dolara, P., Slow-release pellets of sodium butyrate increase apoptosis in the colon of rats treated with azoxymethane, without affecting aberrant crypt foci and colonic proliferation, *Nutr. Cancer*, 30, 175, 1998.

92. McIntyre, A., Gibson, P. R., and Young, G. P., Butyrate production from dietary fibre and protection against large bowel cancer in a rat model, *Gut*, 34, 386, 1993.

93. Giovannucci, E., Insulin and colon cancer, *Cancer Causes Control*, 6, 164, 1995.

94. McKeown-Eyssen, G., Epidemiology of colorectal cancer revisited: are serum triglycerides and/or plasma glucose associated with risk?, *Cancer Epidemiol. Biomarkers Prev.*, 3, 687, 1994.

95. Bruce, W. R. and Corpet, D. E., The colonic protein fermentation and insulin resistance hypothesis for colon cancer etiology: experimental tests using precursor lesions, *Eur. J. Cancer Prev.*, 2, 41, 1996.

96. Thompson, L. U., Nutritional and physiological effects of phytic acid, in *Food Proteins*, Kinsella, J. E. and Soucie, W. G., Eds., American Oil Chemists Society, Champaign, IL, 1989, 410.

97. Graf, E. and Eaton, J. W., Antioxidant functions of phytic acid, *Free Radical Biol. Med.*, 8, 61, 1990.

98. O'Haloran, T. V., Transition metals in control of gene expression, *Science*, 261, 715, 1993.

99. Erhardt, J. G., Lim, S. S., Bode, J. C., and Bode, C., A diet rich in fat and poor in dietary fiber increases the in vitro formation of reactive oxygen species in human feces, *J. Nutr.*, 127, 706, 1997.

100. Nelson, R. L., Dietary iron and colorectal cancer risk, *Free Rad. Biol. Med.*, 12, 161, 1992.

101. Graf, E. and Eaton, J. W., Suppression of colonic cancer by dietary phytic acid, *Nutr. Cancer*, 19, 11, 1993.

102. Babbs, C. F., Free radicals and the etiology of colon cancer, *Free Rad. Biol. Med.*, 8, 191, 1990.

103. Owen, R. W., Spiegelhalder, B., and Bartsch, H., Phytate, reactive oxygen species and colorectal cancer, *Eur. J. Cancer Prev.*, suppl. 2, S41, 1998.

104. Rimbach, G. and Pallauf, J., Phytic acid inhibits free radical formation in vitro but does not affect liver oxidant or antioxidant status in growing rats, *J. Nutr.*, 128, 1950, 1998.

105. Porres, J. M., Stahl, C. H., Cheng, W. H., Fu, Y., Roneker, K. R., Pond, W. G., and Lei, X.G., Dietary intrinsic phytate protects colon from lipid peroxidation in pigs with a moderately high dietary iron intake, *Proc. Soc. Exp. Biol. Med.*, 221, 80, 1999.

106. Vucenik, I. and Shamsuddin, A. M., [^{3}H]Inositol hexaphosphate (phytic acid) is rapidly absorbed and metabolized by murine and human malignant cells in vitro, *J. Nutr.*, 124, 861, 1994.

107. Barker, C. J., Wright, J., Kirk, C. J., and Mitchell, R. H., Inositol 1,2,3-trisphosphate is a product of InsP^6 dephosphorylation in WRK-1 rat mammary epithelial cells and exhibits transient concentration changes during the cell cycle, *Biochem. Soc. Trans.*, 23, 169s, 1995.

108. Wattenberg, L. W. and Estensen, R. D., Chemopreventive effects of myo-inositol and dexamethasone on benzo[a]pyrene and 4-(methylnitrosoamino)-1(3-pyridyl)-butanone-induced pulmonary carcino-genesis in female A/J mice, *Cancer Res.*, 56, 5132, 1996.

109. Shamsuddin, A. M., Metabolism and cellular functions of IP^6: a review, *Anticancer Res.*, 19, 3733, 1999.

110. Jenab, M. and Thompson, L. U., Phytic acid in wheat bran affects colon morphology, cell differentiation and apoptosis, *Carcinogenesis*, 21, 1547, 2000.

111. Chang, W. C. L., Chapkin, R. S. and Lupton, J. R., Predictive value of proliferation, differentiation and apoptosis as intermediate markers for colon tumorigenesis, *Carcinogenesis*, 18, 721, 1997.

112. Nickel, K. P. and Belury, M. A., Inositol hexaphosphate reduces 12-O-tetradecanoylphorbol-13-acetate-induced ornithine decarboxylase independent of protein kinase C isoform expression in kera-tinocytes, *Cancer Lett.*, 140, 105, 1999.

113. Dong, Z., Huang, C., and Ma, W.-Y., PI-3 kinase in signal transduction, cell transformation, and as a target for chemoprevention of cancer, *Anticancer Res.*, 19, 3743, 1999.

114. Baten, A., Ullah, A., Tomazic, V. J., and Shamsuddin, A. M., Inositol-phosphate-induced enhancement of natural killer cell activity correlates with tumor suppression, *Carcinogenesis*, 10, 1595, 1989.

115. Kar, S., Quirion, R., and Parent, A., An interaction between inositol hexakisphosphate (IP^6) and insulin-like growth factor II receptor binding sites in the rat brain, *Neuroreport*, 5, 625, 1994.

116. Sullivan, K. A., Castle, V. P., Hanash, S. M., and Feldman, E. L., Insulin-like growth factor II in the pathogenesis of human neuroblastoma, *Am. J. Pathol.*, 147, 1790, 1995.

117. Lamonerie, T., Lavialle, C., Degalle, B., Binoux, M., and Brison, O., Constitutive or inducible overexpression of the IGF-2 gene in cells of a human colon carcinoma cell line, *Exp. Cell. Res.*, 216, 342, 1995.

118. Manousos, O., Souglakos, J., Bosetti, C., Tzonou, A., Chatzidakis, V., Trichopoulos, D., Adami, H. O., and Mantzoros, C., IGF-I and IGF-II in relation to colorectal cancer, *Int. J. Cancer*, 83, 15, 1999.

119. Morrison, R. S., Shi, E., Kan, M., Yamaguchi, F., McKeehan, W., Rudnicka-Nawrot, M., and Palczewski, K., Inositol hexaphosphate (InsP^6): an antagonist of fibroblast growth factor receptor binding and activity, *In Vitro Cell. Dev. Biol.*, 30A, 783, 1994.

120. Hiasa, Y., Kitahori, Y., Morimoto, J., Konishi, N., Nakaoka, S., and Nishioka, H., Carcinogenicity study in rats of phytic acid 'Daiichi', a natural food additive, *Food Chem. Toxicol.*, 30, 117, 1992.

Definitions and Consumption

Consumption of Dietary Fiber 1992–2000

Julie M. Jones

Prior to 1965, fiber was given no more than a single line in nutrition textbooks and was simply referred to as "roughage" and measured as crude fiber. Dietary fiber was not commonly found as an item in Medline prior to 1970 but was described by Hipsley in 1953.[1] In 1970 the dietary fiber hypothesis was born with the return from practicing in rural Africa of three British physicians, Burkitt, Painter, and Trowell. These men observed that the rural Africans did not have many of the diseases that plagued the West, and they theorized that the high-fiber diet not only exerted positive effects on the gut directly but had many other systemic effects, as well.[2] Thus, fiber was launched from merely being roughage to a substance with many possible therapeutic and preventative roles. In the 30 years since this hypothesis was proposed, there have been nearly 8000 Medline entries on the subject of dietary fiber.

During this time, fiber's popularity with the public, the scientific community, and industry has waxed and waned. In the 1970s and 1980s, there were several attempts by the industry to increase the fiber content of the diet through addition of fiber to products. In 1984, Kellogg's took the bold move of using advice on the intake of dietary fiber from the US National Cancer Institute and placing it on the back of its bran cereal boxes. This campaign to increase consumer awareness and increase bran cereal sales was highly effective. The messages not only increased consumption of Kellogg's cereals, but it also had the effect of increasing consumption of all bran cereals.[3,4] Furthermore, it eventually ushered in the era of allowed health claims and nutrition label changes.[5]

In this same time frame in which wheat brans and bran cereals were touted as a cancer preventative, news about the soluble fibers in oat bran also reached the public. Claims were disseminated through advertising and through a best-seller entitled *The 8-Week Cholesterol Cure*.[6] Oat bran became sought by the public and was being added to a vast array of food products in a wide range of doses from the insignificant to the efficacious. However, when excerpts from a study published in the *New England Journal of Medicine*[7] appeared on the front page of the *New York Times* and showed that the addition of oat bran to the diets was ineffectual, the so-called "oat bran craze" was crushed instantly, probably for all the wrong reasons. Unfortunately, the widely touted study had used subjects with stellar diets and normal blood lipids. All previous studies carried out on populations with elevated serum lipids were summarily discounted and forgotten by the public.

In a like manner, fiber's role in the prevention of colon cancer has been seriously eroded by three recently published studies[8,9,10] which said that fiber did not affect polyp recurrence and did not prevent cancer in women.

Thus, there has been a change in consumer beliefs about including fiber in the diet, despite the fact that most health promotion groups and government agencies recommend that fiber intake be at the very minimum 20 g/day and some recommend up to 35 g/day (Table 7.1.1).

Table 7.1.1   North American Organizations and Their Fiber Recommendations

---

Organizations Which Specify a Fiber Amount

American Dietetics Association — Americans should eat 20–35 g of fiber each day, including both soluble and insoluble fiber.[80] The average American currently eats 12–17 g of fiber a day. Only about 1/4 of this is soluble fiber; therefore, the average American is eating only 3–4 g of soluble fiber — below the recommended amount of 5–10 g. Eating 3 g a day of soluble fiber from oats or 7 g a day of soluble fiber from psyllium has been shown to lower blood cholesterol levels.
American Diabetes Association — Daily consumption of a diet containing 20–35 g of dietary fiber from a wide variety of food sources is recommended.[81]
American Heart Association — 25 to 30 g per day from foods, not supplements, to ensure nutrient adequacy.[82]
American Cancer Society — Choose most of the foods you eat from plant sources.[83] Eat five or more servings of fruits and vegetables each day. Eat other foods from plant sources, such as breads, cereals, grain products, rice, pasta, or beans several times each day (no specified quantity).
National Cancer Institute (NCI)[84] — 25 to 35 g/d.

Organizations Which Recommend Fiber-Containing Foods But Do Not Specify Amounts

USDA Dietary Guidelines 2000[85] — Choose a variety of grains daily, especially whole grains.
Dietary Guidelines for Australians[86] — Eat plenty of breads and cereals (preferably whole grain), vegetables (including legumes), and fruits.
The US Preventive Services Task Force — Recommends that Americans increase fiber and fruit/vegetables intake as well as lower dietary fat and cholesterol to reduce prevalence of heart disease, cancer, stroke, hypertension, obesity, and non-insulin-dependent diabetes mellitus in the United States.[87]

FIBER DEFINITION

While there is agreement that fiber is important nutritionally because of its physiological function and its non-absorbability, there has been no agreement as to its definition. Part of the difficulty stems from lack of agreement on what is to be included, how it can be measured, and what most closely approximates what actually happens in the human gut. Thus, definitions as well as methods of analysis vary from country to country. (This fact is important, as fiber data for various countries may not be comparable.)

When the fiber hypothesis was in its infancy, the only measure of dietary fiber was "crude fiber." After the advent of the fiber hypothesis, there were many attempts to develop methods that would accurately measure what was not digested in the human small intestine. In the 1970s the agreed-upon definition in the US was as follows: *Dietary fiber was defined as the remnants of edible plant cells including polysaccharides, lignin, and associated substances that are resistant to digestion in the alimentary tract of humans.* This definition defined a macro constituent of foods which includes cellulose, hemicellulose, lignin, gums, modified cellulose, mucilages, oligosaccharides, and pectins and associated minor substances such as waxes, cutin, and suberin. The definition then came to be limited to those materials measured by AOAC method 985.29.[11] In 1976 the definition was widened to include all indigestible polysaccharides. This added materials such as modified celluloses. In 2000 a committee of members of the American Association of Cereal Chemists (AACC) agreed upon a definition that expanded somewhat the various compounds that are not absorbed and exert a physiological effect. Thus, the latest definition includes all nonstarch polysaccharides resistant to digestion in the small intestine and fermentable in the large intestine. Non-starch polysaccharides include celluloses, hemicelluloses such as arabinoxylans and arabinoga-lactans, pectins, modified celluloses, oligosaccharides, and polyfructans such as inulin, gums, and mucilages. Oligosaccharides of various lengths are also included in this definition. As with the earlier definition, non-polysaccharide material that is bound to the plant cell wall is also part of the definition. Such material includes lignin waxes, cutin, and suberin. The new definition allowed for materials that behave analogously to dietary fiber to be included. Thus, the term "analogous carbohydrates" was added to the 2000 definition.

The other important difference between the earlier definitions and the AACC definition is that a physiological component is included. The AACC definition is as follows:

> Dietary fiber is the edible parts of plants or analogous carbohydrates that are resistant to digestion and absorption in the human intestine with complete or partial fermentation in the large intestine. Dietary fiber includes polysaccharides, oligosaccharides, lignin, and associated plant substances. Dietary fibers promote beneficial physiological effects including laxation, and/or blood cholesterol attenuation, and/or blood glucose attenuation.

The committee wanted the physiological measures to be included, because that way any newly formed analogous substance would not only need to be structurally similar to existing substances but would also need to have a beneficial physiological effect in order to be included in the fiber label analysis.

Fiber may have more functions than those listed in the current definition, but the evidence for these other functions is still inconclusive. Other functions can be added in subsequent iterations when the data present a clearer picture. The wider definition will require a change in the method in order to capture substances such as the oligosaccharides.

FIBER INTAKES

Fiber Intake as a Marker

Many studies indicate that fiber is a marker of a good diet. In fact, one of the reasons that teasing out the role of fiber in disease prevention is so difficult is that there are too many confounders. Any natural food diet that is high in fiber is also high in plant foods, fruits, vegetables, and cereals. Furthermore, it may mean that the diet is low in saturated fats and higher in fats deemed beneficial. Diets high in fiber usually have more vitamins, minerals, and phytochemicals. Also, those individuals with high intakes of fiber or whole grain diets are more likely to exercise, more likely to use supplements, and less likely to smoke. Thus, attributing that fiber itself is a preventative agent is indeed difficult. Despite overwhelming data that diets high in fiber and plant foods are useful, most populations fail to meet the recommendations.

US General Population

Depending on the specific population group and the actual method of calculating dietary fiber, the average dietary fiber intake for adults in the US is 11 to 15 g/d.[12] Analysis of data[13] from The National Food Consumption Survey (NCFS) of 1987–1988 showed an average intake from 3-day food records of over 9000 respondents at 12–13 g/day. A nearly identical value was determined for intakes in the National Health and Examination Study (NHANES II), which showed that the average American woman ate 13.2 g/d.[14] Likewise, studies conducted by the National Cancer Institute (NCI) determined the mean dietary fiber intake in the US adult population (>19 years of age) to be 13.3 g/d, using Southgate values. Lower mean intakes of 11.1 g/d were determined if fiber values compiled from the literature were used.[15] Intakes did not vary across age groups in NCFS.[13] In contrast, the NCI data showed some differences in intake by group. On a per 1000 kcal basis, women consumed more dietary fiber (6.5 g/1000 kcal) than men (5.5 g/1000 kcal) at every age.[15]

The net analysis of all these studies is best captured by a histogram analysis of the NCI data, which showed that 90% of the population failed to meet the bare minimum fiber intake of 20 g/d. NHANES II data showed that vegetables, especially potatoes, were the principal sources of dietary fiber, followed by bread and fruit. Legumes were important sources for some populations and ranked first for several age–sex–race categories. Breakfast cereals made a smaller contribution to the total fiber intake.

Elderly

In a sample specifically assessing fiber intakes of free-living elderly aged 60–78 years, the mean reported fiber intake was 18.3 g/d.[16] In this sample, the overall mean intake appears to be slightly higher than the population as a whole and would not be consistent with the finding that there was little difference in intakes across population age groups as indicated by the NCFS data. A factor may be that these individuals were free-living and perhaps were healthier and had greater control over their food choices than the segment of elderly in institutions.

The rank-order of sources of fiber for the free-living elderly also varied from that of all adults sampled in NCFS. Breads and cereals contributed 33% of the fiber intake; vegetables, 22%; fruits, 21%; legumes, 7%; and nuts and seeds, 3% in the free-living elderly. As anticipated, those who ate the recommended minimum of 20 g or more of dietary fiber per day had diets that contained more iron, copper, magnesium, selenium, potassium, and zinc.[17]

Fiber Intake in Institutions and Restaurants

Those living in situations of institutional feeding or using food service outlets may have differing fiber intakes. Data gathered for the US Army showed that although higher fiber choices are possible, they are not selected. US Army recruits ate approximately 4.1 g of fiber per 1000 kcal, according to data derived from analysis of a 6-day weighed military ration. It was noted that it would be possible to more than double this amount to 9.5 g/1000 kcal if all whole grain choices were made.[18,19]

Eating food not prepared at home may also be a contributor to the low fiber intakes. Currently over half of the food dollar is spent on food eaten away from home. A recent study[20] showed that there was no increase in fiber, despite often gargantuan portion sizes which delivered an average of nearly 300 more calories, 20 g more fat, and 400 mg more sodium in the high-eating-out group (6–13 times per week) (Table 7.1.2).

Table 7.1.2   Comparison of Intakes of Selected Nutrients of Consumers Who Dine Out Frequently vs. Those Who Don't

	Eat Out Often	Eat Out Seldom
Mean calories	2057	1769
Mean fat (g)	79.5	60.6
Mean sodium	3299	2903

Source: Clemens et al.[20]

Despite the common occurrence that eating away from home has become, many diners tenaciously hold onto the idea that eating out is a treat and that it is not necessary to be concerned about nutrition.[21]

Data from Specific US Cohorts

Fiber intakes of various population segments have been assessed by a variety of methods. In epidemiological data from 43,000 male health professionals who filled out food frequency questionnaires of 131 foods, fiber intake was calculated to range from a median of 12.4 g/d in the lowest quintile to 28.9 g/d in the highest quintile.[22] As was seen in the NCI data for the general population, vegetables provided the most fiber, with the lowest quintile ingesting a median of 3.2 g/d and the highest quintile 11.1 g/d. Cereal foods provided 2.2 g/d in the lowest quintile and 9.7 g/d in the highest quintile. Fruit provided the least dietary fiber, with intakes varying from 1.2 g/d in the lowest quintile to 7.9 g/d in the highest quintile. Similar patterns were seen in the Nurses' Health Study with over 88,000 subjects, but the total amount of fiber was lower, with median daily dietary fiber intake ranging between 9.8 g and 24.8 g and cereal fiber contributing 1.0 g to 4.8 g.

In the National Cancer Institute (NCI) Polyp Prevention Trial,[23] the average baseline dietary fiber intake was reported to be 10–20 g/d, or an average of 9.7 g/1000 kcal. The intervention goal was to increase this number to 18 g/1000 kcal. In this cohort, the participants ate on average 3.7 servings of fruit and vegetable per day.

Obese

Fiber intake and obesity seem to be inversely related. In one study, fiber intake as assessed by dietary records[24] in the normal weight group was 18.8 g/d, while it was lower in both the moderately obese (13.3 g/d) and the severely obese (13.7 g/d). Another study showed the same trend but higher fiber intakes for all groups. Lean women consumed 22.7 g/d and lean men consumed 27.0 g/d. Their obese counterparts consumed 15.7 g/d and 20.9 g/d, respectively.[25] Another study of 203 men showed that those weighing the most ate more fat, less fiber, and less carbohydrate.[26]

Children and Adolescents

The American Academy of Pediatrics recommends 0.5 g of dietary fiber per kg of body weight for children and adolescents. The American Health Foundation (AHF) recommends that children follow the *age + 5 rule* for the minimum dietary fiber intake and no more than *age + 10* for the safe range.[27] For example, an 8-year-old should try to get 8 + 5 or 13 g/d of dietary fiber.

As seen in adults, the fiber intake of US children also fails to meet the various recommendations. According to analysis of data from NFCS on over 2500 children,[28] 55 to 90% of American children failed to meet AHF requirements for dietary fiber. Large cohorts of various-age children in the Bogalusa Heart Study found the average fiber intake by 24-hour recalls was 12 g/d, or 5 g of dietary fiber per 1000 kcal.[29]

Several studies show that the diet contains a smaller percentage of fiber as children age. While 60.2% of the children aged 2–5 years in the NFCS study failed to meet the age + 5 rule, over 90.3% of the girls aged 12–18 years failed to meet this rule.[28] The 1991 US Department of Agriculture Continuing Survey of Food Intakes by Individuals (CSFII) generated similar findings.[29] In this case, 45% of the 4–6-year-olds met the age + 5 rule and only 32% of the 7–10-year-olds.[30] In the Bogalusa study the actual intakes varied from 10.65 to 13.48 g/d for 10–17-year-olds. While the total intake increased slightly from age 10 to 15 years, the total amount of fiber decreased by 17 years of age. Thus, the dietary fiber intake decreased as the body weight increased.[28]

In the North Dakota 15-year-olds,[31] the Bogalusa Heart Study[29] and the NFCS sample[28] males were more likely than females to have higher fiber intakes. The intake gap between males and females widened as age increased. Black children, aged 10 to 17, had higher fiber intakes per 1000 kcal than white children. Comparison with past data on fiber intake showed a decrease in intake from the 1977–1978 CSFII survey to the survey 10 years later.[28] In that time period, there was a decrease in the consumption of fruits and vegetables. Grains and ready-to-eat cereal consumption did increase during this period. However, many of the newer, more popular cereals do not offer significant increases in dietary fiber. A similar trend with respect to changing food patterns was seen in the NFCS, where vegetables and fruits provided the most fiber in 1977–78 and bread provided the most in 1987–88.[29]

Several studies have shown that those children who met the fiber recommendations had better diets than those who failed to meet the recommendations. Those who ate according to the age + five rule consumed more breads, cereals, fruits, vegetables, legumes, nuts, and seeds. These diets were shown to be higher in vitamins A and E, folate, magnesium, and iron.[31] Similar results occurred in North Dakota teens participating in the 24-hour recall collection, where just over a fifth of the respondents reported consuming more than 20 g dietary fiber daily. Over half consumed less than 15 g of fiber daily. In the group with higher fiber intakes, diets were more nutrient dense and were associated with greater likelihood of adequate intake of several key nutrients, including vitamins A, B6, B12, and C; niacin; thiamin; riboflavin; folacin; magnesium; iron; zinc; phosphorus; and calcium.[31]

Surveys of college students do not show that they fare much better.[32] Of those surveyed, 45% failed to meet the fiber recommendations. Only 8% of the students consumed the minimum recommended number of servings for all food groups in the Food Guide Pyramid (FGP), but diets that satisfied FGP recommendations also tended to satisfy nutrient requirements.

Family behavior also impacted fiber intake. In the families involved in the Nurses' Health Study, of the 8677 girls and 7525 boys aged 9 to 14 years, 17% ate together with their families never or only on some days. This group of children and adolescents ate foods with higher glycemic loads, ate fewer fruits and vegetables, and consumed less fiber.[33]

Fiber Intakes in Europe

It should be pointed out that values for fiber are defined differently in various countries, according to the European Prospective Investigation into Cancer and Nutrition (EPIC), which includes Denmark, France, Germany, Greece, Great Britain, Italy, the Netherlands, Spain, and Sweden.[34] Differing methods of measurement may also be used, so values are not always comparable.

UK and Ireland

Until 2000, fiber in the UK was measured as nonstarch polysaccharide (NSP). The NSP intake of a sample of 739 men aged 40–69 was 15.5–16.4 g/d using a validated food-frequency questionnaire that focused on carbohydrates. For women aged 25–69 years, the NSP intake was 14.3–15.3 g/d. In this sample there were no clear differences by age group. These NSP intakes were reported as higher than those from a 1977 survey but fell short of the recent government-recommended population mean of 18 g/d.[35] However, the values are far lower than values reported in 1985 based on a 7-day food record from a small sample of omnivores and vegetarians.[36] In this sample omnivores consumed an average of 23 g of dietary fiber per day. Vegetarians were reported to eat an average of 37 g/d and vegans 47 g/d. These substantially higher values may reflect differences in the sample and measurement techniques and changes in dietary patterns.

Mean intakes in the UK are higher than mean intakes in the US Part of the reason for a higher intake is the tendency to eat more bread and cereal products. A small difference may also be due to differences in the extraction rates commonly used for bread flour. In the UK a 78% extraction rate is used rather than a 70% extraction rate used in the US Some differences may be due to measurement.

Fiber intake of dietitians and members of their households was reportedly much higher than of the population as a whole. A study in the UK using 7-day weighed food records showed that the fiber intake of 472 dietitians and adult members of their households was 38 g/d.[37]

There appeared to be a difference in the readiness of various subgroups to adopt nutrition information and change their fiber intake. Black housewives living in the UK were more likely to respond to various public health programs and messages and report change in dietary fiber intake than their white counterparts. Asians were least likely to change their dietary intake of components such as fiber with public health campaigns and publicity.[38]

Teens and Children in the UK and Ireland

In a study of Irish secondary school youths (ages 12–18), the mean dietary fiber intakes were approximately 19.6–25 g/d for boys and 17 g/d for girls.[39] Thus, these diets would have higher mean fiber intakes than UK adults. However, the story for children seems to be different in England, Scotland, and Wales. Dietary data collected in 1992 and 1993 on nearly 500 children were compared with records on diets of children collected in the 1950s. Children of the 1950s ate substantially more bread and vegetables and less sugar and soft drinks. Thus, the diets of children 50 years ago had higher starch and fiber contents, making those diets more in line with current recommendations on healthy eating.[40]

Special Populations

According to the findings of the Irish National Nutrition Survey, Irish diabetics ate more dietary fiber than the general population, but this is lower than recommended by the European Association for the Study of Diabetes (EASD). The foods that were predominant contributors of dietary fiber were bread and potatoes.[41] Although a survey of Irish attitudes about diet placed nutrition/healthy eating in the top five most frequently selected factors affecting food choice, actual diets selected were not congruent with nutrition and health as being among the most important factors.[42]

Continental Europe

France

Using the statistical data on French food consumption published by the French National Institute of Economic Studies, the average daily consumption of dietary fiber of French adults is about 16 g, below the recommended range of 30–40 g for French adults.[43] In France, the first national dietary survey, called ASPCC, was done in 1993–1994. The intake of fruit and vegetables was particularly low for younger people and manual workers, making the fiber intake in this group low.[44]

Some studies have compared fiber intake of those in Europe with those in the UK. One study compared diets of nearly 500 men and women in the UK and France. Respondents in the UK reported eating more beans and pulses than French respondents but less cereal and fewer fruits and vegetables. In both countries, women had healthier diets in both countries. Overall, the southern French diet was healthier, as French respondents scored significantly better for indices for fat, fruits and vegetables, and dietary fiber.[45]

Finland

Finland appears to have the highest fiber intakes of any Western diet. The median intake of dietary fiber was 26 g/d in the cohort of 22,000 Finnish smokers in the Alpha-Tocopherol Beta Carotene Study. The cohort with the highest intake consumed a median intake of 35 g/d and the quintile with the lowest intake consumed 16.1 g/d.[46] Increased socioeconomic status in Finland did not improve diets or fiber intake.[47] While those in higher socioeconomic groups ate more fruits and vegetables, they ate less bread.

Sweden

Intakes in Sweden appeared to be higher than in the US or some studies in the UK but were less than those observed in Finland. In Sweden the estimated mean consumption of dietary fiber was 19.0 g/d based on the 7-day weighed record and 18.3 g/d based on the food-frequency

questionnaire for 92 randomly selected middle-aged Swedish men.[48] Thus, the method of determining the mean dietary fiber intake had only a small effect on the values. Intake of dietary fiber
in this population correlated with antioxidant intake and inversely correlated with meat intake.
Individuals with low fiber intakes ate less fruit, bread, poultry, fish, and cheese. In teens, the average
daily dietary fiber intake was 1.8 g/MJ.

The Netherlands

The average intake of dietary fiber in the Netherlands of 22 g/d was higher than in some other
European countries. According to the Dutch National Food Consumption Survey of 1987–1988 of
5595 subjects, about 20% of the men and 27% of the women ate the recommended levels of dietary
fiber.[49] There was a difference in fiber intake by education in the Rotterdam study (a cohort of over
5000 men and women over 55), with lower intakes among the less educated (1.88/2.17 vs. 2.03/2.29
g/MJ). In 10-year-old boys, fiber intake was below the desirable level.[51]

Germany

According to the German National Health Interview and Examination Survey of 4030 participants, fiber intake was deemed suboptimal.[52] However, studies of food offered in 20 nursing homes
in the German state of Hessan had dietary fiber contents over 30 g/d. These values exceeded that
recommended by the German Association for Nutrition (Deutsche Gesellschaft für Ernährung).[53]
In a survey of over 10,000 East Germans aged 35–65 years, higher fiber intakes were associated
with supplement use. Those ingesting higher amounts of fiber also ate more fruits and vegetables,
antioxidants, and other markers of a healthy diet.[54]
A study of 627 healthy German children and adolescents between the ages of 1 and 18 years
found the mean fiber intake was 1.9 g/MJ. In this cohort, high sugar intake was associated with
low dietary fiber intakes.[56]
In a study with German insulin-dependent diabetics (EURODIAB IDDM Complications Study),
dietary fiber intakes ranged from 23.0 g/d in the highest quartile to 13.7 g/d in the lowest quartile.[58]

Austria

Diets of 63 youth with insulin-dependent diabetes mellitus were compared with those of other
Austrian youth and were found to be very similar. Dietary fiber intakes were near the recommendations, but the total carbohydrate was too low and fat and cholesterol were deemed too high.[57]

Poland

In Poland, dietary fiber content of 12 standard hospital diets showed that fiber was derived
mainly from grains and gave a mean dietary fiber intake of 11.5 g/d in winter and 8.5 g/d in summer.
Studies of diets in three villages showed that dietary fiber and carbohydrate were 29–35% below
recommended levels.[59] A study of over 4000 adults in Warsaw showed that fiber intake met the
RDA for men but not for women.[60]

Spain

Fiber intakes in Spain were reported as highly variable according to region and other factors.
For example, diets of adolescents in Valencia offer an excess of proteins and saturated fat, while
complex carbohydrates and dietary fiber are scarce.[61]

The differences in fiber intake between men and women were observed in the six countries studied in EURALIM. Dietary fiber density was significantly higher in women than in men.[62]

Some Data from Latin America, Africa, and the South Pacific

Mexico

Dietary fiber intakes in some parts of Mexico are extremely high for both children[63] and adults[64] and have been recorded as high as 94 g/d. For example, the typical Sonoran diet is high in dietary fiber (7.8%) and the majority of this fiber (71%) is insoluble.[65] The very high dietary fiber intake could be attributed to the intake of tortillas and beans and is not related to high intakes of fruits and vegetables. The diet is particularly high in insoluble fiber and phytate.

Thus, the low colon cancer rates (20/100,000 in 1991 to 1995) may be attributed to components of the grains and legumes, as fruit and vegetable consumption is fairly limited.[66] In general, Mexican-Americans born in Mexico consumed significantly less fat and significantly more fiber than those born in the US.[67]

Brazil

Dietary fiber intake of 559 adults (>20 years old) in Sao Paulo was assessed by the dietary history.[68] The average consumption of dietary fiber was 24 g/d, with an average consumption of insoluble fiber of 17 g/d and soluble fiber of 7 g/d. Among women, the average consumption was 20 g/d and among men 29 g/day. Beans were the most important dietary fiber source in the population diet. A study of 52 children (mean age of 6.8 years) with chronic constipation was age- and gender-matched with 52 children with normal intestinal habits. The fiber content of the diet was evaluated with a 24-hour dietary recall. The children with normal bowel habits ate a median of 12.6 g/d using AOAC values and 17.3 g/d using Brazilian food tables. Constipated children consumed less, 9.7 g/d using AOAC values and 13.8 g/d using Brazilian food tables.

South Africa

Nearly 800 free-living Indian men and women (15–69 years of age) living in Durban were interviewed using a 24-hour dietary recall. Median dietary fiber intakes were low and varied between 8.0 and 11.0 g per 4.2 kJ.

Australia and New Zealand

The average Australian consumes 22 g/d of dietary fiber, with vegetarians consuming more than omnivores.[69] In New Zealand, females consumed an average intake of 19 g/d and males 25 g/d.[70] About 33% came from cereals, 31% from vegetables, and 20% from fruits. Seventh-Day Adventists in New Zealand consumed 27–40 g of dietary fiber per day.

Japan

The average adult in Japan was reported to have a dietary fiber intake of 22–24 g/d,[71] according to 351 1-day weighed diet records. In Japanese diets, vegetables were the primary fiber source. A study of 686 Japanese medical students showed the intake to be less that the average Japanese adult.[72] Furthermore, this study showed that the method of analysis made a difference in the actual numbers reported. For male Japanese medical students, the dietary fiber intake was 19.4 g/d by the

Southgate method and 15.9 g/d by the Prosky method; for females, the fiber intake was 18.3 g/d and 16.9 g/d, respectively.

REASONS FOR FAILURE TO MEET FIBER INTAKES

One reason for the low fiber intakes in the US and in other countries is the fact that many fail to eat according to country recommendations or according to food guides such as the USDA Food Guide Pyramid (FGP). If individuals followed the FGP, fiber intakes from the 6–11 servings of the bread and cereals group could range from 6 to 30 g/d. From the meat group, 0–6 g/d of dietary fiber could be obtained if just one serving of nuts or legumes was selected from the meat group. From the five servings of fruits and vegetables, 4–12 g/d of dietary fiber could come from fruit and 4–12 g/d of dietary fiber could come from vegetables.

According to NHANES II data, the survey population failed to eat according to the FGP. Only 3–6% of the US population consumed diets that fulfilled the USDA Pyramid recommendations on any survey day.[73] Only 10% of the population ate at least five servings of fruits and vegetables. On any survey day, 5% of the population failed to consume any foods from the grain group, 46% of the population failed to consume any foods from the fruit group, and 18% of the population failed to consume any foods from the vegetable group.[74] The proportion of the population consuming at least the desired number of servings from each of these food groups was 29% for the grain group, 29% for the fruit group, and 61% for the vegetable group.

Furthermore, diets do not seem to be improving over time. Between 1987 and 1992, the National Health Interview Survey, with 10,000 respondents, showed that the consumption of fruits and vegetables remained constant over that time period.[75] Some studies show that diets are actually getting worse.

Another reason for a poor showing in terms of fiber intake is that many popular, good-tasting foods contain < 2 g of dietary fiber per serving.[76] Increasing the median fiber intake by an average of 9–12 g to the level at which it could be protective would require selection of at least three to four more servings of high-fiber products. While surveys suggest that the average consumer believes that high-fiber foods, especially coarse brown breads, are good for them, many also prefer the taste and texture of their low-fiber counterparts.

Another reason for low fiber intakes is that Americans and Europeans responded that their diets are quite good and do not need changing.[77] Furthermore, many responded that they did not want to give up the foods they liked, preferred the low-fiber foods, or simply did not wish to change.

The strength of the associations between attitudes, knowledge, and dietary behavior varied in some cases according to level of education and perceived barriers to eating a healthful diet. Of the perceived barriers to eating a healthful diet, ease of eating a healthful diet was most strongly and consistently predictive of intake. Knowledge did affect dietary fiber intake in some people. Specifically, fat, fiber, and fruit and vegetable intakes more closely approximated dietary recommendations for persons with more cancer-prevention knowledge.[78]

CONCLUSIONS

Individuals living in Western countries have fiber intakes below recommended levels. Countries such as Mexico and Brazil have higher fiber intakes. Among the Western countries, Finland has the highest intakes and the US has the lowest. While it is not clear that fiber itself is preventative of many diseases, it is clear that the intake of fiber-containing foods is very beneficial in the prevention of disease. Thus, health professionals need to use every means possible to institute programs that can increase the fiber content of the diet. The new dietary fiber definition is just one way to raise consumer and industry awareness so that steps may be taken to encourage the eating of more fiber-containing foods and to strengthen the demand for more fiber in food products.

REFERENCES

1. Hipsley, E. H., Dietary "fibre" and pregnancy toxemia, *Brit. Med. J.*, 2, 240, 1953.
2. Burkitt, D. P., Walker, A. R., and Painter, N. S., Dietary fiber and disease, *JAMA*, 229, 1068, 1974.
3. Levy, A. S. and Stokes, R. C., Effects of a health promotion advertising campaign on sales of ready-to-eat cereals, *Public Health Rep.*, 102, 398, 1987.
4. Freimuth, V. S., Hammond, S. L., and Stein, J. A., Health advertising: prevention for profit, *Am. J. Public Health*, 78, 557, 1988.
5. McNamara, S. H., The brave new world of FDA nutrition regulation — some thoughts about current trends and long-term effects, *Crit. Rev. Food Sci. Nutr.*, 34(2), 215, 1994.
6. Kowalski, R. E., *8 Week Cholesterol Cure*, Harper & Row, 1987.
7. Swain, J. F., Rouse, I. L., Curley, C. B., and Sacks, F. M., Comparison of the effects of oat bran and low-fiber wheat on serum lipoprotein levels and blood pressure, *N. Engl. J. Med.*, 322, 147, 1990.
8. Fuchs, C. S., Giovannucci. E. L., Colditz, G. A., Hunter, D. J., Stampfer, M. J., Rosner, B., Speizer, F. E., and Willett, W. C., Dietary fiber and the risk of colorectal cancer and adenoma in women, *N. Engl. J. Med.*, 340, 169, 1999.
9. Schatzkin, A., Lanza, E., Corle, D., Lance, P., Iber, F., Caan, B., Shike, M., Weissfeld, J., Burt, R., Cooper, M. R., Kikendall, J. W., and Cahill, J., Lack of effect of a low-fat, high-fiber diet on the recurrence of colorectal adenomas, Polyp Prevention Trial Study Group, *N. Engl. J. Med.*, 342, 1149, 2000.
10. Bonithon-Kopp, C., Kronborg, O., Giacosa, A., Rath, U., and Faivre, J., Calcium and fibre supplementation in prevention of colorectal adenoma recurrence: a randomised intervention trial, European Cancer Prevention Organization Study Group, *Lancet*, 14, 356, 1300, 2000.
11. DeVries, J., Dietary Fiber Symposium, Inst. Food Tech. Annual Meeting, Chicago, 1999.
12. Slavin, J., Implementation of dietary modifications, *Am. J. Med.*, 106, 46, discussion 50, 1999.
13. Ganji, V. and Betts, N., Fat, cholesterol, fiber and sodium intakes of US population: evaluation of diets reported in 1987-88 Nationwide Food Consumption Survey, *Eur. J. Clin. Nutr.*, 49, 915, 1995.
14. Kant, A. K., Schatzkin, A., Block, G., Ziegler, R. G., and Nestle, M., Food group intake patterns and associated nutrient profiles of the US population, *J. Am. Diet Assoc.*, 91, 1532, 1991.
15. Lanza, E., Jones, D. Y., Block, G., and Kessler, L., Dietary fiber intake in the US population, *Am. J. Clin. Nutr.*, 46, 790, 1987.
16. Salmerón, J., Ascherio, A., Rimm, E. B., Colditz, G. A., Spiegelman, D., Jenkins, D. J., Stampfer, M. J., Wing, A. L., and Willett, W. C., Dietary fiber, glycemic load, and risk of NIDDM in men, *Diabetes Care*, 20, 545, 1997.
17. Hermann, J. R., Hanson, C. F., and Kopel, B. H., Fiber intake of older adults: relationship to mineral intakes, *J. Nutr. Elder.*, 11, 21, 1992.
18. Warber, J., Haddad, E., Hodgkin, G., and Lee, J., Dietary fiber content of a six-day weighed military ration, *Mil. Med.*, 160, 438, 1995.
19. Warber, J. P., Boquist, S. H., and Cline, A. D., Fruit and vegetables in the service member's diet: data from military institutional feeding studies, *Mil. Med.*, 162, 468, 1997.
20. Clemens, L. H., Slawson, D. L., and Klesges, R. C., The effect of eating out on quality of diet in premenopausal women, *J. Am. Diet Assoc.*, 99, 442, 1999.
21. Sheridan, M., Matters of choice, *Restaurants and Institutions*, 22, 73, 2000.
22. Rimm, E. B., Ascherio, A., Giovannucci, E., Spiegelman, D., Stampfer, M. J., and Willett, W. C., Vegetable, fruit, and cereal fiber intake and risk of coronary heart disease among men, *JAMA*, 275, 447, 1996.
23. Lanza, E., Schatzkin, A., Ballard-Barbash, R., Corle, D., Clifford, C., Paskett, E., Hayes, D., Bote, E., Caan, B., Shike, M., Weissfeld, J., Slattery, M., Mateski, D., and Daston, C., The polyp prevention trial II: dietary intervention program and participant baseline dietary characteristics, *Cancer Epidemiol. Biomarkers Prev.*, 5, 385, 1996.

24. Alfieri, M. A., Pomerleau, J., Grace, D. M., and Anderson, L., Fiber intake of normal weight, moderately obese and severely obese subjects, *Obes. Res.*, 3, 541, 1995.
25. Miller, W. C., Niederpruem, M. G., Wallace, J. P., and Lindeman, A. K., Dietary fat, sugar, and fiber predict body fat content, *J. Am. Diet Assoc.*, 94, 612, 1994.
26. Nelson, L. H. and Tucker, L. A., Diet composition related to body fat in a multivariate study of 203 men, *J. Am. Diet Assoc.*, 96, 771, 1996.
27. Williams, C. L., Bollella, M., and Wynder, E. L., A new recommendation for dietary fiber in childhood, *Pediatrics*, 96, 985, 1995.
28. Saldanha, L. G., Fiber in the diet of US children: results of national surveys, *Pediatrics*, 96, 994, 1995.
29. Nicklas, T. A., Myers, L., and Berenson, G. S., Dietary fiber intake of children: the Bogalusa Heart Study, *JADA*, 95, 209; *Pediatrics* 96, 988, 1995.
30. Hampl, J. S., Betts, N. M., and Benes, B. A., The 'age+5' rule: comparisons of dietary fiber intake among 4- to 10-year-old children, *J. Am. Diet Assoc.*, 98, 1418, 1998.
31. Nicklas, T. A., Myers, L., O'Neil, C., and Gustafson, N., Impact of dietary fat and fiber intake on nutrient intake of adolescents, *Pediatrics*, 105, 21, 2000.
32. Tavelli, S., Beerman, K., Shultz, J. E., and Heiss, C., Sources of error and nutritional adequacy of the food pyramid, *J. Am. Coll. Health*, 47, 77, 1998.
33. Gillman, M. W., Rifas-Shiman, S. L., Frazier, A. L., Rockett, H. R., Camargo, C. A., Jr., Field, A. E., Berkey, C. S., and Colditz, G. A., Family dinner and diet quality among older children and adolescents, *Arch. Fam. Med.*, 9, 235, 2000.
34. Deharveng, G., Charrondière, U. R., Slimani, N., Southgate, D. A., and Riboli, E., Comparison of nutrients in the food composition tables available in the nine European countries participating in EPIC. European Prospective Investigation into Cancer and Nutrition, *Eur. J. Clin. Nutr.*, 53, 60, 1999.
35. Emmett, P. M., Symes, C. L., and Heaton, K. W., Dietary intake and sources of nonstarch polysaccharide in English men and women, *Eur. J. Clin. Nutr.*, 47, 20, 1993.
36. Davies, G. J., Crowder, M., and Dickerson, J. W., Dietary fiber intakes of individuals with different eating patterns, *Hum. Nutr. Appl. Nutr.*, 39, 139, 1985.
37. Cole-Hamilton, I., Gunner, K., Leverkus, C., and Starr, J., A study among dietitians and adult members of their households of the practicalities and implications of following proposed dietary guidelines for the UK British Dietetic Association Community Nutrition Group Nutrition Guidelines Project, *Hum. Nutr. Appl. Nutr.*, 40, 365, 1986.
38. Lip, G. Y., Luscombe, C., McCarry, M., Malik, I., and Beevers, G., Ethnic differences in public health awareness, health perceptions and physical exercise: implications for heart disease prevention, *Ethn. Health*, 1, 47, 1996.
39. Hurson, M. and Corish, C., Evaluation of lifestyle, food consumption and nutrient intake patterns among Irish teenagers, *Ir. J. Med. Sci.*, 166, 225, 1997.
40. Prynne, C. J., Paul, A. A., Price, G. M., Day, K. C., Hilder, W. S., and Wadsworth, M. E., Food and nutrient intake of a national sample of 4-year-old children in 1950: comparison with the 1990s, *Public Health Nutr.*, 2, 537, 1997.
41. Humphreys, M., Cronin, C. C., Barry, D. G., and Ferriss, J. B., Are the nutritional recommendations for insulin-dependent diabetic patients being achieved?, *Diabet Med.*, 11, 79, 1994.
42. Kearney, M., Kearney, J., Dunne, A., and Gibney, M., Sociodemographic determinants of perceived influences on food choice in a nationally representative sample of Irish adults, *Public Health Nutr.*, 3, 219, 2000.
43. Bagheri, S. M. and Debry, G., Estimation of the daily dietary fiber intake in France, *Ann. Nutr. Metab.*, 34, 69, 1990.
44. Volatier, J. L. and Verger, P., Recent national French food and nutrient intake data, *Br. J. Nutr.*, 81, 2, 57, 1999.
45. Holdsworth, M., Gerber, M., Haslam, C., Scali, J., Beardsworth, A., Avallone, M. H., and Sherratt, E., A comparison of dietary behaviour in central England and a French Mediterranean region, *Eur. J. Clin. Nutr.*, 54, 530, 2000.
46. Pietinen, P., Rimm, E. B., Korhonen, P., Hartman, A. M., Willett, W. C., Albanes, D., and Virtamo, J., Intake of dietary fiber and risk of coronary heart disease in a cohort of Finnish men, The Alpha-Tocopherol, Beta-Carotene Cancer Prevention Study, *Circulation*, 94, 2720, 1996.

47. Roos, E., Prättälä, R., Lahelma, E., Kleemola, P., and Pietinen, P., Modern and healthy? Socioeconomic differences in the quality of diet, *Eur. J. Clin. Nutr.*, 50, 753, 1996.

48. Persson, P. G., Carlsson, S., Grill, V., Hagman, U., Lundgren, A. C., Ostenson, C. G., Perers, M., and Wallen, A., Food frequency questionnaire versus 7-day weighed dietary record information on dietary fiber and fat intake in middle-aged Swedish men, *Scand. J. Soc. Med.*, 26, 75, 1998.

49. Hulshof, K. F., Löwik, M. R., Kistemaker, C., Hermus, R. J., ten Hoor, F., and Ockhuizen, T., Comparison of dietary intake data with guidelines: some potential pitfalls (Dutch nutrition surveillance system), *J. Am. Coll. Nutr.*, 12, 176, 1993.

50. van Rossum, C. T., van de Mheen, H., Witteman, J. C., Grobbee, E., and Mackenbach, J. P., Education and nutrient intake in Dutch elderly people, The Rotterdam Study, *Eur. J. Clin. Nutr.*, 54, 159, 2000.

51. Van Poppel, G., Schneijder, P., Löwik, M. R., Schrijver, J., and Kok, F. J., Nutritional status and food consumption in 10-11 year old Dutch boys (Dutch Nutrition Surveillance System), *Br. J. Nutr.*, 66, 161, 1991.

52. Mensink, G. B., Thamm, M., and Haas, K., Nutrition in Germany 1998, *Gesundheitswesen*, 61, 200, 1999.

53. Stelz, A., Winter, S., Gareis, C., Taschan, H., and Muskat, E., Nutritional intake of daily diets in nursing homes for the aged. I — Energy, protein, fat, carbohydrate and fiber, *Z. Ernahrungswiss*, 35, 163, 1996.

54. Klipstein-Grobusch, K,. Kroke, A., Voss, S., and Boeing, H., Influence of lifestyle on the use of supplements in the Brandenburg nutrition and cancer study, *Z. Ernahrungswiss*, 37, 38, 1998.

55. Kersting, M., Sichert-Hellert, W., Alexy, U., Manz, F., and Schoch, G., Macronutrient intake of 1 to 18 year old German children and adolescents, *Z. Ernahrungswiss*, 37, 252, 1998.

56. Linseisen, J., Gedrich, K., Karg, G., and Wolfram, G., Sucrose intake in Germany, *Z. Ernahrungswiss*, 37, 303, 1998.

57. Schober, E., Langergraber, B., Rupprecht, G., and Rami, B., Dietary intake of Austrian diabetic children 10 to 14 years of age, *J. Pediatr. Gastroenterol. Nutr.*, 29, 144, 1999.

58. Buyken, A. E., Toeller, M., Heitkamp, G., Vitelli, F., Stehle, P., Scherbaum, W. A., and Fuller, J. H., Relation of fiber intake to HbA1c and the prevalence of severe ketoacidosis and severe hypoglycaemia, EURODIAB IDDM Complications Study Group, *Diabetologia*, 41, 882, 1998.

59. Pietruszka, B., Brzozowska, A., and Puzio-Dbska, A., Dietary assessment of adults in three villages in Warsaw, Radom and Biaa Podlaska districts, *Rocz. Panstw. Zakl. Hig.*, 49, 219, 1998.

60. Pardo, B., Sygnowska, E., Rywik, S., Kulesza, W., and Waskiewicz, A., Dietary habits of the middle-aged Warsaw population in 1984 relative to nutritional guidelines, *Appetite*, 16, 11, 1991.

61. Farre, R. R., Frasquet, P. I., Martinez, M. I., and Roma, S. R., The usual diet of a group of adolescents from Valencia, *Nutr. Hosp.*, 14, 223, 1999.

62. Beer-Borst, S., Hercberg, S., Morabia, A., Bernstein, M. S., Galan, P., Galasso, R., Giampaoli, S., McCrum, E., Panico, S., Preziosi, P., Ribas, L., Serra-Majem, L., Vescio, M. F., Vitek, O., Yarnell, J., and Northridge, M. E., Dietary patterns in six European populations: results from EURALIM, a collaborative European data harmonization and information campaign, *Eur. J. Clin. Nutr.*, 54, 253, 2000.

63. Wyatt, C. J. and Triana Tejas, M. A., Nutrient intake and growth of preschool children from different socioeconomic regions in the city of Oaxaca, Mexico, *Ann. Nutr. Metab.*, 44, 14, 2000.

64. Ballesteros-Vasquez, M. N., Cabrera-Pacheco, R. M., Saucedo-Tamayo, M. S., and Grijalva-Haro, M. I., Intake of dietary fiber, sodium, potassium, and calcium and its relation with arterial blood pressure in normotensive adult men, *Salud. Publica. Mex.*, 40, 241, 1998.

65. Wyatt, C. J., Dorado, I., Valencia, M. E., and Navarro, E., Colon cancer in rats and diet in the Sonoran desert region of Mexico, *Arch. Latinoam. Nutr.*, 46, 33, 1996.

66. Wyatt, C. J., Evaluation of the composition of the regional diet in Sonora, México: incidence of colon cancer, *Arch. Latinoam. Nutr.*, 48, 225, 1998.

67. Dixon, L. B., Sundquist, J., and Winkleby, M., Differences in energy, nutrient, and food intakes in a US sample of Mexican-American women and men: findings from the Third National Health and Nutrition Examination Survey, 1988-1994, *Am. J. Epidemiol.*, 152, 548, 2000.

68. Mattos, L. L. and Martins, I. S., Dietary fiber consumption in an adult population, *Rev. Saude Publica.*, 34, 50, 2000.

69. Ball, M. J. and Bartlett, M. A., Dietary intake and iron status of Australian vegetarian women, *Am. J. Clin. Nutr.*, 70, 353, 1999.

70. Baghurst, K. I. and Baghurst, P. A., Dietary fibre, *Supplement Food Austral.*, 48, 1996.

71. Imaeda, N., Tokudome, Y., Ikeda, M., Kitagawa, I., Fujiwara, N., and Tokudome, S., Foods contributing to absolute intake and variance in intake of selected vitamins, minerals and dietary fiber in middle-aged Japanese, *J. Nutr. Sci. Vitaminol.* (Tokyo), 45, 519, 1999.

72. Aoki, S., Endo, T., Hasegawa, H., Nakaji, S., Sugawara, K., and Totsuka, M., Dietary patterns and intake of nutrients, energy, and dietary fiber in medical students, *Nippon Koshu Eisei Zasshi*, 43, 632, 1996.

73. Block, G., Dietary guidelines and the results of food consumption surveys, *Am. J. Clin. Nutr.*, 53, 356S, 1991.

74. Kant, A. K., Block, G., Schatzkin, A., Ziegler, R. G., and Nestle, M., Dietary diversity in the US population, NHANES II, 1976-1980, *J. Am. Diet. Assoc.*, 91, 1526, 1991.

75. Breslow, R. A., Subar, A. F., Patterson, B. H., and Block, G., Trends in food intake: the 1987 and 1992 National Health Interview Surveys, *Nutr. Cancer*, 28, 86, 1997.

76. Marlett, J. A. and Cheung, T. F., Database and quick methods of assessing typical dietary fiber intakes using data from 228 commonly consumed foods, *J. Am. Diet. Assoc.*, 97, 1139, 1997.

77. Kearney, J. M. and McElhone, S., Perceived barriers in trying to eat healthier — results of a pan-EU consumer attitudinal survey, *Br. J. Nutr.*, 81, suppl. 2, 133, 1999.

78. Harnack, L., Block, G., Subar, A., Lane, S., and Brand, R., Association of cancer prevention-related nutrition knowledge, beliefs, and attitudes to cancer prevention dietary behavior, *J. Am. Diet. Assoc.*, 97, 957, 1997.

79. *http://www.eatright.org/nfs/nfs88.html*

80. *http://www.diabetes.org/diabetescare/supplement/s16.htm*

81. Van Horn, L., Fiber, lipids, and coronary heart disease, a statement for healthcare professionals from the Nutrition Committee, American Heart Association, *Circulation*, 95, 2701, 1997.

82. American Cancer Society, *Diet, Nutrition, and Cancer Prevention Guidelines*.

83. Butrum, R. R., Clifford, C. K., and Lanza, E., NCI dietary guidelines: rationale, *Am. J. Clin. Nutr.*, 48, 888, 1988.

84. United States Department of Agriculture, *USDA, Dietary Guidelines for Americans*, United States Department of Health and Human Services, 2000.

85. National Health and Medical Research Council, *Dietary Guidelines for Australians*, Australian Government Publishing Service, Canberra, 1994.

85a. National Health and Medical Research Council, *Eat Well for Life, Dietary Guidelines for Older Australians*, Australian Government Publishing Service, Canberra, 1999.

86. Block, G., Gillespie, C., Rosenbaum, E. H., and Jenson, C., A rapid food screener to assess fat and fruit and vegetable intake, *Am. J. Prev. Med.*, 18, 284, 2000.

Patterns of Dietary Fiber Consumption in Humans to 1992

Sheila Bingham

INTRODUCTION

In recent years, the majority of expert committees have recommended an increase in the fiber content of Western diets because there is accumulating evidence that fiber is important in the prevention of a large number of bowel disorders.[1-3] However, although it is assumed that fiber intakes are greater in areas where these disorders are rare, in fact little is known of the patterns of fiber consumption worldwide. This is largely due to methodological problems in both the collection of food consumption data from representative population samples and in converting that data into grams of fiber eaten per day, using tables of food composition.

METHODS

Analytical

There are various methods in existence for the measurement of "fiber" in foods, all of which give different values for particular foods, especially cooked foods. Hence, incorporation of "fiber" values into food tables is a difficult problem and most government-sponsored food tables do not include values for it. Crude fiber analyses are not relevant to human population studies.

UK food tables published in 1978[4] included values for fiber using mainly the Southgate method, and the majority of information about fiber consumption worldwide is based on these analyses. However, recent supplements and editions now incorporate the analysis of nonstarch polysaccharides (NSP) from the analyses of Englyst.[33,36] These do not suffer from analytical problems encountered from the cooking, storage, and preservation of food, which can introduce artifactual increases in "fiber" seen in some other methods. Some information on NSP consumption is beginning to emerge, showing a reduced level using these figures compared with former estimates. In the US, estimates based on the table of Lanza and Butrum,[7,8] which incorporate data using four different methods, are also lower than formerly. Although the data on these new estimates are limited, they are doubtless more accurate and therefore are discussed first in this chapter.

0-8493-2387-8/01/$0.00+$1.50

Food Consumption

In some countries, per capita data on food consumption from national statistics and household surveys are available for the re-analysis of long-term trends in dietary fiber consumption over this century, but these statistics are not available for earlier years. They are also only valid indicators of trends in countries with stable and well-documented population bases, and they give no indication of the amounts of fiber consumed by different age, sex, and occupational groups within the population. National per capita statistics also overestimate food consumption, probably by different amounts in different populations. In Britain, for example, estimates of energy consumption from national statistics are some 25% greater than the estimated energy requirement.[9] Nevertheless, published estimates of dietary fiber consumption are available for some countries using these data and are reported below.

Definitive information on food consumption is obtained from studies of individuals where the amount of food eaten is determined directly. There are many different ways in which this is done,[10] and the data from individuals can be aggregated into group estimates. It should be borne in mind, however, that the estimation of the food intake of free-living individuals is no easy undertaking since all methods rely on information supplied by the subjects themselves, which may not be correct. There are many sources of error, and average intakes estimated on the same population using one method may be up to 30% greater or less than those obtained using a different method.[10] The correct result is usually open to debate, unless actual food intakes can be observed by investigators in certain limited situations, or an independent index, such as 24-h urine N from validated urine collections, is used. Urine N should be 80 ± 5% of calculated dietary N intake in populations consuming amounts of fiber commonly found in Western-type diets.[11]

A second validity check for populations is to calculate basal metabolic rate (BMR) from body weight using published equations and to compare energy intake from the dietary survey with estimated energy expenditure, which is 1.4 to 1.6 times the BMR in sedentary populations.[12] Energy intake to BMR ratios of 1.2 or less, which have been reported in some populations, with no apparent loss of body weight is unphysiological, and hence the validity of this dietary data is questionable. The use of these markers in nutritional epidemiology is discussed elsewhere.[11,12]

NEW ESTIMATES OF NONSTARCH POLYSACCHARIDE (NSP) CONSUMPTION

Estimates of NSP and fiber using newer values are currently available for seven countries; see Table 7.2.1. All of these except one, that based on the US NHANES II study, used the Englyst values for the NSP content of foods. In the NHANES II study,[7] several different methods were used to compile a table of fiber values for foods, and these included the AOAC method, neutral detergent fiber, and Englyst values.[8] The food consumption values in the table also incorporate different methods of obtaining food consumption data, ranging from 7-day weighed records in UK men and women,[16] 16-day weighed records in UK women volunteers,[17] interviews in South African urban blacks,[20] and 24-h recalls in the US NHANES II[7] and Canadian students study.[19] Recalculated data[21] from the US food balance sheets, using the publication of Heller and Hackler for 1973 to 1975 to NSP, are also shown. A figure for Finnish NSP intakes, calculated from food balance sheets, is also shown.[13] In the remaining studies — in Scandinavia,[14] the UK National Household Food Survey,[15] Loma Linda University volunteers,[22] and Japan[18] — duplicate diets were analyzed directly for NSP.

Overall, there is only a small range in average intakes worldwide, from 11 g in the US and Japan to 18 g in men in rural Finland. Insoluble fiber is consumed in rather greater quantities than soluble, and supplies from vegetables usually predominate over cereals. The Japanese diet seems to differ from that of the West with its low content of pentose (xylose and arabinose) polysaccharides

Table 7.2.1 Nonstarch Polysaccharide and Fiber Intake (grams per day)

Country	Total	SD	Range	Soluble	Insoluble	Cellulose	Hexoses	Pentoses	Uronic Acids	From Cereals	From Vegetables	Ref.
Finland	16.0	—	—	4.8	11.2	3.8	—	—	—	9.8	3.5	13
Rural Finland	18.4	7.8	—	—	—	4.2	5.3	7.4	1.9	—	—	14
Rural Denmark	18.0	6.4	—	—	—	3.7	5.5	6.6	2.2	—	—	14
Helsinki	14.5	5.4	—	—	—	3.4	3.7	5.5	2.0	—	—	14
Copenhagen	13.2	4.8	—	—	—	3.2	3.6	4.5	1.9	—	—	14
UK— National Food Survey	12.4	—	—	—	—	2.6	3.4	4.5	1.8	—	—	15
UK— Men	11.2	3.5	5–19	5.2	6.1	3.1	2.2	4.0	1.7 }	.4	5.6	16
UK— Women	12.5	4.1	7–25	5.4	7.2	3.3	2.2	4.8	2.0			
UK— Women volunteers	15.8	5.1	1–68[a]	6.7	9.1	—	—	—	—	—	—	17
Japan	10.9	—	—	4.1	6.8	3.0	2.9	1.8	3.1	—	—	18
Canada — students	12	—	1–81[a]	5	7	—	—	—	—	—	—	19
South Africa — urban black M	14	5	—	—	—	—	—	—	—	—	—	20
urban black F	13	5	—	—	—	—	—	—	—	—	—	
US — National Statistics 1973–75	17	—	—	—	—	—	—	—	—	5.6	6.6	21
US — NHANES II Men	13	—	—	1–48[a]	—	—	—	—	—	—	—	7
Women	9	—	—		—	—	—	—	—	—	—	
US — volunteers Loma Linda Univ. Men	17	—	—	9	8	—	—	—	—	—	—	22
Women	12	—	—	6	6	—	—	—	—	—	—	22

[a] = daily range.

and higher intake of uronic acids. Men generally seem to consume more NSP than women, with the exception of the small study in the UK. South African blacks consume remarkably little NSP compared with previous estimates using Southgate's analyses. However, starch consumption in this area is high and would have led to an overestimate in previous analyses.

There is a very large individual range in NSP intake, up to 81 g/d in Canadian students, for example. However, this is probably due to the fact that single-day estimates are reported in these studies, while other estimates are used in UK volunteers and in the US NHANES study. In the small UK study, individual intakes were averaged over 7 days, when the apparent range was reduced; see Figure 7.2.1. Nevertheless, the individual range in NSP intake, from 7 to 25 g/d, is still greater than the range in average intake worldwide.

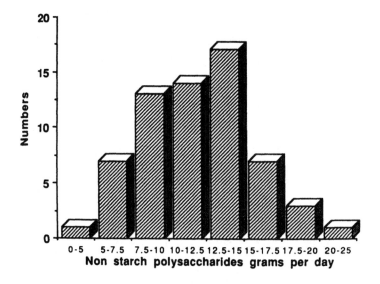

Figure 7.2.1   Distribution of individual nonstarch polysaccharide intakes in 63 men and women. (From Bingham et al., *J. Hum. Nutr. Dietet.*, 3, 333, 1990. With permission.)

DIETARY FIBER (SOUTHGATE ANALYSIS) CONSUMPTION

Europe

National Statistics

In Table 7.2.2, data on 23 countries from Bright-See and McKeown-Eyssen[23] have been collated into 4 regions of Europe. These data, based on food analyses of Southgate, show that fiber intakes are greatest in the Mediterranean countries, with an equal contribution from vegetables and cereals. East European intakes follow a similar pattern. In Scandinavia, intakes are lowest, mainly due to the low intake of 14 g found in Iceland, and cereals contribute more than vegetables. In North and Central Europe, vegetables are the major source.

Individual Surveys

Table 7.2.3 summarizes results from a number of surveys of between 30 and 2200 individuals that have been carried out in Europe. Comparisons are possible because the samples were all randomly selected from population or electoral registers and response rates were high, usually around 80%. In all these surveys, food consumption was assessed by asking subjects to keep records

Table 7.2.2   Per Capita Dietary Fiber Supply in Europe 1972–1974 (grams per day)[23]

Area		Total	From Cereal	From Vegetable	From Fruit
Scandinavia[a]	(5)	21	10	7	4
North/Central[b]	(8)	25	9	11	5
Mediterranean[c]	(5)	38	16	16	6
East[d]	(5)	30	14	12	4

[a] Denmark, Finland, Iceland, Norway, Sweden.
[b] Austria, Belgium, France, Germany, Ireland, Switzerland, Netherlands, U. K.
[c] Greece, Italy, Portugal, Spain, Yugoslavia.
[d] Bulgaria, Czechoslovakia, Hungary, Poland, Romania.

of food actually consumed, and the amounts of food eaten were in most cases weighed by the subjects themselves. Most subjects were asked to keep a record for 1 week, but in one survey in Scotland, each individual was studied for 1 month. The majority of the results were calculated using Southgate's method of analysis in the British food tables, although this was supplemented in Denmark and Finland with Englyst's values for rye flour[26] and in the Netherlands with data from the method of Hellendoorn[37] and Karen.[38] Fiber intakes in the UK were measured at around the 20-g mark, with lowest intakes recorded in Scotland. The largest survey, of over 2000 individuals, recorded an intake as high as 25 g in men.[24] However, modified values for the fiber content of bread were used in these surveys.[39] Intakes in rural Finland and Denmark and in Holland and Yugoslavia were rather greater, whereas intakes in urban areas were also around 20 g/d.

Individual Variation

In some of these surveys in Europe, data on the distribution of dietary fiber intakes of individuals within the overall average are published, and these are summarized in Table 7.2.3. Coefficients of variation (standard deviation/mean %) are on average 35% and the range between individuals is greater than that found between populations, for example, from 8 to 32 g/d in the Welsh and British surveys. Thus, as with NSP, even though dietary fiber intakes in Europe are comparatively low, individuals appear to vary markedly within a population.

Household Surveys

A commonly used method of assessing the dietary intake of populations is the household survey, whereby food entering a household over a certain period, usually 1 week, is estimated and the total food available is divided by the number of people living in the household. This does not give information about the distribution of intakes between different individuals, but additional information about dietary fiber consumption in European populations is provided from a survey carried out in the EEC from 1963 to 1965 to assess levels of radioactive contamination.[40] In this survey, each family weighed all their food after preparing it, thus eliminating the need to make corrections for inedible wastage. All the areas studied were rural, and approximately 30 families were studied per month over a period of 3 years. Table 7.2.4 summarizes fiber intakes calculated from the published values on food consumption, using values for British foods together with data from another household survey, the National Food Survey, which has been carried out every year in Britain since 1940. In this, about 6500 households are studied per year, randomly selected from each of the nine standard regions in England, Wales, and Scotland. Food entering the household is not weighed, but it is estimated from records of food purchases kept by the housewife for 1 week. Total dietary fiber intakes in Britain, a largely urban area, estimated from this survey in a comparative year, 1966, were 21 g/d. This is less than the rural areas of Europe with only 32% derived from cereals, compared with an average of 45% in the EEC, although the staple food in all of the areas was white bread.

TABLE 7.2.3 Dietary Fiber Consumption in Europe: Individual Surveys

Country	Sample	Cooperation Rate (%)	No.	Survey Method	Analytical Method	Total DF (g/d)	Cereal DF (d/f)	Vegetable DF (g/d)	Fruit DF (g/d)	TDF (CV %)	Range (g)	Ref.
Great Britain	Randomly selected from electoral registers, 16–64 years	70										
	Men		1087	7-d weighed record	SM	25	—	—	—	36	10–45	24
	Women		1110			19	—	—	—	36	7–33	24
England	Randomly selected from electoral registers, 20–80 years											
	Men	82	32	7-d weighed record	S	19.8	5.7	8.8	2.0	27	10–32	25
	Women	58	31			20.1	6.6	7.6	2.6	26	18–32	
Wales	Randomly selected men from prevalence study of heart disease	89	119	7-d weighed record	S	19.9	9.0	—	—	34	8–32	26
Scotland	Randomly selected men aged 40 years	78	107	7-d weighed record	S	17.5	7.6	—	—	32	6–36	27
Scotland	Randomly selected men and women aged 21–69 years	84										
	Men		16	28-d estimated record	S	16.5	—	—	—	—	—	28
	Women		27			15.0	—	—	—	—	—	

Country	Description	Subgroup		n	Method	Code						Range	Ref
N. Ireland	Randomly selected from electoral registers, 16–64 years	Men	74	258	7-d weighed record	S	21	—	—	—	37	—	
		Women		334			23	—	—	—	32	—	29
Netherlands	Randomly selected from electoral registers, 25–65 years	Men	67	44	7-d estimated record	K	27.5	7.7	9.8	3.6	28	—	30
		Women		56		S	21.3	—	—	—	22	—	
		Men, Zutphen	—	871	Diet history	H ?	30.4	—	—	—	32	—	32
Finland	Randomly selected from population registers, men aged 50–89 years	Rural	83	30	4-d weighed record	S	26.6	19.5	4.6	1.6	42	5–45	32, 33
		Helsinki	74	29		E	21.5	12.8	6.1	1.6	42	10–40	
Denmark	Randomly selected from population registers, men aged 50–59 years	Rural	63	30	4-d weighed record	S	23.4	13.5	6.5	2.7	37	10–55	32, 33
		Copenhagen	75	30		E	18.0	10.6	4.7	1.7	36	2–30	
Yugoslavia	Randomly selected men; 7 countries heart study		—	49	7-d weighed record	S	25.5	8.7	13.3	3.4	29	9–46	34, 35

Note: S[4], H[37], K[38], E[36], SM[39].

Table 7.2.4 Sources of Dietary Fiber in 11 Regions of the European Economic Community[a]

Area[b]	Cereal	Vegetable	Fruit, Nuts	Potato	Total
Friesland (H)	8.2	5.6	2.6	6.3	22.6
Gent (B)	10.9	4.1	1.7	12.3	28.9
Liege (B)	8.0	6.0	2.3	10.5	26.8
Luxembourg	7.3	6.5	2.1	13.2	29.1
Hessen (G)	11.6	4.9	2.6	8.2	27.3
Normandy (F)	9.1	5.7	2.2	7.8	24.8
Bretagne (F)	10.2	4.9	1.8	6.9	23.8
Vendee (F)	10.1	12.7	2.8	4.0	29.6
Fruili (I)	14.7	5.1	1.3	3.8	24.9
Campania (I)	13.4	7.7	4.3	1.6	26.9
Basilicata (I)	13.5	5.7	3.9	0.7	23.8
Britain (1966)	6.7	10.3[c]	2.3	—	21.1

[a] Values are given as grams per person per day.
[b] H, Holland; B, Belgium; G, Germany; F, France; I, Italy.
[c] Includes potato.

Seasonal variations in dietary fiber estimated from these two surveys have been reported elsewhere.[34] In the rural areas, seasonal changes from month to month were substantial and, in some cases, greater than the variations between areas. Possible seasonal variations need, therefore, to be taken into account when comparing dietary fiber intake of individuals or populations, although in largely urban countries, such as Britain, quarterly seasonal variations are not as marked and are related to consumption of different types of vegetables.[34]

Long-Term Trends

In Britain[42] and the Netherlands,[30] some long-term trends in dietary fiber consumption over the 20th century have been calculated from national statistics. These are summarized in Table 7.2.5, together with calculations of the dietary fiber content of diets consumed by farming households in Denmark.[42] In all three European countries, cereal dietary fiber intake has probably declined, although by only 2 to 3 g since 1909 in Britain. Cereal fiber intakes may have been greater in 1860,[34] although there are no national statistics available earlier than 1909. The decline in cereal fiber consumption has been offset somewhat by increases in vegetable sources of dietary fiber, and the most striking change in Britain was the doubling of fiber intakes during the period 1940 to 1953. This was the result of the raising of flour extraction rates, thus more than doubling the fiber content of bread and cereal fiber intakes during and after World War II. At the same time, bread and vegetable consumption was encouraged while other foods such as meat and cheese were in short supply, so that more bread was eaten.

Africa

While much has been written about dietary fiber intakes in Africa, in fact, very little is known about it. No dietary surveys have been done specifically to measure fiber intake and nothing is therefore known of its main sources and composition. Dietary surveys to quantitate intakes of other nutrients have been done, and these have been used as a basis for obtaining some preliminary figures for fiber intakes. These are summarized in Table 7.2.6. Studies on dietary fiber intake, using 7-day weighed records and values for the NDF content of foods in 300 young Nigerian women, suggest intakes of 63 g in urban areas and 69 g in rural ones.[50]

Previous data[44] showing intakes of 150 g in Uganda and 130 g in the Kikuyu resulted from food analyses of 6% in plantain and 10% in maize flour.[4] These high values were almost certainly

Table 7.2.5   Long-Term Trends in Dietary Fiber Consumption in Europe (grams per head per day)

Year	Britain[42]		Netherlands[30]		Denmark[43]	
	Total	Cereal	Total	Cereal	Total	Cereal
1909–1913	24	11	—	—	—	—
1927	—	—	—	—	34	—
1933	—	—	—	—	32	—
1938	22	9	—	—	—	—
1944	32–40	19–25	—	—	37	—
1950–1951	—	—	27	14	31	—
1957–1960	23	9	24	10	25	—
1970–1976	23	8	25	8	23	—

[30] Van Staveren et al., *J. Am. Dietet. Assoc.*, 80, 324, 1982.
[42] Southgate et al., *Nature (London)*, 274, 51, 1978.
[43] Helms et al., *Nutr. Cancer*, 4, 23, 1982.

Table 7.2.6   Dietary Fiber Intakes in Africa and India (grams per head per day)

	Total	Cereal	Vegetable	Fruit, nuts	Ref.
Africa					
Kenya					
Kikuyu	86	32	54	—[a]	45
Masai					
Warriors	0	0	0	0	
Women	25	25	—	—	
Malawi (foothill village)	55	40	10	4	46
Swaziland (middle veld)	60	40	19	1	47, 48
Uganda (Buganda)	70	0	67	3	
Nigeria (urban)	63	23	40	— }	49
(rural)	69	10	59	—	
India					
Andhra	23	18	—	—	50
Karnataka	42	36	—	—	
Kerala	22	10	—	—	
Tamil Nadu	32	22	—	—	

[a] Not available.

contaminated with starch, and recently published values are much lower, 2% and 4%, respectively.[5,6] The data have therefore been recalculated and result in intakes of 70 g and 90 g, respectively, in these areas (Table 7.2.6).

Intakes are still comparatively high, however, compared with present day estimates of 14 g in 76 urban Sowetan black males and 13 g in 113 females, obtained by Segal and Walker[20] (Table 7.2.1). They state that fiber intake in the past was higher, 40 to 50 g daily in rural blacks, and that the current intake from unpublished surveys is 25 to 35 g/d. In Soweto, an urban area, refined maize meal is consumed, although there is a trend for increased consumption of brown bread. Legume consumption has decreased, and consumption of vegetables is low due to their high cost. Despite these low fiber intakes, bowel disease is rare. However, starch (including resistant starch) intakes are high and may account for the absence of Western bowel diseases.

Data from another African country, Mauritius, were obtained from food balance sheets by Bright-See and McKeown-Eyssen[23] and are shown in Table 7.2.7. The staple cereal in Mauritius is rice, so that country's intakes of cereal dietary fiber are similar to those of other rice-eating areas, such as Japan, about 10 g/d. Intakes of vegetables and fruit dietary fiber are, however, much lower so that total intakes are apparently some of the lowest in the world, with only Iceland having a lower value at 14 g/d.[23]

Table 7.2.7   Per Capita Dietary Fiber Supply 1972–1974 (grams per day)

Area	Total	From Cereal	From Vegetables	From Fruit
Australasia Australia and New Zealand (wheat)	24	9	10	5
Japan, Hong Kong, Singapore (rice)	28	10	14	4
America Chile, Cuba, Trinidad, Uruguay (wheat and rice)	25	12	10	3
Costa Rica, Mexico (maize)	33	19	9	5
North America United States	23	6	11	6
Canada	22	6	11	5
Other Israel	36	16	12	8
Mauritius	17	10	6	1

India

Dietary fiber intakes have been calculated using data from a number of dietary surveys carried out by the National Nutritional Monitoring Bureau in 1980 in India.[49] These show a twofold range in fiber intake from 22 g/d in predominantly rice-eating states such as Kerala to 42 g/d in Karnataka, where additional cereals such as millet are eaten. In Kerala, 9.8 g/d of dietary fiber came from cereals, compared with 35.9 g/d in Karnataka (Table 7.2.6).

Australasia

A number of reports of the dietary fiber intake in New Zealand, Polynesia, and Australia are available and are summarized in Table 7.2.7. All suggest that dietary fiber intakes are low and similar to those of Europe, around 20 g/d in New Zealand women and in Australia. Intakes are three times higher in Tongan women, 65% of the dietary fiber coming from taro, cassava, and breadfruit, but surprisingly low on another Polynesian island, Tokelau (Table 7.2.8).

Table 7.2.8 Dietary Fiber Intakes in Australasia (grams per head per day)

	Total	Cereal	Vegetable	Fruit	Ref.
New Zealand					
Europeans[a]	18 ± 5	6	8	4	51, 52, 53
Maori[a]	16 ± 6	6	8	3	51, 52
New Zealand Tongans[a]	19 ± 6	5	10	4	51, 52
Polynesia					
Tonga[a]	72 ± 29	1	48	22	51, 52
Tokelau[a]	15	—	—	—	54
Tokelau[b]	16	—	—	—	54
Australia					
Adelaide[a]	20–22	—	—	—	55
Adelaide[b]	19–20	—	—	—	55

[a] Women.
[b] Men.

Japan

With its highly urbanized society yet a disease pattern which contrasts with Western countries, Japan is of special interest to the epidemiologist, particularly since these patterns of disease change within one or two generations in Japanese who migrate.[56] Traditional Japanese diets are known to be low in fat and high in carbohydrate, on which basis dietary fiber intakes might be expected to be high. However, since rice contains so little dietary fiber,[5] it might be predicted that the fiber intake of populations where rice is the staple cereal would be low. The Japanese diet was thus reported to contain only 19.4 g/d in 1979.[57]

Mori, using his own technique for analyses of Japanese foods, reported the dietary fiber content of two student meals to be 14.8 and 19.5 g/d.[58] Estimates from food balance sheet data are rather greater, 32 g/d.[23] The estimates of Far East countries are shown in Table 7.2.7. These estimates using Southgate values for fiber are less than those for NSPs, which are 11 g/d (Table 7.2.1).

Long-Term Trends

In Japan, yearly nationwide household surveys are carried out, and this data has been used to calculate dietary fiber intakes using the British Food Tables together with neutral detergent fiber plus pectin values for some seaweed-based foods.[52,53] Total dietary fiber from rice has fallen from 7.7 g/d in 1965 to 5.1 g/d in 1979, and overall total dietary fiber intake has fallen from 21.2 g/d in 1965 to 19.4 g/d in 1979 (Table 7.2.9). These changes are small compared with a 70 g/d decline in carbohydrate intake since 1965, a threefold increase in fat intake, and a 25% increase in the amount of protein derived from animal products since 1950.

Table 7.2.9 Secular Changes in Major Nutrient Intakes, 1950–1979, (per capita per day) in Japan

Year	Fat (g)	Carbohydrate (g)	Dietary Fiber		Protein from Animal Food (g)
			Total (g)	From Rice (g)	
1950	18	418	—[a]	—	25.0
1955	20.3	411	—	—	32.0
1960	24.7	399	—	—	35.4
1965	36.0	384	21.2[b]	7.7[b]	40.0
1970	46.5	368	20.2	7.0	44.1
1975	52.0	337	20.2	5.7	48.6
1979	54.8	315	19.4	5.1	50.3

[a] Data not available.
[b] 1966.

There are no household statistics available prior to 1950, but a dietary record of an artist's family (all adults) in 1925 showed that on a typical day, rice was eaten three times a day, together with pickles, salted fish, soybean curd, radishes, spring onions, and soy sauce. Only 12 g/d of fat was eaten, but the dietary fiber content was the same as today, 18.2 g/d, although at that time rice supplied 11.3 g/d.[57]

Present-Day Intakes

Geographic comparisons within Japan show that these changes in diet have been most marked in the urban areas.[57] In the ten largest cities in 1979, 57.5 g/d of fat were eaten, and 52% of protein was derived from animal foods. Carbohydrate and dietary fiber intakes were also lower, 296 and 17.7 g/d in these areas. This compares with less fat, 50.6 g/d; less protein from animal sources,

48.2%; more carbohydrate, 332 g; and more dietary fiber, 20.2 g, in towns and villages. There is a clear trend between these extremes, depending on the size of the city.

North America

Fiber intakes calculated using Southgate analyses from the food balance sheets of Canada and the US show almost identical intakes of 22 to 23 g per capita per day, 6 g from cereals and 11 g from vegetables (Table 7.2.7). Previous studies suggested an intake of about 20 g/d from individual surveys (Table 7.2.10), although the recent reanalysis of the NHANES II suggests intakes lower than this, 11 g for women and 16 g for men, 13 g on average.[7] Intakes assessed by a questionnaire of the third quintile of 88,751 American female nurses ranged from 14 to 17 g/d, with 5 to 7 g obtained from vegetables and 4 to 5 g from cereals.[60] Intakes of 8000 American-Japanese men were lower, 12 g/d, and range (from 24-h recall data) from 1 to 46 g/d.[61]

Table 7.2.10 Dietary Fiber Intake in North America (grams per head per day)

	Total	Cereal	Vegetable	Fruit	Ref.
U. S.					
Men	20 ± 10	7[a]	9	5	60
Women	13 ± 6	4[a]	5	3	60
Simulated diet	19	—	—	—	61
NHANES II					
Men[b]	16	—	—	—	7
Women[b]	11	—	—	—	
Female nurses					
Third quintile	14–17	4–5	5–7	2–3	64
American-Japanese men	12	(range 1–46 g)			65
Canada					
Men[b]	18 ± 9	9 ± 6	—	—	62
Women	19 ± 7	—	—	—	63

[a] Includes fiber from legumes. [b] Food consumption estimated for 24-h recall.

NSP estimates (Table 7.2.1) are some 25% lower for food balance sheet estimates, 17 g/d in the US, of which 7 g is derived from vegetables and 6 g from cereals. NHANES estimates using the fiber table of Lanza and Butrum are 20% less, 11 g on average compared with 13 g using Southgate analyses alone.[7,8] Recalculations of data on long-term trends in food intake showed a 33% decrease in total dietary fiber and a 55% decrease in cereal dietary fiber in the US from 1909 to 1975.[21,34]

South America

No individual surveys to measure dietary fiber consumption have been published in South American countries, although Bright-See and McKeown-Eyssen[23] calculated fiber intakes from food balance sheets which are summarized in Table 7.2.7. Calculated intakes were higher in the two maize-eating areas, Costa Rica and Mexico. In wheat and rice areas, fiber intakes were similar to North America, although there was a wide variation; Uruguayan intakes were 20 g/d, whereas those in Chile were 35 g.[23]

The Middle East

Data from food balance sheets and individual surveys are available for Israel. Food balance sheet data suggest that intakes are comparatively high, at 38 g/d (Table 7.2.7). Intakes assessed by interviews of 250 adults aged over 40 years were lower, 19 ± 6 g in Tel Aviv, and 31 ± 11 g and 23 ± 8 g in two rural Kibbutz areas.[66]

CONCLUSIONS

Current evidence indicates that average dietary fiber intake is in the range of 20 to 40 g/d in the majority of populations studied throughout the world. Evidence from Japan and India suggests that in areas where rice is the staple cereal, intakes of dietary fiber are likely to be similar to those in the West. The most accurate data using newer values for the fiber analysis of foods confirm this, with average intakes of 11 to 12 g in Japan, the US, and the UK. Worldwide, newer analyses show that there is only a small range in intake to a maximum of 16 to 18 g/d in Finland.

Trends in dietary fiber intake in Holland, Denmark, and Japan are similar to those reported in the US and Britain, namely a decline in cereal fiber consumption which has been offset to some extent by an increase in vegetable consumption. Relatively little data is available, however, and for some areas, such as parts of Asia, most of the Middle East, and Russia, there is no data at all due partly to continuing problems in the analysis of dietary fiber and the assessment of food consumption. More carefully standardized and validated studies to assess dietary fiber intake worldwide are clearly needed.

REFERENCES

1. WHO, *Diet, Nutrition and Chronic Diseases*, Tech. Rep. Set. 797, World Health Organization, Geneva, 1990.
2. *COMA Report on DRV for Food Energy and Nutrients for the UK*, D. H. Rep. Health Soc. Subj. 41, Her Majesty's Stationery Office, London, 1991.
3. *Recommended Dietary Allowances 10th Edition*, Food and Nutrition Board Sub-Committee on the Tenth Edition of the RDAs, National Academic Press, 1989.
4. Paul, A. A. and Southgate, D. A. T., *McCance and Widdowson's The Composition of Foods*, 4th ed., MRC Spec. Rep. 297, Her Majesty's Stationery Office, London, 1978.
5. Holland, B., Unwin, I. D., and Buss, D. H., *Cereals and Cereal Products*, 3rd Suppl., Royal Society of Chemistry, Letchworth, UK, 1988.
6. Holland, B., Unwin, I. D., and Buss, D. H., *Vegetables, Herbs and Spices*, 5th Suppl., Royal Society of Chemistry, Letchworth, UK, 1991.
7. Lanza, E., Jones, Y., Block, G., and Kessler, L., Dietary fiber intakes in the US population, *Am. J. Clin. Nutr.*, 46, 790, 1987.
8. Lanza, E. and Butrum, R., A critical review of fiber analysis and data, *J. Am. Diet. Assoc.*, 86, 732, 1986.
9. Ministry of Agriculture, Fisheries and Food, *Household Food Consumption and Expenditure 1966*, Annual Reports of National Food Survey Committee, Her Majesty's Stationery Office, London, 1968.
10. Bingham, S., The dietary assessment of individuals, *Nutr. Abs. Rev.*, 57, 705, 1987.
11. Bingham, S., Validations of dietary assessment through biomarkers, in *Biomarkers of Dietary Exposure,* Kok, F. J. and van't Voer, P., Eds., Smith-Gordon, London, 1991.
12. Bingham, S. and Westerterp, K. R., Energy expenditure as a biomarker of energy intake: workshop report, in *Biomarkers of Dietary Exposure*, Kok, F. J. and van't Voer, P., Eds., Smith-Gordon, 1991.
13. Varo, P., Laine, R., Veijalainen, K., Pero, K., and Koivistoinen, P., Dietary fibre and available carbohydrates in Finnish cereal products, vegetables and fruits, *J. Agric. Sci. Finland*, 56, 39, 1984.
14. IARC, Report of the Second IARC Coordinated International Study on Diet and Large Bowel Cancer in Denmark and Finland, *Nutr. Cancer*, 4, 3, 1982.
15. Bingham, S. A., Williams, D. R. R., and Cummings, J. H., Dietary fibre consumption: new estimates and their relation to large bowel cancer mortality in Britain, *Br. J. Cancer*, 52, 399, 1985.
16. Bingham, S. A., Pett, S., and Day, K. C., Non-starch polysaccharide intake of a representative sample of British adults, *J. Hum. Nutr. Dietet.*, 3, 333, 1990.

17. Bingham, S. A., unpublished.
18. Kuratsune, M., Honda, T., Englyst, H. N., and Cummings, J. H., Dietary fiber in the Japanese diet as investigated in connection with colon cancer risk, *Jpn. J. Cancer Res.*, 77, 736, 1986.
19. Stephen, A. M., New perspectives on carbohydrates, *Can. Pharm. J.*, October, 443, 1990.
20. Segal, I. and Walker, A. R. P., Low fat intake with falling fiber intake in Soweto, *Nutr. Cancer*, 8, 185, 1986.
21. Heller, S. N. and Hackler, L. R., Changes in the crude fibre content of the American diet, *Am. J. Clin. Nutr.*, 31, 1510, 1978. (Data recalculated by S. Kingman, personal communication.)
22. Rider, A. A., Arthur, R. S., and Calkins, B. M., Laboratory analysis of 3 day composite food samples, *Am. J. Clin. Nutr.*, 40, 914, 1984. Reanalysis of composites, with Englyst method (Englyst, personal communication).
23. Bright-See, E. and McKeown-Eyssen, G. E., Estimates of dietary fibre supply in 38 countries, *Am. J. Clin. Nutr.*, 39, 821, 1985; 41, 824, 1985.
24. Gregory, J., Foster, K., Tyler, H., and Wiseman, M., The dietary and nutritional survey of British adults, OPCS: Her Majesty's Stationery Office, London, 1990.
25. Bingham, S., Cummings, J. H., and McNeil, N. I., Intakes and sources of dietary fiber in the British population, *Am. J. Clin. Nutr.*, 32, 1313, 1979.
26. Yarnell, J. W. G., Fehilly, A. M., Milbank, J. E., Sweetnam, P. M., and Walker, C. L., A short dietary questionnaire for use in an epidemiological study, *Hum. Nutr. Appl. Nutr.*, 37A, 103, 1983.
27. Thompson, M., Logan, R. L., Sharman, M., Lockerbie, L., Riemersma, R. A., and Oliver, M. F., Dietary survey in 40 year old Edinburgh men, *Hum. Nutr. Appl. Nutr.*, 36A, 272, 1982.
28. Bull, N. L., Smart, G. A., and Judson, H., Food and nutrient intakes on Westray in the Orkney Islands, *Ecol. Food. Nutr.*, 12, 97, 1982.
29. Barker, M. E. et al., Diet, lifestyle and health in Northern Ireland, University of Ulster, N. Ireland, 1989.
30. Van Staveren, W. A., Hautvast, J. G. A., Katan, M. B., van Montfort, M. A., and van Oosten-van der Goes, H. G. C., Dietary fiber consumption in an adult Dutch population, *J. Am. Dietet. Assoc.*, 80, 324, 1982.
31. Kromhout, D., Bosschieter, E. B., and Coulander, C., Dietary fiber and 10 year mortality in the Zutphen study, Lancet, 2, 518, 1982.
32. Bingham, S., Cummings, J. H., Cole, T. J., Helms, P., and Seppanen, R., Individual variation in dietary fibre intake in different populations, in *Fibre Hum. Nutr.*, Bulletin 20, Royal Society of New Zealand, Wellington, N.Z., 1983, 33.
33. Englyst, H. N., Bingham, S. A., Wiggins, H. S., Southgate, D. A. T., Seppanen, R., Helms, P., Anderson, V., Day, K. C., Choolun, R., Collinson, E., and Cummings, J. H., Non-starch polysaccharide consumption in four Scandinavian populations, *Nutr. Cancer*, 4, 50, 1982.
34. Bingham, S. and Cummings, J. H., Intakes and sources of dietary fibre in man, in *Medical Aspects of Dietary Fibre*, Spiller, G. A. and Kay, R. M., Eds., Plenum Press, New York, 1980, 261.
35. Buzina, R., Ferber, E., Keys, A., Brodavec, A., Agneletto, B., and Horvat, A., Diets of rural families and heads of families in two regions of Yugoslavia, *Voeding*, 25, 629, 1964.
36. Englyst, H., The determination of carbohydrate and its composition in plant material, in *The Analysis of Dietary Fibre in Food*, James, W. P. T. and Theander, O., Eds., Marcel Dekker, New York, 1981.
37. Hellendoorn, E. W., Noordhoff, M. G., and Slagman, J., Enzymatic determination of the indigestible residue content of human food, *J. Sci. Food Agric.*, 26, 1461, 1975.
38. Katan, N. and van de Bovenkamp, P., Determination of total dietary fiber by difference and of pectin by titration or copper titration, in *The Analysis of Dietary Fiber in Food*, James, W. P. T. and Theander, O., Eds., Marcel Dekker, New York, 1981.
39. Wenlock, R. W., Sivell, L. M., and Agater, J. B., Dietary fiber fractions in cereal products in Britain, *J. Sci. Food Agric.*, 36, 113, 1985.
40. Cresta, M., Ledermann, S., Gardiner, A., Lombardo, E., and Lacourly, G., A dietary survey of 11 areas of the E.E.C. in order to determine levels of radioactive contamination, *Euratom*, EUR.4218F, 1969.
41. Ministry of Agriculture, Fisheries and Food, *Household Food Consumption and Expenditure, 1950–1981.* Annual reports of the National Food Survey Committee, Her Majesty's Stationery Office, London, 1953-1983.
42. Southgate, D. A. T., Bingham, S., and Robertson, J., Dietary fibre in the British diet, *Nature (London)*, 274, 51, 1978.

43. Helms, P., Jorgensen, I. M., Paerregaard, A., Bjerrum, L., Poulson, L., and Mosbech, J., Dietary patterns in Them and Copenhagen, Denmark, *Nutr. Cancer*, 4, 23, 1982.

44. Bingham, S., Patterns of dietary fiber consumption in humans, in *CRC Handbook of Dietary Fiber in Human Nutrition*, Spiller, G., Ed., CRC Press, Boca Raton, FL, 1986.

45. Orr, J. B. and Gilks, J. L., *Studies of Nutrition, The Physique and Health of Two African Tribes*, M. R. C. Spec. Rep. Ser. 155, Her Majesty's Stationery Office, London, 1931.

46. Platt, B. S., Unpublished report on Nyasaland held at London School of Hygiene and Tropical Medicine, London, 1938/39.

47. Jones, S., *A Study of Swazi Nutrition*, Report for the University of Natal for the Swaziland Government (not dated).

48. Ruitishauser, I., personal communication, 1977.

49. Mbofung, C. N., Atinmo, T., and Omolulu, A., Dietary fiber in the diets of urban and rural Nigerian women, *Nutr. Res.*, 4, 225, 1984.

50. Shetty, P. S., Dietary fibre intakes in India, Proc. Annual Conf. Ind. Soc. Gastrol., Trivandrum, 1981.

51. Stace, N. H., Pomare, E. W., Peters, S., Thomas, L., and Fisher, A., *Gastroenterology*, 89, 1291, 1981.

52. Pomare, E. W., Stace, N. H., Peters, S. G., and Fisher, A., Dietary intakes, stool characteristics and biliary bile acid composition in four South Pacific populations, in *Fibre in Human and Animal Nutrition*, Bulletin 20, Royal Society of New Zealand, Wellington, N.Z., 1983, 33.

53. Hillman, L. C., Stace, N. J., Fisher, A., and Pomare, E. W., Dietary intakes and stool characteristics of patients with the irritable bowel syndrome, *Am. J. Clin. Nutr.*, 36, 626, 1982.

54. Prior, I. A., Davidson, F., Salmond, C. E., and Czochanska, Z., The Pukapuka and Tokelau Island studies, *Am. J. Clin. Nutr.*, 34, 1552, 1981.

55. Potter, J. D., McMichael, A. J., and Bonnett, A. J., A case control study of colorectal cancer in South Australia, in *Fibre in Human and Animal Nutrition*, Bulletin 20, Royal Society of New Zealand, Wellington, N.Z., 1983, 35.

56. Haenszel, W. and Kurihara, M., Studies of Japanese migrants mortality from cancer and other diseases among Japanese in the United States, *J. Natl. Cancer Inst.*, 40, 43, 1968.

57. Minowa, M., Bingham, S., and Cummings, J. H., Dietary fibre intake in Japan, *Hum. Nutr.*, 37A, 113, 1983.

58. Mori, B. and Aragane, K., On the determination of dietary fibre, *Nutr. Food*, 34, 97, 1981.

59. Nakamura, H., Tamura, A., Tanaka, H., Natsushita, C., Yamamoto, F., Yoshi, S., and Izumi, D., Dietary fibre content of foodstuffs for diabetes, *Nutr. Food*, 34, 71, 1981.

60. Marlett, J. A. and Bokram, R. L., Relationship between calculated and crude fiber intakes of 200 college students, *Am. J. Clin. Nutr.*, 34, 335, 1981.

61. Ahrens, E. H. and Boucher, C. A., The composition of a simulated American diet, *J. Am. Dietet. Assoc.*, 73, 613, 1978.

62. Kay, R. M., Sabry, Z. I., and Csima, A., Multivariate analysis of diet and serum lipids in normal men, *Am. J. Clin. Nutr.*, 33, 2566, 1980.

63. Gibson, R. S. and Scythes, C. A., Trace element intakes of women, *Br. J. Nutr.*, 48, 241, 1982.

64. Willett, W. C., Stampfer, M. J., Colditz, G. A., Rosner, B. A., and Speizer, F. E., Relation of meat, fat and fiber intake to risk of colon cancer, *New Engl. J. Med.*, 323, 1664, 1990.

65. Heilbrun, L. K., Nomura, A., Hankin, J., and Stemmerman, G. N., Diet and colorectal cancer with special reference to fiber intake, *Int. J. Cancer*, 44, 1, 1989.

66. Rozen, P., Horwitz, C., Takenkin, C., Ron, E., and Katz, L., Dietary habits and colorectal cancer incidence in a second-defined Kibbutz population, *Nutr. Cancer*, 9, 177, 1987.

Dietary Fiber, Nonstarch Polysaccharide, and Resistant Starch Intakes in Australia

Katrine I. Baghurst, Peter A. Baghurst, and Sally J. Record

INTRODUCTION

Until the early to mid-1980s, the only nationally based information about dietary fiber intake in the Australian population came from the apparent consumption or food disappearance data collected by the Australian Bureau of Statistics. The only data available from direct survey of individuals was on selected, and usually small, subpopulations and, furthermore, Australian databases were limited, so survey analyses relied on British food databases.

In 1987, the Life Sciences Research Office of the Federation of American Societies for Experimental Biology[1] adopted a definition of dietary fiber as "the endogenous components of plant materials in the diet which are resistant to digestion by enzymes produced by humans." As pointed out by Southgate,[2] this definition is virtually identical to that for "unavailable carbohydrates" as originally defined by McCance and Lawrence in 1929.[3] It can be considered to include some components of what is now known as "resistant starch." One difficulty with the word "endogenous" in this definition is that it excludes, for example, those forms of resistant starch that arise as a consequence of cooking and processing techniques. It also excludes substances which are intimately associated with the major components of dietary fiber and which are capable of having important nutritional and/or physiological effects such as phytates, lectins, saponins, non-polymeric polyphenols, and inorganic constituents.

In the absence of a consensus, a *de facto* working definition of the term "dietary fiber" appears to be emerging which includes all nonstarch polysaccharides and lignin from plants.

The earlier surveys of the Australian population[4-16] were limited to an estimate of total dietary fiber using the definition of the time. Since 1983, several national or statewide, randomized surveys of the Australian population have been undertaken[17-23] and, where assessed, the data is given for dietary fiber, nonstarch polysaccharide, and resistant starch intake.

METHODOLOGIES

The subjects and methodologies employed in the surveys described here are shown in the relevant tables alongside the relevant intake data. Many of the studies used traditional techniques such as 24-hour recall or record, 3-day records, or diet history which will not be detailed here, but a large number of the surveys employed a variation of the quantitative food-frequency technique developed by the CSIRO Division of Human Nutrition.[24] As with the methodologies used, the techniques for sampling varied widely, as detailed in the tables. Many of the random surveys, in particular those conducted by the CSIRO, used a random selection procedure based on the Electoral Rolls of the States of the Commonwealth.

RESULTS AND DISCUSSION

Tables 7.3.1 and 7.3.2 show the dietary fiber intakes and the group mean fiber-to-energy ratios from selected non-randomized surveys from the late 1970s and early 1980s,[4–16] and from randomized population surveys carried out by the Commonwealth Government and the CSIRO Division of Health Sciences and Nutrition since 1983.[17–23] Assessment of trends over time is difficult because of the non-random nature of earlier surveys and the variety of measurement techniques employed. However, if the more generally representative data from the earlier period are used for comparative purposes, it does appear that dietary fiber intake has increased over the past 20 years or so by about 50%, from 17–18 g/day in the late 1970s to 24–28 g/day in the mid-1990s.

Data from the CSIRO National Dietary Surveys (adults only, aged 18 yr plus) of 1988 and 1993 showed that, while fiber continued to increase over the period, the increases were much smaller than had been observed from the late 1970s to late 1980s. In the 1993 survey, intakes of women increased with age and occupational status, but this was not evident in men. Between 1988 and 1993, there was a small increase in the number of people reaching the target of 30 g/day recommended by the Commonwealth Department of Health. The increase was most marked in the older age groups, for women in the highest occupational group, and for men from the lowest occupational group. However, well under half the population still failed to reach recommended intakes.

Figure 7.3.1 shows the percentiles of intake of dietary fiber as well as NSP and resistant starch in the 1993 CSIRO survey.

The more recent random surveys of adults indicate that approximately 33% of dietary fiber is currently provided by cereals, 31% by vegetables, and 20% by fruit (Table 7.3.3). When comparing the CSIRO National Dietary Surveys of 1988 and 1993, the percentage of fiber provided by vegetables had decreased, particularly for people in the top occupational group, while the yield from breakfast cereal, fruit and fruit juice, and the processed meat categories increased. Breakfast cereals were a more important source of dietary fiber in older people and for people of upper-occupational status.

The figures for adults indicate an increasing relative contribution to total fiber intake from the cereal group over the last decade and a lessening of the relative contribution of vegetables and, to a lesser extent, fruit.

Until recently, there was a paucity of data on dietary fiber intakes of young children in Australia apart from smaller, non-random population groups. However, the 1995/6 National Nutrition Survey of the Commonwealth Department of Health and Aged Care showed intakes of 13.4 g/day in 2–3-year-olds rising to 16.0 g at 4–7 years, 18.8 g at 8–11 years, 21.4 g at 12–15 years, and 23.0 g/day at 16–18 years of age.

NONSTARCH POLYSACCHARIDES

Tables 7.3.4 and 7.3.5 show the intakes and major food sources of total nonstarch soluble and insoluble polysaccharides in the CSIRO National Dietary Surveys of Adults (1988 and 1993). In general, the intake of NSP mirrored that of total dietary fiber, as assessed using the Southgate

Table 7.3.1   Mean Daily Fiber and Energy Intakes in Selected, Non-Random Australian Population Samples from 1977 to 1995

Survey	Sex	No.	Method	Energy (MJ/day)	Fiber (g/day)	Fiber/Energy Ratio[a]
Urban community[4]	M	481	FFQ	9.9	20.2	20.4
(random within age bands)	F	441		7.5	19.5	26.0
Fitness intervention group[5]	M	581	FFQ	9.0	21.8	24.2
	F	454		7.2	22.7	31.5
Public servants[6]	M	142	FFQ	8.8	22.4	25.4
	F	60		7.3	22.8	31.2
Parents of 10-yr-olds[7]	M	300	FFQ	10.1	24.2	24.2
	F	300		7.83	23.5	30.0
10-yr-old children of above group[7]	M and F	300	FFQ	7.76	21.5	27.7
Children, urban SA[8]						
11 yr	M	124	4-day record	8.5	17.0	20.4
	F	106		7.4	15.0	20.0
13 yr	M	121		9.0	19.0	21.3
	F	116		7.2	15.0	21.1
15 yr	M	104		9.9	21.0	21.6
	F	104		6.9	15.0	21.3
Children urban WA[9]						
11 yr	M		24-hr. record	8.4	18.0	21.4
	F			7.6	15.0	19.7
12 yr	M			8.6	19	22.1
	F			7.5	17	22.7
Rural children SA[10]	M	161	FFQ	10.5	24.9	23.7
aged 13 yr	F	172		9.8	24.4	25.0
Urban adolescents SA	M	72	FFQ	12.0	19.5	16.3
14–15 yr[4]	F	69		9.4	18.9	20.1
Pregnant women[11]	F	91	3-day record	9.1	22.0	24.2
Elderly						
Community[12]	M and F	27	Hist.	8.0	20.9	26.1
Institutionalized[13]	M and F	87	3-day record	7.4	11.8	15.9
Nursing home[14]	M and F	30		6.5	13.7	21.1
Religious groups[15]						
Adventist (vegetarian)	M ⎫ F ⎭	98	24-hr. record	⎧ 11.0 ⎩ 8.6	44.3 32.6	40.3 37.9
Adventist (omnivore)	M ⎫ F ⎭	82	24-hr. record	⎧ 10.5 ⎩ 8.0	41.4 27.1	39.4 33.9
Mormon (omnivore)	M ⎫ F ⎭	113	24-hr. record	⎧ 11.6 ⎩ 8.4	24.3 19.7	20.9 23.4
Vietnamese migrants[16]	F	200	24-hr. record	7.53	15.5	20.6

[a] Group mean ratio g fiber/10 MJ.

method, with a mean intake in 1993 of some 21 g/day for both adult men and women. Insoluble NSP accounted for about 12 g of the total, and soluble accounted for some 9 g.

RESISTANT STARCH

To estimate current resistant starch intakes in Australia, a food database was constructed using analytical data presented at the EURESTA[25] meeting and from published figures. Because of the small amount of available data, the varying techniques used to assess resistant starch, and a number of inconsistencies in existing databases, care should be taken in interpreting the data. It is likely

Table 7.3.2   Random Surveys of Australian Population Samples from 1983 to 1995

Survey	Sex	No.	Method	Energy (MJ/day)	Fiber (g/day)	Fiber/Energy Ratio[a] (fiber/10 MJ)
Commonwealth Government Surveys						
National Adults Survey[b]	M	3021	24-hr. recall	11.0	23.2	21.1
1983 (25–64 yr.)[16]	F	3234		7.4	18.7	25.3
National schoolchildren's	M (10–11 yr)	912	24-hr. record	8.3	18.0	21.7
survey 1985[17]	M (12–15 yr)	1719		10.3	21.5	20.9
	F (10–11 yr)	925		7.2	15.4	21.4
	F (12–15 yr)	1668		7.7	17.0	22.0
National Nutrition Survey	M	5079	24-hr. recall	11.0	25.9	23.3
1995/6 (19+ yr.)[18]	F	5770		7.48	20.3	27.1
CSIRO Surveys						
Victorian State surveys (18+ yr.)[19]						
1985	M	1321	FFQ	9.4	23.6	25.1
	F	1595		7.6	24.2	31.9
1990	M	1321	FFQ	10.0	27.3	27.3
	F	1595		8.1	27.1	33.5
South Australian State surveys (18+ yr.)[20]						
1988	M	445	FFQ	10.5	26.4	25.3
	F	456		8.0	26.0	32.4
1990	M	445	FFQ	10.3	26.8	25.9
	F	456		8.3	27.2	32.8
1993	M	445	FFQ	10.3	28.3	27.5
	F	456		7.9	26.0	34.3
National Dietary Surveys (18+ yr.)[21]						
1988	M	1115	FFQ	10.4	27.9	26.8
	F	1200		8.2	26.7	32.4
1993	M	736	FFQ	10.1	32.7	32.4
	F	997		8.0	28.0	34.8
National Elderly Survey	M	606	FFQ	9.1	28.2	31.1
(55–75 yr.) 1989/90[22]	F	707		7.9	29.7	37.8

[a] Group mean ratio.
[b] Metropolitan sample only.

that some of the analyses based on chemical assessment of resistance might underestimate resistance in the human gut and that much individual variation will occur with respect to physiological functions such as degree of chewing foods, etc. The composite food database was used to estimate intakes using data collected from the CSIRO Food & Nutrition Surveys of 1988 and 1993 and the Commonwealth Department of Health's National Dietary Survey of Adults undertaken in 1983 and of Schoolchildren undertaken in 1985.

The analysis of the 1988 and 1993 CSIRO National Dietary Surveys gave a mean figure of about 5.3 g/day of resistant starch for men and 5.0 g/day for women in 1993, rising from 4.9 g in 1988 for men and 4.4 g in 1988 for women (Table 7.3.6). There was little evidence of any age- or occupation-related trends in the density of resistant starch in the diet. Resistant starch density in 1993 was some 5.4 g per 10 MJ in men and 6.3 g per 10 MJ in women, with approximately 4% of starch in men and 4.7% in women being resistant.

Table 7.3.7 shows the estimate of NSP plus resistant starch from the 1993 survey, showing an average for these combined components of 26.7 g/day in men and 26.2 g in women. The main

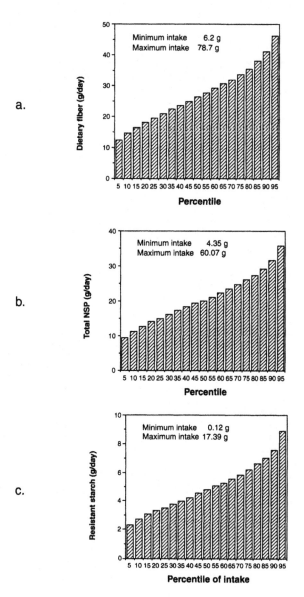

Figure 7.3.1 Percentiles of intake for dietary fiber, nonstarch polysaccharides, and resistant starch in the Australian population.

sources of resistant starch found in the 1988 and 1993 CSIRO surveys of adults are shown in Table 7.3.8. About 42% of resistant starch was provided by cereals, with 26% from vegetables and 22% from fruit and fruit juice. A re-analysis of the 1983 and 1985 CDH National Dietary Surveys of Adults and Schoolchildren gave estimates of resistant starch intakes ranging from 5.2 g/day in younger men to 4.0 g in older men and from 3.2 g/day in younger women to 2.7 g/day in older women in 1983. At that time, for adults, the density of resistant starch seems to have approximated 4.2 g per 10 MJ or 3.1 g per 100 g starch.

For children, intakes rose from 4 g/day in 10-year-old boys to 5.6 g/day in 15-year-old boys. In girls, there was no consistent age trend, with intakes ranging from 3.4 to 3.7 g/day across age categories. This equated in both girls and boys to about 3.2% of starch being resistant, with a resistant starch density of some 4.7–4.8 g per 10 MJ energy.

Table 7.3.3 Sources of Dietary Fiber in the Australian Population

| | Percentage of Total Dietary Fiber Derived from Food Groups | | | | | |
| | Cereals | Vegetables | | | Fruit | Other[a] |
Survey		Brassica and Green-Leafy	Legumes, Peas, and Beans	Total		
Urban community samples 1978–83 (CSIRO)	32.8	4.7	13.2	37.2	23.3	6.7
DCSH National Adults 1983	37.2	6.9	8.6	32.9	20.0	9.9
DCSH National School-children's 1985	39.0	2.3	8.5	26.3	17.4	17.3
CSIRO National Survey 1993	33.2	4.5	5.9	30.6	20.2	15.9

[a] Includes composite dishes such as pies, pizzas, etc.; snack foods; beverages; nuts; and seeds.

Source: Department of Community Services and Health (DCSH).

Table 7.3.4 CSIRO National Dietary Surveys — Dietary Fiber[a] and Nonstarch Polysaccharide (NSP) Intakes and Densities

| | Men | | Women | |
	1988	1993	1988	1993
Intake (g/day)				
Dietary fiber	27.0	27.7	25.9	27.3
Total NSP	20.7	21.4	20.1	21.2
Soluble NSP	8.9	9.2	8.6	9.1
Insoluble NSP	11.8	12.1	11.5	12.1
Density (g/10 MJ)				
Dietary fiber	26.8	28.4	32.4	34.8
Total NSP	20.6	22.0	25.2	27.1
Soluble NSP	8.8	9.5	10.8	11.6
Insoluble NSP	11.8	12.5	14.5	15.5

[a] As measured by Southgate method.

Table 7.3.5 Food Sources of Nonstarch Polysaccharides from CSIRO National Dietary Surveys of Australian Adults 1993 (percentage contribution of food groups)

Food Sources	Total NSP	Soluble NSP	Insoluble NSP
Breakfast cereals	8	7	9
Breads and crackers	18	16	20
Rice and pasta	5	3	6
Fruit and fruit juice	20	24	17
Vegetables	34	24	34
Processed meats and cooked meat dishes	5	5	5
Confectionery, cakes, and biscuits	7	7	7
Takeaways and snacks	3	4	3

Table 7.3.6   Resistant Starch Intakes and Densities by Demographics from CSIRO National Surveys

	Intake (g/day)					Density (g/10 MJ)			
	M 1988	M 1993	F 1988	F 1993		M 1988	M 1993	F 1988	F 1993
Age									
18–29	5.20	6.11	4.41	5.06		4.63	5.38	5.17	6.36
30–39	4.66	5.28	4.50	5.10		4.85	5.26	5.30	6.12
40–49	4.91	4.98	4.61	5.05		4.95	5.26	5.40	6.25
50–59	5.30	4.99	3.94	4.81		5.25	5.41	5.3	6.57
60+	4.63	4.88	4.34	4.70		5.01	5.76	5.73	6.12
Occupation									
Top	4.92	4.96	4.53	5.45		5.13	5.19	5.40	6.63
2nd	4.73	5.58	4.38	4.78		4.51	5.48	5.31	5.87
3rd	5.05	5.63	4.69	4.91		4.94	5.35	5.16	6.46
4th	4.52	5.57	4.17	4.92		4.72	5.26	5.16	6.08
5th	5.12	5.67	4.09	5.05		4.74	5.30	5.35	6.56

Table 7.3.7   Sum of Intake of Resistant Starch and NSPs from CSIRO National Survey 1993

	Men (g/day)	Women (g/day)
Total	26.7	26.2
Age		
18–29	28.5	24.5
30–39	26.5	26.2
40–49	25.8	26.6
50–59	25.2	26.1
60+	26.5	27.5
Occupation		
Top	26.7	28.7
2nd	26.8	26.6
3rd	27.9	24.3
4th	25.4	24.8
5th	28.1	24.4

Table 7.3.8   Sources of Resistant Starch % Contribution to Total Intake

	1988	1993
Breads and crackers	26.9	24.7
Vegetables	26.6	26.1
Fruit and fruit juice	21.8	22.3
Rice and pasta	8.7	11.6
Breakfast cereals	4.8	5.7
Takeaways and snacks	4.2	3.6
Processed meats +	3.8	2.6
Confectionery +	2.1	2.2
Dairy and ice cream	0.5	0.5
Chicken and fish +	0.4	0.4
Drinks	0.1	0.0
Spreads and sauces	0.0	0.3
Red and organ meat	0.0	0.0

COMPARISONS OF AUSTRALIAN RS INTAKE WITH OTHER COUNTRIES

Estimates of resistant starch intake in developed countries vary widely in the literature, with figures ranging from 3–4 g/day to 15–20 g/day. Estimates for developing countries range from 9–10 g/day to 30–40 g/day for countries with high starch intake. The range of estimates reflects the fact that some estimates relate only to retrograded starch; others attempt to include an estimate of all possible forms of resistant starch. A recent data-based analysis reported at the EURESTA summary meeting in 1994 gave intakes ranging from 3.5 to 6.0 g/day for a number of European countries. The estimates of Australian intakes show them to be at the upper end of the European range.

A more detailed review of dietary fiber, nonstarch polysaccharide, and resistant starch intakes in Australia and New Zealand was published in 1996 and is available from the authors.[26]

REFERENCES

1. Life Sciences Research Office, *Physiological Effects and Health Consequences of Dietary Fibre*, Federation of American Societies for Experimental Biology, Bethesda, MD, 1987.
2. Southgate, D. A. T., *Determination of Food Carbohydrates*, Elsevier Science, Essex, U.K., 1991.
3. McCance, R. A. and Lawrence, R. D., *The Carbohydrate Content of Foods*, MRC Special Report Series no. 135, HMSO, London, 1929.
4. Baghurst, K. I. and Record, S. J., Intake and sources, in selected Australian subpopulations, of dietary constituents implicated in the aetiology of chronic disease, *J. Food Nutr.*, 40, 1, 1983.
5. Baghurst, K. I., Sedgwick, A. W., and Strohm, K., Nutritional profile of recruits to a fitness program, *Med. J. Aust.*, 143, 188, 1985.
6. Baghurst, K. I. and Record, S. J., Dietary intakes of public servants, unpublished data, 1983.
7. Syrette, J. A. and Baghurst, K. I., Dietary intake of ten-year-old children and their parents with respect to occupational status, *Proc. Nutr. Soc. Aust.*, 12, 160, 1987.
8. Magarey, A. and Boulton, J., The Adelaide Nutrition Study. 2. Macronutrient and micronutrient intakes at ages 11, 13, and 15 years: age and sex differences, *Aust. J. Nutr. Diet*, 51:3, 111, 1994.
9. Jenner, D. and Miller, M., Intakes of selected nutrients in Year 7 Western Australian schoolchildren; comparisons between weekdays and relationships with socioeconomic status, *Aust. J. Nutr. Diet*, 48 (9), 50, 1991.
10. Baghurst, K. I., Baghurst, P. A., and Record, S. J., Dietary intakes of children in Port Pirie, unpublished data, 1988.
11. Ash, S., unpublished data.
12. Flint, D. M., Wahlquist, M., Parish, A. E., and Smith, T. J., Dietary fiber intakes of elderly Australians, in *Fibre in Human and Animal Nutrition*, Wallace, G. and Bell, L., Eds., Royal Society of New Zealand, 1983, 33.
13. Flint, D. M., unpublished data.
14. Baghurst, K. I., Hope, A., and Down, E., Dietary fibre intake in a group of institutionalised elderly and the effect of a fibre supplementation program on nutrient intake and weight gain, *Comm. Hlth. Stud.*, 9, 99, 1985.
15. Rouse, I. L., Armstrong, B. K., and Beilin, L. J., The relationship of blood pressure to diet and lifestyle in two religious populations, *J. Hypertension*, 1, 65, 1983.
16. Baghurst, K. I., Syrette, J. A., and Tran, M. M., Dietary profile of Vietnamese migrant women in Australia, *Nutr. Res.*, 11, 715, 1991.
17. English, R., Cashel, K., Bennett, S., Berzins, J., Waters, A.-M., and Magnus, P., *National Dietary Survey of Adults: 1983. 2. Nutrient Intakes*, AGPS, Canberra, Australia, 1987.
18. English, R., Cashel, K., Lewis, J., Waters, A.-M., and Bennett, S., *National Dietary Survey of School-children (Aged 10-15 Years): 1985. 2. Nutrient Intakes*, AGPS, Canberra, Australia, 1989.
19. Commonwealth Department of Health and Aged Care and Australian Bureau of Statistics, *National Nutrition Survey 1995. Nutrient Intakes and Physical Measurements*, ABS, Canberra, Australia, 1998.
20. Baghurst, K. I., Record, S. J., and Syrette, J. A. et al., *What are Australians eating? Results from the 1985 and 1990 Victorian Nutrition Surveys*, CSIRO, Adelaide, Australia, 1993.

21. Baghurst, K. I., Record, S. J., Syrette, J. A., and Baghurst, P. A., *Nutrition in South Australia from 1988 to 1993*, CSIRO, Adelaide, Australia, 1989.

22. Baghurst, K. I., Record, S. J., Baghurst, P. A., Syrette, J. A., and Powis, G., *Food and Nutrition in Australia — Does Five Years Make a Difference. Results from the CSIRO Australian Food and Nutrition Surveys, 1988 and 1993*, CSIRO, Adelaide, Australia, 1995.

23. Baghurst, K. I., Record, S. J., and Baghurst, P. A., *National Dietary Survey of the Elderly*, CSIRO, Adelaide, Australia, 1991.

24. Baghurst, K. I. and Record, S. J., A computerized dietary analysis system for use with diet diaries or food frequency questionnaires, *Comm. Health Stud.*, 8, 11, 1984.

25. EURESTA summary meeting, France, 1994.

26. Baghurst, P. A., Baghurst, K. I., and Record, S. J., Dietary fibre, nonstarch polysaccharides and resistant starch: a review, *Food Australia*, March suppl., s1-36, 1996.

Consumption of Dietary Fiber–Rich Foods in China

Zhi-Ping Shen and Su-Fang Zheng

China is a big country with great varieties of foodstuffs. However, the most important components of the daily diets are grains and cereals, which provide about 80% of the daily caloric intake. In south China, the predominant grain is rice and in the north, the main staple foods are wheat and coarse grains including corn, millet, sorghum, etc. The amount and varieties of plant subsidiary foods are dependent on the climate. In general, Chinese diets are rich in vegetables. The supply of staple and nonstaple food varies in amount and varieties with season. National nutrition surveys carried out in China in 1959 and 1982 indicate that the consumption pattern of plant foods and crude fiber intake differ in different parts of China, as shown in Table 7.4.1. Crude fiber is mainly from cereal grains and vegetables. The data in Table 7.4.2 indicate the contribution of crude fiber from various foods in north China peasant diets[1] as calculated by Zheng from the annual dietary surveys in 1979. The crude fiber content of the Chinese daily diet is much higher than the daily crude fiber intake in England, which was estimated to be about 4 g per capita.[2] The age-adjusted death rate for colorectal cancer in China was 5.49 per 100,000 in 1979, the second-lowest in the world.[3]

The Chinese government has stipulated the standard of rice milling and wheat flour extraction in order to retain more nutrients. Table 7.4.3 lists the crude fiber contents of processed rice and wheat.[4]

The comparison between crude fiber and neutral detergent fiber contents in selected Chinese foods is listed in Table 7.4.4.[5]

0-8493-2387-8/01/$0.00+$1.50

Table 7.4.1 Consumption Pattern of Fiber-Containing Foods and Crude Fiber Intake in Different Parts of China (Grams/Day/Capita)

	Beijing North	Shanghai South	Jiangxi South	Hebei North	Shanxi North	Gansu Northwest
Food						
Rice	90	463	558	13	11	3
Wheat flour	314	44	13	350	173	610
Coarse grains	125	—	—	252	344	49
Starchy tubers	35	43	110	97	352	149
Legumes, dried	8	4	9	3	21	5
Vegetables	440	326	383	280	305	147
Fruits	82	9	1	30	13	34
Nuts	4	1	1	2	1	—
Crude fiber	8.5	6.9	7.7	9.3	11.3	6.6

Table 7.4.2　Contribution of Crude Fiber from Various Foods in North China Peasant Daily Diets

	Linxian County, Henan			Xianxiang County, Henan		
Food	Consumption (g)	Crude Fiber (g)	Contribution (%)	Consumption (g)	Crude Fiber (g)	Contribution (%)
Rice	13	0.06	0.5	66	0.29	2.7
Wheat flour	250	1.46	11.2	456	2.66	24.4
Coarse grains	300	4.47	34.2	225	0.02	26.3
Starchy tubers	646	2.76	21.1	11	0.42	0.2
Legumes	21	0.81	6.2	20	4.06	3.8
Vegetables	583	3.44	26.2	830	0.52	37.2
Fruits	3	0.03	0.2	85	—	4.8
Nuts	1	0.02	0.2	—	0.07	—
Seaweeds	—	—	—	1	—	0.6

Table 7.4.3　Crude Fiber Contents of Processed Cereal Grains in China

Rice, Long Grains		Wheat Flour	
Grade	Crude Fiber (g/100 g)	Extraction	Crude Fiber (g/100 g)
Husked	0.7	Whole	2.4
Fine	0.3	75% extraction	0.2
Standard, 1st	0.4	81% extraction	0.4
Standard, 2nd	0.5	85% extraction	0.6

Table 7.4.4 Comparison Between Crude Fiber and Neutral
Detergent Fiber Contents in Selected Chinese Foods

Food	C F	N D F
	(g/100 g dried edible portion)	
Cereals		
Corn	1.70	8.42
Corn meal	0.88	4.50
Millet	0.24	1.54
Sorghum	0.28	3.19
Rice, glutinous	0.13	0.49
Rice, long-grain	0.17	0.70
Rice, round-grain	0.11	0.24
Whole wheat flour	2.12	9.70
Legumes, dried		
Adsuki bean	3.90	8.41
Kidney bean	4.04	7.81
Mung bean	3.74	7.16
Soybean, green	3.74	10.43
Soybean, yellow	3.50	10.03
Vegetables		
Cabbage, celery	8.37	14.53
Cabbage, Chinese	10.94	18.21
Cabbage, common	7.90	18.55
Celery stem	11.79	18.20
Chive	8.99	14.30
Garlic green	11.42	17.40
Garlic shoot	8.89	10.38
Onion shallot	6.57	11.66
Spinach	8.04	21.38
Roots		
Carrot	6.57	11.66
Lotus root	2.36	7.03
Potato	1.59	3.48
Yam	1.23	4.09

REFERENCES

1. Zheng, S., The crude fiber intake of peasants in north China, unpublished.
2. Trowell, H., Definition of dietary fiber and hypothesis that it is a protective factor in certain diseases, *Am. J. Clin. Nutr.,* 29, 417, 1976.
3. Dai, X., Colorectal cancer, in *The Investigation of The Cancer Mortality in China* (in Chinese), The National Cancer Control Office of the Ministry of Health, Ed., People's Medical Publishing House, Beijing, 1979.
4. Institute of Health, Chinese Academy of Medical Sciences, *Food Composition Table* (in Chinese), 3rd ed., People's Medical Publishing House, Beijing, 1981.
5. Zao, Z., Comparison between crude fiber and dietary fiber contents in foods, *Acta Nutrimenta Simica,* 9, 333, 1989.

Consumption of Dietary Fiber in France (1950–1981)

Yves Le Quintrec

INTRODUCTION

Little has been published about the consumption of dietary fiber in France and, more generally, about food consumption. In this chapter we will make a distinction between direct and indirect methods for evaluating this consumption.

DIRECT METHOD OF EVALUATION

This method is based on dietary recall in a sample of people as representative as possible of the general population. The dietary fiber consumption can then be calculated by tables using the Paul-Southgate method[1] to obtain the total fiber consumption and not just the crude fiber consumption.

Three studies of this type have been published in France (Table 7.5.1). The results are identical in two studies, but in the third[4] the consumption of dietary fibers is far more important. This difference can be partly explained: in the first and second studies, the calculation of the dietary fiber content was made with Southgate's table,[1] which is based on English alimentation and, in particular, English bread; in the third study, the content of dietary fiber was calculated with a new analysis of fiber content carried out by Southgate himself on French bread and flour which showed a higher proportion of fiber in French products (Table 7.5.2). Therefore, while the consumption of cereal fiber is virtually the same in the three studies, the total consumption of fiber is higher in the study by Macquart-Moulin et al.[4]

Table 7.5.1 Average Daily Consumption of Dietary Fiber in France Calculated from Dietary Recall

	Total Dietary Fiber (g/day)	Cereal Fiber (g/day)	Ref.
Females	12.7 ± 5.8	3.6 ± 0.8	2
Females			
May	11.81 ± 1.88		
October	8.64 ± 0.70		3
Males			
May	10.61 ± 0.70		
October	8.34 ± 1.08		
Females	28.0 ± 7.0	6.6 ± 4.0	4
Males	28.0 ± 8.3	11.6 ± 6.4	

Table 7.5.2 Dietary Fiber Content (g/%) of Bread and Flour from Southgate

French Bread[4]	English Bread[1]	French Flour[4]	English Flour[1]
5.67–5.96	2.7	3.71–3.93	3.0

INDIRECT METHODS OF EVALUATION

These methods consist of measuring the total consumption of a given food in a given population and then dividing it by the number of individuals to obtain an evaluation of the average per capita consumption. We have, therefore, two major sources of information in France:

1. Inquiries by INSEE (National Institute of Statistic and Economic Studies[5]); 10,000 households, statistically representative of the total French population, are each examined for 1 week, the study being completed in the course of 1 year. Unfortunately, only the "at-home" consumption is estimated and not the away-from-home consumption (including restaurants, canteens, etc.). Therefore, food consumption is always underestimated; still, interesting comparisons between different population subgroups can be made.
2. Agricultural Statistics of the CEE (European Economic Community) or Eurostat.[6] Here, consumption means the gross amount of foodstuffs made available at the wholesale stage, in all forms: direct, preserved, and processed products. Consequently the consumption is overestimated, because no account is taken of losses at the retail trade stage or at the household level.

CEREAL CONSUMPTION (TABLES 7.5.3 TO 7.5.7)

The total cereal consumption has been quite stable for the last 10 years. The major cereal in France is wheat (soft wheat). The consumption of rice is increasing but is still very low.

The consumption of bread has been decreasing for many years, but this tendency seems to have now stopped. Still, bread remains the chief source of cereal fiber in the French diet. Bread consumption appears to be higher in the agricultural population than in the urban (Table 7.5.6), but this result may be due to the lack of information about away-from-home consumption (lunch is frequently taken in a restaurant or a canteen by the urban population).

CONSUMPTION OF FRUITS AND VEGETABLES (TABLES 7.5.8 TO 7.5.12)

The consumption of potatoes has been steadily decreasing for many years. Nevertheless, it remains high in the agricultural population and constitutes a large percentage of the total away-from-home consumption of vegetables. The consumption of dried pulses is very small.

The consumption of other vegetables and fresh fruits, except for citrus fruits, is no longer on the rise. There is a great discrepancy between the data on this consumption collected by Eurostat (Table 7.5.9) and INSEE (Table 7.5.11). The estimation by Eurostat probably is more realistic because it reflects all forms of consumption including preserves, jam, etc. It also includes the away-from-home consumption, which represents at least 10% of the total consumption of vegetables and about 15% of the fruit consumption.[7]

According to the data of INSEE, the consumption of fruits (including bananas and citrus fruits) is certainly higher in the urban population than in the highest classes of society (Table 7.5.11).

Table 7.5.3 Total Human Consumption of Cereals in France (1000 t/year) (Eurostat's Data[6])

Year	Total Cereals (excluding rice)	Total Wheat	Soft Wheat	Other Cereals (excluding wheat and rice)	Rice
1970–1971	5089	4978	4444	111	160
1975–1976	5016	4898	4426	118	211
1980–1981	5344	5180	4650	164	278

Table 7.5.4 Average Annual Consumption of Cereal (Kilograms per Capita) in Flour Equivalent (= Grain × 0.77) (Eurostat's Data[6])

Year	Total Cereals (excluding rice)	Total Wheat	Soft Wheat	Other Cereals (excluding wheat and rice)	Rice
Before 1970	80	78	70	2	2
1975–1976	73	79	64	2	4
1980–1981	76	75	67	1	4

Table 7.5.5 Average Daily Consumption of Wheat and Rice (Grams per Capita) Calculated from Annual Consumption

Year	Total Wheat	Wheat in Flour Equivalent	Bread	Rice
1970–1971	268	206	199	5.5
1975–1976	257	198	182	11
1980–1981	261	201	148	12.5

Table 7.5.6 Average Annual At-Home Consumption of Cereal Foods (Kilograms per Capita) (INSEE's Data 1980[5])

	Bread (total)	Noodles	Wheat Flour	Rice
Total population	48.57	5.49	4.16	3.86
Agricultural population	78.57	7.41	5.78	2.58
Nonagricultural population	45.32	5.28	3.98	4.00
Population of the greater Paris area	37.72	4.65	3.37	5.93

INTAKE OF DIETARY FIBER

An estimate of average daily fiber consumption can be made from these data, with a large margin of error. From Eurostat (Table 7.5.13), the "average Frenchman's" total dietary fiber intake ranges from 17.85 to 24.60 g/day, including 116 g of cereal fiber. From INSEE, the at-home consumption is surprisingly not much lower: 16 to 20 g/day. If one calculates the quantity of dietary fiber in the diets of farm owners and the unemployed (Table 7.5.14), who probably take the greatest number of meals at home, the values are a little higher: 22 to 26 g/day and 19 to 24 g/day.

For the last century (Figure 7.5.1), the consumption of bread and potatoes has been decreasing to a considerable extent. Conversely, the consumption of fruits and vegetables has been increasing, but this increase cannot compensate for the lack of cereal fiber. Therefore, the intake of dietary fiber currently is a great deal lower than in the years 1900 to 1930.[9]

Table 7.5.7 Average Annual Consumption of Cereal Foods by Occupation Group (Kilograms per Capita) (INSEE's Data 1980[5])

	Farm Owners	Farm Laborers	Self-Employed Professionals	Upper-Level Executives	Medium-Level Executives	White-Collar Workers	Blue-Collar Workers	Unemployed
Bread	81.11	64.03	42.43	32.38	38.53	39.17	51.22	48.75
Noodles	6.96	6.50	4.39	3.92	4.53	4.87	5.63	5.41
Wheat flour	4.65	5.27	3.32	2.58	3.49	2.99	4.52	4.12
Rice	2.12	2.55	2.97	3.85	3.00	3.86	4.75	5.13

Table 7.5.8   Total Human Consumption of Fruits and Vegetables (100 t/Year) (Eurostat's Data[6])

Year	Potatoes	Dried Pulse	Other Vegetables	Total Fresh Fruits	Citrus Fruits
1970–1971	4897	—	6632	2819	856
1975–1976	4790	113	6257	2890	998
1980–1981	3970	73	6168	2779	1015

Table 7.5.9   Average Annual Consumption of Fruits and Vegetables (Kilograms per Capita) (Eurostat's Data[6])

Year	Potatoes	Dried Pulse	Other Vegetables	Total Fresh Fruits	Citrus Fruits
Before 1970	97	—	129	56	17
1975–1976	81	2.1	118	55	19
1980–1981	74	1.4	115	52	19

Table 7.5.10   Average Daily Consumption of Fruits and Vegetables (Grams per Capita) Calculated from Annual Consumption

Year	Potatoes	Dried Pulse	Other Vegetables	Total Fresh Fruits	Citrus Fruits
1970–1971	266	—	353	153	47
1975–1976	222	5.7	323	151	52
1980–1981	202	3.8	315	142	52

Table 7.5.11   Average Annual At-Home Consumption of Fruits and Vegetables (Kilograms per Capita) (INSEE's Data 1980[5])

	Potatoes	Dried Pulse	Other Vegetables	Metropolitan Fresh Fruits	Bananas and Citrus Fruits
Total population	55.5	1.47	64.64	40.55	22.50
Agricultural population	62.79	2.45	77.46	37.44	14.54
Nonagricultural population	54.69	1.38	63.29	40.87	22.39
Population of the greater Paris area	40.93	1.69	63.81	45.82	29.38

DIETARY FIBER INTAKE AND MORBIDITY

Statistics on this problem are very rare in France. We did not find any difference in the dietary fiber intake between two groups of women, one consisting of women suffering from constipation and the other of controls. In both groups, the total dietary fiber intake (12.4 and 12.7 g/day) and the cereal fiber intake (3.3 and 3.6 g/day) were virtually the same.[10] Therefore, the lack of dietary fiber in alimentation cannot be considered the only cause of constipation.

Meyer found a negative correlation between consumption of fruits and mortality due to colonic cancer[8] but did not calculate the total dietary fiber intake or even the crude fiber intake. Recently, Macquart-Moulin et al.[4] found that, among other dietary factors, an increased intake of dietary fiber was correlated with a diminished relative risk of colorectal cancer.

Table 7.5.12 Average Consumption of Fruits and Vegetables by Occupation Group (Kilograms per Capita) (INSEE's Data 1980[5])

	Farm Owners	Farm Laborers	Self-Employed Professionals	Upper-Level Executives	Medium-Level Executives	White-Collar Workers	Blue-Collar Workers	Unemployed
Potatoes	57.83	50.42	48.12	29.24	44.34	42.68	64.74	69.03
Dried pulse	2.24	2.35	1.24	0.88	1.01	1.45	1.54	1.77
Vegetables	73.70	58.41	58.20	60.12	60.68	57.29	54.97	83.70
Fresh fruits	35.55	28.50	33.71	42.42	40.42	34.24	36.13	52.18
Bananas and citrus fruits	13.13	17.12	20.77	27.85	21.71	23.78	21.63	24.85

Table 7.5.13 Average Daily Fiber Intake (Eurostat's Data[6])

	Cereals in Flour Equivalent	Potatoes	Vegetables	Fruits	Citrus Fruits	Total
% of total that is dietary fiber	3.8	2	1.5–3	0.5–2	2	
(g/day)	200	200	300	145	52	
Dietary fiber (g/day)	7.6	4	4.5–9	0.75–3	1	17.85–24.6

Table 7.5.14 Average Daily Fiber Intake by Occupation Groups (INSEE's Data) Calculated from Southgate's Analyses

	Bread	Noodles	Wheat Flour	Rice	Potatoes	Dried Pulse	Vegetables	Fruits	Bananas	Total
% of total that is dietary fiber	5.8	?	3.8	2	2	15	1.5–3	0.5–2	2	
Farm owners (g/day)	222	19	13	5.8	160	6	200	97	35	
Dietary fiber	12.8	?	0.5	0.1	3.2	0.9	4–6	0.5–2	0.7	22.7–26.1
Unemployed (g/day)	133	15	11	14	190	5	230	140	68	
Dietary fiber	7.8	?	0.4	0.3	3.8	0.75	4.6–6.9	0.7–2.8	1.3	19.65–24.0
General average (g/day)	133	15	11	9.5	150	4	175	110	60	
Dietary fiber	7.8	?	0.4	0.2	3	0.6	2.6–5.2	0.55–2.2	1.2	16.35–20.6

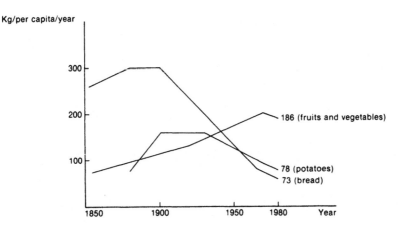

Figure 7.5.1 Evolution of dietary fiber in France.[9]

REFERENCES

1. Paul, A. A. and Southgate, D. A. T., *McCance and Widdowson's: The Composition of Foods*, Vol. 1, Her Majesty's Stationery Office, London, 1978.
2. Meyer, F. and Le Quintrec, Y., Rapports entre fibres alimentaires et constipation, *Nouv. Presse Med.*, 10, 2479, 1981.
3. Frexinos, J. and Allegret, M., Evaluation de la ration en fibres alimentaires dans la région Midi-Pyrénéés et en Nouvelle Calédonie, *Gastroenterol. Clin. Biol.*, 4, 739, 1980.
4. Macquart-Moulin, G., Durbec, J. P., Corvee, J., Berthezene, P., and Southgate, D. A. T., Alimentation et cancer recto-colique, *Gastroenterol. Clin. Biol.*, 7, 277, 1983.
5. Mercier, M. A., Consommation et lieux d'achat des produits alimentaires en 1980, Vol. 1, INSEE (Ser. M, No. 99), 1983.
6. EUROSTAT, Statistiques de production agricole de la Communauté Européenne, Publiees par O.F.C.E., 1970 a 1980.
7. Vlandas, S., Les fruits et légumes frais dans la restauration collective et communale. Centre technique interprofessionel des fruits et légumes, *Documents*, 27, 9, 1982.
8. Meyer, F., Relations alimentation—cancer en France, *Gastroenterol. Clin. Biol.*, 1, 971, 1977.
9. Meyer, F., Evolution de l'alimentation des Français 1781–1972, *Gastroenterol. Clin. Biol.*, 1, 1043, 1977.
10. Le Quintrec, Y. and Meyer, F., Fibres alimentaires et constipation, *Gastroenterol. Clin. Biol.*, 4, 174A (summary), 1980.

Fiber Consumption in Italy

Ottavio Bosello, Fabio Armellini, and Mauro Zamboni

INTRODUCTION

Epidemiological and alimentary studies on the population of Italy from 1954 to 1978[1] have shown a substantial increase in daily energy intake, a doubling of animal-origin proteins and animal and plant fats, and a clear drop in carbohydrate consumption (Table 7.6.1). Research by the Istituto Nazionale della Nutrizione (National Institute of Nutrition: INN) for the period 1980 to 1984 (Table 7.6.4) has shown a further increase in consumption of animal-origin products and a reduction in those of plant origin. Caloric intake, on the other hand, has dropped to 1964–1966 values.

This gradual change in Italy's traditional eating habits, going from the Mediterranean model[2] to a Western diet, has also involved a decrease in dietary fiber consumption and is more accentuated in northern Italy and less so in the south.[8]

SUBJECTS AND METHODS

The Trento Study (Table 7.6.2)

This research,* carried out in 1989, considered a representative sample of the city of Trento in northern Italy: 1697 people, 809 males and 888 females, between 25 and 69 years of age. Systematic sampling was performed on the resident population in the city and each of its suburbs. Food consumption was monitored by simultaneous recording of the food consumed during meals, with total quantity evaluation for a 7-day period.[3] The diary, previously sent to the subject's residence, was then checked and discussed with the subject by a dietitian when the diary was picked up. Nutritional and fiber values were calculated using the food composition tables published by the INN.[4]

Italian INN Study (Table 7.6.4)

The INN, in the period from 1980 to 1984, carried out sample monitoring and registration[5] of family food consumption in many zones of Italy (180 towns and cities, distributed over 9 regions). Research involved about 10,000 families selected by random sampling of the civic lists of voters.

---

* Unpublished information from an epidemiological cross-sectional study by M. Miori (Departmentof Internal Medicine, Trento Hospital) on a randomly selected sample of the population of Trento (northeast Italy) in 1989.

Table 7.6.1   Changes in Food Consumption from 1954 to 1978 in Italy[1]

		1954–1956	1964–1966	1976–1978
Proteins g/day	Plant	45.8	54.9	48.0
	Animal	24.8	33.6	49.4
	Total	70.6	88.5	97.4
Lipids g/day	Plant	32.6	52.1	65.8
	Animal	26.1	37.2	48.4
	Total	58.7	89.3	114.2
Carbohydrates g/day	Total	389.9	451.5	428.1
Energy MJ/day	Total	9.4	11.9	13.3

Data were collected by a mixed weight and inventory method, employing specifically trained dietitians. Nutritional and dietary fiber values were calculated using the INN tables.[4]

European Economic Community Survey (Table 7.6.3)

For the European Economic Community (EEC) Dietary Survey, research was performed in Europe between 1963 and 1965, as part of studies to determine environmental radioactive contamination levels.[6] The weekly eating habits of 30 family units were studied each month for 3 years. Research in Italy involved three regions: Friuli Venezia Giulia in northeastern Italy, Campania in south-central Italy, and Basilicata in southern Italy. Each family weighed the food after preparation but before cooking, thus avoiding the need to make corrections for waste. Fiber intake was calculated, using British food composition tables,[7] on the food intakes as measured.

Verona Vegetarian Study (Table 7.6.7)

This study* was performed in 1989 on 11 members of the vegetarian community in Verona (northeastern Italy). Comparisons were made on a one-to-one basis with a group of subjects of equal age, weight, body mass index, degree of physical activity, and sociocultural level. Nutritional parameters were obtained using a diary with simultaneous registration of foods consumed during meals, measured by quantity, for 7 days.[3] Data were subsequently checked by a dietitian. Nutritional and dietary fiber values were calculated using the INN tables.[4]

CONSUMPTION PATTERNS

Table 7.6.2 gives a few results from the Trento study, separately for males and females and for three age groups. Fiber intake is indicated. The table also includes both total and percentage values for daily energy intake from each of the three main nutrients. There is a tendency for greater fiber consumption in older age groups, both for males (21 ± 9 g/day in the oldest age group, 17 ± 8 g/day in the youngest) and for females (20 ± 9 g/day in the oldest, 17 ± 8 g/day in the youngest).

Table 7.6.3 gives total and food-group fiber consumption measured during the EEC study. These results show that Italian fiber intake from potatoes is low (0.7 to 3.8 g per person per day) and that from grains is high (13.4 to 14.7 g per person per day). Other European countries show a totally opposite picture.[8]

---

* Unpublished information from a case-control study by M. Zamboni about dietary fiber consumption in lacto-ovo-vegetarians and omnivores living in Verona (northeast Italy) in 1989.

Table 7.6.2 Mean (± SD) Daily Energy, Nutrient (as % Daily Energy), and Dietary Fiber Consumption in an Urban Northern Italian Population by Sex and Age, in 1989[a]

Sex	Age (Years)	Number of Subjects	Energy MJ/day	Carbohydrates (% Daily Energy)	Lipids (% Daily Energy)	Proteins (% Daily Energy)	Dietary Fiber (g/day)
Males	25–39	227	9.7 ± 2.8	48 ± 10	35 ± 9	16 ± 4	17 ± 8
	40–54	204	9.3 ± 3.1	45 ± 10	34 ± 9	16 ± 3	20 ± 9
	55–69	177	9.5 ± 2.6	44 ± 11	35 ± 10	16 ± 3	21 ± 9
Females	25–39	256	8.2 ± 2.8	45 ± 10	39 ± 9	15 ± 4	17 ± 8
	40–54	172	8.0 ± 2.6	44 ± 10	38 ± 10	16 ± 4	17 ± 8
	55–69	222	7.9 ± 2.3	45 ± 10	38 ± 9	16 ± 3	20 ± 9

[a] Unpublished information from an epidemiological cross-sectional study by M. Miori (Department of Internal Medicine, Trento Hospital) on a randomly selected sample of the population of Trento (northeast Italy) in 1989.

Table 7.6.3 Dietary Fiber Intake from Food (g per person per day), in Three Italian Regions, 1963–1965[6]

Region	Cereals	Vegetables	Fruits and Nuts	Potatoes	Total
Friuli Venezia Giulia (northeast)	14.7	5.1	1.3	3.8	24.9
Campania (central)	13.4	7.7	4.3	1.6	26.9
Basilicata (south)	13.5	5.7	3.9	0.7	23.8

Table 7.6.4   Mean (± SE) Fiber, Nutrients, and Energy Intake in Italy, 1980–1984[5]

Fiber (g/day)	20.9 ± 0.04
Protein (g/day)	
Animal	59.7 ± 0.12
Plant	38.1 ± 0.07
Total	97.8 ± 0.15
Lipids (g/day)	
Animal	53.6 ± 0.13
Plant	54.5 ± 0.16
Total	108.1 ± 0.22
Carbohydrates (g/day)	
Available	325.6 ± 0.54
Soluble	89.1 ± 0.21
Alcohol (g/day)	17.8 ± 0.09
Energy (MJ/day)	11.3 ± 0.02

Table 7.6.4 gives mean values for fiber consumption and total and percentage energy intake per nutrient for Italians as indicated by the Italian INN study. A look at four geographic areas shows moderate variations (Table 7.6.5) from one area to another of Italy.[9] Table 7.6.5 gives interesting data regarding energy and nutrients. Whereas average total protein and lipid consumption values show only small percentage differences with respect to totals between geographic areas, these same consumption values vary much more when they are subdivided into plant and animal protein and lipid values. Percentage differences in animal protein consumption, compared to the national average (59.7 g/day) given in Table 7.6.4, range from +9% in northeastern Italy to –8% in southern Italy. Plant protein consumption compared with the national average (38.1 g/day) ranges from +8% in southern Italy to –13% in northwestern Italy. For animal fats, when compared with the national average (53.6 g/day), consumption varies from +21% in northeastern Italy to –16% in southern Italy, whereas plant fat consumption compared with the national average (54.5 g/day) ranges from +7% in southern Italy to –17% in northwestern Italy. Data on fiber consumption compared with the national average (20.9 g/day) show greater consumption in central (+4%) and southern (+6%) Italy than in the north (–12 and –13 %). Table 7.6.6 illustrates this same territorial variability phenomenon in terms of consumptions expressed as food preferences.

Table 7.6.7 gives results from a study on vegetarians (lacto-ovo-vegetarians) and nonvegetarians (omnivores) living in a northern Italian town. The latter demonstrate eating habits practically identical to the population at large, and this is true for fiber intake, as well. The vegetarians, on the other hand, showed about twice the fiber intake (31.9 ± 4.4 g/day) compared to the nonvegetarians (17.3 ± 2.3 g/day). The fiber intake of these northern Italian vegetarians is greater even than that measured in 1980 to 1984 in the southern regions of Italy (22.2 g/day); see Table 7.6.5.

Table 7.6.5 Percentage Intake of Fiber, Nutrients, and Energy in Four Geographic Areas, Compared with the Whole of Italy (intake = 100), 1980–1984; Actual Fiber Intake, g/day, Given in Parentheses[9]

Fiber	Northwest 88 (18.4)	Northeast 87 (18.2)	Center 104 (21.7)	South 106 (22.2)
Protein				
Animal	106	109	104	92
Plant	87	89	100	108
Total	99	101	102	98
Lipids				
Animal	120	121	103	84
Plant	83	95	100	107
Total	102	108	102	95
Carbohydrates				
Available	95	99	99	103
Soluble	98	109	100	97
Alcohol	97	121	105	88
Energy	98	103	101	99

FIBER CONSUMPTION AND CARDIOVASCULAR DISEASE IN ITALY

In Italy, it is practically impossible to evaluate mortality trends for cardiovascular diseases and ischemic heart diseases, in particular. This is because many risk factors have undergone simultaneous changes. Starting in 1970, for example, a continuous increase in fat consumption and cigarette smoking has been counterbalanced by better control of high blood pressure, increased physical activity, and improved health care for patients with coronary disease.[10] On the other hand, there have been studies in Italy that show the beneficial effects that fiber has on the main coronary risk factors.[11,12]

FIBER CONSUMPTION AND CANCER IN ITALY

One study[13] performed on 206 women with endometrial cancer and on 206 controls showed that the risk for contracting this disease is higher for subjects consuming the more fat-rich diets that are also poor in green vegetables, fruits, and whole foods. The risk for contracting endometrial cancer appears inversely correlated to beta-carotene and fiber intake. The same authors[14] have performed a similar case-control study on stomach cancer; foods that are especially rich in fiber and complex carbohydrates, such as whole wheat bread and whole wheat pasta, have a protective effect with regard to stomach cancer.

CONCLUSIONS

Fiber consumption in Italy is higher in central than in northern regions of Italy and is even greater in the south. These southern and central areas seem to still be fairly well tied to the Mediterranean alimentary model, where the source of proteins and lipids is predominantly from plants and where there is an evident preference for the consumption of vegetables, bread, pasta, and pizza, in comparison with other Italian regions. In northern Italy, on the other hand, the influence of the Western diet is much stronger and fiber intake is low. A recent study that shows that, in the same northern-Italian urban environment, there is lower fiber consumption in the younger age groups compared to the elderly, who are presumably still tied to older, but healthier, eating habits gives further confirmation of this change toward the so-called Western diet which is relatively low in fiber.

Table 7.6.6 Food Preferences in Four Italian Geographical Areas, 1980–1984[9]

Northwest	Northeast	Center	South
More Frequently Consumed Food			
Rice	Cereals[a]	Tomatoes	Pizza
Fresh fruit	Potatoes	Vegetables	Pasta
Salted meats	Dry fruit	Citrus fruit	Dry legumes
Giblets	Fresh pork	Beef	Meat
Yogurt	Poultry	Preserved fish	Fresh fish
Medium-fat cheese	Milk	Animal fats	Low-fat cheese
High-fat cheese	Plant fats and oils	Soup preparations	
Biscuits and cakes	Pasta sauces		
Artificial sweeteners	Sugar		
Dietetic products	Soft drinks		
Soft drinks	Wine		
	Beer		
	Spirits		
Less Frequently Consumed Food			
Pasta	Bread and pizza	Rice	Cereals[a]
Dry legumes	Tomatoes for	Potatoes	Citrus fruit
Vegetables	sauces	Giblets	Dry fruit and nuts
Fresh fish	Fresh fruit	Low-fat cheese	Beef
Preserved fish	Meat	Plant fats and oils	Pork
Whole milk	Low-fat cheese	Sugar and honey	Salted meats
	Eggs	Soft drinks	Poultry
	Olive oil	Beer	Nonfat milk
	Snacks		Low-fat milk
			Yogurt
			Medium-fat cheese
			Animal fats
			Pasta sauces
			Soup preparations
			Biscuits and cakes
			Wine
			Spirits

[a] Excluding bread, pizza, and pasta.

Table 7.6.7   Mean (± SE) Fiber, Nutrients, and Energy Intake by Lacto-ovo-vegetarians and Omnivores Living in a Northern Italian Town, 1989[a]

	Lacto-Ovo-Vegetarians	Omnivores
Protein (g/day)		
Animal	17.9 ± 3.8	48.6 ± 6.0
Plant	42.2 ± 4.8	29.1 ± 9.3
Total	60.1 ± 5.7	77.7 ± 7.8
Lipids (g/day)		
Monounsaturated	32.8 ± 5.3	32.6 ± 4.7
Polyunsaturated	13.3 ± 4.3	7.6 ± 1.1
Saturated	23.2 ± 3.5	28.5 ± 4.3
Total	69.0 ± 9.5	75.7 ± 10.6
Carbohydrates (g/day)		
Total	378.0 ± 37.4	320.1 ± 42.4
Fiber	31.9 ± 4.4	17.3 ± 2.3
Energy (MJ/day)	9.8 ± 0.9	9.6 ± 1.2

[a] Unpublished information from a case-control study by M. Zamboni about dietary fiber consumption in lacto-ovo-vegetarians and omnivores living in Verona (Northeast Italy) in 1989.

REFERENCES

1. Cialfa, E. and Mariani Costantini, A., Situazione ed evoluzione dei consumi alimentari in Italia, in *Nutrizione Umana,* Fidanza, F. and Liguori, G., Eds., Idelson, Napoli, 1981.
2. Spiller, A. G., *The Mediterranean Diet in Health and Disease,* Van Nostrand Reinhold, New York, 1991.
3. Fidanza, F., Tecniche di rilevamento delle abitudini e dei consumi alimentari, in *Nutrizione Umana,* Fidanza, F. and Liguori, G., Eds., Idelson, Napoli, 1981.
4. Istituto Nazionale della Nutrizione, *Tabelle di composizione degli alimenti,* edizione 1988, Litho Delta, Milano, 1989.
5. Saba, A., Turrini, A., Mistura, G., and Cialfa, E., Indagine nazionale sui consumi alimentari delle famiglie 1980–84. Alcuni importanti risultati, *La Rivista della Societa Italiana di Scienza dell' Alimentazione,* 19(4), 53, 1990.
6. Cresta, M., Ledermann, S., Gardiner, A., Lombardo, E., and Lacourly, G., A dietary survey of 11 areas of the E.E.C. in order to determine levels of radioactive contamination, *Euratom,* EUR.4218F, 1969.
7. Ministry of Agriculture, Fisheries and Food, Household Food Consumption and Expenditure, 1950–1981, Annual reports of the National Food Survey Committee, Her Majesty's Stationery Office, London, 1953–1983.
8. Bingham, S., Patterns of Dietary Fiber Consumption in Humans, in *CRC Handbook of Dietary Fiber in Human Nutrition,* Spiller, G. A., Ed., CRC Press, Boca Raton, FL, 1986.
9. Cialfa, E., Turrini, A., and Lintas, C., A national food survey. Food balance sheets and other methodologies: a critical overview, *Human Nutrition Reviews* (ILSI), MacDonald, I., Ed., 1991, 24.
10. Menotti, A., Capocaccia, R., Farchi, F., and Pasquali, M., Recent trends in coronary heart disease and other cardiovascular diseases in Italy, *Cardiology,* 72, 88, 1985.
11. Bosello, O., Ostuzzi, R., Armellini, F., Micciolo, R., and Scuro, L. A., Glucose tolerance and blood lipids in bran fed patients with impaired glucose tolerance, *Diabetes Care,* 3, 46, 1980.
12. Rivellese, A., Riccardi, G., Giacco, A., et al., Reduction of risk factors for atherosclerosis in diabetic patients treated with high-fiber diet, *Prev. Med.,* 12(1), 128, 1983.
13. La Vecchia, C., De Carli, A., Fasoli, M., and Gentile, A., Nutrition and diet in the etiology of endometrial cancer, *Cancer,* 57, 1248, 1986.
14. La Vecchia, C., Negri, E., De Carli, A., D'Avanzo, B., and Franceschi, S., A case-control study of diet and gastric cancer in northern Italy, *Int. J. Cancer,* 40, 484, 1987.

APPENDIX

Tables of Dietary Fiber and Associated Substances Content in Food

Appendix — Table A.1
Dietary Fiber Values for Common Foods

Sally F. Schakel, Janet Pettit, and John H. Himes

The dietary fiber table developed by the Nutrition Coordinating Center (NCC) contains values compiled from scientific literature; the USDA Nutrient Database for Standard Reference;[135] manufacturer's information; and estimated data. Estimated values were derived from (1) a different form of the same food (e.g., raw to cooked), (2) a similar food, or (3) calculation of recipes or formulations.

Where only two of the three fiber values were known for a food, the third was calculated using the following formula: Total Dietary Fiber = Insoluble Fiber + Soluble Fiber. For some foods, the three fiber values were obtained from different references and, therefore, the sum of the insoluble and soluble fractions may not equal the value for total dietary fiber.

Table A.1 Dietary Fiber Values for Common Foods

	Amount[a]	Weight (g)	Total Dietary Fiber (g)	Insoluble Fiber (g)	Soluble Fiber (g)
Bread and Other Related Products					
Bagel, egg	1 Medium	57.00	1.31	0.54	0.78
Bagel, oat bran	1 Medium	57.00	2.06	0.99	0.94
Bagel, pumpernickel	1 Medium	57.00	2.61	1.58	0.92
Bagel, rye	1 Medium	57.00	2.61	1.58	0.92
Bagel, white flour	1 Medium	57.00	1.31	0.80	0.51
Bagel, whole wheat	1 Medium	57.00	2.58	1.76	0.71
Biscuit, baking powder or buttermilk	1 Medium	37.00	0.59	0.22	0.31
Bread crumbs, plain	1 T	6.75	0.16	0.09	0.07
Bread, Boston brown	1 Slice	45.00	2.11	1.62	0.49
Bread, cheese	1 Slice	31.10	0.49	0.18	0.26
Bread, cinnamon swirl	1 Slice	26.00	0.60	0.34	0.26
Bread, cracked wheat	1 Slice	25.00	1.03	0.76	0.27
Bread, cracked wheat, reduced-calorie and high-fiber	1 Slice	28.00	3.36	1.67	1.40
Bread, egg	1 Slice	23.00	0.40	0.15	0.22
Bread, focaccia	1 Slice	70.50	1.35	0.47	0.69
Bread, French	1 Slice	25.00	0.67	0.25	0.42
Bread, hovis	1 Slice	28.35	0.59	0.35	0.23
Bread, Italian	1 Slice	20.00	0.54	0.20	0.34
Bread, multigrain or granola	1 Slice	26.00	1.79	1.48	0.31
Bread, multigrain or granola, reduced-calorie and high-fiber	1 Slice	26.00	3.12	1.55	1.30
Bread, oat bran	1 Slice	26.00	1.15	0.65	0.41
Bread, oatmeal	1 Slice	27.00	1.08	0.51	0.57
Bread, pumpernickel	1 Slice	26.00	1.51	0.73	0.78
Bread, raisin	1 Slice	26.00	1.12	0.86	0.26
Bread, rye (light or dark)	1 Slice	26.00	1.51	0.73	0.78
Bread, sourdough	1 Slice	25.00	0.67	0.25	0.42
Bread, wheat	1 Slice	25.00	1.03	0.76	0.27
Bread, wheat, reduced-calorie and high-fiber	1 Slice	28.00	3.36	1.67	1.40
Bread, white	1 Slice	25.00	0.57	0.32	0.25
Bread, white, reduced-calorie and high-fiber	1 Slice	29.00	3.48	1.73	1.45
Bread, whole wheat	1 Slice	28.35	1.96	1.62	0.34
Breadsticks, bread type	1 Medium	32.00	0.86	0.32	0.54
Coffee cake, quick-bread or crumb type	1 Square	84.00	0.92	0.30	0.45

Bread and Other Related Products

Item	Serving				
Coffee cake, yeast type	1 Square	39.00	0.64	0.23	0.33
Cornbread	1 Piece	60.00	1.27	1.07	0.19
Crepe, plain	1 Medium	54.90	0.42	0.17	0.25
Croissant	1 Medium	57.00	0.89	0.34	0.49
Croutons	1 C	30.00	1.53	0.86	0.66
Danish pastry	1 Medium	65.00	1.03	0.36	0.52
Doughnut, cake	1 Medium	47.00	0.59	0.23	0.32
Doughnut, raised or yeast	1 Medium	60.00	0.93	0.30	0.43
French toast	1 Slice	59.00	0.60	0.32	0.25
Muffins, blueberry	1 Medium	57.00	0.89	0.50	0.38
Muffins, bran	1 Medium	57.00	2.64	2.26	0.38
Muffins, carrot	1 Medium	57.00	0.95	0.41	0.48
Muffins, corn	1 Medium	57.00	1.23	1.00	0.23
Muffins, English muffin, white	1 Each	57.00	1.54	1.08	0.46
Muffins, English muffin, whole wheat	1 Each	66.00	4.42	3.58	0.62
Muffins, oat bran or oatmeal	1 Medium	57.00	1.21	0.59	0.63
Pancake, white flour, frozen	1 Each	36.00	0.64	0.37	0.27
Pancake, white flour, prepared from a mix	1 Each	38.00	0.53	0.29	0.24
Pancake, white flour, prepared from a recipe	1 Each	38.00	0.38	0.15	0.22
Pancake, whole wheat	1 Each	44.00	1.83	1.56	0.27
Pita, white	1 Medium	45.00	0.99	0.45	0.54
Pita, whole wheat	1 Medium	45.00	3.33	2.62	0.45
Popover	1 Each	62.90	0.56	0.23	0.33
Rolls, cracked wheat	1 Medium	36.00	1.49	1.10	0.39
Rolls, crescent (refrigerated dough)	1 Each	28.00	0.45	0.17	0.24
Rolls, French or Vienna	1 Medium	45.00	1.21	0.45	0.76
Rolls, hamburger, wheat	1 Medium	43.00	1.78	1.32	0.46
Rolls, hamburger, white	1 Medium	43.00	1.16	0.77	0.39
Rolls, hamburger, whole wheat	1 Medium	43.00	2.97	2.45	0.52
Rolls, hard	1 Medium	50.00	1.15	0.83	0.31
Rolls, hot dog	1 Regular	43.00	1.16	0.77	0.39
Rolls, Kaiser	1 Medium	50.00	1.15	0.83	0.31
Rolls, multigrain	1 Medium	36.00	1.49	1.10	0.39
Rolls, oat bran	1 Medium	36.00	1.53	0.65	0.66
Rolls, oatmeal	1 Medium	36.00	1.08	0.47	0.52
Rolls, pumpernickel	1 Medium	36.00	2.09	1.01	1.08
Rolls, rye	1 Medium	36.00	2.09	1.01	1.08

Table A.1 (Continued) Dietary Fiber Values for Common Foods

	Amount[a]	Weight (g)	Total Dietary Fiber (g)	Insoluble Fiber (g)	Soluble Fiber (g)
Bread and Other Related Products					
Rolls, sourdough	1 Medium	45.00	1.21	0.45	0.76
Rolls, submarine or hoagie	1 Medium	94.00	2.82	2.01	0.81
Rolls, wheat	1 Medium	36.00	1.49	1.10	0.39
Rolls, white	1 Medium	36.00	1.08	0.68	0.40
Rolls, whole wheat	1 Medium	36.00	2.48	2.05	0.43
Scone	1 Medium	42.00	0.74	0.38	0.35
Sweet roll	1 Medium	57.00	1.06	0.28	0.42
Taco shell, hard	1 Regular	13.30	1.00	0.88	0.12
Toaster pastry or Pop-Tart	1 Regular	52.00	1.09	0.51	0.59
Tortilla, corn	1 Each	26.00	1.35	1.14	0.21
Tortilla, white flour	1 Each	43.00	1.42	0.99	0.43
Waffles, white flour, frozen	1 Each – 4 in. diameter	39.00	0.53	0.22	0.32
Waffles, white flour, home recipe	1 Each – 7 in. diameter	95.00	0.97	0.39	0.57
Cereals — Cooked					
Cornmeal	1 C	240.00	2.64	2.62	0.02
Cracked wheat	1 C	242.00	6.39	5.44	0.94
Cream of rice	1 C	244.00	0.32	0.29	0.05
Cream of wheat, multigrain flavored	1 C	241.00	3.08	1.64	1.30
Creamed wheat, instant cooking	1 C	241.00	1.06	0.60	0.46
Creamed wheat, quick cooking	1 C	239.00	0.93	0.53	0.38
Creamed wheat, regular cooking	1 C	251.00	1.25	0.73	0.53
Grits	1 C	242.00	0.63	0.48	0.17
Mix 'N Eat Cream of Wheat, flavored	1 C	241.00	1.37	0.51	0.87
Mix 'N Eat Cream of Wheat, plain	1 C	241.00	0.82	0.48	0.36
Oat bran	1 C	219.00	5.67	3.02	2.65
Oatmeal, instant cooking, flavored	1 C	234.00	3.14	1.64	1.47
Oatmeal, instant cooking, plain	1 C	234.00	3.84	2.06	1.78
Oatmeal, quick cooking	1 C	234.00	3.98	2.13	1.85
Oatmeal, regular cooking	1 C	234.00	3.98	2.13	1.85
Rolled wheat	1 C	242.00	3.85	3.27	0.58

Cereals — Ready-to-Eat

100% Bran (Nabisco)	1 C	87.09	24.78	22.40	2.37
All-Bran (Kellogg's)	1 C	62.00	20.03	18.44	1.59
All-Bran Bran Buds (Kellogg's)	1 C	90.09	35.95	28.20	7.51
All-Bran with Extra Fiber (Kellogg's)	1 C	52.00	26.57	24.67	1.40
Alpha-Bits (Post)	1 C	32.00	1.73	1.14	0.59
Amaranth Flakes (Arrowhead Mills)	1 C	34.00	3.29	2.12	1.16
Apple & Cinnamon Toasty O's (Malt-O-Meal)	1 C	40.00	2.24	1.19	1.04
Apple Cinnamon Cheerios (General Mills)	1 C	40.00	2.12	1.10	1.02
Apple Jacks K-sentials (Kellogg's)	1 C	33.00	0.63	0.37	0.25
Apple Zaps (Quaker)	1 C	30.00	1.42	1.34	0.07
Basic 4 (General Mills)	1 C	55.00	3.35	2.60	0.77
Berry Berry Kix (General Mills)	1 C	40.00	0.24	0.14	0.10
Berry Colossal Crunch (Malt-O-Meal)	1 C	40.00	0.44	0.29	0.15
Betty Crocker Cinnamon Streusel (General Mills)	1 C	40.00	1.47	1.21	0.25
Betty Crocker Dutch Apple (General Mills)	1 C	55.00	1.65	1.04	0.61
Bite Size Shredded Wheat, Sweetened (Arrowhead Mills)	1 C	55.00	5.25	4.47	0.77
Bite Size Shredded Wheat (Arrowhead Mills)	1 C	49.00	6.24	5.32	0.92
Body Buddies (General Mills)	1 C	30.00	0.93	0.68	0.21
Booberry (General Mills)	1 C	30.00	0.39	0.38	0.00
Bran Cereal with Apples & Cinnamon (Health Valley)	1 C	65.33	11.39	9.75	1.64
Bran Flakes (Arrowhead Mills)	1 C	29.00	4.35	3.69	0.64
Bran Flakes (Malt-O-Meal)	1 C	40.00	6.67	6.01	0.65
Bran Flakes (Post)	1 C	40.00	6.72	6.04	0.69
Cap'n Crunch (Quaker)	1 C	36.00	1.15	1.07	0.09
Cap'n Crunch's Crunch Berries (Quaker)	1 C	34.67	1.11	1.03	0.08
Cap'n Crunch's Peanut Butter Crunch (Quaker)	1 C	36.00	1.04	0.69	0.35
Cheerios (General Mills)	1 C	30.00	3.03	2.17	0.87
Cinnamon Life (Quaker)	1 C	50.00	2.95	2.23	0.70
Cinnamon Toast Crunch (General Mills)	1 C	40.00	2.00	1.70	0.30
Cocoa Blasts (Quaker)	1 C	33.00	1.41	1.34	0.06
Cocoa Comets (Malt-O-Meal)	1 C	40.00	1.52	1.40	0.08
Cocoa Frosted Flakes K-sentials (Kellogg's)	1 C	41.33	0.33	0.21	0.07
Cocoa Krispies K-sentials (Kellogg's)	1 C	41.33	0.54	0.41	0.12

Table A.1 (Continued) Dietary Fiber Values for Common Foods

	Amount[a]	Weight (g)	Total Dietary Fiber (g)	Insoluble Fiber (g)	Soluble Fiber (g)
Cereals — Ready-to-Eat					
Cocoa Pebbles (Post)	1 C	38.67	0.64	0.49	0.13
Cocoa Puffs (General Mills)	1 C	30.00	0.18	0.14	0.04
Colossal Crunch (Malt-O-Meal)	1 C	40.00	1.77	1.57	0.20
Complete Oat Bran Flakes (Kellogg's)	1 C	40.00	4.83	3.25	1.58
Complete Wheat Bran Flakes (Kellogg's)	1 C	38.67	6.15	5.52	0.63
Corn Bursts (Malt-O-Meal)	1 C	31.00	1.00	0.99	0.01
Corn Chex (General Mills)	1 C	30.00	1.05	0.96	0.09
Corn Flakes (Arrowhead Mills)	1 C	35.00	1.99	1.78	0.17
Corn Flakes (Kellogg's)	1 C	28.00	0.78	0.66	0.06
Corn Flakes (Malt-O-Meal)	1 C	30.00	1.00	0.89	0.06
Corn Pops K-sentials (Kellogg's)	1 C	31.00	0.43	0.35	0.04
Count Chocula (General Mills)	1 C	30.00	0.45	0.35	0.10
Country Corn Flakes (General Mills)	1 C	30.00	0.45	0.29	0.10
Cracklin' Oat Bran (Kellogg's)	1 C	65.33	7.77	6.28	1.48
Crispix (Kellogg's)	1 C	29.00	0.64	0.51	0.13
Crispy Puffs (Arrowhead Mills)	1 C	20.00	1.40	1.11	0.29
Crispy Rice (Malt-O-Meal)	1 C	30.00	0.66	0.51	0.15
Crispy Wheaties 'N Raisins (General Mills)	1 C	55.00	3.41	2.87	0.54
Crunchy Bran (Quaker)	1 C	36.00	6.41	6.11	0.18
Double Chex (General Mills)	1 C	24.00	0.43	0.34	0.10
Erewhon Apple Stroodles (U.S. Mills)	1 C	40.00	2.36	1.31	1.04
Erewhon Aztec (U.S. Mills)	1 C	30.00	1.17	0.83	0.34
Erewhon Banana-O's (U.S. Mills)	1 C	40.00	2.12	1.28	0.83
Erewhon Corn Flakes (U.S. Mills)	1 C	36.00	0.59	0.44	0.15
Erewhon Crispy Brown Rice, No Salt Added (U.S. Mills)	1 C	30.00	0.97	0.82	0.14
Erewhon Crispy Brown Rice (U.S. Mills)	1 C	30.00	1.29	1.10	0.19
Erewhon Fruit'n Wheat (U.S. Mills)	1 C	70.67	8.00	6.97	1.04
Erewhon Galaxy Grahams (U.S. Mills)	1 C	37.33	2.93	2.48	0.44
Erewhon Kamut Flakes (U.S. Mills)	1 C	50.98	5.77	5.03	0.75
Erewhon Poppets (U.S. Mills)	1 C	30.00	1.18	1.01	0.17
Erewhon Raisin Bran (U.S. Mills)	1 C	52.00	6.01	5.26	0.74
Erewhon Wheat Flakes (U.S. Mills)	1 C	53.00	6.00	5.23	0.78
Fat-Free 10 Bran O's, Apple Cinnamon (Health Valley)	1 C	36.00	4.16	3.12	0.99

Fat-Free Honey Clusters & Flakes, Almond (Health Valley)	1 C	41.33	5.63	4.76	0.81
Fat-Free Honey Clusters & Flakes, Apple Cinnamon (Health Valley)	1 C	41.33	5.63	4.76	0.81
Fat-Free Honey Clusters & Flakes, Honey Crunch (Health Valley)	1 C	41.33	5.63	4.76	0.81
Fiber One (General Mills)	1 C	60.00	28.50	26.59	1.29
Frankenberry (General Mills)	1 C	30.00	0.39	0.38	0.00
French Toast Crunch (General Mills)	1 C	40.00	1.84	1.83	0.01
Froot Loops K-sentials (Kellogg's)	1 C	32.00	0.61	0.42	0.18
Frosted Cheerios (General Mills)	1 C	30.00	1.36	0.82	0.54
Frosted Flakers (Quaker)	1 C	41.33	1.97	1.95	0.01
Frosted Flakes (Malt-O-Meal)	1 C	40.00	1.45	1.44	0.01
Frosted Flakes K-sentials (Kellogg's)	1 C	41.33	0.83	0.69	0.08
Frosted Oats (Quaker)	1 C	28.00	1.06	0.57	0.49
Frosted Shredded Wheat Bite Size (Nabisco)	1 C	52.00	4.08	3.48	0.60
Frosted Toasty O's (Malt-O-Meal)	1 C	30.00	1.42	0.96	0.45
Fruit & Fiber — Dates, Raisins & Walnuts (Post)	1 C	55.00	5.00	4.30	0.69
Fruitangy Oh's (Quaker)	1 C	31.00	1.41	1.31	0.10
Fruity Pebbles (Post)	1 C	36.00	0.59	0.46	0.13
Golden Crisp (Post)	1 C	36.00	0.47	0.19	0.28
Golden Flax (Health Valley)	1 C	100.00	12.94	9.40	3.48
Golden Grahams (General Mills)	1 C	40.00	1.24	1.15	0.09
Golden Puffs (Malt-O-Meal)	1 C	36.00	1.27	1.08	0.19
Grainfield's Brown Rice (Weetabix)	1 C	30.00	1.38	1.18	0.20
Grainfield's Corn Flakes (Weetabix)	1 C	30.00	1.71	1.53	0.15
Grainfield's Crispy Rice (Weetabix)	1 C	30.00	0.72	0.56	0.16
Grainfield's Raisin Bran (Weetabix)	1 C	44.00	6.14	5.36	0.77
Grape-Nuts (Post)	1 C	116.00	9.88	8.11	1.40
Grape-Nuts Flakes (Post)	1 C	38.67	4.00	3.24	0.76
Healthy Choice Almond Crunch with Raisins (Kellogg's)	1 C	58.00	4.22	3.62	0.55
Healthy Choice Golden Multi-Grain Flakes (Kellogg's)	1 C	41.33	3.89	3.46	0.41
Healthy Choice Toasted Brown Sugar Squares (Kellogg's)	1 C	54.00	4.66	3.94	0.72
Honey & Nut Toasty O's (Malt-O-Meal)	1 C	30.00	1.94	1.07	0.88
Honey Bunches of Oats Honey Roasted (Post)	1 C	40.00	1.33	1.04	0.29
Honey Bunches of Oats with Almonds (Post)	1 C	41.33	1.34	1.02	0.32
Honey Crunch Corn Flakes (Kellogg's)	1 C	40.00	0.88	0.78	0.10
Honey Frosted Wheaties (General Mills)	1 C	40.00	1.99	1.95	0.04
Honey Graham Oh's (Quaker)	1 C	36.00	0.94	0.84	0.09
Honey Nut Cheerios (General Mills)	1 C	30.00	1.56	1.01	0.55
Honey Nut Clusters (General Mills)	1 C	55.00	3.00	2.52	0.46
Honey Nut Oats (Quaker)	1 C	28.00	1.31	0.72	0.59

Table A.1 (Continued) Dietary Fiber Values for Common Foods

	Amount[a]	Weight (g)	Total Dietary Fiber (g)	Insoluble Fiber (g)	Soluble Fiber (g)
Cereals — Ready-to-Eat					
Honey Nut Shredded Wheat - Bite Size (Nabisco)	1 C	52.00	4.05	3.44	0.61
Honeycomb (Post)	1 C	21.76	0.28	0.20	0.07
Just Right Fruit & Nut (Kellogg's)	1 C	60.00	3.00	2.45	0.56
Just Right with Crunchy Nuggets (Kellogg's)	1 C	56.00	2.86	2.43	0.41
Kaboom (General Mills)	1 C	24.00	1.20	0.74	0.45
Kamut Flakes (Arrowhead Mills)	1 C	32.00	2.99	2.50	0.48
King Vitaman (Quaker)	1 C	20.67	0.79	0.56	0.22
Kix (General Mills)	1 C	22.51	0.61	0.39	0.22
Kretschmer Honey Crunch Wheat Germ (Quaker)	1 C	134.37	14.81	11.14	3.67
Life (Quaker)	1 C	42.67	2.73	1.75	0.99
Lucky Charms (General Mills)	1 C	30.00	1.20	0.64	0.55
Maple Corns (Arrowhead Mills)	1 C	53.00	6.04	5.85	0.11
Marshmallow Alpha-Bits (Post)	1 C	29.00	1.01	0.56	0.44
Marshmallow Blasted Froot Loops K-sentials (Kellogg's)	1 C	30.00	0.77	0.66	0.10
Marshmallow Mateys (Malt-O-Meal)	1 C	30.00	1.23	0.65	0.56
Marshmallow Safari (Quaker)	1 C	40.00	1.39	0.73	0.63
Mini-Wheats - Apple Cinnamon (Kellogg's)	1 C	73.33	6.45	5.49	0.95
Mini-Wheats - Blueberry (Kellogg's)	1 C	72.00	6.34	5.39	0.93
Mini-Wheats - Frosted Bite Size (Kellogg's)	1 C	55.00	5.88	5.02	0.86
Mini-Wheats - Frosted Original (Kellogg's)	1 C	55.00	5.88	5.02	0.86
Mini-Wheats - Raisin (Kellogg's)	1 C	70.67	6.64	5.59	1.05
Mini-Wheats - Strawberry (Kellogg's)	1 C	66.67	5.87	4.99	0.86
Morning Traditions Banana Nut Crunch (Post)	1 C	59.00	4.00	3.03	0.98
Morning Traditions Blueberry Morning (Post)	1 C	44.00	1.60	1.39	0.22
Morning Traditions Cranberry Almond Crunch (Post)	1 C	55.00	3.00	2.40	0.60
Morning Traditions Great Grains Crunchy Pecan (Post)	1 C	79.46	6.00	4.60	1.41
Morning Traditions Great Grains Raisins, Dates & Pecans (Post)	1 C	80.96	6.00	4.81	1.21
Mueslix — Apple & Almond Crunch (Kellogg's)	1 C	70.67	6.01	4.56	1.46
Mueslix — Raisin & Almond Crunch with Dates (Kellogg's)	1 C	82.46	5.61	4.44	1.17
Multi Grain Cheerios Plus (General Mills)	1 C	30.00	1.92	1.52	0.39
Multi Grain Flakes (Arrowhead Mills)	1 C	35.00	2.88	2.25	0.63
Multi-Bran Chex (General Mills)	1 C	46.40	5.60	5.35	0.24
Nature O's (Arrowhead Mills)	1 C	32.00	3.00	1.92	1.07

Nutri-Grain — Almond Raisin (Kellogg's)	1 C	39.20	3.14	2.87	0.27
Nutri-Grain — Golden Wheat (Kellogg's)	1 C	40.00	5.04	4.63	0.41
Oat Bran Flakes (Arrowhead Mills)	1 C	34.00	3.46	1.87	1.61
Oat Bran Ready-To-Eat (Quaker)	1 C	45.60	4.79	2.78	2.01
Oatmeal Crisp — Almond (General Mills)	1 C	55.00	4.34	3.13	1.21
Oatmeal Crisp — Apple Cinnamon (General Mills)	1 C	55.00	4.45	2.78	1.68
Oatmeal Crisp — Raisin (General Mills)	1 C	55.00	3.52	2.49	1.03
Oatmeal Squares — Cinnamon (Quaker)	1 C	60.00	4.56	2.54	2.02
Oatmeal Squares (Quaker)	1 C	56.00	4.26	2.54	1.71
Oreo O's (Post)	1 C	36.00	0.92	0.56	0.31
Organic Amaranth Flakes (Health Valley)	1 C	37.33	5.56	4.85	0.67
Organic Blue Corn Flakes (Health Valley)	1 C	37.33	5.50	5.29	0.11
Organic Bran with Raisins (Health Valley)	1 C	66.67	9.10	7.97	1.12
Organic Crisp Brown Rice (Health Valley)	1 C	42.67	2.24	1.93	0.32
Organic Fiber 7 Flakes (Health Valley)	1 C	37.33	5.56	4.85	0.67
Organic Healthy Fiber Flakes (Health Valley)	1 C	37.33	5.73	4.77	0.96
Organic Oat Bran Flakes (Health Valley)	1 C	37.33	4.10	2.53	1.57
Organic Oat Bran Flakes with Raisins (Health Valley)	1 C	41.33	5.29	4.01	1.20
Organic Oat Bran O's (Health Valley)	1 C	37.33	3.07	2.03	1.04
Organic Raisin Bran Flakes (Health Valley)	1 C	44.00	5.26	4.58	0.68
Post Toasties (Post)	1 C	28.00	0.45	0.34	0.11
Product 19 (Kellogg's)	1 C	30.00	0.99	0.66	0.33
Puffed Corn (Arrowhead Mills)	1 C	22.00	0.35	0.26	0.09
Puffed Corn (Health Valley)	1 C	32.00	1.74	1.72	0.01
Puffed Kamut (Arrowhead Mills)	1 C	16.00	1.52	1.30	0.22
Puffed Millet (Arrowhead Mills)	1 C	25.00	2.57	2.22	0.35
Puffed Rice (Arrowhead Mills)	1 C	23.00	0.55	0.43	0.12
Puffed Rice (Malt-O-Meal)	1 C	15.00	0.39	0.30	0.09
Puffed Rice (Quaker)	1 C	14.00	0.24	0.18	0.06
Puffed Wheat (Arrowhead Mills)	1 C	25.00	2.37	2.02	0.35
Puffed Wheat (Malt-O-Meal)	1 C	15.00	1.42	1.21	0.21
Puffed Wheat (Quaker)	1 C	12.00	1.13	0.60	0.53
Raisin Bran (Arrowhead Mills)	1 C	54.00	8.06	7.04	0.95
Raisin Bran (Kellogg's)	1 C	61.00	8.17	7.15	1.02
Raisin Bran (Malt-O-Meal)	1 C	61.00	7.99	7.09	0.89
Raisin Bran (Post)	1 C	59.00	8.14	7.26	0.88
Raisin Nut Bran (General Mills)	1 C	55.00	5.06	4.41	0.65
Real Oat Bran — Almond Crunch (Health Valley)	1 C	96.00	9.62	5.22	4.36
Reese's Peanut Butter Puffs (General Mills)	1 C	40.00	0.52	0.40	0.12

Table A.1 (Continued) Dietary Fiber Values for Common Foods

	Amount[a]	Weight (g)	Total Dietary Fiber (g)	Insoluble Fiber (g)	Soluble Fiber (g)
Cereals — Ready-to-Eat					
Rice Chex (General Mills)	1 C	31.00	0.75	0.58	0.17
Rice Krispies K-sentials (Kellogg's)	1 C	26.40	0.29	0.21	0.08
Rice Krispies Treats (Kellogg's)	1 C	40.00	0.40	0.28	0.11
Shredded Wheat (Nabisco)	1 BIS	23.00	2.25	1.89	0.37
Shredded Wheat (Quaker)	1 BIS	21.00	2.06	1.72	0.34
Shredded Wheat Spoon Size (Nabisco)	1 C	49.00	4.80	4.02	0.78
Shredded Wheat'n Bran (Nabisco)	1 C	47.20	6.18	5.34	0.84
Skinner's Corn Flakes (U.S. Mills)	1 C	41.98	2.98	2.96	0.03
Skinner's Raisin Bran (U.S. Mills)	1 C	55.00	7.21	6.38	0.82
Smacks (Kellogg's)	1 C	36.00	1.26	1.01	0.25
Smart Start (Kellogg's)	1 C	50.00	2.35	1.83	0.38
S'Mores Grahams (General Mills)	1 C	40.00	1.12	1.09	0.03
Special K (Kellogg's)	1 C	31.00	0.96	0.54	0.15
Spelt Flakes (Arrowhead Mills)	1 C	30.00	3.12	2.75	0.36
Sweet Crunch (Quaker)	1 C	27.00	1.00	0.94	0.07
Toasted Oatmeal — Honey Nut (Quaker)	1 C	49.00	3.33	2.32	1.00
Toasted Oatmeal — Original (Quaker)	1 C	41.33	2.97	2.05	0.92
Toasty O's (Malt-O-Meal)	1 C	30.00	2.43	1.31	1.12
Tootie Fruities (Malt-O-Meal)	1 C	30.00	1.00	0.73	0.28
Total (General Mills)	1 C	40.00	3.52	3.00	0.52
Total Corn Flakes (General Mills)	1 C	22.51	0.56	0.54	0.00
Total Raisin Bran (General Mills)	1 C	55.00	5.00	4.39	0.62
Trix (General Mills)	1 C	30.00	0.72	0.70	0.01
Uncle Sam (U.S. Mills)	1 C	55.00	9.87	7.88	1.99
Waffle Crisp (Post)	1 C	30.00	1.45	1.06	0.40
Wafflers — Cinnamon (U.S. Mills)	1 C	44.98	1.89	1.58	0.31
Wafflers — Maple (U.S. Mills)	1 C	44.98	1.89	1.58	0.31
Wafflers — Original (U.S. Mills)	1 C	44.98	1.89	1.58	0.31
Wafflers — Vanilla Nut (U.S. Mills)	1 C	44.98	1.89	1.58	0.31
Weetabix (Weetabix)	1 BIS	17.50	1.98	1.69	0.29
Wheat Bran (Arrowhead Mills)	1 C	64.00	27.39	25.22	2.18
Wheat Chex (General Mills)	1 C	66.67	5.65	4.83	0.83
Wheaties (General Mills)	1 C	30.00	2.10	1.38	0.72

Granola and Muesli

Product	Serving				
100% Natural Granola — Oats & Honey (Grist Mill)	1 C	110.00	7.94	5.32	2.64
100% Natural Granola — Oats, Honey & Raisins (Grist Mill)	1 C	110.00	8.00	5.33	2.66
100% Natural Low Fat Granola with Raisins (Quaker)	1 C	82.46	4.16	2.93	1.21
98% Fat-Free Granola — Date Almond (Health Valley)	1 C	82.46	7.74	4.72	3.01
98% Fat-Free Granola — Raisin Cinnamon (Health Valley)	1 C	82.46	7.74	4.72	3.01
98% Fat-Free Granola — Tropical (Health Valley)	1 C	82.46	7.74	4.72	3.01
Alpen (Weetabix)	1 C	90.09	7.07	5.01	2.09
Erewhon #9 Granola with Bran (U.S. Mills)	1 C	144.14	15.08	9.20	5.94
Erewhon New England Style Granola — Date Nut (U.S. Mills)	1 C	144.14	12.14	6.92	5.13
Erewhon New England Style Granola — Honey Almond (U.S. Mills)	1 C	138.14	11.63	6.63	4.92
Erewhon New England Style Granola — Maple (U.S. Mills)	1 C	150.15	12.64	7.21	5.35
Erewhon Spiced Apple Granola (U.S. Mills)	1 C	141.14	11.88	6.77	5.02
Erewhon Sunflower Crunch Granola (U.S. Mills)	1 C	147.15	12.39	7.06	5.24
Familia Swiss Muesli — No Added Sugar	1 C	114.00	9.50	6.93	2.56
Familia Swiss Muesli — Original Recipe	1 C	120.00	10.00	7.30	2.70
Fat-Free Granola O's — Almond (Health Valley)	1 C	41.33	3.67	2.48	1.19
Fat-Free Granola O's — Apple Cinnamon (Health Valley)	1 C	41.33	3.67	2.48	1.19
Fat-Free Granola O's — Honey Crunch (Health Valley)	1 C	41.33	3.67	2.48	1.19
Heartland Granola — Original (Pet)	1 C	128.00	8.84	5.20	3.64
Heartland Granola — Raisin (Pet)	1 C	128.00	8.84	5.20	3.64
Low Fat Alpen (Weetabix)	1 C	90.09	7.43	5.22	2.18
Low Fat Granola (Kellogg's)	1 C	98.00	5.78	4.04	1.73
Low Fat Granola with Raisins (Kellogg's)	1 C	89.96	5.40	3.73	1.64
Mountain House Granola with Blueberries (Oregon Freeze Dry)	1 C	110.00	7.94	4.76	3.20
Nature Valley Low Fat Fruit Granola (General Mills)	1 C	82.46	5.11	2.90	2.19
Sun Country Granola with Almonds (Quaker)	1 C	114.00	5.93	3.52	2.41
Sun Country Granola with Raisins & Dates (Quaker)	1 C	120.00	7.20	4.24	2.93
Vita Crunch Granola — Almond (Organic Milling Company)	1 C	73.33	5.28	3.49	1.80
Vita Crunch Granola — Light & Crunchy 7 Grain (Organic Milling Company)	1 C	73.33	4.88	3.21	1.69
Vita Crunch Granola — Raisin (Organic Milling Company)	1 C	73.33	4.88	3.21	1.69
Vita Crunch Granola — Tropical (Organic Milling Company)	1 C	73.33	5.28	3.49	1.80

Table A.1 (Continued) Dietary Fiber Values for Common Foods

	Amount[a]	Weight (g)	Total Dietary Fiber (g)	Insoluble Fiber (g)	Soluble Fiber (g)
Crackers					
Butter	1 Round	3.00	0.05	0.02	0.03
Cheese	1 Round	3.00	0.07	0.04	0.03
Crispbread — rye	1 Wafer	10.00	0.27	0.11	0.16
Flatbread	1 Each	5.80	0.16	0.06	0.09
Matzo or matzoh, plain	1 Each	28.35	0.85	0.37	0.37
Matzo or matzoh, egg	1 Each	28.35	0.77	0.30	0.47
Matzo or matzoh, whole wheat	1 Each	28.35	0.85	0.37	0.37
Melba toast	1 Rectangle	5.00	0.13	0.05	0.08
Oyster	1 Each	1.00	0.04	0.03	0.01
Rye wafer, plain	1 Wafer	11.00	0.30	0.12	0.18
Rye wafer, seasoned	1 Wafer	11.00	0.50	0.25	0.25
Saltine or soda, white	1 Each	3.00	0.12	0.08	0.04
Saltine or soda, whole wheat	1 Each	3.00	0.11	0.07	0.04
Wheat	1 Square	2.00	0.09	0.07	0.02
Whole wheat	1 Each	4.00	0.15	0.09	0.06
Zwieback	1 Each	7.00	0.08	0.03	0.05
Snacks and Chips					
Bagel chip	1 oz	28.35	1.05	0.36	0.39
Cereal bar	1 Bar	37.00	1.00	0.60	0.41
Cereal party mix, commercial	1 C	44.78	1.80	1.44	0.36
Cereal party mix, homemade	1 C	70.50	4.05	3.13	0.92
Cheese balls, puffs or twists	1 oz	28.35	1.38	1.37	0.01
Corn chip	1 oz	28.35	1.36	1.35	0.01
Corn nuts	1 C	84.08	5.80	5.75	0.05
Fried pork rinds	1 oz	28.35	0.00	0.00	0.00
Fruit bar	1 Bar	15.00	1.55	0.72	0.83
Granola bars, chocolate-coated	1 Bar	27.80	1.17	0.89	0.27
Granola bars, plain bar (no coating), flavors other than peanut butter	1 Bar	23.50	0.99	0.75	0.23
Granola bars, plain bar (no coating), peanut butter	1 Bar	23.50	1.14	0.65	0.50
Onion flavored rings	1 oz	28.35	1.66	1.64	0.01
Popcorn cake	1 Each	10.00	0.42	0.39	0.03

Popcorn, caramel or sugar-coated	1 C	35.20	1.13	1.00	0.12
Popcorn, cheese-flavored	1 C	11.00	1.13	1.09	0.04
Popcorn, commercially popped (prepopped), not "buttered"	1 C	11.00	1.22	1.18	0.04
Popcorn, home-popped, hot-air-popped	1 C	8.00	1.21	1.17	0.04
Popcorn, home-popped, popped in fat	1 C	12.80	1.21	1.17	0.04
Popcorn, microwave popped from package	1 C	9.00	0.83	0.80	0.02
Potato chip	1 oz	28.35	1.31	0.56	0.75
Potato sticks	1 oz	36.00	1.22	0.52	0.70
Pretzels, hard type	1 oz	28.35	0.91	0.65	0.26
Rice cake	1 Each	9.00	0.38	0.36	0.03
Taco or tortilla chips	1 oz	28.35	1.68	1.67	0.01
Pasta, Rice, and Other Grains					
Amaranth, dry	1 C	195.00	29.64	20.16	9.48
Barley, cooked	1 C	157.00	8.53	6.67	1.85
Barley, dry	1 C	200.00	31.20	24.40	6.80
Bran, corn, dry	1 C	76.00	64.96	61.60	1.60
Bran, oat bran, dry	1 C	94.00	14.48	7.71	6.77
Bran, rice, dry	1 C	118.00	24.78	21.59	3.19
Bran, wheat (unprocessed)	1 C	58.00	24.80	22.88	1.92
Buckwheat groats, dry	1 C	164.00	16.89	14.55	2.31
Bulgur, dry	1 C	140.00	25.62	21.31	4.28
Bulgur, canned	1 C	135.00	5.87	4.89	0.99
Bulgur, home-cooked	1 C	182.00	7.94	6.59	1.33
Corn grits, dry	1 C	156.00	2.50	1.87	0.62
Cornmeal, dry	1 C	138.00	10.21	10.13	0.08
Couscous, cooked	1 C	157.00	2.68	2.07	0.61
Couscous, dry	1 C	173.00	8.65	6.71	1.94
Flour, arrowroot	1 C	128.00	4.35	4.22	0.13
Flour, baking mix	1 C	113.40	1.47	1.10	0.37
Flour, barley	1 C	148.00	14.95	11.69	3.26
Flour, barley bran	1 C	148.00	99.97	95.70	4.29
Flour, barley malt	1 C	162.00	11.50	8.99	2.51
Flour, buckwheat	1 C	120.00	12.00	10.34	1.66
Flour, cake or pastry	1 C	137.00	2.33	0.95	1.38
Flour, chickpea	1 C	92.00	9.94	7.84	2.09
Flour, corn	1 C	114.00	10.94	6.09	4.86
Flour, peanut, defatted	1 C	60.00	9.48	6.87	2.61
Flour, peanut, low-fat	1 C	60.00	9.48	6.87	2.61

Table A.1 (Continued) Dietary Fiber Values for Common Foods

	Amount[a]	Weight (g)	Total Dietary Fiber (g)	Insoluble Fiber (g)	Soluble Fiber (g)
Pasta, Rice, and Other Grains					
Flour, potato	1 C	160.00	9.44	4.32	5.12
Flour, rice, brown	1 C	158.00	7.27	6.19	1.07
Flour, rice, white	1 C	158.00	3.79	2.95	0.84
Flour, rye	1 C	102.00	14.89	10.91	3.98
Flour, soy, defatted	1 C	100.00	17.50	9.63	7.88
Flour, soy, full-fat	1 C	84.00	8.06	4.44	3.63
Flour, soy, low-fat	1 C	88.00	8.98	3.43	5.54
Flour, triticale, whole grain	1 C	130.00	18.98	15.48	3.48
Flour, white all-purpose	1 C	125.00	3.37	1.37	2.00
Flour, whole wheat	1 C	120.00	14.64	12.48	2.16
Hominy, canned	1 C	165.00	4.13	2.34	1.78
Kasha, cooked	1 C	168.00	5.29	4.57	0.72
Millet, dry	1 C	200.00	17.00	13.82	3.18
Millet, cooked	1 C	240.00	6.48	5.26	1.22
Oatmeal, dry	1 C	81.00	8.59	4.62	3.97
Pasta, macaroni noodles, white, cooked	1 C	140.00	1.82	0.70	1.12
Pasta, macaroni noodles, whole wheat, cooked	1 C	140.00	3.92	3.08	0.84
Pasta, noodles, cellophane, cooked	1 C	160.00	1.60	1.23	0.34
Pasta, noodles, Chinese, soft type, cooked	1 C	176.00	2.29	0.88	1.41
Pasta, noodles, chow fun rice, cooked	1 C	160.00	1.60	1.23	0.34
Pasta, noodles, chow mein, crisp type	1 C	45.00	1.75	0.71	1.04
Pasta, noodles, egg, cooked	1 C	160.00	1.76	0.96	0.80
Pasta, noodles, rice, cooked	1 C	176.00	1.76	1.36	0.37
Pasta, noodles, whole wheat, cooked	1 C	160.00	4.48	3.52	0.96
Pasta, spaghetti noodles, white, cooked	1 C	140.00	1.82	0.70	1.12
Pasta, spaghetti noodles, whole wheat, cooked	1 C	140.00	3.92	3.08	0.84
Quinoa, cooked	1 C	158.00	9.32	8.06	1.26
Quinoa, dry	1 C	170.00	10.03	8.67	1.36
Rice, brown, cooked	1 C	195.00	3.51	3.28	0.23
Rice, white, instant (precooked), cooked	1 C	165.00	0.66	0.48	0.18
Rice, white, parboiled (converted), cooked	1 C	175.00	0.70	0.51	0.19
Rice, white, regular cooking, cooked	1 C	158.00	0.63	0.46	0.17
Sorghum	1 C	192.00	26.53	18.47	8.06

Tapioca, dry	1 C	152.00	1.37	1.22	0.15
Teff, dry	1 C	198.00	26.73	21.72	5.01
Wheat, cracked whole wheat	1 C	135.00	16.47	14.04	2.43
Wheat, germ	1 C	113.00	14.58	10.96	3.62
Wheat, gluten	1 C	413.99	12.42		
Wheat, spelt	1 C	120.00	13.68	12.12	1.56
Wheat, sprouted	1 C	108.00	1.19	0.98	0.19
Wild rice, cooked	1 C	164.00	2.95	2.62	0.33

Fruit

Apple, fresh, with skin	1 Medium	138.00	3.73	2.76	0.97
Apple, fresh, without skin	1 Medium	128.00	2.43	1.66	0.77
Apple, baked or scalloped, with skin, sweetened	1 C	190.00	4.94	3.61	1.33
Apple, baked or scalloped, with skin, unsweetened	1 C	187.00	5.42	4.02	1.40
Apple, dried, uncooked	1 C	86.00	7.48	3.44	4.04
Applesauce or stewed apples, canned, sweetened	1 C	255.00	3.06	2.09	0.97
Applesauce or stewed apples, canned, unsweetened	1 C	244.00	2.93	2.00	0.93
Apricot, fresh	1 C	155.00	3.72	1.70	2.01
Apricot, canned, water pack	1 C	243.00	3.89	2.21	1.68
Apricot, canned, heavy syrup pack	1 C	258.00	4.13	2.58	1.55
Apricot, dried, uncooked	1 C	130.00	11.70	5.98	5.72
Apricot, dried, cooked, unsweetened	1 C	250.00	8.00	3.85	4.15
Avocado, black skin, California type	1 Each	173.00	8.65	5.54	3.11
Banana, fresh or ripe	1 Medium	118.00	2.83	2.12	0.71
Blackberries, fresh	1 C	144.00	7.63	6.19	1.44
Blueberries, fresh	1 C	145.00	3.91	3.48	0.43
Cantaloupe, fresh	1 C	160.00	1.28	0.96	0.32
Carambola (starfruit), fresh	1 C	108.00	2.92	1.62	1.30
Cherries, fresh	1 C	145.00	3.33	2.32	1.01
Cherries, canned, heavy syrup pack	1 C	253.00	3.79	2.66	1.14
Cherries, maraschino cherries	1 C	161.00	1.45	1.01	0.43
Cranberries, fresh	1 C	95.00	3.99	2.94	1.04
Cranberries, dried (Craisins)	1 C	120.12	6.01	4.44	1.56
Dates	1 C	178.00	13.35	11.21	2.14
Elderberries, fresh	1 C	145.00	10.15	8.24	1.91
Figs, fresh	1 C	177.00	5.84	2.83	3.01
Figs, canned, heavy syrup pack	1 C	259.00	5.70	2.77	2.93
Figs, dried, uncooked	1 C	199.00	24.28	16.32	7.96
Fruit cocktail, canned, water pack	1 C	237.00	2.37	1.47	0.90

Table A.1 (Continued) Dietary Fiber Values for Common Foods

	Amount[a]	Weight (g)	Total Dietary Fiber (g)	Insoluble Fiber (g)	Soluble Fiber (g)
Fruit					
Fruit cocktail, canned, juice pack	1 C	237.00	2.37	0.95	1.42
Fruit cocktail, canned, heavy syrup pack	1 C	248.00	2.48	0.99	1.49
Gooseberries, fresh	1 C	150.00	6.45	5.10	1.35
Gooseberries, canned	1 C	252.00	6.05	4.03	2.02
Grapefruit, fresh, white	1 Medium	256.00	2.82	0.51	2.30
Grapefruit, fresh, pink or red	1 Medium	256.00	2.82	0.51	2.30
Grapefruit, canned, water pack	1 C	244.00	0.98	0.37	0.61
Grapefruit, canned, syrup pack	1 C	254.00	1.02	0.18	0.84
Grapes, fresh	1 C	160.00	1.60	0.96	0.64
Guava, fresh common	1 C	165.00	8.91	7.42	1.48
Honeydew melon, fresh	1 C	170.00	1.02	0.68	0.34
Kiwi	1 Medium	76.00	2.58	1.98	0.61
Kumquat, fresh	1 Each	19.00	1.25	0.80	0.46
Lemon, fresh	1 Medium	58.00	1.62	0.61	1.01
Loganberries, fresh	1 C	147.00	7.20	6.47	0.73
Mandarin orange, fresh	1 C	195.00	4.48	2.73	1.75
Mandarin orange, canned, syrup pack	1 C	252.00	1.76	1.26	0.50
Mango, fresh	1 Each	207.00	3.73	2.19	1.53
Nectarine, fresh	1 Medium	136.00	2.18	1.36	0.82
Orange, fresh	1 Medium	131.00	3.14	1.31	1.83
Papaya, fresh	1 C	140.00	2.52	1.27	1.25
Passion fruit, fresh	1 Each	18.00	1.87	0.53	1.34
Peach, fresh	1 Medium	98.00	1.96	1.18	0.78
Peach, canned, water pack	1 C	244.00	3.17	1.98	1.20
Peach, canned, heavy syrup pack	1 C	262.00	3.41	2.04	1.36
Peach, dried, uncooked	1 C	160.00	13.12	7.04	6.08
Peach, dried, cooked, unsweetened	1 C	258.00	6.97	3.74	3.22
Pear, fresh	1 Medium	166.00	3.98	1.83	2.16
Pear, canned, water pack	1 C	244.00	3.90	3.12	0.78
Pear, canned, heavy syrup pack	1 C	266.00	4.26	1.97	2.29
Pear, dried, uncooked	1 C	180.00	13.50	8.10	5.40
Pear, dried, cooked, unsweetened	1 C	255.00	16.32	7.47	8.82
Persimmon, fresh	1 Each	168.00	6.05	5.26	0.79

Food	Amount	Weight			
Pineapple, fresh	1 C	155.00	1.86	1.70	0.15
Pineapple, canned, juice pack	1 C	249.00	1.99	1.49	0.50
Pineapple, canned, light syrup pack	1 C	252.00	2.02	1.51	0.50
Plantains, ripe, boiled or baked	1 C	154.00	3.54	2.77	0.77
Plum, fresh	1 C	165.00	2.47	1.15	1.32
Plum, canned, heavy syrup pack	1 Each	258.00	2.58	1.21	1.37
Pomegranate	1 Each	154.00	0.92	0.75	0.17
Prune, dried, uncooked	1 C	170.00	12.07	5.61	6.46
Prune, dried, cooked, unsweetened	1 C	248.00	16.37	12.15	4.22
Raisins, uncooked	1 C	155.00	6.20	4.49	1.70
Raspberries, fresh	1 C	123.00	8.36	7.50	0.86
Raspberries, frozen, sweetened	1 C	250.00	11.00	9.75	1.25
Rhubarb, cooked from fresh, sweetened	1 C	240.00	4.80	3.60	1.20
Rhubarb, cooked from fresh, unsweetened	1 C	240.00	3.36	2.16	1.20
Sapodilla, fresh	1 Each	170.00	13.94	9.01	4.93
Strawberries, fresh	1 C	144.00	3.31	2.45	0.86
Strawberries, frozen, sweetened	1 C	255.00	4.84	3.57	1.27
Watermelon, fresh	1 Slice	286.00	1.43	0.86	0.57

Juices

Food	Amount	Weight			
Apple juice	1 C	248.00	0.25	0.17	0.07
Apricot nectar	1 C	251.00	1.51	0.75	0.75
Black currant juice	1 C	250.00	1.50	0.52	0.97
Carrot juice	1 C	236.00	1.89	1.37	0.52
Cranberry juice	1 C	253.00	0.25	0.18	0.08
Cranapple juice	1 C	245.00	0.24	0.15	0.05
Grape juice	1 C	253.00	0.25	0.00	0.25
Grapefruit juice	1 C	250.00	0.25	0.05	0.20
Lemon juice	1 C	244.00	0.98	0.24	0.73
Orange juice	1 C	249.00	0.50	0.25	0.25
Papaya juice	1 C	247.00	1.48	0.79	0.69
Passion fruit juice	1 C	247.00	0.49	0.15	0.35
Peach nectar	1 C	249.00	1.49	0.40	1.10
Pineapple juice	1 C	250.00	0.50	0.25	0.25
Prune juice	1 C	256.00	2.56	1.28	1.28
Tomato juice	1 C	243.00	0.97	0.44	0.53
Vegetable juice	1 C	242.00	1.94	1.45	0.48

Table A.1 (Continued) Dietary Fiber Values for Common Foods

	Amount[a]	Weight (g)	Total Dietary Fiber (g)	Insoluble Fiber (g)	Soluble Fiber (g)
Vegetables and Legumes					
Artichoke, regular globe, cooked	1 C	168.00	9.07	2.47	6.60
Arugula, raw	1 C	20.00	0.32	0.27	0.05
Asparagus, cooked	1 C	180.00	2.88	1.44	1.44
Asparagus, canned, drained	1 C	242.00	3.87	2.90	0.97
Bamboo shoots, canned, drained	1 C	131.00	1.83	1.31	0.52
Basil, fresh	1 T	2.65	0.10		
Beans, baked beans with pork in tomato sauce	1 C	253.00	12.14	7.08	5.06
Beans, baked beans with pork in brown sugar	1 C	253.00	13.16	8.10	5.06
Beans, baked beans, vegetarian	1 C	254.00	12.55	7.57	4.39
Beans, bayo, cooked	1 C	172.00	5.76	3.49	2.27
Beans, garbanzo, cooked from dried	1 C	164.00	12.46	9.84	2.62
Beans, green or string, cooked from fresh	1 C	125.00	3.75	2.12	1.62
Beans, green or string, cooked from frozen	1 C	135.00	4.05	2.29	1.75
Beans, green or string, canned, drained	1 C	135.00	2.56	1.62	0.94
Beans, kidney, cooked from dried	1 C	177.00	11.33	5.66	5.66
Beans, lima, cooked from dried	1 C	188.00	13.16	6.20	6.96
Beans, lima, cooked from frozen	1 C	170.00	9.86	7.14	2.72
Beans, navy, cooked from dried	1 C	182.00	11.65	7.28	4.37
Beans, northern, cooked from dried	1 C	177.00	11.15	8.32	2.83
Beans, pinto, cooked from dried	1 C	171.00	14.71	10.94	3.76
Beans, refried beans, canned	1 C	252.00	13.36	9.20	4.18
Beans, soybeans, cooked from dried	1 C	172.00	10.32	5.68	4.64
Beans, soybeans, green or immature, cooked	1 C	180.00	7.56	4.16	3.40
Beans, soybeans, roasted	1 C	172.00	30.44	16.75	13.69
Beans, tepary, cooked	1 C	262.00	13.36		
Beans, wax or yellow, cooked from fresh	1 C	125.00	3.75	2.12	1.62
Beans, wax or yellow, cooked from frozen	1 C	135.00	4.05	2.29	1.75
Beans, wax or yellow, canned, drained	1 C	135.00	1.75	0.81	0.94
Beets, cooked from fresh	1 C	170.00	3.40	1.36	2.04
Beets, canned. drained	1 C	170.00	2.89	1.53	1.36
Beet greens, raw	1 C	38.00	1.41	0.99	0.42
Beet greens, cooked	1 C	144.00	4.18	2.29	1.89
Broccoflower (green cauliflower), raw	1 C	64.00	2.05	1.02	1.02

Food	Unit	Weight			
Broccoflower (green cauliflower), cooked	1 C	82.00	2.71	1.53	1.18
Broccoli, raw	1 C	88.00	2.64	1.69	0.95
Broccoli, cooked from fresh	1 C	156.00	4.68	2.34	2.34
Broccoli, cooked from frozen	1 C	184.00	5.52	2.76	2.76
Brussels sprouts, cooked	1 C	155.00	6.35	2.48	3.88
Cabbage, green, raw	1 C	89.00	2.05	1.33	0.71
Cabbage, green, cooked	1 C	150.00	3.45	1.90	1.54
Cabbage, red, raw	1 C	89.00	1.78	0.96	0.82
Cabbage, red, cooked	1 C	150.00	3.00	1.68	1.32
Carrots, raw	1 C	110.00	3.30	1.65	1.65
Carrots, cooked from fresh	1 C	156.00	5.15	2.96	2.18
Carrots, cooked from frozen	1 C	146.00	4.82	2.77	2.04
Carrots, canned, drained	1 C	146.00	2.19	0.73	1.46
Cassava (yuca), cooked	1 C	132.00	1.53	0.92	0.61
Cauliflower, raw	1 C	100.00	2.50	1.60	0.90
Cauliflower, cooked from fresh	1 C	125.00	3.37	2.50	0.87
Cauliflower, cooked from frozen	1 C	180.00	4.86	3.60	1.26
Celeriac or celery root, cooked	1 C	155.00	1.86	0.98	0.88
Celery, raw	1 C	120.00	2.04	1.32	0.72
Celery, cooked	1 C	150.00	2.40	1.65	0.75
Chard, cooked	1 C	175.00	3.67	3.66	0.61
Chinese cabbage, Pak-choi, raw	1 C	70.00	0.70	0.38	0.32
Chinese cabbage, Pak-choi, cooked	1 C	170.00	2.72	1.70	1.02
Chinese cabbage, Pe-tsai, raw	1 C	76.00	2.36	1.90	0.46
Chinese cabbage, Pe-tsai, cooked	1 C	119.00	3.21	1.49	1.73
Chinese vegetables, canned, drained	1 C	125.49	1.42	0.88	0.53
Chives, raw	1 T	3.00	0.07	0.05	0.02
Collards, raw	1 C	36.00	1.30	0.51	0.78
Collards, cooked	1 C	190.00	5.32	2.09	3.23
Coriander leaf, fresh	1 T	2.88	0.08	0.03	0.05
Coriander leaf, dried	1 TS	0.60	0.06	0.02	0.04
Corn, cooked from fresh, cob	1 Medium	100.00	2.80	2.30	0.50
Corn, cooked from frozen, whole kernel	1 C	164.00	3.94	3.44	0.49
Corn, canned, drained	1 C	164.00	3.28	2.95	0.33
Cucumber, raw with peel	1 C	104.00	0.83	0.62	0.21
Cucumber, raw without peel	1 C	119.00	0.83	0.62	0.21
Dill weed, fresh	1 T	0.56	0.01	0.01	0.00
Eggplant, cooked	1 C	99.00	2.47	1.78	0.69
Endive (curly), raw	1 C	29.00	0.90	0.64	0.26

Table A.1 (Continued) Dietary Fiber Values for Common Foods

	Amount[a]	Weight (g)	Total Dietary Fiber (g)	Insoluble Fiber (g)	Soluble Fiber (g)
Vegetables and Legumes					
Endive (curly), cooked	1 C	130.00	5.19	3.68	1.51
Fennel bulb, raw	1 C	87.00	2.70	1.74	0.96
Garlic, fresh	1 TS	2.83	0.06	0.01	0.05
Ginger root, raw	1 C	96.00	1.92		
Hearts of palm, canned	1 C	146.00	3.50		
Jicama or yambean, raw	1 C	130.00	6.37	3.07	3.30
Jicama or yambean, cooked	1 C	135.20	2.57	1.46	1.11
Kale, cooked	1 C	130.00	2.60	1.17	1.43
Kohlrabi, raw	1 C	135.00	4.86	1.48	3.38
Kohlrabi, cooked	1 C	165.00	1.81	0.56	1.25
Lentils, cooked from dried	1 C	198.00	15.64	14.45	1.19
Lettuce, iceberg	1 C	55.00	0.77	0.66	0.11
Lettuce, romaine or cos	1 C	56.00	0.95	0.62	0.34
Mixed vegetables (corn, lima beans, peas, green beans, and carrots), cooked from frozen	1 C	182.00	8.01	4.19	3.82
Mixed vegetables (corn, lima beans, peas, green beans, and carrots), cooked from frozen	1 C	182.00	5.46	4.37	1.09
Mixed vegetables (corn, lima beans, peas, green beans, and carrots), canned, drained					
Mixed vegetables (peas and carrots), cooked from frozen	1 C	160.00	4.96	3.26	1.70
Mixed vegetables (peas and carrots), canned, drained	1 C	160.00	4.48	3.28	1.20
Mushrooms, raw	1 C	70.00	0.84	0.70	0.14
Mushrooms, cooked from fresh	1 C	156.00	3.43	3.12	0.31
Mushrooms, canned, drained	1 C	156.00	3.74	3.43	0.31
Okra, cooked	1 C	184.00	5.15	3.13	2.02
Onion, white, yellow, or red, raw	1 C	160.00	2.88	1.12	1.76
Onion, white, yellow, or red, cooked	1 C	210.00	2.94	0.84	2.10
Parsley, fresh	1 T	3.75	0.12	0.02	0.10
Parsnip, cooked	1 C	156.00	6.24	2.65	3.59
Peas, green peas, cooked	1 C	160.00	8.80	6.24	2.56
Peas, green peas, canned, drained	1 C	170.00	6.97	6.12	0.85
Peas, cowpeas, cooked from dried	1 C	172.00	11.18	9.80	1.38
Peas, cowpeas, cooked from fresh	1 C	165.00	8.25	7.36	0.89
Peas, snow peas or edible pea pods, cooked	1 C	160.00	4.48	3.36	1.12
Peas, split peas, yellow or green, cooked from dried	1 C	196.00	16.27	14.11	2.16

Peas, split peas, yellow or green, canned, drained	1 C	196.00	16.27	14.11	2.16
Peppers, green pepper — sweet, raw	1 C	149.00	2.68	1.64	1.04
Peppers, green pepper — sweet, cooked	1 C	184.00	2.21	0.74	1.47
Peppers, red — sweet, raw	1 C	149.00	2.98	1.94	1.04
Peppers, red — sweet, cooked	1 C	184.00	2.21	0.92	1.29
Peppers, yellow — sweet, raw	1 C	149.00	1.34	0.85	0.49
Peppers, yellow — sweet, cooked	1 C	184.00	1.73	1.09	0.63
Peppers, hot chili, green, raw	1 C	150.00	2.25	1.38	0.87
Peppers, hot chili, green, cooked from fresh	1 C	136.00	2.04	0.68	1.36
Peppers, hot chili, green, canned, drained	1 C	139.00	2.36	0.79	1.57
Peppers, hot chili, red, raw	1 C	150.00	2.25	1.38	0.87
Peppers, hot chili, red, cooked from fresh	1 C	136.00	2.12	1.31	0.82
Peppers, hot chili, red, canned, drained	1 C	136.00	1.77	0.60	1.17
Peppers, hot chili, sun-dried	1 C	37.00	10.62		
Peppers, jalapeno pepper, raw	1 C	90.00	2.52	1.54	0.98
Peppers, jalapeno pepper, cooked from fresh	1 C	136.00	3.96	2.42	1.54
Peppers, jalapeno pepper, canned, drained	1 C	136.00	3.54	1.18	2.35
Potato, baked, skin eaten	1 C	122.00	2.93	1.71	1.22
Potato, baked, skin not eaten	1 C	127.00	1.90	0.60	1.31
Potato, boiled, with skin	1 C	156.00	3.01	1.76	1.25
Potato, boiled, without skin	1 C	156.00	2.81	1.20	1.61
Potato, canned, drained	1 C	180.00	4.52	0.99	3.53
Pumpkin, canned	1 C	245.00	7.10	6.13	0.98
Radicchio, raw	1 C	40.00	0.36	0.18	0.18
Radish, raw	1 C	116.00	1.86	1.39	0.46
Rutabaga, cooked	1 C	170.00	3.06	2.55	0.51
Sauerkraut	1 C	236.00	5.90	3.85	2.05
Scallions or spring onions, raw	1 C	100.00	2.60	1.01	1.59
Scallions or spring onions, cooked	1 C	219.00	5.50	2.63	2.87
Spinach, raw	1 C	30.00	0.81	0.57	0.24
Spinach, cooked from fresh	1 C	180.00	5.40	4.32	1.08
Spinach, cooked from frozen	1 C	205.00	6.15	4.92	1.23
Spinach, canned, drained	1 C	214.00	5.14	3.85	1.28
Sprouts, alfalfa	1 C	33.00	0.82	0.63	0.20
Sprouts, mung bean, cooked from fresh	1 C	124.00	0.99	0.37	0.62
Sprouts, mung bean, canned, drained	1 C	125.00	1.00	0.52	0.47
Sprouts, soybean, raw	1 C	70.00	0.77	0.41	0.36
Squash, acorn, cooked	1 C	245.00	10.78	4.63	6.15
Squash, butternut, cooked	1 C	240.00	3.36	1.92	1.44

Table A.1 (Continued) Dietary Fiber Values for Common Foods

	Amount[a]	Weight (g)	Total Dietary Fiber (g)	Insoluble Fiber (g)	Soluble Fiber (g)
Vegetables and Legumes					
Squash, chayote, cooked	1 C	160.00	4.48	3.52	0.96
Squash, hubbard, cooked	1 C	236.00	6.61	2.83	3.78
Squash, spaghetti, cooked	1 C	155.00	2.17	0.93	1.24
Squash, zucchini, raw	1 C	113.00	1.36	0.79	0.56
Squash, zucchini, cooked	1 C	180.00	2.52	1.44	1.08
Squash, summer-type (green or yellow), raw	1 C	113.00	1.58	1.24	0.34
Squash, summer-type (green or yellow), cooked	1 C	180.00	2.52	1.98	0.54
Squash, winter-type (dark green or orange), cooked	1 C	240.00	6.72	2.88	3.84
Sweet potato, cooked	1 C	255.00	7.65	4.84	2.80
Sweet potato, canned, syrup-packed, drained	1 C	196.00	5.88	2.25	3.63
Sweet potato, canned, vacuum-packed	1 C	200.00	3.60	2.22	1.38
Tomatillo, raw	1 C	132.00	2.51	2.28	0.22
Tomato, raw	1 C	180.00	1.98	1.80	0.18
Tomato, canned	1 C	240.00	2.40	1.44	0.96
Tomato, green, raw	1 C	180.00	1.98	1.80	0.18
Tomato, orange, raw	1 C	158.00	1.42	1.30	0.13
Tomato, paste	1 C	262.00	10.74	8.59	2.15
Tomato, puree	1 C	250.00	5.00	3.00	2.00
Tomato, sun-dried, dry pack	1 C	54.00	6.64	6.04	0.60
Tomato, sun-dried, oil pack, drained	1 C	110.00	6.38	5.80	0.58
Tomato, yellow, raw	1 C	139.00	0.97	0.89	0.08
Turnip, cooked	1 C	155.00	3.10	1.98	1.12
Turnip greens, cooked	1 C	144.00	5.04	2.76	2.28
Water chestnuts, canned	1 C	140.00	3.08	1.83	1.25
Watercress, raw	1 C	34.00	0.51	0.24	0.27
Yams, cooked	1 C	255.00	7.65	4.84	2.80
Yams, canned, syrup-packed, drained	1 C	196.00	5.88	2.25	3.63
Yams, canned, vacuum-packed	1 C	200.00	3.60	2.22	1.38
Meat Substitutes					
Bacon bits, textured vegetable protein	1 T	7.00	0.56	0.40	0.16
Breakfast strips, textured vegetable protein	1 Strip	8.00	0.21	0.12	0.09

Canadian-style bacon, soy product	1 oz	28.35	0.13	0.05	0.04
Hamburger/ground beef substitute — meatless	1 oz	28.35	0.18	0.00	0.00
Hot dogs, frankfurters, or wieners substitute — meatless	1 oz	28.35	1.73	0.93	0.80
Sausage, breakfast or brown-and-serve, substitute — meatless, link	1 oz	28.35	0.20	0.08	0.07
Sausage, breakfast or brown-and-serve, substitute — meatless, patty	1 oz	28.35	0.24	0.10	0.08
Tempeh (fermented soybean product)	1 oz	28.35	2.92	1.61	1.32
Textured vegetable protein, from dry	1 C	94.05	9.21	6.63	2.59
Textured vegetable protein, from frozen	1 oz	28.35	0.21	0.12	0.09
Tofu (soybean curd)	1 oz	28.35	0.06	0.03	0.03
Vegetable burger	1 oz	28.35	0.68	0.42	0.27
Nuts and Seeds					
Almonds	1 C	142.00	15.90	14.34	1.56
Almond butter	1 T	15.63	0.58	0.52	0.06
Almond paste	1 T	14.19	0.77	0.70	0.08
Brazil nuts	1 C	140.00	7.56	5.74	1.82
Cashews	1 C	130.00	4.94	4.50	0.44
Cashew butter	1 T	16.00	0.32	0.29	0.03
Chestnuts	1 C	143.00	16.73	13.16	3.57
Coconut, dried (shredded or flaked), sweetened	1 C	74.00	3.33	3.05	0.28
Coconut, dried (shredded or flaked), unsweetened	1 C	80.00	13.04	11.92	1.12
Coconut, fresh	1 Medium	397.00	35.73	31.76	3.97
Filberts or hazelnuts	1 C	135.00	8.23	4.86	3.38
Flax seeds	1 C	114.00	25.46	11.57	13.89
Trail mix (nuts, seeds, and dried fruit)	1 C	150.00	11.13	9.09	2.05
Hickory nuts	1 C	120.00	7.68	5.88	1.80
Macadamia nuts	1 C	134.00	12.46	9.92	2.55
Mixed nuts with peanuts	1 C	142.00	12.78	10.22	2.56
Mixed nuts without peanuts	1 C	144.00	7.92	6.61	1.31
Peanuts	1 C	144.00	13.25	10.51	2.74
Peanut butter	1 T	16.13	0.95	0.69	0.26
Pecans	1 C	108.00	8.21	6.59	1.62
Pine nuts — pignolias	1 C	136.00	14.55	13.06	1.50
Pine nuts — pinyon	1 C	130.00	13.91	12.48	1.43
Pistachio nuts	1 C	128.00	13.82	10.37	3.46
Poppy seeds	1 C	140.80	14.08		
Pumpkin or squash seeds	1 C	227.00	8.85	6.42	2.43
Sesame seeds	1 C	150.00	11.68	8.83	2.85
Tahini (sesame butter)	1 T	15.00	1.39	1.10	0.29

Table A.1 (Continued) Dietary Fiber Values for Common Foods

	Amount[a]	Weight (g)	Total Dietary Fiber (g)	Insoluble Fiber (g)	Soluble Fiber (g)
Nuts and Seeds					
Sunflower seeds	1 C	128.00	13.44	10.75	2.69
Sunflower butter	1 T	16.00	1.28	0.79	0.49
Walnuts	1 C	120.00	5.76	3.96	1.80
Soup					
Bean with bacon, ham, or pork, prepared from ready-to-serve can	1 C	238.00	5.31	3.95	1.38
Bean with bacon, undiluted	1 C	256.00	10.65	7.88	2.74
Beef with noodles or pasta, prepared from ready-to-serve can	1 C	241.00	0.80	0.51	0.29
Beef with noodles or pasta, undiluted	1 C	252.00	0.76	0.43	0.35
Black bean, prepared from ready-to-serve can	1 C	242.00	5.30	3.94	1.38
Black bean, undiluted	1 C	252.00	6.80	5.07	1.76
Broccoli cheese, undiluted	1 C	248.00	3.92	1.96	2.01
Cheese, undiluted	1 C	248.00	0.27	0.10	0.15
Chicken with noodles or pasta, prepared from ready-to-serve can	1 C	238.00	0.38	0.21	0.17
Chicken with noodles or pasta, prepared from ready-to-serve can, chunky-style	1 C	240.00	0.67	0.38	0.26
Chicken with noodles or pasta, undiluted	1 C	252.00	0.76	0.43	0.35
Chicken with rice, prepared from ready-to-serve can	1 C	238.00	0.33	0.21	0.12
Chicken with rice, undiluted	1 C	252.00	0.71	0.45	0.25
Chicken with vegetables, prepared from ready-to-serve can	1 C	240.00	1.22	0.67	0.55
Chicken with vegetables, undiluted	1 C	252.00	2.44	1.36	1.13
Clam chowder, Manhattan (tomato base), prepared from ready-to-serve can	1 C	239.00	1.03	0.55	0.45
Clam chowder, Manhattan (tomato base), undiluted	1 C	252.00	2.02	1.13	0.93
Clam chowder, New England (cream base), prepared from ready-to-serve can	1 C	240.00	1.61	0.70	0.91
Clam chowder, New England (cream base), undiluted	1 C	252.00	2.12	0.66	0.88
Cream of broccoli, undiluted	1 C	248.00	1.24	0.57	0.67
Cream of celery, undiluted	1 C	248.00	2.01	1.26	0.72
Cream of chicken, undiluted	1 C	248.00	0.47	0.15	0.22
Cream of mushroom, undiluted	1 C	248.00	0.62	0.40	0.25
Cream of onion, undiluted	1 C	248.00	0.97	0.30	0.67

Food	Serving	Weight (g)			
Lentil, prepared from ready-to-serve can	1 C	245.00	7.52	6.44	1.08
Minestrone, prepared from ready-to-serve can	1 C	245.00	3.33	2.20	1.10
Minestrone, undiluted	1 C	252.00	6.60	4.41	2.19
Onion, clear (French style), undiluted	1 C	252.00	3.10	0.68	1.66
Pea (green), undiluted	1 C	256.00	17.56	15.18	2.38
Split pea with bacon, ham, or pork, prepared from ready-to-serve can	1 C	243.00	8.21	7.05	1.17
Split pea with ham or bacon, undiluted	1 C	256.00	16.46	14.13	2.36
Split pea, vegetarian, prepared from ready-to-serve can	1 C	244.00	8.76	7.56	1.20
Tomato, prepared from ready-to-serve can	1 C	241.00	1.08	0.77	0.31
Tomato, undiluted	1 C	248.00	2.18	1.56	0.62
Vegetable beef, prepared from ready-to-serve can	1 C	245.00	1.57	1.10	0.44
Vegetable beef, prepared from ready-to-serve can, chunky-style	1 C	245.00	3.28	2.20	1.15
Vegetable beef, undiluted	1 C	252.00	3.15	2.19	0.96
Vegetable, plain (vegetarian), prepared from ready-to-serve can	1 C	241.00	3.18	1.61	0.89
Vegetable, undiluted	1 C	252.00	3.28	2.07	1.18

Candy and Sweets

Food	Serving	Weight (g)			
Bridge mix	1 oz	28.35	0.78	0.63	0.15
Candy-coated almonds	1 oz	28.35	1.33	1.20	0.13
Candy-coated chocolate	1 oz	28.35	0.71	0.57	0.12
Candy-coated peanuts and chocolate	1 oz	28.35	0.96	0.74	0.23
Caramel, plain	1 oz	28.35	0.34	0.00	0.34
Carob	1 oz	28.35	1.08	0.29	0.79
Carob-coated peanuts	1 oz	28.35	1.77	0.67	1.11
Carob-coated raisins	1 oz	28.35	0.71	0.39	0.32
Chocolate-covered almonds	1 oz	28.35	2.45	2.18	0.27
Chocolate-covered caramel	1 oz	28.35	0.23	0.22	0.01
Chocolate-covered caramel and nougat	1 oz	28.35	0.48	0.39	0.09
Chocolate-covered caramel and peanuts	1 oz	28.35	0.99	0.80	0.20
Chocolate-covered caramel, peanuts, and nougat	1 oz	28.35	0.82	0.61	0.21
Chocolate-covered cherry	1 oz	28.35	0.33	0.27	0.07
Chocolate-covered coconut	1 oz	28.35	1.65	1.53	0.13
Chocolate-covered cream	1 oz	28.35	0.43	0.41	0.02
Chocolate-covered fondant	1 oz	28.35	0.43	0.41	0.02
Chocolate-covered marshmallow	1 oz	28.35	0.31	0.23	0.05
Chocolate-covered peanut butter	1 oz	28.35	0.91	0.69	0.21
Chocolate-covered peanuts	1 oz	28.35	1.33	1.03	0.31
Chocolate-covered raisins	1 oz	28.35	1.19	1.00	0.18
Chocolate-covered toffee	1 oz	28.35	0.71	0.59	0.12

Table A.1 (Continued) Dietary Fiber Values for Common Foods

	Amount[a]	Weight (g)	Total Dietary Fiber (g)	Insoluble Fiber (g)	Soluble Fiber (g)
Candy and Sweets					
Chocolate-covered toffee with nuts	1 oz	28.35	1.45	1.28	0.17
Dark chocolate	1 oz	28.35	1.67	1.60	0.07
Fruit leather or rolls	1 oz	28.35	0.48	0.26	0.18
Fruit snacks	1 oz	28.35	0.06	0.00	0.01
Halvah, plain	1 oz	28.35	1.28	1.01	0.27
Licorice	1 oz	28.35	0.37	0.15	0.22
Malted milk balls	1 oz	28.35	1.05	0.53	0.52
Marshmallow	1 C	50.00	0.05	0.00	0.00
Milk chocolate with almonds	1 oz	28.35	1.76	1.50	0.26
Milk chocolate with cereal	1 oz	28.35	0.88	0.72	0.16
Milk chocolate with peanuts	1 oz	28.35	0.99	0.78	0.21
Milk chocolate, plain	1 oz	28.35	0.96	0.79	0.17
Salted nut roll	1 oz	28.35	1.62	1.28	0.33
White chocolate	1 oz	28.35	0.00	0.00	0.00
Yogurt-covered almonds	1 oz	28.35	1.39	1.25	0.14
Yogurt-covered peanuts	1 oz	28.35	0.39	0.28	0.10
Yogurt-covered raisins	1 oz	28.35	0.57	0.41	0.16
Spices, Condiments, and Miscellaneous					
Allspice (ground)	1 TS	2.00	0.43		
Anise seed	1 TS	2.23	0.33		
Baking chocolate	1 oz	28.35	4.37	4.19	0.18
Basil (ground)	1 TS	1.50	0.61		
Bay leaf	1 TS	0.60	0.16		
Caraway seed	1 TS	2.23	0.85		
Cardamom (ground)	1 TS	1.93	0.54		
Carob powder	1 TS	2.33	0.93	0.25	0.68
Catsup	1 T	15.00	0.19	0.15	0.04
Celery seed	1 TS	2.17	0.26		
Chervil (dried)	1 TS	0.63	0.07		

Chili powder	1 TS	2.50	0.85		
Cinnamon (ground)	1 TS	2.27	1.23		
Cloves (ground)	1 TS	2.20	0.75		
Cocoa powder, unsweetened	1 TS	1.79	0.59	0.47	0.13
Coriander seed	1 TS	1.67	0.70		
Cumin seed	1 TS	2.00	0.21		
Curry powder	1 TS	2.10	0.70		
Dill seed	1 TS	2.20	0.46	0.28	0.18
Dill weed, dried	1 TS	1.03	0.16	0.10	0.06
Fennel seed	1 TS	1.93	0.77		
Fenugreek seed	1 TS	3.70	0.91		
Garlic, powder	1 TS	2.80	0.28	0.06	0.22
Ginger (ground)	1 TS	1.80	0.22		
Hot chili pepper — mature red (dried), with seeds	1 TS	2.00	0.19		
Hot chili pepper — mature red (dried), without seeds	1 TS	2.00	0.22		
Mace (ground)	1 TS	1.77	0.36		
Marjoram (dried)	1 TS	0.57	0.23		
Miso (soybean paste)	1 TS	5.73	0.31	0.16	0.15
Mustard	1 TS	5.21	0.14		
Mustard, powder	1 TS	1.50	0.02		
Nutmeg	1 TS	2.33	0.49		
Olives, black	1 Medium	4.00	0.13	0.12	0.01
Olives, green	1 Medium	3.40	0.03	0.03	0.00
Olives, stuffed	1 Medium	4.00	0.04	0.04	0.00
Onion powder	1 TS	2.17	0.12	0.05	0.08
Oregano (ground)	1 TS	1.50	0.64		
Paprika	1 TS	2.30	0.48		
Parsley (dried)	1 TS	0.43	0.13		
Pepper (ground), black	1 TS	2.13	0.57	0.07	0.07
Pepper (ground), red	1 TS	1.77	0.48		
Pepper (ground), white	1 TS	2.37	0.62		
Pickles, bread-and-butter	1 C	160.00	1.76	1.36	0.40
Pickles, dill	1 C	143.00	1.72	1.36	0.36
Pickles, sweet — gherkins	1 C	160.00	1.76	1.36	0.40
Pimiento	1 T	12.00	0.23	0.09	0.13
Rosemary, dried	1 TS	1.10	0.47		
Rosemary, fresh	1 TS	0.57	0.08		
Saffron	1 TS	0.70	0.03		
Sage (ground)	1 TS	0.67	0.27		

Table A.1 (Continued) Dietary Fiber Values for Common Foods

	Amount[a]	Weight (g)	Total Dietary Fiber (g)	Insoluble Fiber (g)	Soluble Fiber (g)
Spices, Condiments, and Miscellaneous					
Savory (ground)	1 TS	1.47	0.67		
Tarragon (ground)	1 TS	1.60	0.12		
Thyme, fresh	1 T	2.40	0.34		
Thyme (ground)	1 TS	1.43	0.53		
Turmeric (ground)	1 TS	2.27	0.48		
Yeast, baking — compressed	1 Cake	17.00	1.38		
Yeast, baking — active dry	1 T	12.00	2.52		
Yeast, Brewers	1 T	15.00	3.00		

Note: Includes both analytic and estimated values. This table has been revised since the 1994 2nd edition, based on the availability of improved data. For further information regarding specific values, contact The Nutrition Coordinating Center, Division of Epidemiology, School of Public Health, 1300 South Second Street, Suite 300, Minneapolis, Minnesota 55454-1015.

[a] Abbreviations: T = tablespoon, C = cup, oz = ounce, BIS = biscuit, TS = teaspoon.

REFERENCES

1. Aalto, T., Lehtonen, M., and Varo, P., Dietary fiber content of barley grown in Finland, *Cereal Chem.*, 65, 284, 1988.
2. Alaoui, L. and Essatara, M., Dietary fiber and phytic acid levels in the major food items consumed in Morocco, *Nutr. Rep. Int.*, 31, 469, 1985.
3. Anderson, J. W., *Plant Fiber in Foods*, HCF Nutrition Research Foundation, Lexington, KY, 1990.
4. Anderson, J. W. and Bridges, S.R., Dietary fiber content of selected foods, *Am. J. Clin. Nutr.*, 47, 440, 1988.
5. Anderson, J. W., Bridges, S. R., Tietyen, J., and Gustafson, N. J., Dietary fiber content of simulated American diet and selected research diets, *Am. J. Clin. Nutr.*, 49, 352, 1989.
6. Anderson, J. W., Gustafson, N. J., Byrant, C. A., and Tietyen-Clark, J., Dietary fiber and diabetes: a comprehensive review and practical application, *J. Am. Dietet. Assoc.*, 87, 1189, 1987.
7. Anderson, J. W. and Ward, K., Long-term effects of high-carbohydrate, high-fiber diets on glucose and lipid metabolism: a preliminary report on patients with diabetes, *Diabetes Care*, 1, 77, 1978.
8. Anderson, N. E. and Clydesdale, F. M., Effects of processing on the dietary fiber content of wheat bran, pureed green beans, and carrots, *J. Food Sci.*, 45, 1533, 1980.
9. Angus, R., Sutherland, T. M., and Farrell, D. J., Insoluble dietary fibre content of some local foods, *Proc. Nutr. Soc. Aust.*, 6, 161, 1981.
10. Asp, N.-G., Johansson, C.-G., Hallmer, H., and Siljestrom, M., Rapid enzymatic assay of insoluble and soluble dietary fiber, *J. Agric. Food Chem.*, 31, 476, 1983.
11. Babcock, D., Rice bran as a source of dietary fiber, *Cereal Foods World*, 32, 538, 1987.
12. Baker, D., The determination of fiber in processed cereal foods by near-infrared reflectance spectroscopy, *Cereal Chem.*, 60, 217, 1983.
13. Baker, D., Fiber in wheat foods, *Cereal Foods World*, 23, 557, 1978.
14. Baker, D. and Holden, J. M., Fiber in breakfast cereals, *J. Food Sci.*, 46, 396, 1981.
15. Baker, R.A., Reassessment of some fruit and vegetable pectin levels, *J. Food Sci.*, 62, 225, 1997.
16. Balasubramaniam, K., Polysaccharides of the kernel of maturing and matured coconuts, *J. Food Sci.*, 41, 1370, 1976.
17. Bell, B. M., A rapid method of dietary fibre estimation in wheat products, *J. Sci. Food Agric.*, 36, 815, 1985.
18. Belo, P. S. and de Lumen, B. O., Pectic substance content of detergent-extracted dietary fibers, *J. Agric. Food Chem.*, 29, 373, 1981.
19. Best, D., Building fiber into foods, *Prep. Foods*, July, 112, 1987.
20. Bittner, A. S., Burritt, E. A., Moser, J., and Street, J. C., Composition of dietary fiber: neutral and acidic sugar composition of the alcohol insoluble residue from human foods, *J. Food Sci.*, 47, 1469, 1982.
21. Boothby, D., Pectic substances in developing and ripening plum fruits, *J. Sci. Food Agric.*, 34, 1117, 1983.
22. Brandt, L. M., Jeltema, M. A., Zabik, M. E., and Jeltema, B. D., Effects of cooking in solutions of varying pH on the dietary fiber components of vegetables, *J. Food Sci.*, 49, 900, 1984.
23. Brillouet, J.-M., Rouau, X., Hoebler, C., Barry, J.-L., Carre, B., and Lorta, E., A new method for determination of insoluble cell walls and soluble nonstarchy polysaccharides from plant materials, *J. Agric. Food Chem.*, 36, 969, 1988.
24. Candlish, J. K., Gourley, L., and Lee, H. P., Dietary fiber and starch in some Southeast Asian fruits, *J. Food Comp. Anal.*, 1, 81, 1987.
25. Cardozo, M. S. and Eitenmiller, R. R., Total dietary fiber analysis of selected baked and cereal products, *Cereal Foods World*, 33, 414, 1988.
26. Cardozo, M. S. and Li, B. W., Total dietary fiber content of selected nuts by two enzymatic-gravimetric methods, *J. Food Comp. Anal.*, 7, 37, 1994.
27. Chen, H., Rubenthaler, G. L., Leung, H. K., and Baranowski, J. D., Chemical, physical, and baking properties of apple fiber compared with wheat and oat bran, *Cereal Chem.*, 65, 244, 1988.
28. Chen, M. L., Chang, S. C., and Guoo, J. Y., Fiber contents of some Chinese vegetables and their in vitro binding capacity of bile acids, *Nutr. Rep. Int.*, 26, 1053, 1982.

29. Chen, W.-J. L. and Anderson, J. W., Soluble and insoluble plant fiber in selected cereals and vegetables, *Am. J. Clin. Nutr.*, 34, 1077, 1981.

30. Claye, S. S., Idouraine, A., and Weber, C. W., Extraction and fractionation of insoluble fiber from five fiber sources, *Food Chem.*, 57, 305, 1996.

31. Dong, F. M. and Rasco, B. A., The neutral detergent fiber, acid detergent fiber, crude fiber, and lignin contents of distillers' dried grains with solubles, *J. Food Sci.*, 52, 403, 1987.

32. Dreher, M. L., Breedon, C., and Orr, P. H., Percent starch hydrolysis and dietary fiber content of chipped and baked potatoes, *Nutr. Rep. Int.*, 28, 687, 1983.

33. Englyst, H., Determination of carbohydrate and its composition in plant materials, in *The Analysis of Dietary Fibers in Food*, James, W. P. T. and Theander, O., Eds., Marcel Dekker, New York, 1981.

34. Englyst, H. N., Anderson, V., and Cummings, J. H., Starch and non-starch polysaccharides in some cereal foods, *J. Sci. Food Agric.*, 34, 1434, 1983.

35. Englyst, H. N. and Cummings, J. H., Improved method for measurement of dietary fiber as nonstarch polysaccharides in plant foods, *J. Assoc. Off. Anal. Chem.*, 71, 808, 1988.

36. Faulks, R. M. and Timms, S. B., A rapid method for determining the carbohydrate component of dietary fibre, *Food Chem.*, 17, 273, 1985.

37. Femenia, A., Robertson, J. A., Waldron, K. W., and Selvendran, R. R., Cauliflower (*Brassica oleracea L.*), globe artichoke (*Cynara scolymus*) and chicory witloof (*Cichorium intybus*) processing by-products as sources of dietary fibre, *J. Sci. Food Agric.*, 77, 511, 1998.

38. Fleming, S. E., A study of relationships between flatus potential and carbohydrate distribution in legume seeds, *J. Food Sci.*, 46, 794, 1981.

39. Foy, W. L., Evans, J. L., and Wohlt, J. E., Detergent fiber analyses on thirty foodstuffs ingested by man, *Nutr. Rep. Int.*, 24, 575, 1981.

40. Frolich, W. and Asp, N.-G., Dietary fiber content in cereals in Norway, *Cereal Chem.*, 58, 524, 1981.

41. Frolich, W. and Hestangen, B., Dietary fiber content of different cereal products in Norway, *Cereal Chem.*, 60, 82, 1983.

42. Garcia-Lopez, S. and Wyatt, C. J., Effect of fiber in corn tortillas and cooked beans on iron availability, *J. Agric. Food Chem.*, 30, 724, 1982.

43. Graham, H., Rydberg, M.-B. G., and Aman, P., Extraction of soluble dietary fiber, *J. Agric. Food Chem.*, 36, 494, 1988.

44. Greenberg, N. A. and Sellman, D., Partially hydrolyzed guar gum as a source of fiber, *Cereal Foods World*, 43, 703, 1996.

45. Harada, T., Tirtohusodo, H., and Paulus, K., Influence of the composition of potatoes on their cooking kinetics, *J. Food Sci.*, 50, 463, 1985.

46. Hardinge, M. G., Swarner, J. B., and Crooks, H., Carbohydrates in foods, *J. Am. Dietet. Assoc.*, 46, 197, 1965.

47. Heckman, M. M. and Lane, S. A., Comparison of dietary fiber methods for foods, *J. Assoc. Off. Anal. Chem.*, 64, 1339, 1981.

48. Hellendoorn, E. W., Noordhoff, M. G., and Slagman, J., Enzymatic determination of the indigestible residue (dietary fibre) content of human food, *J. Sci. Food Agric.*, 26, 1461, 1975.

49. Herranz, J., Vidal-Valverde, C., and Rojas-Hidalgo, E., Cellulose, hemicellulose and lignin content of raw and cooked processed vegetables, *J. Food Sci.*, 48, 274, 1983.

50. Herranz, J., Vidal-Valverde, C., and Rojas-Hidalgo, E., Cellulose, hemicellulose and lignin content of raw and cooked Spanish vegetables, *J. Food Sci.*, 46, 1927, 1981.

51. Holloway, W. D., Composition of fruit, vegetable and cereal dietary fibre, *J. Sci. Food Agric.*, 34, 1236, 1983.

52. Holloway, W. D., Monro, J. A., Gurnsey, J. C., Pomare, E. W., and Stace, N. H., Dietary fiber and other constituents of some Tongan foods, *J. Food Sci.*, 50, 1756, 1985.

53. Holloway, W. D., Tasman-Jones, C., and Maher, K., Towards an accurate measurement of dietary fibre, *N.Z. Med. J.*, 85, 420, 1977.

54. Horvath, P. J., The measurement of dietary fiber and the effects of fermentation, Thesis, Cornell University, 1984.

55. Jeltema, M. A. and Zabik, M. E., Revised method for quantitating dietary fibre components, *J. Sci. Food Agric.*, 31, 820, 1980.

56. Jeraci, J. L., Lewis, B. A., Van Soest, P. J., and Robertson, J. B., Urea enzymatic dialysis procedure for determination of total dietary fiber, *J. Assoc. Off. Anal. Chem.*, 72, 677, 1989.

57. Johnston, D. E., Kelly, D., and Dorrian, P. P., Losses of pectic substances during cooking and the effect of water hardness, *J. Sci. Food Agric.*, 34, 733, 1983.

58. Johnston, D. E. and Oliver, W. T., The influence of cooking technique on dietary fibre of boiled potato, *J. Food Technol.*, 17, 99, 1982.

59. Jones, G. P., Briggs, D. R., Wahlqvist, M. L., and Flentje, L. M., Dietary fibre content of Australian foods. 1. Potatoes, *Food Technol. Aust.*, 37, 81, 1985.

60. Jones, G. P., Briggs, D. R., Wahlqvist, M. L., Flentje, L. M., and Shiell, B. J., Dietary fibre content of Australian foods. 2. Vegetables, *Food Aust.*, 42, 26, 1990.

61. Jones, G. P., Briggs, D. R., Wahlqvist, M. L., Flentje, L. M., and Shiell, B. J., Dietary fibre content of Australian foods. 3. Fruits and fruit products, *Food Aust.*, 42, 143, 1990..

62. Jwuang, J. W.-L. and Zabik, M. E., Enzyme neutral detergent fiber analysis of selected commercial and home-prepared foods, *J. Food Sci.*, 44, 924, 1979.

63. Kamath, M. V. and Belavady, B., Unavailable carbohydrates of commonly consumed Indian foods, *J. Sci. Food Agric.*, 31, 194, 1980.

64. Katan, M. B. and Van de Bovenkamp, P., Analyse van het totale voedingsvezlgehalte en van het pectine-aandeel hierin in Nederlandse voedingsmillelen, *Voeding*, 5, 153, 1982.

65. Kayisu, K., Hood, L. F., and VanSoest, P. J., Characterization of starch and fiber of banana fruit, *J. Food Sci.*, 46, 1885, 1981.

66. Kays, S. E., Barton, F. E., Windham, W. R., and Himmelsbach, D. S., Prediction of total dietary fiber by near-infrared reflectance spectroscopy in cereal products containing high sugar and crystalline sugar, *J. Agric. Food Chem.*, 45, 3944, 1997.

67. Knuckles, B. E., Hudson, C. A., Chiu, M. M., and Sayre, R. N., Effect of β-glucan barley fractions in high-fiber bread and pasta, *Cereal Foods World*, 42, 94, 1997.

68. Kunerth, W. H. and Youngs, V. L., Effect of variety and growing year on the constituents of durum bran fiber, *Cereal Chem.*, 61, 350, 1984.

69. Lanza, E. and Butrum, R. R., A critical review of food fiber analysis and data, *J. Am. Dietet. Assoc.*, 86, 732, 1986.

70. Lanza, E., Jones, D. Y., Block, G., and Kessler, L., Dietary fiber intake in the U.S. population, *Am. J. Clin. Nutr.*, 46, 790, 1987.

71. Leeds, A. R., Psyllium — a superior source of soluble dietary fibre, *Food Aust.*, 47 (suppl.), S2, 1995.

72. Li, B. W., Comparison of three methods and two cooking times in the determination of total dietary fiber content of dried legumes, *J. Food Comp. Anal.*, 8, 27, 1995.

73. Li, B. W. and Cardozo, M. S., Simplified enzymatic-gravimetric method for total dietary fiber in legumes compared with a modified AOAC method, *J. Food Sci.*, 58, 929, 1993.

74. Lintas, C. and Cappelloni, M., Dietary fiber content of Italian fruit and nuts, *J Food Comp. Anal.*, 5, 146, 1992.

75. Longe, O. G., Effect of boiling on the carbohydrate constituents of some non-leafy vegetables, *Food Chem.*, 6, 1, 1981.

76. Longe, O. G., Fetuga, B. L., and Akenova, M. E., Changes in the composition and carbohydrate constituents of okra (*Abelmoschus esculentus*, Linn) with age, *Food Chem.*, 8, 27, 1982.

77. Luh, B. S., Sarhan, M. A., and Wang, Z., Pectins and fibres in processing tomatoes, *Food Technol. Aust.*, 36, 70, 1984.

78. Lund, E. D. and Smoot, J. M., Dietary fiber content of some tropical fruits and vegetables, *J. Agric. Food Chem.*, 30, 1123, 1982.

79. Lund, E. D., Smoot, J. M., and Hall, N. T., Dietary fiber content of eleven tropical fruits and vegetables, *J. Agric. Food Chem.*, 31, 1013, 1983.

80. Manthey, F. A., Hareland, G. A. and Huseby, D. J., Soluble and insoluble dietary fiber content and composition in oat, *Cereal Chem.*, 76, 417, 1999.

81. Marlett, J. A., Content and composition of dietary fiber in 117 frequently consumed foods, *J. Am. Dietet. Assoc.*, 92, 175, 1992.

82. Marlett, J. A. and Chesters, J. G., Measuring dietary fiber in human foods, *J. Food Sci.*, 50, 410, 1985.

83. Marlett, J. A. and Cheung, T.-F., Database and quick methods of assessing typical dietary fiber intakes using data for 228 commonly consumed foods, *J. Am. Dietet. Assoc.*, 97, 1139, 1997.

84. Marlett, J. A. and Lee, S. C., Dietary fiber, lignocellulose and hemicellulose contents of selected foods determined by modified and unmodified Van Soest procedures, *J. Food Sci.*, 45, 1688, 1980.
85. Marlett, J. A. and Navis, D., Comparison of gravimetric and chemical analyses of total dietary fiber in human foods, *J. Agric. Food. Chem.*, 36, 311, 1988.
86. Marlett, J. A. and Vollendorf, N. W., Dietary fiber content and composition of different forms of fruits, *Food Chem.*, 51, 39, 1994.
87. Matthee, V. and Appledorf, H., Effect of cooking on vegetable fiber, *J. Food Sci.*, 43, 1344, 1978.
88. McCormick, R., Function and nutrition guide fiber ingredient selections, *Prep. Foods*, November, 83, 1988.
89. McQueen, R. E. and Nicholson, J. W. G., Modification of the neutral-detergent fiber procedure for cereals and vegetables by using a-amylase, *J. Assoc. Off. Anal. Chem.*, 62, 676, 1979.
90. Mongeau, R. and Brassard, R., A rapid method for the determination of soluble and insoluble dietary fiber: comparison with AOAC total dietary fiber procedure and Englyst's method, *J. Food Sci.*, 51, 1333, 1986.
91. Mongeau, R. and Brassard, R., Determination of neutral detergent fiber in breakfast cereals: pentose, hemicellulose, cellulose and lignin content, *J. Food Sci.*, 47, 550, 1982.
92. Mongeau, R., Brassard, R., and Verdier, P., Measurement of dietary fiber in a total diet study, *J. Food Comp. Anal.*, 2, 317, 1989.
93. Monro, J. A., Harding, W. R., and Russell, C. E., Dietary fibre of coconuts from a Pacific atoll: Soluble and insoluble components in relation to maturity, *J. Sci. Food Agric.*, 36, 1013, 1985
94. Mori, B., Contents of dietary fiber in some Japanese foods and the amount ingested through Japanese meals, *Nutr. Rep. Int.*, 26, 159, 1982.
95. Neilson, M. J. and Marlett, J. A., A comparison between detergent and nondetergent analyses of dietary fiber in human foodstuffs, using high-performance liquid chromatography to measure neutral sugar composition, *J. Agric. Food Chem.*, 31, 1342, 1983.
96. Nishimune, T., Yakushiji, T., Sumimoto, T., Taguchi, S., Konishi, Y., Nakahara, S., Ichikawa, T., and Kunita, N., Glycemic response and fiber content of some foods, *Am. J. Clin. Nutr.*, 53, 414, 1991.
97. Park, G. L., Byers, J. L., Pritz, C. M., Nelson, D. B., Navarro, J. L., Smolensky, D. C., and Vandercook, C. E., Characteristics of California navel orange juice and pulpwash, *J. Food Sci.*, 48, 627, 1983.
98. Patrow, C. J. and Marlett, J. A., Variability in the dietary fiber content of wheat and mixed-grain commercial breads, *J. Am. Dietet. Assoc.*, 86, 794, 1986.
99. Paul, A. A. and Southgate, D. A. T., McCance and Widdowson's "The Composition of Foods": Dietary fibre in egg, meat and fish dishes, *J. Hum. Nutr.*, 33, 335, 1979.
100. Plaami, S. and Kumpulainen, J., Soluble and insoluble dietary fiber contents of various breads, pastas, and rye flours on the Finnish market, 1990–1991, *J. Food Comp. Anal.*, 7, 134, 1994.
101. Plaami, S. P., Kumpulainen, J. T., and Tahvonen, R. L., Total dietary fibre contents in vegetables, fruits and berries consumed in Finland, *J. Sci. Food Agric.*, 59, 545, 1992.
102. Plessi, M. Bertelli, D., Monzani, A., Simonetti, M. S., Neri, A., and Damiani, P., Dietary fiber and some elements in nuts and wheat brans, *J. Food Comp. Anal.*, 12, 91, 1999.
103. Prosky, L., Asp, N.-G., Furda, I., Devries, J. W., Schweizer, T. F., and Harland, B. F., Determination of total dietary fiber in foods, food products, and total diets: interlaboratory study, *J. Assoc. Off. Anal. Chem.*, 67, 1044, 1984.
104. Prosky, L., Asp, N.-G., Furda, I., Devries, J. W., Schweizer, T. F., and Harland, B. F., Determination of total dietary fiber in foods and food products: Collaborative study, *J. Assoc. Off. Anal. Chem.*, 68, 677, 1985.
105. Prosky, L., Asp, N.-G., Schweizer, T. F., DeVries, J. W., and Furda, I., Determination of insoluble, soluble, and total dietary fiber in foods and food products: interlaboratory study, *J. Assoc. Off. Anal. Chem.*, 71, 1017, 1988.
106. Przybyla, A. E., Formulating fiber into foods, *Food Eng.*, October, 77, 1988.
107. Ranhotra, G. and Gelroth, J., Soluble and insoluble fiber in soda crackers, *Cereal Chem.*, 65, 159, 1988.
108. Ranhotra, G. and Gelroth, J., Soluble and total dietary fiber in white bread, *Cereal Chem.*, 65, 155, 1988.
109. Reddy, N. N. and Sistrunk, W. A., Effect of cultivar, size, storage, and cooking method on carbohydrates and some nutrients of sweet potatoes, *J. Food Sci.*, 45, 682, 1980.
110. Reinhold, J. G. and Garcia L. J. S., Fiber of the maize tortilla, *Am. J. Clin. Nutr.*, 32, 1326, 1979.

111. Reistad, R., Andelic, I., Steen, M., and Rogeberg, E. S., Dietary fibre in some Norwegian plant foods during storage, *Food Chem.*, 17, 265, 1985.
112. Reistad, R. and Hagen, B. F., Dietary fibre in raw and cooked potatoes, *Food Chem.*, 19, 189, 1986.
113. Ross, J. K., Dietary fiber values for various breads are higher using enzymatic analysis rather than detergent analysis, *J. Am. Dietet. Assoc.*, 94, 166, 1994.
114. Ross, J. K., English, C., and Perlmutter, C. A., Dietary fiber constituents of selected fruits and vegetables, *J. Am. Dietet. Assoc.*, 85, 1111, 1985.
115. San Buenaventura, M. L., Dong, F. M., and Rasco, B. A., The total dietary fiber content of wheat, corn, barley, sorghum, and distillers' dried grain with solubles, *Cereal Chem.*, 64, 135, 1987.
116. Sanchez-Castillo, C. P., Englyst, H. N., Hudson, G. J., Lara, J. J., de Lourdes Solano, M., Munguia, J. L., and James, W. P. T., The non-starch polysaccharide content of Mexican foods, *J. Food Comp. Anal.*, 12, 293, 1999.
117. Schaller, D., Fiber content and structure in foods, *Am. J. Clin. Nutr.*, 31, S99, 1978.
118. Schneeman, B. O., Dietary fiber: physical and chemical properties, methods of analysis and physiological effects, *Food Technol.*, February, 104, 1986.
119. Schweizer, T. F. and Wursch, P., Analysis of dietary fibre, *J. Sci. Food Agric.*, 30, 613, 1979.
120. Seibert, S. E., Oat bran as a source of soluble dietary fiber, *Cereal Foods World*, 32, 552, 1987.
121. Selvendran, R. R., The plant cell wall as a source of dietary fiber: chemistry and structure, *Am. J. Clin. Nutr.*, 39, 320, 1984.
122. Selvendran, R. R. and DuPont, M. S., Simplified methods for the preparation and analysis of dietary fibre, *J. Sci. Food Agric.*, 31, 1173, 1980.
123. Siddiqui, I. R., Studies on vegetables: fiber content and chemical composition of ethanol-insoluble and -soluble residues, *J. Agric. Food Chem.*, 37, 647, 1989.
124. Skurray, G. R., Wooldridge, D. A., and Nguyen, M., Rice bran as a source of dietary fibre in bread, *J. Food Technol.*, 21, 727, 1986.
125. Slavin, J. L., Dietary fiber: classification, chemical analyses and food sources, *J. Am. Dietet. Assoc.*, 87, 1164, 1987.
126. Somogyi, L. P., Prunes, a fiber-rich ingredient, *Cereal Foods World*, 32, 541, 1987.
127. Southgate, D. A. T., Dietary fiber: analysis and food sources, *Am. J. Clin. Nutr.*, 31, S107, 1978.
128. Southgate, D. A. T., Bailey, B., Collinson, E., and Walker, A. F., A guide to calculating intakes of dietary fibre, *J. Human Nutr.*, 30, 303, 1976.
129. Southgate, D. A. T., Hudson, G. J., and Englyst, H., The analysis of dietary fibre — the choices for the analyst, *J. Sci. Food Agric.*, 29, 979, 1978.
130. Suhasini, A. W., Muralikrishna, G., and Malleshi, N. G., Free sugars and non-starch polysaccharide contents of good and poor malting varieties of wheat and their malts, *Food Chem.*, 60, 537, 1997.
131. Theander, O. and Aman, P., Studies on dietary fibres 1. Analysis and chemical characterization of water-soluble and water-insoluble dietary fibres, *Swedish J. Agric. Res.*, 9, 97, 1979.
132. Theander, O. and Aman, P., Studies on dietary fibre. A method for the analysis and chemical characterisation of total dietary fibre, *J. Sci. Food Agric.*, 33, 340, 1982.
133. Theander, O. and Westerlund, E. A., Studies on dietary fiber. 3. Improved procedures for analysis of dietary fiber, *J. Agric. Food Chem.*, 34, 330, 1986.
134. Torp, J., Variation in the concentration of major carbohydrates in the grain of some spring barleys, *J. Sci. Food Agric.*, 31, 1354, 1980.
135. *USDA Nutrient Database for Standard Reference, Release 13*, Agricultural Research Service, Nutrient Data Laboratory, U. S. Department of Agriculture, 1999.
136. Varo, P., Laine, R., Veijalainen, K., Pero, K., and Koivistoinen, P., Dietary fibre and available carbohydrates in Finnish cereal products, *J. Agric. Sci. Fin.*, 56, 39, 1984.
137. Varo, P., Veijalainen, K., and Koivistoinen, P., Effect of heat treatment on the dietary fibre contents of potato and tomato, *J. Food Technol.*, 19, 485, 1984.
138. Vidal-Valverde, C., Blanco, I., and Rojas-Hidalgo, E., Pectic substances in fresh, dried, desiccated and oleaginous Spanish fruits, *J. Agric. Food Chem.*, 30, 832, 1982.
139. Vidal-Valverde, C., Herranz, J., Blanco, I., and Rojas-Hidalgo, E., Dietary fiber in Spanish fruits, *J. Food Sci.*, 47, 1840, 1982.
140. Vidal-Valverde, C., Lopez, M. P., and Rojas-Hidalgo, E., Pectic substances in raw and cooked, fresh or processed Spanish vegetables, *J. Agric. Food Chem.*, 31, 949, 1983.

141. Visser, F. R. and Gurnsey, C., Inconsistent differences between neutral detergent fiber and total dietary fiber values of fruits and vegetables, *J. Assoc. Off. Anal. Chem.*, 69, 565, 1986.

142. Vollendorf, N. W. and Marlett, J. A., Comparison of two methods of fiber analysis of 58 foods, *J. Food Comp. Anal.*, 6, 203, 1993.

143. Waslien, C., What is dietary fiber and what is starch?, *Cereal Foods World*, 33, 312, 1988.

144. Wenlock, R. W., Sivell, L. M., and Agater, I. B., Dietary fibre fractions in cereal and cereal-containing products in Britain, *J. Sci. Food Agric.*, 36, 113, 1985.

145. Wills, R. B. H., Composition of Australian fresh fruit and vegetables, *Food Technol. Aust.*, 39, 523, 1987.

146. Wills, R. B. H., Evans, T. J., Lim, J. S. K., Scriven, F. M., and Greenfield, H., Composition of Australian foods. 25. Peas and beans, *Food Technol. Aust.*, 36, 512, 1984.

147. Wills, R. B. H., Lim, J. S. K., and Greenfield, H., Composition of Australian foods. 23. Brassica vegetables, *Food Technol. Aust.*, 36, 176, 1984.

148. Wills, R. B. H., Lim, J. S. K., and Greenfield, H., Composition of Australian foods. 38. Tuber, root and bulb vegetables, *Food Technol. Aust.*, 39, 384, 1987.

149. Wills, R. B. H., Lim, J. S. K., and Greenfield, H., Composition of Australian foods. 39. Vegetable fruits, *Food Technol. Aust.*, 39, 488, 1987.

150. Wills, R. B. H., Lim, J. S. K., and Greenfield, H., Composition of Australian foods. 42. Canned fruits, *Food Technol. Aust.*, 40, 223, 1988.

151. Wills, R. B. H., Wong, A. W. K., Scriven, F. M., and Greenfield, H., Nutrient composition of Chinese vegetables, *J. Agric. Food Chem.*, 32, 413, 1984.

152. Zyren, J., Elkins, E. R., Dudek, J. A., and Hagen, R. E., Fiber contents of selected raw and processed vegetables, fruits and fruit juices as served, *J. Food Sci.*, 48, 600, 1983.

Appendix — Table A.2
Dry Matter, Ash, Crude Protein, Total Dietary Fiber, Soluble Fiber, Neutral Detergent Residue, Hemicellulose, Cellulose, and Lignin Content of Selected Foods

James B. Robertson

0-8493-2387-8/01/$0.00+$1.50

Table A.2 Dry Matter Content of Selected Foods

Description	Maker	% DM	ASH	CP	TDF	SF	NDR	HC	CE	Ls
Breads, Crackers, etc.										
Apple honey wheat, toasted	Brownberry	76.64	ND	13.23	5.50	-0.54	8.19	4.06	2.52	1.61
Apple honey wheat	Brownberry	64.82	ND	12.64	5.76	-0.08	6.43	4.10	1.22	1.10
Bagel		69.89	2.17	16.32	4.41	ND	2.63	1.39	0.58	0.66
Bagel, plain	Cornell	67.37	2.24	16.11	4.35	1.83	3.25	2.17	0.50	0.57
Biscuit mix, buttermilk	Quaker	89.53	5.21	ND	5.67	ND	1.14	1.00	0.28	-0.13
Biscuits, reg. recipe, baked		92.96	4.84	9.20	4.22	-1.60	7.51	5.72	0.58	1.21
Bread mix, corn, white	Quaker	88.79	5.95	ND	10.76	ND	7.55	5.20	1.98	0.38
Bread mix, corn, yellow	Quaker	88.41	5.41	ND	6.02	ND	4.06	2.68	1.13	0.25
Bread, corn	Homemade	62.39	2.85	9.99	5.43	-0.25	6.05	3.33	1.37	1.35
Bread, French		64.34	3.17	14.52	4.99	-0.37	5.96	3.87	0.92	1.18
Bread, wheat	Less	51.22	3.67	18.71	19.42	3.30	17.65	3.79	12.85	1.00
Bread, white	Millbrook	59.65	2.82	14.33	5.29	3.41	2.64	1.69	0.49	0.46
Bread, white	Less	52.63	3.74	20.21	19.07	1.80	18.22	3.11	13.66	1.46
Bread, white		62.13	3.40	14.06	5.48	4.81	1.15	0.87	0.03	0.25
Bread, whole wheat	Pepperidge Farm	57.30	3.90	17.13	13.99	1.89	14.32	8.73	2.25	3.35
Cake, yellow	Homemade	72.01	2.09	7.40	3.36	2.97	0.68	0.46	0.06	0.16
Cookie, plain		95.62	1.56	6.29	2.99	1.99	1.53	1.08	0.07	0.38
Cookies, ginger snaps		95.77	1.94	6.18	4.31	1.01	3.97	2.47	0.31	1.19
Cookies, Oreo		93.89	2.11	5.09	14.72	ND	3.33	0.61	0.72	2.01
Cookies, shortbread		92.81	1.52	6.26	9.76	ND	2.22	1.55	0.24	0.46
Fibre Goodness Bread	Stroehmann	56.01	2.98	20.21	11.19	3.31	8.70	2.28	5.77	0.65
Fibread	Dr. Olindo	52.08	4.39	19.99	26.24	6.13	27.52	18.33	19.03	3.07
Flour, enriched, self-rising	Quaker	89.21	4.50	ND	3.46	ND	1.17	0.98	0.06	0.13
Flour, white		90.20	0.69	12.70	3.70	2.76	1.31	0.98	0.19	0.14
Graham crackers		94.31	2.35	7.15	3.52	3.94	2.69	1.26	1.29	0.13
Muffin mix, blueberry	Quaker	91.78	2.63	ND	4.12	ND	0.57	0.42	0.19	-0.04
Muffin mix, corn	Quaker	91.06	3.17	ND	5.19	ND	2.33	1.56	0.54	0.22
Muffins, plain		70.23	2.49	8.39	3.75	-0.33	4.94	3.05	0.71	1.18
Natural bran	Brownberry	63.19	0.00	13.51	10.09	-0.97	11.60	8.44	1.95	1.20
Natural bran, toasted	Brownberry	73.72	0.00	13.96	9.47	-1.05	12.24	8.13	2.34	1.77
Norwegian flatbread	Kavli	91.99	2.44	9.33	15.32	5.16	11.71	8.17	1.26	2.28
Oatmeal bread	Pepperidge Farm	61.25	3.62	14.22	9.39	7.30	3.25	2.17	0.50	0.57
Pancake mix		90.39	6.40	10.10	4.36	0.70	3.95	2.24	0.52	1.18

Pancake mix, buckwheat	Quaker	90.57	6.64	ND	11.64	ND	9.45	3.39	3.46	2.61
Pancake mix, whole wheat	Quaker	90.78	6.81	ND	9.55	ND	6.89	4.79	1.48	0.62
Premium saltines	Nabisco	96.71	3.53	9.40	5.55	3.88	2.63	1.69	0.06	0.88
Pretzels, hard	Wege	95.79	4.79	10.91	4.58	2.94	3.49	2.55	0.30	0.64
Pretzels, whole wheat	Wege	96.04	1.12	10.50	8.11	4.06	7.20	4.87	1.18	1.15
Prograin bread	Friehofer	63.92	4.03	18.96	13.10	5.92	8.92	4.96	2.35	1.61
Rice cakes	Quaker	93.77	0.00	9.67	4.05	-0.98	5.53	4.04	1.17	0.32
Rolls, sweet, cinnamon		69.96	1.92	10.72	5.76	1.57	4.66	2.88	0.66	1.12
Rye cakes	Quaker	94.61	0.00	16.09	12.21	5.45	7.37	5.14	1.78	0.47
Saltine crackers		96.84	3.36	10.05	3.77	2.11	1.66	0.78	0.92	-0.04
Sesame crackers	Ak-Mak	95.60	3.50	16.36	12.64	2.25	13.74	8.90	2.27	2.57
Snackbread	Ryvita	92.44	1.71	11.25	5.61	2.16	3.82	3.30	0.35	0.17
Snackbread, whole wheat	Ryvita	95.26	2.46	12.67	12.18	3.28	10.10	7.85	1.57	0.68
Swedish rye crispbread	Siljans	90.78	2.27	10.03	17.86	5.46	15.29	12.15	2.00	1.14
Taco shells	Old El Paso	93.76	2.78	6.55	12.42	2.51	11.30	8.14	1.67	1.49
Taco shells		94.42	1.85	6.61	7.49	2.07	6.73	3.63	2.73	0.37
Triscuit	Nabisco	97.19	2.69	8.28	12.43	2.49	10.84	8.70	1.86	0.28
Wheat cakes	Quaker	94.88	0.00	16.41	9.77	3.31	7.07	5.29	1.33	0.50
Wheat thins	Nabisco	97.92	2.57	7.54	8.12	3.69	5.16	3.42	0.50	1.24
White extra fiber, toasted	Arnold's	73.86	0.00	15.50	6.15	-1.03	8.55	2.80	4.56	1.20
White extra fiber	Arnold's	60.92	0.00	15.40	7.33	0.60	7.01	2.54	3.92	0.57

Pasta

Macaroni		97.01	0.59	15.54	5.07	1.47	4.32	1.44	2.25	0.63
Macaroni, Cooked		28.18	0.42	16.80	4.41	2.50	2.35	1.84	0.37	0.13
Noodles, egg, cooked		30.94	1.22	19.45	3.41	1.72	1.87	1.17	0.53	0.18
Spaghetti	Goia	90.02	0.87	16.68	3.47	1.27	2.47	1.57	0.53	0.37
Spaghetti, cooked		37.12	0.74	15.67	4.34	2.57	2.07	1.62	0.31	0.14
Spaghetti w/sauce, cooked		26.38	3.95	13.96	6.88	ND	3.49	1.77	1.26	0.46
Spaghetti, whole wheat	Goia	91.33	1.80	15.87	10.44	1.07	9.82	7.36	1.70	0.76

Cereals

100% Bran	Nabisco	95.42	6.45	12.30	35.67	5.90	33.16	24.16	6.55	2.45
100% Bran	Nabisco	96.60	6.19	12.42	34.16	5.87	32.63	22.18	7.21	3.24
100% Bran	Nabisco	95.79	6.75	13.45	36.89	5.36	32.67	22.50	6.05	3.64
100% Natural	Quaker	96.41	2.01	12.93	9.78	5.58	4.55	2.70	0.93	0.69
40% Bran Flakes		95.53	4.79	12.02	19.75	9.76	11.76	7.21	2.89	1.41
Bran Flakes		95.93	4.60	11.87	19.90	4.26	21.44	11.76	5.20	4.48
All Bran	Kellogg's	96.86	7.18	12.75	38.13	5.40	37.65	27.63	7.30	2.72

Table A.2 (Continued) Dry Matter Content of Selected Foods

Description	Maker	% DM	ASH	CP	TDF	SF	NDR	HC	CE	Ls
						In Dry Matter (%)				
Cereals										
All Bran	Kellogg's	94.98	6.74	12.78	37.76	6.28	35.41	22.28	8.55	4.59
All Bran	Kellogg's	98.39	7.29	13.47	40.26	10.34	38.10	25.09	8.72	4.30
All Bran w/ Extra Fiber	Kellogg's	95.84	6.03	10.80	50.46	7.00	47.46	34.14	10.76	2.56
All Bran w/ Extra Fiber	Kellogg's	96.20	6.09	11.82	49.61	6.57	47.45	33.26	11.30	2.90
Bran Flakes	Kellogg's	96.66	4.65	12.00	16.93	6.40	15.18	8.74	4.08	2.36
Cap'n Crunch	Quaker	96.35	2.45	ND	2.79	ND	3.67	2.27	1.22	0.19
Cheerios	General Mills	94.48	5.04	14.38	11.04	ND	6.46	4.33	0.95	1.19
Cheerios	General Mills	94.47	4.40	16.63	13.03	8.95	5.06	3.25	0.71	0.94
Cheerios		93.59	4.21	12.78	11.35	6.54	12.76	7.03	2.69	3.04
Choco Crunch	Quaker	95.59	1.94	ND	3.59	ND	4.69	2.99	0.71	0.78
Corn Bran	Quaker	97.73	3.07	ND	18.03	ND	20.35	15.66	3.88	0.82
Corn Flakes	Kellogg's	94.63	3.37	7.60	3.30	3.38	0.81	0.43	0.19	0.14
Corn Flakes	Kellogg's	94.24	2.90	6.87	3.62	3.60	1.59	0.78	0.35	0.47
Corn Flakes	Kellogg's	95.45	3.04	7.24	3.68	ND	2.74	1.19	0.46	1.09
Corn Flakes	Kellogg's	96.19	3.15	6.73	3.24	2.21	4.97	2.12	1.34	1.52
Corn Flakes	General Mills	95.39	5.94	6.59	2.69	0.44	2.73	1.10	0.39	1.24
Cream of Wheat, cooked		11.33	1.74	11.96	6.30	-2.65	9.50	6.70	1.66,	1.14
Creamy Wheat, quick	Quaker	87.42	0.49	ND	3.47	ND	4.49	3.87	-0.09	0.71
Crunchberries	Quaker	96.82	2.23	ND	3.17	ND	4.33	2.78	0.72	0.83
Crunchy Nut Oh's	Quaker	97.15	1.70	ND	5.72	ND	4.65	2.99	0.84	0.82
Double Chex	Ralston Purina	97.36	0.00	7.62	5.08	2.54	3.74	1.91	1.35	0.48
Fibre One	General Mills	95.38	6.56	11.66	48.42	7.39	44.76	33.22	9.50	2.04
Fibre One	General Mills	96.09	6.58	12.92	48.12	6.91	45.94	33.18	10.08	2.68
Grits		89.97	0.43	8.30	7.32	3.54	4.56	2.39	1.95	0.21
Grits, instant	Quaker	90.43	4.25	ND	9.12	ND	6.55	5.21	1.06	0.27
Honey Graham Oh's	Quaker	97.40	2.22	ND	3.34	ND	5.14	2.47	0.46	2.22
King Vitamin	Quaker	95.93	2.75	ND	4.99	ND	4.98	3.41	0.64	0.93
Life	Quaker	95.82	4.13	21.59	10.10	8.07	2.47	1.28	0.46	0.50
Life	Quaker	94.61	4.14	ND	9.77	ND	4.98	3.32	0.87	0.79
Life, Cinnamon	Quaker	95.07	4.14	ND	9.76	ND	5.75	3.87	0.95	0.82
Natural Cereal	Quaker	96.93	1.97	ND	10.78	ND	6.98	4.61	1.25	1.11
Natural Cereal, Apple Cinnamon	Quaker	95.44	1.76	ND	10.30	ND	7.32	4.81	1.51	1.01
Natural Cereal, Raisin Date	Quaker	94.83	1.93	ND	9.31	ND	8.08	4.78	1.39	1.91

Natural Cereal, Whole Wheat	Quaker	88.81	1.79	ND	12.39	ND	12.59	7.35	2.56	1.08
Nature Valley Granola	General Mills	94.35	1.73	9.86	10.47	6.04	7.18	5.56	0.83	0.79
Nature's Harvest Granola		96.12	2.24	16.28	22.08	14.40	8.51	4.57	1.50	1.80
Nutrigrain	Kellogg's	96.45	2.74	8.97	10.71	2.16	11.30	7.62	1.77	1.91
Oat Bran	Kellogg's	97.83	3.61	10.32	17.30	2.28	17.87	11.34	3.45	3.08
Oat Bran Creamy Hot Cereal	Quaker	91.22	3.39	ND	19.64	ND	16.29	12.77	1.82	1.84
Oats, Instant	Quaker	90.57	5.38	ND	11.81	ND	6.64	4.64	1.00	1.00
Oats, Instant, Apple Cinnamon	Quaker	92.30	4.26	ND	9.41	ND	5.77	3.61	1.28	0.88
Oats, Instant, Apple Raisin	Quaker	92.86	2.40	ND	9.98	ND	6.04	3.13	2.05	0.85
Oats, Instant, Blueberries and Cream	Quaker	93.65	3.21	ND	6.87	ND	5.80	3.76	0.66	1.38
Oats, Instant, Peaches and Cream	Quaker	91.62	3.21	ND	9.45	ND	5.76	3.98	1.12	0.66
Oats, Instant, Raisin Date Walnut	Quaker	92.36	3.71	ND	10.82	ND	6.42	3.67	1.10	1.66
Oats, Instant, Raisin Walnut	Quaker	91.12	3.50	ND	9.75	ND	4.66	3.13	0.90	0.63
Oats, Instant, Strawberries and Cream	Quaker	92.41	3.49	ND	8.25	ND	4.07	2.98	0.78	0.31
Oats, Old Fashioned	Quaker	90.02	2.17	ND	11.90	ND	7.50	5.60	0.89	1.00
Oats, One-Minute, Apple Raisin Spice	Quaker	90.25	1.88	ND	9.24	ND	5.10	3.35	1.04	0.71
Oats, One-Minute, Raisin Cinnamon	Quaker	89.41	1.88	ND	7.80	ND	6.12	3.28	0.54	2.30
Peanut Butter Crunch	Quaker	97.08	2.50	ND	4.56	ND	5.11	2.82	0.93	1.36
Popeye Sweet Puffs	Quaker	97.79	1.23	ND	4.14	ND	4.79	2.47	1.39	0.93
Post Toasties	General Foods	94.12	2.76	8.08	3.75	3.61	1.88	1.16	0.25	0.37
Product 19	Kellogg's	95.43	3.81	9.42	6.08	6.38	1.73	1.23	0.25	0.12
Product 19	Kellogg's	95.83	3.48	8.12	4.27	0.81	7.09	2.79	1.39	2.91
Puffed Rice	Quaker	95.10	0.48	ND	1.23	ND	4.68	3.86	0.66	0.17
Puffed Rice	Quaker	93.19	0.39	ND	2.13	ND	0.80	0.47	0.13	0.16
Puffed Wheat	Quaker	95.17	1.57	ND	9.50	ND	9.99	5.56	1.26	3.15
Puffed Wheat	Quaker	93.94	0.88	ND	12.24	ND	5.71	3.16	1.35	0.97
Rice Krispies	Kellogg's	95.37	3.42	6.82	1.90	2.20	3.31	2.05	0.38	0.89
Rice Krispies	Kellogg's	95.28	3.26	7.35	2.01	ND	5.74	3.45	0.76	1.52
Rice Krispies	Kellogg's	94.95	3.38	6.64	2.02	1.50	2.21	1.50	0.23	0.35
Shredded Wheat	Nabisco	91.85	1.69	10.43	13.21	1.21	13.51	10.91	2.23	0.37
Shredded Wheat		92.21	1.71	13.80	12.96	2.62	13.65	8.72	4.01	0.93
Shredded Wheat	Nabisco	94.70	1.72	13.13	13.49	5.70	10.02	6.81	1.69	0.97
Shredded Wheat N' Bran	Nabisco	95.30	0.00	12.10	14.38	4.81	10.61	6.36	0.15	1.21
Special K	Kellogg's	93.74	2.54	20.30	3.15	2.91	2.35	1.78	0.18	0.38
Sweet Crunch	Quaker	96.20	2.33	ND	3.20	ND	2.92	2.01	0.68	0.24

Table A.2 (Continued) Dry Matter Content of Selected Foods

Description	Maker		% DM	ASH	CP	TDF	In Dry Matter (%)				
							SF	NDR	HC	CE	Ls
Cereals											
Team	Nabisco		95.45	2.10	7.43	4.17	3.28	2.04	1.22	0.35	0.35
Total	General Mills		95.28	4.82	12.35	10.66	4.35	7.64	5.25	1.24	0.69
Wheat Germ	Kretschmer		96.27	4.80	30.35	18.10	7.81	10.73	6.49	2.56	1.35
Wheat Germ			95.77	5.11	32.58	17.70	3.37	15.91	9.87	3.38	2.66
Wheaties	General Mills		94.77	5.06	11.82	10.79	7.10	6.04	3.86	1.38	0.71
Fruits											
Apple Juice	Cornell		10.85	2.25	0.50	2.14	ND	1.27	0.14	0.38	0.75
Apple Sauce			18.13	0.95	0.63	8.36	ND	4.90	1.53	2.54	0.83
Apple, Red Delicious, cored			14.79	3.41	1.19	14.72	7.84	7.06	1.63	4.46	0.97
Apple, Red Delicious, cored and peeled			13.90	2.11	0.32	11.40	4.49	6.91	2.03	4.15	0.73
Avocado, California			21.73	7.92	10.65	25.60	-1.78	27.66	7.25	10.79	9.63
Banana			22.56	3.24	5.14	8.54	3.37	5.83	1.25	1.83	2.75
Blueberries			13.71	1.27	3.25	20.12	ND	17.75	5.24	5.54	6.98
Blueberries	Fresh		11.83	1.51	2.68	22.15	7.12	15.43	3.27	8.06	4.10
Cantaloupe	Fresh		9.82	11.33	8.79	9.22	4.55	4.74	0.66	3.31	0.77
Cherries, tart	Canned		7.70	2.96	8.62	13.26	8.25	5.67	1.19	2.53	1.96
Grapes, Thomson	Fresh		17.98	5.64	5.00	6.02	2.20	4.29	0.43	2.35	1.52
Orange juice	Cornell		10.81	13.97	5.22	4.57	ND	1.32	0.02	0.61	0.70
Orange, Florida, peeled	Fresh		11.72	3.69	4.68	17.95	11.76	6.25	1.15	4.19	0.91
Orange, navel, peeled	Fresh		12.76	3.48	7.21	16.39	10.88	5.51	0.88	3.63	1.01
Oranges, mandarin	Canned		11.96	1.85	3.63	4.85	ND	2.26	0.31	0.83	1.12
Peaches	Canned		12.77	1.85	3.68	8.75	ND	4.91	0.94	2.51	1.46
Pear, Bartlett, cored	Fresh		13.74	1.87	1.81	26.28	13.25	13.16	2.20	8.35	2.61
Pears	Canned		9.73	1.16	2.07	17.59	5.78	12.00	2.32	7.80	1.88
Pineapple	Canned		14.83	1.92	2.93	5.05	0.54	4.73	1.99	2.33	0.41
Plum, friar	Fresh		10.97	5.78	4.32	15.59	10.13	5.98	1.05	3.02	1.91
Raisins, seedless	Wegmans		85.78	2.13	3.88	ND	ND	4.32	1.06	1.09	2.17
Strawberries	Fresh		26.11	0.95	1.63	6.32	ND	4.25	0.94	1.83	1.47

Strawberries	Fresh	8.76	4.45	7.53	19.50	7.16	13.53	2.01	6.27	5.25
Tangerine, peeled	Fresh	13.30	4.14	6.17	15.21	9.68	5.59	1.05	3.67	0.86
Watermelon	Fresh	8.69	17.19	6.40	4.32	1.59	2.79	0.61	1.58	0.60

Vegetables

Artichoke hearts, frozen	General Foods	12.10	ND	20.40	48.98	ND	12.50	3.10	8.10	1.50
Asparagus, frozen	General Foods	8.50	ND	36.10	25.17	ND	12.60	2.40	9.10	1.10
Asparagus spears, canned		6.14	17.93	36.08	23.31	10.17	17.51	3.22	10.81	3.48
Bean sprouts, canned		3.49	5.01	32.20	30.83	9.26	29.64	6.63	16.65	6.36
Beans, green, cooked		8.83	5.91	15.22	32.42	ND	18.43	6.52	9.95	1.96
Beans, green, canned		5.29	14.93	16.18	34.69	19.73	22.69	4.29	14.52	3.88
Beans, green, frozen		10.79	ND	ND	32.41	ND	18.76	7.68	10.08	1.01
Beans, green, frozen	General Foods	7.70	ND	18.10	30.09	ND	17.60	3.30	11.20	3.10
Beans, green, boiled		9.24	ND	ND	34.11	ND	24.69	10.78	12.42	1.49
Beans, kidney, canned		21.93	5.64	23.41	23.91	10.40	17.22	4.18	11.12	1.93
Beans, kidney, boiled		39.58	ND	ND	28.86	ND	54.83	43.08	9.50	2.24
Beans, lima, boiled		40.36	ND	ND	27.12	ND	43.97	35.78	7.57	0.62
Beans, lima, canned		24.30	5.31	20.71	18.85	3.94	15.66	3.58	10.83	1.25
Beans, lima, frozen	General Foods	33.20	ND	19.30	20.32	ND	11.90	3.70	7.40	0.80
Beans, navy, microwaved		47.08	ND	ND	35.10	ND	45.62	37.07	8.21	0.34
Beans, pork, canned		23.62	7.01	18.49	22.22	12.36	14.50	0.77	10.49	3.25
Beans, wax, frozen	General Foods	8.50	ND	18.90	37.66	ND	18.70	2.30	14.30	2.10
Beans, wax, microwaved		9.31	ND	ND	37.73	ND	24.27	7.57	14.85	1.85
Beet root, canned		7.17	11.62	10.92	25.26	10.29	15.99	6.92	8.83	0.24
Broccoli, frozen	General Foods	7.30	ND	33.60	35.60	ND	18.40	2.00	13.60	2.70
Broccoli, cooked		9.12	6.74	39.61	36.30	15.68	22.20	4.89	13.43	3.88
Broccoli, cooked		9.18	7.10	29.91	34.84	ND	18.53	5.37	11.38	1.78
Brussels sprouts, frozen	General Foods	12.41	ND	ND	33.86	ND	28.35	12.19	14.61	1.54
Brussels sprouts, frozen		10.20	ND	23.90	35.23	ND	21.90	7.40	13.00	1.80
Cabbage, boiled		20.91	ND	ND	28.98	ND	18.33	5.74	11.42	1.16
Cabbage		6.01	10.82	20.89	28.70	15.26	13.77	2.05	11.18	0.54
Cabbage, red, microwaved		12.87	ND	ND	30.19	ND	15.89	3.80	11.51	0.58
Carrots, peeled		11.64	6.75	9.17	24.25	14.18	10.31	1.47	8.48	0.36
Carrots, boiled		11.70	ND	ND	27.53	ND	10.15	1.96	7.67	0.52
Carrots, cooked		11.63	4.66	6.46	34.18	ND	11.64	2.13	9.01	0.50
Cauliflower, cooked		5.43	6.59	27.34	36.49	16.37	21.75	4.76	15.34	1.64
Cauliflower, cooked		5.43	6.59	27.34	36.49	16.37	21.75	4.76	15.34	1.64
Cauliflower, frozen	General Foods	6.20	ND	24.70	27.67	ND	16.00	4.10	10.80	1.50
Cauliflower		8.03	ND	ND	34.89	ND	23.89	8.07	13.47	2.35

Table A.2 (Continued) Dry Matter Content of Selected Foods

Description	Maker	% DM	In Dry Matter (%)							
			ASH	CP	TDF	SF	NDR	HC	CE	Ls
Vegetables										
Celery		5.17	16.96	11.24	40.12	19.55	21.04	1.80	17.95	1.29
Collard greens, frozen	General Foods	9.60	ND	27.80	32.83	ND	18.60	3.20	12.10	3.10
Corn, canned		21.96	3.98	10.94	7.87	1.43	7.58	5.00	2.01	0.58
Corn, frozen	General Foods	20.40	ND	13.80	11.65	ND	7.90	3.40	2.60	1.90
Cucumber, with skin		3.66	10.74	18.43	27.21	10.14	17.83	2.09	11.57	4.17
Cucumber, peeled		3.36	10.31	16.13	19.49	7.17	12.44	2.56	9.09	0.79
Kale, frozen	General Foods	8.40	ND	27.70	34.91	ND	16.50	2.00	12.30	2.30
Lentils, boiled		40.28	ND	ND	32.95	ND	43.90	33.93	7.69	2.28
Mushrooms		9.85	ND	ND	20.83	ND	21.65	12.10	9.31	0.24
Mustard greens, frozen	General Foods	7.60	ND	31.20	36.21	ND	21.70	4.10	14.40	3.10
Okra, frozen		9.07	ND	ND	40.08	ND	24.51	7.22	9.74	7.55
Okra, frozen	General Foods	7.50	ND	20.60	40.91	ND	14.10	3.30	9.20	1.60
Olives, black		18.88	10.52	5.50	14.68	-6.93	26.00	7.90	5.16	12.95
Olives, green, stuffed		23.24	25.16	3.67	13.30	-5.18	20.96	6.98	4.88	9.15
Onions, boiled		8.96	ND	ND	19.48	ND	11.05	3.09	7.02	0.93
Onions, frozen	General Foods	6.60	ND	9.20	18.65	ND	7.60	0.90	6.20	0.60
Onions, peeled		9.05	4.39	8.96	16.35	8.84	7.64	1.93	5.47	0.24
Onions, green		6.69	11.00	20.24	28.58	12.86	15.72	3.29	10.65	1.78
Peas, black-eyed, canned		20.75	6.23	26.86	18.86	-2.20	27.65	18.91	7.02	1.73
Peas, black-eyed, frozen	General Foods	35.00	ND	27.00	19.34	ND	9.00	0.90	6.30	1.80
Peas, black-eyed, boiled		41.71	ND	ND	32.54	ND	19.10	13.66	4.07	1.36
Peas, green, microwaved		44.26	ND	ND	31.75	ND	11.71	6.77	4.00	0.94
Peas, green, canned		17.58	5.00	23.34	26.49	8.17	19.28	4.25	14.87	0.16
Peas, green, frozen	General Foods	20.70	ND	30.90	20.51	ND	13.30	2.80	10.00	0.50
Pepper, green seeded		5.58	6.03	11.68	29.36	8.97	20.39	2.09	11.63	6.67
Pickles, dill		4.95	61.05	6.39	23.09	8.88	14.21	1.10	11.10	2.01
Potatoes, french fries	Ore-Ida	30.62	3.21	7.83	7.11	2.90	4.40	1.41	2.37	0.62
Potatoes, boiled, mashed		18.84	3.07	7.61	13.73	ND	4.89	2.21	1.97	0.71
Potatoes, peeled, boiled		19.38	3.40	10.91	9.61	5.69	3.92	0.88	2.99	0.06
Potatoes, w/skins, baked		25.23	4.55	11.74	9.29	3.17	6.41	1.43	4.18	0.79
Radishes		5.32	12.96	14.86	25.32	12.26	13.06	1.35	10.93	0.79
Rice, cooked		27.40	0.68	7.49	1.49	1.08	1.25	0.69	0.31	0.25
Rice, boiled		26.85	0.95	7.32	7.09	ND	3.75	1.80	1.11	0.83

Rutabaga, boiled		11.14	ND	ND	28.67	ND	14.11	2.91	10.60	0.60
Spinach, microwaved		9.70	ND	ND	29.27	ND	26.56	12.93	9.93	3.70
Squash, frozen	General Foods	11.20	ND	20.60	21.48	ND	15.14	3.58	11.43	0.13
Squash, cooked		9.80	ND	20.60	19.28	ND	13.60	2.40	10.50	0.70
Squash, summer, frozen	General Foods	5.00	ND	ND	21.41	ND	11.40	1.60	8.10	1.70
Squash, summer, microwaved		14.86	11.77	19.43	20.83	11.96	13.82	4.15	8.21	1.46
Squash, summer, zucchini		4.89	ND	18.90	22.42	ND	10.46	1.87	7.77	0.82
Squash, zucchini, frozen	General Foods	4.60	2.12	4.81	23.51	1.82	12.50	2.10	8.80	1.60
Sweet potatoes		23.36	ND	ND	7.85	ND	7.91	1.46	4.47	1.99
Sweet potatoes, baked		21.86	11.90	4.32	14.48	ND	8.16	2.67	4.59	0.90
Tomato catsup		27.96	21.63	16.48	5.09	2.32	2.98	0.38	2.11	0.49
Tomatoes, canned		5.46	ND	ND	13.63	4.58	10.33	1.74	6.28	2.32
Turnip		8.28	13.47	29.47	29.24	ND	15.23	2.02	12.52	0.69
Turnip greens, frozen		6.65	ND	34.90	37.39	17.93	21.12	3.34	15.15	2.63
Turnip greens, frozen	General Foods	6.60	13.33	12.48	35.51	ND	19.40	1.40	15.20	2.80
Vegetable soup, canned		16.53	ND	ND	12.27	0.94	14.29	8.19	5.05	1.05
Yams		26.15	ND	ND	11.36	ND	11.09	7.21	3.48	0.40
Nuts										
Peanuts		95.50	3.40	29.57	9.18	3.88	10.27	4.16	4.35	1.76
Walnuts		99.05	1.64	16.72	6.30	2.27	4.30	1.47	2.35	0.48
Other										
Fruit Wrinkles (Fruit Punch)	Fresh	95.64	0.00	0.00	1.27	1.27	0.00	0.00	0.00	0.00
Fruit Wrinkles (Strawberry)	Fresh	93.15	0.00	0.00	1.15	0.99	0.16	0.00	0.00	0.16
Fiber Supplements										
Fiber 88	Natrol	94.88	8.38	6.32	48.80	1.12	48.28	21.12	21.36	5.80
Fiber Diet	Puritan's Pride	95.45	5.92	6.94	54.12	10.54	47.27	6.57	39.47	1.23
Fiber Diet	Vitamin World	94.10	6.52	9.31	52.73	9.63	45.55	8.08	35.77	1.70
Fiber Diet	BQE Vit & Suppl.	96.16	28.91	17.86	53.57	2.45	51.12	14.95	33.27	2.90
Fiber Filler	Your Life	94.70	2.08	1.45	83.39	3.47	80.80	3.49	74.90	2.42
Fiber Full	Solar Nutrition	93.63	6.84	9.96	64.34	8.73	58.77	20.36	31.04	7.37
Fiber-Off	Nutrition Headquarters	95.18	5.60	13.00	47.86	8.00	41.00	6.34	33.93	0.73
Fiberall Orange Sugarfree	Rydelle Laboratories	89.07	3.06	6.99	65.57	52.82	12.75	8.48	3.87	0.40
Fiberall Regular Sugarfree	Rydelle Laboratories	89.59	2.91	8.24	84.53	72.28	12.25	7.70	4.23	0.32
Fiberall Wafers	Rydelle Laboratories	93.49	1.62	6.41	28.37	24.10	6.72	4.65	1.51	0.55
Fiberguard	Ayerst	91.79	14.33	14.41	62.74	32.43	33.70	12.99	19.34	1.37

Table A.2 (Continued) Dry Matter Content of Selected Foods

Description	Maker	% DM	ASH	CP	In Dry Matter (%) TDF	SF	NDR	HC	CE	Ls
Fiber Supplements										
Fiberguard	Ayerst	92.13	15.21	13.53	59.04	23.36	40.43	18.33	19.03	3.07
Fibermed Wafers	Purdue Fredrick	92.86	3.57	9.76	30.69	6.45	28.34	21.39	6.20	0.75
Fibretrim	Schering	90.86	5.03	24.86	44.88	8.80	42.71	21.41	15.26	6.03
Fibretrim	Schering	92.71	6.11	23.85	46.00	9.07	48.22	25.18	16.51	6.53
Fibretrim w/Calcium	Schering	92.99	23.26	19.58	41.97	6.85	44.93	25.02	14.77	5.14
Full of Fiber	Jameson Nutritional	95.80	42.27	6.43	14.58	3.36	12.01	2.41	9.08	0.52
Grain 'N Citrus	Hilstone	94.66	38.18	4.18	49.70	16.20	35.72	12.19	17.51	6.02
Hi-Fiber	Walgreen Laboratories	93.83	5.32	9.04	51.96	8.34	45.89	8.40	36.09	1.40
Metamucil Regular	Searle	90.47	1.40	17.40	52.59	44.31	8.28	6.55	1.68	0.05
Metamucil Regular Sugarfree	Searle	89.80	2.76	16.16	98.51	84.51	14.00	10.20	3.92	-0.12
Serutan, Regular	J. W. Williams Co	94.10	1.91	4.66	52.98	44.48	8.50	5.88	2.26	0.36
Serutan, Toasted	J. W. Williams Co	97.05	3.65	11.31	46.82	35.32	11.50	8.85	2.25	0.40
Slim with Fiber	Nature's Bounty	95.18	9.14	10.07	49.65	8.72	43.25	6.58	34.09	2.58
Ultra Plan	Hi-Health	93.10	6.83	12.54	16.95	4.04	13.64	4.54	5.25	3.85

Notes: 1. DM = Dry matter; CP = Crude protein (N × 6.25): TDF = Total dietary fiber; SF = Soluble fiber; NDR = Neutral detergent residue (insoluble fiber); HC = Hemicellulose; CE = Cellulose; Ls = Klason lignin.

2. METHODS: (A) Total dietary fiber values obtained by the methods of: Prosky, L., Asp, N.-G., Furda, I., DeVries, J. W., Schweizer, T. F., and Harland, B., Determination of total dietary fiber in foods, food products and total diets: interlaboratory study, *J. AOAC*, 67, 1044, 1984. Prosky, L., Asp, N.-G., Schweizer, T. F., DeVries, J. W., and Furda, I., Determination of insoluble, soluble, and total dietary fiber in foods and food products. Interlaboratory study, *J. AOAC*, 71, 1017, 1988. (B) Neutral detergent residue and its components by the methods of Van Soest: Robertson, J. B. and Van Soest, P. J., The detergent system of analysis and its application to human foods, in *The Analysis of Dietary Fiber in Food*, James, W. P. T. and Theander, O., Eds., Marcel Deckker, New York, 1981. 123. Jeraci, J. L., Hernandez, T. M., Robertson, J. B., and Van Soest, P. J., New and improved procedure for neutral-detergent fiber, *J. Anim. Sci.*, 66 (Suppl.) 1, 351, 1988. (C) Soluble fiber determined directly or by the difference (TDF-NDF corrected for residual protein).

3. Samples provided mainly by J. A. Marllett, B. A. Lewis, D. H. Hurt, and P. J. Van Soest.

4. The majority of these analyses were supported by the National Cancer Institute Contract N01-CN-45182.

Appendix — Table A.3
Dietary Fiber Content of Selected Foods by the Southgate Methods

David A. T. Southgate

0-8493-2387-8/01/$0.00+$1.50

Table A.3   Dietary Fiber Content of Selected Foods by the Southgate Methods (Grams Per 100 g Edible Part)

	Total Dietary Fiber	Noncellulosic Polysaccharides[a]	Cellulose[b]	Lignin[c]
Flours				
White, bread-making	3.15	2.52	0.60	0.03
Brown	7.87	5.70	1.42	0.75
Whole meal	9.51	6.25	2.46	0.80
Breads				
White	2.72	2.01	0.71	Tr
Brown	5.11	3.63	1.33	0.15
Hovis	4.54	3.19	1.04	0.32
Whole meal	8.50	5.95	1.31	1.24
Breakfast cereals				
All Bran	26.70	17.82	6.01	2.88
Cornflakes	11.00	7.26	2.42	1.32
Grapenuts	7.00	5.14	1.28	0.58
Readibreak	7.60	5.39	0.99	1.22
Rice Krispies	4.47	3.47	0.78	0.22
Puffed Wheat	15.41	10.35	2.59	2.47
Sugar Puffs	6.08	4.00	0.99	1.09
Shredded Wheat	12.26	8.79	2.63	0.84
Special K	5.45	3.68	0.72	1.05
Swiss breakfast (mixed brands)	7.41	5.31	1.36	0.74
Weetabix	12.72	9. 18	2.35	1.19
Cookies and crispbreads				
Chocolate digestive (half-coated)	3.50	2.13	0.59	0.78
Chocolate (fully coated)	3.09	1.36	0.42	1.31
Crispbread, rye	11.73	8.33	1.66	1.74
Crispbread, wheat	4.83	3.34	0.94	0.55
Ginger biscuits	1.99	1.45	0.30	0.24
Matzo	3.85	2.72	0.70	0.43
Oatcakes	4.00	3.16	0.40	0.44
Semisweet	2.31	1.76	0.33	0.22
Short-sweet	1.66	1.42	0.11	0.13
Wafers (filled)	1.62	1.08	0.47	0.07
Leafy vegetables				
Broccoli tops (boiled)	4.10	2.92	1.15	0.03
Brussels sprouts (boiled)	2.86	1.99	0.80	0.07
Cabbage (boiled)	2.83	1.76	0.69	0.38
Cauliflower (boiled)	1.80	0.67	1.13	Tr
Lettuce (raw)	1.53	0.47	1.06	Tr
Onions (raw)	2.10	1.55	0.55	Tr
Legumes				
Beans, baked (canned)	7.27	5.67	1.41	0.19
Beans, runner (boiled)	3.35	1.85	1.29	0.21
Peas, frozen (raw)	7.75	5.48	2.09	0.18
Garden (canned)[d]	6.28	3.80	2.47	0.01
Processed (canned)[d]	7.85	5.20	2.30	0.35
Peanuts	9.30	6.40	1.69	1.21
Root vegetables				
Carrots, young (boiled)	3.70	2.22	1.48	Tr
Parsnips (raw)	4.90	3.77	1.13	Tr
Swedes (raw)	2.40	1.61	0.79	Tr
Turnips (raw)	2.20	1.50	0.70	Tr
Potato				
Main crop (raw)	3.51	2.49	1.02	Tr
Chips (fries)	3.20	2.05	1.12	0.03
Crisps	11.90	10.60	1.07	0.32
Canned	2.51	2.23	0.28	Tr

Table A.3 (Continued)   Dietary Fiber Content of Selected Foods by the Southgate Methods (Grams Per 100 g Edible Part)

	Total Dietary Fiber	Noncellulosic Polysaccharides[a]	Cellulose[b]	Lignin[c]
Peppers (cooked)	0.93	0.59	0.34	Tr
Tomato				
Fresh	1.40	0.65	0.45	0.30
Canned[d]	0.85	0.45	0.37	0.03
Sweet corn				
Cooked	4.74	4.31	0.31	0.12
Canned[d]	5.69	4.97	0.64	0.08
Fruits				
Apples				
Flesh only	1.42	0.94	0.48	0.01
Peel only	3.71	2.21	1.01	0.49
Bananas	1.75	1.12	0.37	0.26
Cherries (flesh and skin)	1.24	0.92	0.25	0.07
Grapefruit (canned)[d]	0.44	0.34	0.04	0.06
Guavas (canned)[d]	3.64	1.67	1.17	0.80
Mandarin oranges (canned)[d]	0.29	0.22	0.04	0.03
Mangoes (canned)[d]	1.00	0.65	0.32	0.03
Peaches (flesh and skin)	2.28	1.46	0.20	0.62
Pears				
Flesh only	2.44	1.32	0.67	0.45
Peel only	8.59	3.72	2.18	2.67
Plums (flesh and skin)	1.52	0.99	0.23	0.30
Rhubarb (raw)	1.78	0.93	0.70	0.15
Strawberries				
Raw	2.12	0.98	0.33	0.81
Canned[d]	1.00	0.48	0.20	0.33
Sultanas	4.40	2.40	0.83	1.17
Nuts				
Brazil	7.73	3.60	2.17	1.96
Preserves				
Jam				
Plum	0.96	0.80	0.14	0.03
Strawberry	1.12	0.85	0.11	0.15
Lemon curd	0.20	0.18	0.02	Tr
Marmalade	0.71	0.64	0.05	0.01
Fruit mincemeat	3.19	2.09	0.60	0.50
Peanut butter	7.55	5.64	1.91	Tr
Pickle	1.53	0.91	0.50	0.12
Dried soups (as purchased)				
Minestrone	6.61	4.60	1.91	0.10
Oxtail	3.84	2.89	0.94	0.01
Tomato	3.32	1.95	1.33	0.04
Beverages (concentrated)				
Cocoa	43.27	11.25	4.13	27.90
Drinking chocolate	8.20	2.61	1.16	4.43
Coffee and chicory essence	0.79	0.73	0.02	0.04
Instant coffee	16.41	15.55	0.53	0.33
Extracts				
Bovril (beef extract)	0.91	0.85	0.03	0.03
Marmite (yeast extract)	2.69	2.60	0.03	0.06

[a] Expressed as the sum of the component monosaccharides.
[b] Expressed as glucose.
[c] This value includes heat-induced artefacts analyzing as lignin.
[d] Drained material.

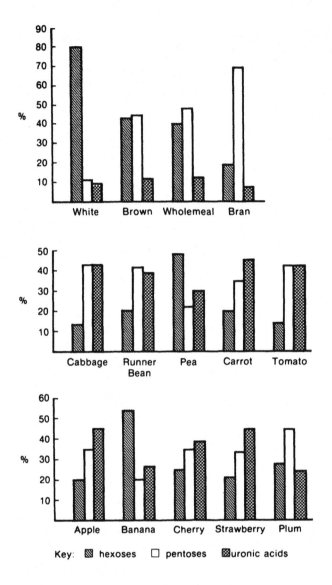

Figure A.3.1 Percentage composition of the noncellulosic polysaccharides in wheat flours, vegetables, and fruits.

REFERENCE

Southgate, D. A. T., Bailey, B., Collinson, E., and Walker, A. F., A guide to calculating intakes of dietary fiber, *J. Hum. Nutr.*, 30, 303, 1976.

Appendix — Table A.4
Dietary Fiber Content of Cereals in Norway

Wenche Frølich

0-8493-2387-8/01/$0.00+$1.50
© 2001 by CRC Press LLC

Table A.4   Dietary Fiber Content of Cereals in Norway

	Dietary Fiber (wet weight %)	Moisture (%)	Dietary Fiber (dry weight %)
White wheat flour (78 to 80% extraction)	3.1	11.2	3.5
Whole grain flour	12.1	11.4	13.6
Rye flour (mixed with 15% white wheat flour)	6.9	10.9	7.7
Whole grain flour, rye	14.1	11.4	15.9
Barley flour (50% extraction)	10.8	10.7	12.1
Barley flour (70% extraction)	13.6	10.4	15.2
Whole grain, barley	21.5	8.5	25.3
Oat flakes	10.7	8.6	11.7
Bran of wheat	50.7	11.4	57.2
Bran-germ of wheat	22.1	8.1	24.0
Germ of wheat	18.4	9.1	20.2
Semolina	2.3	11.7	2.6
Triticale	13.9	7.4	15.0
Everyday breakfast cereal	9.8	6.1	10.2
4-Grain breakfast	10.0	8.0	10.9
Bran-cracker type I	45.8	4.4	47.9
Bran-cracker type II	34.9	2.9	35.9
Bran-cracker type III	42.0	3.5	43.5
Bran-cracker, health shop	36.6	4.9	38.5
Kavli flatbread	17.9	3.4	18.5
Kavli breakfast flatbread	18.6	3.0	19.2
Kavli flatbread with bran	22.0	4.2	23.0
Kavli thin crispbread	21.9	4.8	23.0
Ideal flatbread	7.6	3.0	7.8
Ideal homemade	10.7	3.2	11.1
Ideal fiber flatbread	15.7	3.7	16.2
Spaghetti, wheat flour	4.1	9.6	4.5
Macaroni, wheat flour	4.5	8.9	5.0
Spaghetti, whole wheat flour	9.7	8.7	10.7
Macaroni, whole wheat flour	10.8	8.1	11.0
Rice, porridge	3.0	10.0	3.3
Rice, parboiled	3.1	7.8	3.4
Rice, precooked	3.3	8.9	3.6
Rice, quick rice	2.5	9.0	2.7
Rice, nature rice	4.6	10.7	5.1
Rice, brown rice	9.1	10.2	10.1
Unpolished, round-grain rice (health shop)	3.4	6.8	3.7
Unpolished, long-grain rice (health shop)	4.2	11.6	4.7
Nature, biodynamic-grown rice (health shop)	4.5	10.2	5.0

REFERENCE

Asp, N.-G., Johansson, C.-G., Hallner, H., and Siljeström, M., Rapid enzymatic assay of insoluble and soluble dietary fiber, *Agric. Food Chem.*, 31, 476, 1983.

Appendix — Table A.5
Crude Fiber Values of Typical Samples

Ivan Furda

Table A.5   Crude Fiber Values of Typical Samples[a]

Sample	Crude Fiber (g/100 g)	Moisture (%)	Crude Fiber (moisture-free basis) (%)
Avocados, raw	1.6	74.0	6.2
Artichokes, raw	2.4	85.5	16.5
Apples, fresh, raw	1.0	84.4	6.4
Almonds, dried	2.6	4.7	2.7
Bean flour, lima	2.0	10.5	2.2
Beans, lima, raw	1.0	90.1	10.0
Bananas	1.8	67.5	5.5
Breads			
White	0.2	35.6	0.31
Rye	0.4	35.5	0.6
French	0.2	30.6	0.3
Pumpernickel	1.1	34.0	1.7
Whole wheat	1.6	36.4	2.5
Broccoli, raw	1.5	89.1	13.6
Cabbage, raw	0.8	92.4	10.5
Carob flour	7.7	11.2	8.7
Chocolate, bitter	2.5	2.3	2.6
Cocoa, dry powder	4.3	3.0	4.4
Corn grits, dry	0.4	12.0	0.5
Corn flour	0.7	12.0	0.8
Corn, field, whole grain, raw	2.0	13.8	2.3
Carrots			
Raw	1.0	88.2	8.5
Dehydrated	9.3	4.0	9.7
Cauliflower, raw	1.0	91.0	11.1
Cornmeal, whole-ground	1.6	12.0	1.8
Grapefruit, raw	0.2	88.4	1.7
Grapes, raw	0.6	81.6	3.2
Horseradish, raw	2.4	74.6	9.4
Macadamia nuts	2.5	3.0	2.6
Malt, dry	5.2	5.7	5.5
Mushrooms, raw	0.8	90.4	8.3
Oatmeal, dry	1.2	8.3	1.3
Okra, raw	1.0	88.9	9.0
Olives, green	1.3	78.2	6.0
Onions, raw	0.6	89.1	5.5
Onions, dehydrated	4.4	4.0	4.6
Oranges, raw peeled fruit	0.5	86.0	3.6
Peaches	0.6	89.1	5.4
Peanuts, raw without skins	1.9	5.4	2.0
Peanut flour, defatted	2.7	7.3	2.9
Pears, raw (including skin)	1.4	83.2	8.3
Peas, edible podded, raw	1.2	83.3	7.2
Peppers, sweet, immature, green, raw	1.4	93.4	21.2
Pineapple, raw	0.4	85.3	2.7
Plums, raw prune type	0.4	78.7	1.9
Popcorn, popped, plain	2.2	4.0	2.3
Potatoes, raw	0.5	79.8	2.5
Potato flour	1.6	7.6	1.7
Pumpkin, raw	1.1	91.6	13.1

Table A.5 (Continued) Crude Fiber Values of Typical Samples[a]

Sample	Crude Fiber (g/100 g)	Moisture (%)	Crude Fiber (moisture-free basis) (%)
Rice, white (milled or polished), enriched, raw	0.3	12.0	0.3
Rice, brown, raw	0.9	12.0	1.0
Rice bran	11.5	9.7	12.7
Rye (whole grain)	2.0	11.0	2.2
Rye flour (light)	0.4	11.0	0.4
Rye flour (dark)	2.4	11.0	2.7
Rye wafers (whole grain)	2.2	6.0	2.3
Soybeans (mature seeds), dry, raw	4.9	10.0	5.5
Soybean flour			
(full-fat)	2.4	8.0	2.6
(defatted)	2.3	8.0	2.5
Spinach, raw	0.1	90.7	6.5
Squash, raw	0.6	94.0	10.0
Strawberries, raw	1.3	89.9	12.9
Sweet potatoes, raw	0.7	70.6	2.4
Tomatoes, ripe, raw	0.5	93.5	7.7
Turnips, raw	0.9	91.5	10.6
Walnuts, black	1.7	3.1	1.8
Wheat, whole grain			
Hard Red Spring	2.3	13.0	2.6
White	1.9	11.5	2.1
Wheat flours			
Whole (from hard wheats)			
80% extraction	0.5	12.0	0.6
Straight, soft wheat	0.4	12.0	0.45
Bread flour (enriched)	0.3	12.0	0.3
Wheat bran (crude, commercially milled)	9.1	11.5	10.3
Wheat germ (crude, commercially milled)	2.5	11.5	2.8
Yeast (Brewer's, debittered)	1.7	5.0	1.8
Yam, tuber, raw	0.9	73.5	3.4

[a] Adapted from *Composition of Foods*, Agriculture Handbook No. 8, Watt, B. K. and Merrill, A. L., Eds., Agricultural Research Service, U.S. Department of Agriculture, Washington, D.C., 1963.

Appendix — Table A.6
Comparison of Analyses of Dietary Fiber and Crude Fiber

Gene A. Spiller

Table A.6   Comparison of Analyses of Dietary Fiber and Crude Fiber

Foods	Crude Fiber[1] (%)	Total Dietary Fiber[2] (%)
Vegetables		
Beans, baked	1.50	7.27
Beans, green	1.00	3.35
Carrots, cooked	1.00	3.70
Corn, sweet, cooked	0.70	4.74
Lettuce, raw	0.60	1.53
Onions, raw	0.60	2.10
Parsnips, raw	2.00	4.90
Peas, frozen, raw	1.90	7.75
Peas, canned	1.40	7.07
Potatoes, raw	0.50	3.51
Tomatoes, fresh	0.50	1.40
Fruits		
Apples, flesh only	0.60	1.42
Bananas	0.50	1.75
Cherries, flesh and skin	0.40	1.24
Peaches, flesh and skin	0.60	2.28
Pears, flesh only	1.40	2.44
Plums, flesh and skin	0.50	1.52
Strawberries, raw	1.30	2.12
Nut-like products		
Peanut butter	1.90	7.55
Grains and grain products		
Flour, white	0.30	3.15
Flour, whole wheat	2.30	9.15
Bran	9.41	44.00
Bread, white	0.20	2.72
Bread, whole wheat	1.60	8.50
All Bran cereal	7.80	26.70
Corn Flakes	0.70	11.00

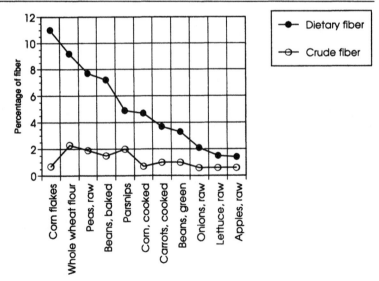

Figure A.6.1   Data for dietary fiber (Southgate method, Chapter 3.4) and crude fiber for various foods showing lack of correlation between the two measurements.

REFERENCES

1. Crude fiber data from *Composition of Foods*, Handbook Number 8, U.S. Department of Agriculture, Washington, D.C., 1963.
2. Dietary fiber data from Southgate, D. A. T., Bailey, B., Collinson, E., and Walker, A. F., A guide to calculating intakes of dietary fiber, *J. Hum. Nutr.*, 30, 303, 1976.

Appendix — Table A.7
Phytate Contents of Foods

Barbara F. Harland

0-8493-2387-8/01/$0.00+$1.50

Table A.7 Phytate Contents of Foods[a]

Food	Moisture[b] (%)	Serving (U[c])	Size (g)	Phytate per Serving (mg)	EP[d], mg	100 g Dry Wt, mg
Almonds (Taylor's Sunshine Colony)	5.0	1/2 c	71	909	1280	347 ± 17[c]
Apples, raw, not pared	84.4	1	150	94	63	404
Artichoke, Jerusalem, boiled	80.2	1 bud	380	110	29	146
Artichoke, Jerusalem, flour	10.9	1 Tbsp	15	70	468	525 ± 24[f]
Artichoke hearts, whole (S & W)	90.0	1	120	11	9	88 ± 2[c]
Avocado	66.1	1	201	2	1	3 ± 2[c]
Bacon chips, imitation (Bacos, Betty Crocker)	5.0	1 Tbsp	15	196	1310	1379 ± 9[e]
Baking mix, buttermilk (Bimix, Martha White)	7.5	1 Tbsp	15	27	180	195 ± 14[e]
Baking mix, buttermilk (Bisquick)	7.5	1 Tbsp	15	11	73	79 ± 7[e]
Barley, infant cereal, instant cooking, dry (Gerber)	10.3	1 oz	28	251	897	1000
Barley, pearl, boiled	69.6	1/2 c	120	197	164	539
Beans, broad, boiled	83.7	1/2 c	120	22	18	110
Beans,[g] green, casserole with cheddar cheese	70.0	1 c	124	112	90	300
Beans, kidney, canned, drained	69.0	1/2 c	92	282	307	990 ± 2[h]
Beans, lima, immature, raw	67.5	1/2 c	55	124	226	695 ± 9[f]
Beans, lima, mature, dry, raw	10.3	1/4 c	40	404	1010	1126
Beans, navy, mature, dry, boiled, drained	69.0	1/2 c	85	294	346	1116
Beans, navy, mature, dry, raw	10.9	1/2 c	62	564	910	1021 ± 18[e]
Beans, pinto, raw	67.5	1/2 c	55	122	222	684 ± 5[f]
Beans, snap, green, canned, drained	91.9	1/2 c	62	56	91	1123
Beets, canned, sliced (Del Monte)	90.7	1/2 c	85	2	3	30 ± 7[e]
Blackberries	82.0	1/2 c	72	7	10	56
Blueberries, sweetened, canned, drained	72.3	1/2 c	115	3	3	11 ± 4[h]
Bouillon cubes, beef-flavored (Wyler's)	4.0	2 cubes	8	7	88	92 ± 2[e]
Bouillon cubes, chicken-flavored (Wyler's)	4.0	2 cubes	8	3	32	33 ± 2[e]
Brazil nuts	8.5	1/2 c	70	1259	1799	1966
Bread, French	30.6	1 sl	35	6	17	24
Bread, high-fiber, wheat (Fresh Horizons)	36.4	1 sl	28	65	232	365 ± 2[h]
Bread, high-fiber, white (Fresh Horizons)	35.8	1 sl	27	21	79	123 ± 1[h]
Bread, Norwegian flat (Kauli)	4.3	1	10	65	654	683 ± 3[h]
Bread, pita (Giant)	25.0	1	35	43	123	164 ± 2[h]
Bread, pumpernickel (Giant)	34.0	1 sl	32	34	107	162
Bread, raisin (Giant)	35.3	1 sl	25	14	58	89
Bread, rye, American (Giant)	35.5	1 sl	25	39	155	240
Bread, wheat (Melba Toast, Borden)	6.0	2 sl	10	18	183	195 ± 5[e]

Bread, white, enriched (Giant)	35.8	1 sl	27	18	69	107
Bread, whole wheat (Giant)	36.4	1 sl	28	109	390	613
Bread, whole wheat (Oroweat)	36.9	1 sl	24	80	334	529 ± 2e
Breading mix (Shake n' Bake)	8.0	1 oz	28	102	365	397 ± 2e
Broccoli, fresh	88.8	1 bud	44	8	18	164 ± 0e
Bun, plain, hamburger (United Premium Quality)	33.3	1	52	43	82	124 ± 0e
Cake, chocolate, without icing (Duncan Hines Swiss Choc. Mix)	24.2	1 sl	120	637	531	701 ± 6h
Cake, white, lightly iced (Duncan Hines Mix)	20.0	1 sl	104	18	17	21
Candy, milk chocolate (Hershey)	0.9	1 oz	28	36	127	128 ± 12h
Caraway seeds	5.5	1 Tbsp	8	81	1019	1078 ± 11h
Carrots, raw	88.2	1	81	8	9	76
Cashew nuts	5.2	1/2 c	70	1306	1866	1968 ± 31h
Cashew nuts, honey-roasted (Eagle Snacks)	5.0	1/2 c	70	665	950	1000 ± 20e
Chestnuts	51.7	1/2 c	80	38	47	97
Chickpeas (garbanzos), dry, raw	10.7	1/2 c	100	730	730	817 ± 9h
Chickpeas or garbanzos, mature seeds, dry, boiled, drained	69.0	1/2 c	62	129	208	670
Chili con carne, no beans (Wolf)	70.7	1 c	225	187	83	284 ± 10e
Chili con carne, w/ beans (Wolf)	73.1	1 c	225	169	75	280 ± 3e
Cocoa, dry powder (Hershey)	4.1	1 Tbsp	5	94	1880	1960
Coconut meat, dried, sweetened, shredded	3.3	1 oz	28	65	230	237
Coffee cake (Butter Streusel, Sara Lee)	22.0	1 sl	42	21	50	64 ± 6h
Coffee, brewed (Folgers Flaked)	98.1	6 oz c	180	12	7	368
Coffee, instant (Tasters Choice 100% Freeze-Dried)	98.1	6 oz c	180	1	0.7	37
Coffee substitute, grain and spice (Celestial Seasonings)	98.1	6 oz c	180	18	10	526
Collard greens, raw	88.9	1 c	80	10	12	112 ± 9f
Cookie, chocolate chip (Chips Ahoy, Nabisco)	8.0	4	60	89	148	161 ± 3e
Cookie, chocolate sandwich cream-filled (Oreos, Nabisco)	2.2	4	40	74	186	190 ± 6h
Cookie, coconut bar (Rippin Good)	3.8	10	90	294	327	340 ± 10h
Cookie, fig bar (Fig Newtons, Nabisco)	12.7	4	56	20	35	40 ± 6h
Cookie (Nilla Wafers, Nabisco)	2.8	2	20	7	37	38 ± 3e
Cookie, oatmeal and raisin (Pepperidge Farm)	2.8	4	52	101	194	200 ± 6h
Cookie (Peanut Butter Nut, Duncan Hines)	11.0	2	28	92	328	368 ± 10e
Cookie (Toddler Biter Biscuits, Gerber)	4.0	2	38	38	100	104 ± 3e
Cookie mix, brownie, baked (Duncan Hines)	11.0	1	20	31	153	161 ± 3e
Cookie mix, peanut butter (Duncan Hines)	10.0	1 oz	28	55	197	219 ± 7e

Table A.7 (Continued) Phytate Contents of Foods[a]

Food	Moisture[b] %	Serving U[c]	Size g	Phytate per Serving mg	EP[d], mg	Dry Wt, mg (100 g)
Cornbread, whole ground corn meal (Washington Cornbread Mix)	53.9	1 sl	78	489	627	1360
Corn, canned, whole-kernel, yellow, drained solids	75.9	1/2 c	82	26	31	129
Corn cereal, ready-to-eat (Corn Bran, Quaker)	3.5	1 oz	28	65	232	240 ± 16[h]
Corn cereal, ready-to-eat (Corn Flakes, Kellogg's)	2.6	1 oz	28	20	70	72 ± 3[e]
Corn cereal, ready-to-eat (Corn Pops, Kellogg's)	3.4	1 oz	28	26	94	97 ± 10[e]
Corn chips (Cheetos)	6.0	1 oz	28	20	73	78 ± 3[e]
Corn chips (Cornquistos, Snack Master)	5.0	1 oz	28	65	232	244 ± 18[e]
Corn chips (Doritos)	3.8	1 oz	28	178	635	660
Corn chips (Fritos)	6.0	1 oz	28	142	506	538 ± 2[e]
Corn chips (Nacho Dorritos)	11.0	1 oz	28	142	507	570 ± 3[e]
Corn germ flour (Quaker)	12.0	1 c	120	2048	1707	1940 ± 6[h]
Corn meal (Quaker)	12.0	1/2 c	80	754	943	1072 ± 6[h]
Cornmeal, unbolted, stoneground (Stone Mountain)	12.0	1 Tbsp	15	107	711	808 ± 0[e]
Corn pudding[j]	34.0	1/2 c	122	20	16	24
Cracker, animal (Barnum's, Nabisco)	6.0	4	10	8	84	89 ± 3[e]
Cracker, graham (Honey Maid, Nabisco)	6.0	4	28	50	179	190 ± 5[e]
Cracker (Ritz, Nabisco)	4.0	4	11	11	103	107 ± 3[e]
Cracker, saltine (Nabisco)	4.3	4	11	19	172	180
Cracker (Wheat Thins, Nabisco)	6.0	2	30	95	317	337 ± 3[e]
Croutons, toasted (Brownberry)	7.0	2 oz	56	79	141	152 ± 2[e]
Cucumber, raw	54.1	1/2 c	52	15	28	62 ± 5[e]
Doughnut, cake, sugar-coated (Mrs. Baird's)	24.0	1	32	117	366	481 ± 15[e]
Farina, regular, cooked (Cream of Wheat)	89.5	1/2 c	122	5	4	38
Figs, dried, uncooked	23.0	1/2 c	89	343	385	500 ± 57[h]
Filberts (hazelnuts), shelled, chopped	5.8	1/2 c	59	956	1620	1720
Granola, coconut, assorted nuts, and raisins (Nature Valley)	3.8	1 oz	28	175	625	650
Hickory nuts	3.3	1/2 c	78	1260	1615	1670
High-protein infant cereal, instant dry form (Gerber)	10.3	1 oz	28	311	1112	1240
Hominy, cooked (corn grits), degermed, enriched	87.1	1/2 c	122	344	282	2186 ± 38[h]
Hot chocolate, instant (Swiss Miss Hot Cocoa Mix)	98.1	6 oz c	180	2	1	53
Kale, raw	88.7	1 c	80	11	14	128 ± 7[f]
Ketchup, tomato (Heinz)	65.9	1 Tbsp	15	1	7	20 ± 3[e]
Lentils, raw	12.2	1/2 c	95	412	434	494

Macaroni, elbow, enriched (Kroger)	10.4	1/2 c	43	112	260	290 ± 5[e]
Millet, dry	11.8	1/4 c	25	124	494	560 ± 8[h]
Mixed grain cereal, ready-to-eat (Alpha Bits, Post)	1.3	1 oz	28	143	510	517 ± 7[e]
Mixed grain cereal, ready-to-eat (Apple Jacks, Kellogg's)	2.3	1 oz	28	50	177	181 ± 0[e]
Mixed grain cereal, ready-to-eat (Froot Loops, Kellogg's)	2.5	1 oz	28	45	162	166 ± 5[e]
Mixed grain cereal, ready-to-eat (Product 19, Kellogg's)	3.2	1 oz	28	76	272	281 ± 2[e]
Mixed grain cereal, ready-to-eat (Special K, Kellogg's)	2.2	1 oz	28	76	272	278 ± 8[e]
Mixed grain cereal, ready-to-eat (Team, Nabisco)	3.2	1 oz	28	65	232	240
Mixed grain cereal, infant, instant, dry form (Gerber)	10.3	1 oz	28	203	726	809
Muffin, English (Thomas)	39.0	1	66	48	73	120 ± 6[h]
Muffin, wheat bran (Duncan Hines Mix)	35.1	1	40	199	498	767 ± 8[h]
Noodles, chow mein (La Choy)	1.0	1 oz	28	114	409	413 ± 2[e]
Oatmeal or rolled oats, cooked (Quaker)	86.5	1/2 c	120	133	111	822
Oatmeal, dry (Quaker)	8.9	1 oz	28	264	943	1035
Oatmeal, infant cereal, instant, dry form (Gerber)	10.3	1 oz	28	251	897	1000
Okra, cooked (Trappey's)	94.8	1/2 c	80	4	5	88 ± 2[e]
Okra, raw	88.9	1/2 c	48	15	32	286 ± 4[e]
Olives, green, Spanish w/pimiento	74.9	2	40	1	3	11 ± 3[e]
Olives, ripe, sliced	85.1	2	48	1	2	15 ± 2[e]
Pancakes, wheat germ (Aunt Jemima Mix plus 1 teaspoon of wheat germ/pancake)	50.6	1	28	244	871	1763
Parsnips, raw	76.9	1 c	67	21	32	137 ± 3[e]
Peach pie (Giant)	47.5	1 sl	118	4	3	6
Peanuts, toasted, salted (Tom's)	6.6	1 oz	28	261	933	999 ± 22[e]
Peanut butter (Jif, extra crunchy)	2.2	1 Tbsp	16	200	1252	1280
Peas, blackeyed, dried, raw	10.5	1/2 c	100	815	815	911 ± 7[h]
Peas, dried, raw	13.3	1/2 c	100	851	851	982
Peas, green, immature, canned, drained solids	81.5	1/2 c	85	24	28	151
Peas, split, dry	11.7	1/2 c	100	664	664	752 ± 2[h]
Pecans, shelled	3.4	1/2 c	54	793	1468	1519
Piecrust stick (Betty Crocker)	19.0	1/6	53	62	117	144 ± 3[e]
Plantain, raw	66.4	1/2 c	50	16	32	95 ± 16[f]
Popcorn, popped, plain	4.0	1 c	6	37	614	640
Popcorn, unpopped (Orville Redenbacher's Gourmet)	9.8	1/8 c	6	34	561	622 ± 13[e]

Table A.7 (Continued) Phytate Contents of Foods[a]

Food	Moisture[b] %	Serving U[c]	Size g	Phytate per Serving mg	EP[d], mg	100 g Dry Wt, mg
Poppy seeds	5.5	1 Tbsp	8	175	2189	2316 ± 13[h]
Potato chips	1.8	1 oz	28	55	196	200 ± 15[h]
Potatoes, boiled in skin, drained, pared	79.8	1/2 c	78	63	81	401
Potatoes, French fries	44.7	10	50	50	100	181 ± 1[h]
Potato salad w/ egg (Giant, Deli)	82.8	1/2 c	75	63	84	488
Pretzels, butter (Seyferts)	5.0	10	60	63	105	111 ± 6[e]
Pumpkin seeds	5.5	1 oz	28	529	1889	1998 ± 15[h]
Radish, fresh	94.4	1	45	3	6	108 ± 15[e]
Rice, brown, dry	10.3	1/4 c	25	130	518	577 ± 22[h]
Rice, long-grain, uncooked (Minute, General Foods)	9.6	1/4 c	45	65	144	159 ± 7[e]
Rice, white, regular, dry form, fully milled or polished	10.3	1/4 c	25	64	255	284
Rice, wild	12.0	1/2 c	100	1936	1936	2200
Rice cereal, ready-to-eat (Cocoa Krispies, Kellogg's)	2.5	1 oz	28	38	136	139 ± 2[e]
Rice cereal, ready-to-eat (Cocoa Pebbles, Post)	2.1	1 oz	28	53	189	193 ± 2[e]
Rice cereal, ready-to-eat (Fruity Pebbles, Post)	2.9	1 oz	28	41	146	150 ± 2[e]
Rice cereal, ready-to-eat (Rice Krispies, Kellogg's)	2.3	1 oz	28	58	207	212 ± 10[e]
Rice cereal, infant, instant, dry form (Gerber)	10.3	1 oz	28	246	879	980
Roll, ready-to-serve, plain (Giant)	31.4	1	28	18	64	93
Rye flour (Pillsbury)	15.0	1 c	128	1176	919	1081
Sesame seeds	5.5	1 Tbsp	8	129	1616	1710 ± 14[h]
Soy-based chicken analog (General Mills)	7.0	1 oz	28	70	251	270
Soy-based ham analog (General Mills)	7.0	1 oz	28	31	112	120
Soy-based infant formula (Advance, Concentrate)	87.0	4 oz	120	10	8	62 ± 2[h]
Soy-based TVP bacon (Archer Daniels Midlands)	7.0	1 oz	28	248	884	951
Soy-based TVP bacon and vitamins (Archer Daniels Midlands)	7.0	1 oz	28	300	1070	1151
Soy-based TVP beef (Archer Daniels Midlands)	7.0	1 oz	28	354	1265	1360
Soy-based TVP ham (Archer Daniels Midlands)	7.0	1 oz	28	328	1172	1260
Soy-based TVP pork (Archer Daniels Midlands)	7.0	1 oz	28	370	1321	1420
Soy-based TVP unflavored and vitamins (Archer Daniels Midlands)	7.0	1 oz	28	424	1516	1630
Soybeans, mature seeds, dry, raw Elton variety	10.0	1/2 c	105	2438	2322	2580

Soy flour (Ralston Purina)	8.0	1 c	137	1915	1398	1520 ± 11^h
Soy isolate (Ralston Purina)	8.0	1 c	137	1689	1233	1340 ± 11^h
Soy, textured concentrate (Patti Pro, General Mills)	5.0	1 oz	28	399	1425	1500
Strawberries, frozen, sweetened, drained	71.3	1/2 c	128	8	6	21 ± 2^h
Sunflower seeds	5.5	1 Tbsp	8	128	1606	1699 ± 4^h
Sweet potato, raw	70.0	1	180	9	5	17
Taco shells (Paco's)	4.0	1	20	110	549	572 ± 8^e
Tea, brewed (Kaffree, dried leaves)	99.4	6 oz c	180	3	2	333
Tea, instant (Nestea 100% Instant)	99.4	6 oz c	180	2	1	167
Tomato seeds	5.5	1 Tbsp	8	148	1847	1955 ± 8^h
Tomato soup (Campbell's)	87.8	1/2 c	122	8	6	49
Tomatoes, canned solids and liquid	93.7	1/2 c	120	8	6	95
Triticale flour	11.0	1 Tbsp	15	90	597	670 ± 0^f
Turnips, raw	87.2	1/2 c	65	4	6	47 ± 3^e
Walnuts, black, shelled	3.1	1/2 c	62	1226	1977	2040
Walnuts, English, shelled	23.5	1/2 c	50	380	760	993
Wheat bran, crude AACC ref.^{j}	10.4	1 oz	28	843	3011	3360
Wheat cereal, ready-to-eat (40% Bran, Post)	3.0	1 oz	28	305	1088	1122 ± 10^e
Wheat cereal, ready-to-eat 100% bran (All Bran, Kellogg's)	3.6	1 oz	28	887	3168	3286 ± 2^h
Wheat cereal, ready-to-eat, Bran Chex (Ralston Purina)	3.5	1 oz	28	375	1341	1390 ± 22^h
Wheat cereal, ready-to-eat (Bran Flakes, Kellogg's)	3.0	1 oz	28	298	1066	1099 ± 2^e
Wheat cereal, ready-to-eat (Frosted Flakes, Kellogg's)	2.5	1 oz	28	16	58	60 ± 2^e
Wheat cereal, ready-to-eat (Grape Nuts Flakes, Post)	3.4	1 oz	28	151	541	560 ± 3^e
Wheat cereal, ready-to-eat (Honey Smacks, Kellogg's)	3.2	1 oz	28	51	182	188 ± v8^e
Wheat cereal, ready-to-eat (Post Toasties)	3.0	1 oz	28	22	80	83 ± 0^e
Wheat cereal, ready-to-eat (Raisin Bran, Kellogg's)	8.3	1 oz	28	184	659	719 ± 2^e
Wheat cereal, ready-to-eat, shredded (Nabisco)	3.2	1 oz	28	415	1481	1530
Wheat cereal, ready-to-eat, fortified (Special K, Kellogg's)	3.5	1 oz	28	186	666	690 ± 10^h
Wheat cereal, ready-to-eat (Super Sugar Crisps, Post)	1.5	1 oz	28	77	274	278 ± 7^e
Wheat cereal, ready-to-eat (Wheaties, General Mills)	3.5	1 oz	28	411	1467	1520

Table A.7 (Continued) Phytate Contents of Foods[a]

Food	Moisture[b] %	Serving U[c]	Size g	Phytate per Serving mg	100 g EP[d], mg	100 g Dry Wt, mg
Wheat flour, all-purpose (General Mills)	12.0	1 c	137	386	282	320
Wheat flour, enriched, unbleached (Gold Medal, General Mills)	12.0	1 Tbsp	15	20	136	154 ± 2[e]
Wheat flour, whole wheat (Pillsbury)	12.0	1 c	120	1014	845	960
Wheat germ (Kretchmer)	11.5	1 Tbsp	6	244	4071	4600
Wheat gluten flour	8.5	1 Tbsp	15	38	252	276 ± 4[f]
Yam, raw	73.0	1	180	94	52	193
Yeast, baker's dry	5.0	1/4 oz	7	35	495	521 ± 7[f]

[a] Table 1 is taken in part from Harland, B. F. and Oberleas, D., *Phytate in Foods*, World Review of Nutrition and Dietetics, Vol. 52, S. Karger, Basel, 1987, 235.
[b] If no value was given, a "best estimate" was calculated from existing data.
[c] c = 8-oz cup, oz = ounce, Tbsp = tablespoon, and sl = slice.
[d] Edible portion.
[e] Mean ± SE of triplicate determinations by Oberleas and Roy (1985).
[f] Mean ± SE of triplicate determinations by Harland et al. (1986).
[g] Two c snap green beans, drained, 1 can Campbell's Cream of Mushroom Soup, 1/2 c grated cheddar cheese. Mix and heat.
[h] Mean ± SE of triplicate determinations by Harland and Oberleas (1986).
[i] One c whole-kernel corn, 2 c cream-style corn, 1/2 c melted butter, 2 beaten eggs, 1 c sour cream, 1 pkg Jiffy cornbread mix. Mix ingredients, bake at 350°F for 30 min.
[j] AACC Certified Food Grade Wheat Bran (10-4-77) used as a reference material during phytate analyses (American Association of Cereal Chemists, 3340 Pilot Knob Road, St. Paul, MN 55121). This food has been certified to contain 3 ± 0.2% or 3348 ± 223 mg phytate/100 g (dry weight).

Appendix — Table A.8
Tartaric Acid Content of Foods

Monica Spiller and Gene A. Spiller

Few foods contain more than minimal quantities of tartaric acid ($C_4H_6O_6$). In temperate climates only grapes and their products have reasonable amounts of tartaric acid, amounts that may have physiological significance. Tartaric acid is of interest in fiber studies and in health, as it affects colon function. In sun-dried raisins all of the tartaric acid of the grape is present, while in wine making some of the tartaric acid is lost.

Food	Amount
Grapes (fresh)	0.55–0.9 g/100 g
Wine	0.5–0.7 g/100 ml
Sun-dried raisins	2.0–3.5 g/100 g
Raisin juice concentrate	1.8–2.2 g/100 ml
Raisin paste	1.5–2.2 g/100 g

Appendix — Table A.9
Plant Foods That Contain Significant Levels of Saponins and Their Estimated Saponin Content

David Oakenfull and John D. Potter

0-8493-2387-8/01/$0.00+$1.50

Table A.9

Plant	Saponin Content (g/kg dry weight)
Alfalfa sprouts (*Medicago sativa*)	80
Asparagus (*Asparagus officinalis*)	15
Broad bean (*Vicia faba*)	3.5
Chickpea (*Cicer arietinum*)	0.7–60
Green pea (*Pisum sativum*)	1.8–11
Kidney bean (*Phaseolus vulgaris*)	2–16
Lentil (*Lens culinaris*)	0.7–1.1
Mung bean (*Phaseolus mungo*)	0.5–6
Navy bean (*Phaseolus vulgaris*)	4.5–21
Oats (*Avena sativa*)	0.2–0.5
Peanut (*Arachis hypogaea*)	0.05–16
Quinoa (*Chenopodium quinoa*)	10–23
Sesame seed (*Sesamum indicum*)	3
Silver beet (*Beta vulgaris*)	58
Soy bean (*Glycine max*)	5.6–56
Spinach (*Spinacea oleracia*)	47
Sweet lupin (*Lupinus augustifolius*)	0.4–0.7

INDEX

A

Acetate, 287–313, 483, *See also* Short-chain fatty acids
Acetyl bromide method, 99
Acid detergent fiber (ADF), 27, 63
  nitrogen excretion and balance effects, 147
  protein digestibility and, 136
  protein utilization effects, 153
Additives, polysaccharide, 23–25, 33
African dietary and morbidity patterns, 363–365, 369, 423, 431, 561, 569, 570, 574–576
Agar, 24, 27
  antitoxic effects, 446
  blood glucose and insulin responses and, 324
  fecal composition studies, 209
  nitrogen excretion and balance effects, 149
  protein digestibility and, 138
Agarose, 27
Agiolax, 306
Alfalfa
  antitoxic effects, 446, 447
  digestive enzymes and, 278, 282
  fecal composition studies, 216
  fecal mutagens and, 318
  sprouts, *See* Sprouts
Algal polysaccharides, 24, 27, *See also* Agar; Alginates; Carrageenans
Alginates, 24, 27
  antitoxic effects, 446
  digestive enzymes and, 278, 279
  protein digestibility and, 138
  protein utilization and, 144, 155
  short-chain fatty acids and, 311
Alginic acid, 27
Almond, 637, 666, 674
Amaranth, 627
American Academy of Pediatrics, 557
American Association of Cereal Chemists (AACC), 554–555
American Cancer Society, 554

American Diabetes Association, 554
American Diatetics Association, 554
American Health Foundation (AHF), 557
American Heart Association, 391, 554
Aminopolysaccharide, 45–46
Amoebic dysentery, 198
Amylases, 52, 54, 55, 64, 90, 277, 278, 280
Amyloglucosidases, 51, 52, 90, 92
Amylopectin, 40
Amylose, 40, *See also* Starch
Amylose, retrograde, 16, 40, *See also* Resistant starch
Analytical methods
  AOAC approved methods, 53–60, 87–105
  detergent systems, 63–65
  Englyst procedure for nonstarch polysaccharides, 70–81, 567, *See also* Englyst procedure
  enzymatic gravimetry, 51–60, 87, *See* Enzymatic gravimetric methods
  historical perspectives, 88
  insoluble and soluble fiber, 52–53
  lignin, 20
  modified carbazole method, 97
  phytate analysis, 113–125, *See also* Phytate, analytical methods
  protein hydrolysis, 55
  reagent toxicity, 64
  sample extraction, 83–84
  sample preparation, 54
  saponins, 127–130
  Southgate method for unavailable carbohydrates, 83–85, 88, 567, *See also* Southgate method
  starch, 84–85, 88, 90–92
  sugar and lipid removal, 90
  Uppsala method for total dietary fiber, 87–105, *See also* Uppsala procedure
Animal connective tissues, 17
Animal fibers (chitin and chitosan), 45–46
Antioxidants, 453–458, 482
  cardiovascular protective effects, 486
  fecal mutagens and, 317
  food product content, 455–456

C

H

Y

Z